AF686320

Biomechanics and Motion Analysis

Biomechanics and Motion Analysis

Guest Editors

Christina Zong-Hao Ma
Hong Fu

MDPI

Basel • Beijing • Wuhan • Barcelona • Belgrade • Novi Sad • Cluj • Manchester

Guest Editors

Christina Zong-Hao Ma
Department of Biomedical Engineering
The Hong Kong Polytechnic University
Hong Kong
China

Hong Fu
Department of Mathematics and Information Technology
The Education University of Hong Kong
Hong Kong
China

Editorial Office
MDPI AG
Grosspeteranlage 5
4052 Basel, Switzerland

This is a reprint of the Special Issue, published open access by the journal *Bioengineering* (ISSN 2306-5354), freely accessible at: https://www.mdpi.com/journal/bioengineering/special_issues/KF1A243LC5.

For citation purposes, cite each article independently as indicated on the article page online and as indicated below:

Lastname, A.A.; Lastname, B.B. Article Title. *Journal Name* **Year**, *Volume Number*, Page Range.

ISBN 978-3-7258-6630-4 (Hbk)
ISBN 978-3-7258-6631-1 (PDF)
https://doi.org/10.3390/books978-3-7258-6631-1

© 2026 by the authors. Articles in this reprint are Open Access and distributed under the Creative Commons Attribution (CC BY) license. The reprint as a whole is distributed by MDPI under the terms and conditions of the Creative Commons Attribution-NonCommercial-NoDerivs (CC BY-NC-ND) license (https://creativecommons.org/licenses/by-nc-nd/4.0/).

Contents

About the Editors

Christina Zong-Hao Ma

Christina Zong-Hao Ma is an Assistant Professor, a Certified Prosthetist and Orthotist (CPO, ISPO Category I), and a Certified Rehabilitation Therapist (CRT) at the Department of Biomedical Engineering, The Hong Kong Polytechnic University (PolyU). Before her appointment at PolyU, she served as a Lecturer, later promoted to Assistant Professor (permanent position), in Prosthetics and Orthotics at the Department of Rehabilitation, Jönköping University, Sweden, from 2018 to 2020. She received her PhD from the Faculty of Engineering, the Hong Kong Polytechnic University (2018), and her BSc from the West China School of Medicine, Sichuan University (2012). She also used to work as a Certified Prosthetist and Orthotist and a Clinical Instructor at the China Rehabilitation Research Center (permanent employment, 2012–2013) and as a Visiting Research Scholar in Mechanical Engineering at the University of Michigan, Ann Arbor (2017). Dr. Ma's research focuses on 1) investigating the mechanisms of human posture and motion control; 2) promoting physical activity and active health; and 3) developing solutions for improving balance and preventing falls in older/disabled people. Her research has been supported by the Health and Medical Research Fund (HMRF) Research Fellowship Scheme, the Chinese Association of Rehabilitation Medicine, and the Hong Kong Research Grants Council (RGC) Early Career Scheme (ECS).

Hong Fu

Hong Fu is an Associate Professor at the Department of Mathematics and Information Technology, the Education University of Hong Kong. She received her PhD from the Hong Kong Polytechnic University (2007) and her M.Eng (2003) and B.Eng and B.Mgt (2000) from Xi'an Jiaotong University. Dr. Fu's research focuses on computer vision algorithms, artificial intelligence in healthcare and education, eye tracking, and motion detection. Her research has been recognized by a number of awards, including a Gold Medal from the International Exhibition of Inventions of Geneva 2023, a Gold Medal and Jury's Choice Award from the International Invention Innovation Competition in Canada (iCAN) 2023, a Silver Medal from the 3rd Asia Exhibition of Innovations and Inventions (2023), and a Bronze Medal from the International Exhibitions of Inventions Geneva 2025.

bioengineering

MDPI

Editorial

Biomechanics and Motion Analysis: From Human Performance to Clinical Practice

Chen He [1], Hong Fu [2] and Christina Zong-Hao Ma [3,4,*]

1 School of Health Science and Engineering, University of Shanghai for Science and Technology, Shanghai 200093, China; hechen@usst.edu.cn
2 Department of Mathematics and Information Technology, The Education University of Hong Kong, Hong Kong SAR 999077, China; hfu@eduhk.hk
3 Department of Biomedical Engineering, The Hong Kong Polytechnic University, Hong Kong SAR 999077, China
4 Research Institute for Smart Ageing, The Hong Kong Polytechnic University, Hong Kong SAR 999077, China
* Correspondence: czh.ma@polyu.edu.hk; Tel.: +852-2766-7671; Fax: +852-2334-2429

1. Introduction

Research in biomechanics and motion analysis quantifies motion, forces, and control strategies, bridging the gap between fundamental science and practical applications. By translating movement into measurable data, it enables performance optimization, injury prevention, and improved clinical outcomes. Recent technological advances have enhanced motion analysis, allowing for more precise and accessible assessment of human movement. Such progress has deepened our understanding of both normal and pathological motion patterns, directly informing the development of targeted interventions from sports training to rehabilitation therapies.

This Special Issue compiles nineteen original research articles and two review articles, examining three different research areas: (1) the biomechanics of performance, adaptation and injury risk in specialized populations; (2) the application of motion analysis in diagnosing movement disorders and guiding rehabilitation; and (3) innovations in measurement technologies that enhance accuracy, accessibility, and privacy. Together, these studies illustrate how biomechanical insights can inform evidence-based practice across sports, occupational, and clinical settings.

2. Contributions to This Special Issue

2.1. Biomechanics of Performance, Adaption and Injury Risk

Conducting motion analysis on professional populations who perform high-intensity tasks provides an evidence base for optimizing performance through individualized training strategies and reducing injury risk via targeted interventions. Regarding athletic populations, Fernández-Baeza et al. [1] used tensiomyography (TMG) to identify imbalances in quadricep muscles in professional football players, linking these asymmetries to injury risk and emphasizing the potential of targeted training to restore muscle balance. Similarly, Liu et al. [2] reported bilateral technical asymmetry among elite speed skaters during sprinting; although it did not hinder performance, this asymmetry could be perceived as an efficient compensatory strategy for high-speed motion. Furthermore, Zhou et al. [3] demonstrated that elite jump rope athletes adjusted to increasing tempos by reducing contact time and joint range of motion. This strategy for optimizing movement control offers practical guidance for improving training efficiency and stability.

Studying occupational participants, Kasović et al. [4] observed that carrying a standard 3.5 kg load significantly increased asymmetry in ground reaction forces and plantar pressures in police recruits, substantiating the associated musculoskeletal injury risks. Conversely, Rožac et al. [5] found that progressively increasing loads up to 45 kg did not significantly affect spatiotemporal gait asymmetry in experienced intervention police officers, indicating that long-term professional training may contribute to adaptive responses that preserve stability under load.

These adaptations are further nuanced by specific individual factors. Wang et al. [6] demonstrated that obstacle height amplified latent gender differences in joint biomechanics during crossing tasks. These findings reveal context-dependent motor control strategies and underscore the importance of considering individual biomechanical profiles in training programs.

2.2. Clinical Biomechanics of Motor Dysfunction and Rehabilitation

Conducting biomechanical analysis in a clinical setting facilitates the detection of subtle movement flaws and alterations that precede or accompany specific pathologies. Zhu et al. [7] compared reactive balance control methods in older adults who had a history of falling and those who did not, finding that the former tended to rely more on suspensory strategies to compensate for deficiencies in ankle and hip strategies, which led to longer recovery times. This provides a new perspective for identifying and implementing interventions for individuals at a high risk of falling. Chang et al. [8] noted significant kinematic alterations in adolescents after treatment for unilateral developmental dysplasia of the hip, suggesting that these changes may increase loading on the contralateral limb and the long-term risk of osteoarthritis. Similarly, Tovaruela-Carrión et al. [9] revealed that hallux limitus induces subtle but significant alterations in stance phase contact, emphasizing the value of early biomechanical detection in preventing functional decline.

Biomechanical analysis also drives the development of targeted, evidence-based treatments from wearables to surgical protocols. Wang et al. [10] demonstrated that wearable focal vibration therapy is a feasible and effective home-based intervention for improving key gait parameters in individuals with multiple sclerosis. Molteni et al. [11] developed and validated a novel upper limb kinematic protocol using a custom marker set (capturing three-plane movement plus trunk/head kinematics), which can be used in clinical applications for conditions such as cerebral palsy. In Jie et al.'s study [12], a new digitalized 3D spinal decompression and correction device (with longitudinal traction and multi-planar forces) was shown to significantly improve in-brace correction and comfort in adolescents with idiopathic scoliosis. A review by He et al. [13] confirmed that next-generation scoliosis braces are biomechanically comparable to traditional designs, but they require better ergonomic refinement and more researches into their long-term value in clinic. Ma et al. [14] analyzed lumbar stability after partial facetectomy, providing crucial biomechanical evidence for optimizing surgical approaches to preserve spinal integrity. Yan et al. [15] introduced an "assist-as-needed" control strategy for rehabilitation robots, enhancing active participation in patients with stroke by dynamically adjusting assistance based on their subjective intent.

2.3. Methodological Innovations in Motion Capture and Analysis

Reliable motion analysis requires continuous methodological refinement. In this Special Issue, several studies address the core technical challenges in this area. Yuhai et al. [16] introduced a deep learning-based method that significantly outperformed traditional approaches in recovering missing motion capture data, thereby enhancing data completeness. Lee et al. [17] demonstrated that machine learning can reliably differentiate genuine hemiplegic gait from mimicked patterns. Their model achieved good discrimination using ten key kinematic and force features, showcasing a pathway to efficient, data-driven clinical assessments. To guide the selection of motion capture systems, Rohrer et al. [18] compared "around-body" and "on-body" systems to provide evidence-based recommendations for choosing the appropriate technology for specific clinical conditions. In an ergonomic assessment, Lind et al. [19] revealed that the common 'N-position' can result in a substantial underestimation of arm elevation, questioning its validity without correction.

Regarding privacy concerns, Su et al. [20] presented a high-fidelity mmWave radar dataset for human pose estimation that inherently preserves privacy, addressing the critical need for monitoring in sensitive environments. Luttmer et al. [21] introduced a unique data library of human–object interactions that combines kinematic data with kinetic measurements of haptic forces, this is an important tool for researchers studying real-world behavior, bridging the fields of biomechanics, robotics, and virtual reality.

3. Conclusions

The studies in this Special Issue demonstrate how movement analysis can improve athletic training, occupational safety, and clinical rehabilitation. The integration of wearable sensors, artificial intelligence, and large-scale biomechanical data increases the precision and personalization of these applications. We hope to inspire continued efforts and collaborations to further advance the biomechanical analysis of human movement and its practical impact.

Author Contributions: Conceptualization, C.H., H.F. and C.Z.-H.M.; writing—original draft preparation, C.H.; writing—review and editing, H.F. and C.Z.-H.M. All authors have read and agreed to the published version of the manuscript.

Funding: This research received no external funding.

Conflicts of Interest: The authors declare no conflicts of interest.

References

1. Fernández-Baeza, D.; Díaz-Ureña, G.; González-Millán, C. Contractile and Mechanical Properties of Quadriceps Muscles Measured by the Method of Tensiomyography (TMG) in Professional Soccer Players: A Systematic Review, Meta-Analysis, and Meta-Regression. *Bioengineering* **2024**, *11*, 1295. [CrossRef]
2. Liu, Z.; Ding, M.; Zhang, M.; Yu, B.; Liu, H. Effects of Technique Asymmetry on 500 m Speed Skating Performance. *Bioengineering* **2024**, *11*, 899. [CrossRef]
3. Zhou, Q.; Liu, Y.; Kang, J.; Wang, X.; Zhang, K.; Shan, G. Biomechanical Analysis of Cycle-Tempo Effects on Motor Control Among Jump Rope Elites. *Bioengineering* **2025**, *12*, 162. [CrossRef] [PubMed]
4. Kasović, M.; Štefan, A.; Štefan, L. Carrying Police Load Increases Gait Asymmetry in Ground Reaction Forces and Plantar Pressures Beneath Different Foot Regions in a Large Sample of Police Recruits. *Bioengineering* **2024**, *11*, 895. [CrossRef] [PubMed]
5. Rožac, D.; Kasović, M.; Knjaz, D. Spatiotemporal Gait Asymmetries Remain Unaffected by Increased Load Carriage in Professional Intervention Police Officers. *Bioengineering* **2024**, *11*, 1140. [CrossRef] [PubMed]
6. Wang, C.; Guo, Y.; Du, W.; Li, Z.; Chen, W. Gender Differences in Joint Biomechanics During Obstacle Crossing with Different Heights. *Bioengineering* **2025**, *12*, 189. [CrossRef]
7. Zhu, R.T.-L.; Hung, T.T.M.; Lam, F.M.H.; Li, J.-Z.; Luo, Y.-Y.; Sun, J.; Wang, S.; Ma, C.Z.-H. Older Fallers' Comprehensive Neuromuscular and Kinematic Alterations in Reactive Balance Control: Indicators of Balance Decline or Compensation? *A Pilot Study. Bioengineering* **2025**, *12*, 66. [CrossRef]
8. Chang, C.-F.; Lu, T.-W.; Hu, C.-H.; Wu, K.-W.; Kuo, C.-C.; Wang, T.-M. Lower Limb Inter-Joint Coordination and End-Point Control During Gait in Adolescents with Early Treated Unilateral Developmental Dysplasia of the Hip. *Bioengineering* **2025**, *12*, 836. [CrossRef]
9. Tovaruela-Carrión, N.; Becerro-de-Bengoa-Vallejo, R.; Losa-Iglesias, M.E.; López-López, D.; Gómez-Salgado, J.; Bayod-López, J. Exploring the Association of Hallux Limitus with Baropodometric Gait Pattern Changes. *Bioengineering* **2025**, *12*, 316. [CrossRef]
10. Wang, H.; Shin, Y.C.; Tester, N.J.; Rempe, T. Feasibility and Preliminary Efficacy of Wearable Focal Vibration Therapy on Gait and Mobility in People with Multiple Sclerosis: A Pilot Study. *Bioengineering* **2025**, *12*, 932. [CrossRef]

11. Molteni, L.E.; Piccinini, L.; Panzeri, D.; Micheletti, E.; Andreoni, G. A Novel Protocol for Integrated Assessment of Upper Limbs Using the Optoelectronic Motion Analysis System: Validation and Usability in Healthy People. *Bioengineering* **2025**, *12*, 905. [CrossRef]
12. Jie, Y.; Li, M.; Dong, A.; Luo, Y.-Y.; Luo, C.-L.; Li, J.; Zheng, P.; Zhang, X.; Wong, M.S.; Ma, C.Z.-H.; et al. Digitalized 3D Spinal Decompression and Correction Device Improved Initial Brace Corrections and Patients' Comfort Among Adolescents with Idiopathic Scoliosis: A Single-Centre, Single-Blinded Randomized Controlled Trial. *Bioengineering* **2024**, *11*, 1246. [CrossRef] [PubMed]
13. He, C.; Xie, J.; Pang, R.; Hu, B.; Ma, C.Z.-H. Could Novel Spinal Braces with Flexibility, Robotic Components, and Individualized Design Generate Sufficient Biomechanical Treatment Efficacy in Patients with Scoliosis? *Bioengineering* **2025**, *12*, 1083. [CrossRef]
14. Ma, T.; Tu, X.; Li, J.; Wu, J.; Nong, L. In Vitro Biomechanical Experiment on the Effect of Unilateral Partial Facetectomy Performed by Percutaneous Endoscopy on the Stability of Lumbar Spine. *Bioengineering* **2025**, *12*, 414. [CrossRef]
15. Yan, H.; Zhang, F.; Li, X.; Zhang, C.; Zhang, Y.; Feng, Y. An Assist-as-Needed Control Strategy Based on a Subjective Intention Decline Model. *Bioengineering* **2024**, *11*, 1113. [CrossRef]
16. Yuhai, O.; Choi, A.; Cho, Y.; Kim, H.; Mun, J.H. Deep-Learning-Based Recovery of Missing Optical Marker Trajectories in 3D Motion Capture Systems. *Bioengineering* **2024**, *11*, 560. [CrossRef]
17. Lee, Y.-u.; Kwon, S.; Kim, C.-H.; Seo, J.-W.; Lee, S. Classification of Hemiplegic Gait and Mimicked Hemiplegic Gait: A Treadmill Gait Analysis Study in Stroke Patients and Healthy Individuals. *Bioengineering* **2025**, *12*, 1074. [CrossRef]
18. Rohrer, K.; De Anda, L.; Grubb, C.; Hansen, Z.; Rodriguez, J.; St Pierre, G.; Sheikhlary, S.; Omer, S.; Tran, B.; Lawendy, M.; et al. Around-Body Versus On-Body Motion Sensing: A Comparison of Efficacy Across a Range of Body Movements and Scales. *Bioengineering* **2024**, *11*, 1163. [CrossRef]
19. Lind, C.M.; Rhen, I.-M.; Forsman, M. Reliability and Accuracy of Standard Reference Procedures for Measurements of Trunk and Arm Postures in Ergonomics. *Bioengineering* **2025**, *12*, 50. [CrossRef]
20. Su, Y.; Hou, H.; Lan, H.; Ma, C.Z.-H. A High-Fidelity mmWave Radar Dataset for Privacy-Sensitive Human Pose Estimation. *Bioengineering* **2025**, *12*, 891. [CrossRef]
21. Luttmer, N.G.; Baum, N.I.; Flores-Gonzalez, J.; Hollerbach, J.M.; Minor, M.A. The Utah Manipulation and Locomotion of Large Objects (MeLLO) Data Library. *Bioengineering* **2025**, *12*, 317. [CrossRef]

Disclaimer/Publisher's Note: The statements, opinions and data contained in all publications are solely those of the individual author(s) and contributor(s) and not of MDPI and/or the editor(s). MDPI and/or the editor(s) disclaim responsibility for any injury to people or property resulting from any ideas, methods, instructions or products referred to in the content.

bioengineering

MDPI

Article

Simulating Real-World Slips: Enhanced Kinematic and Neuromuscular Responses to Experimental Slips in the Early vs. Late Stance Phase in Young and Older Adults

Marina Geissmann [1], Nicole Sarah Holliger [2,3,4], Lennart Carlson Neumann [2,3,4], Antonia Maria Eilfort [2,3,4] and Linard Filli [1,2,4,*]

1 Swiss Center for Movement Analysis (SCMA), Balgrist Campus AG, 8008 Zurich, Switzerland; marina.geissmann@balgristcampus.ch
2 Neuroscience Center Zurich, University of Zurich, 8008 Zurich, Switzerland; nicole.holliger@balgrist.ch (N.S.H.); lennart.neumann@balgrist.ch (L.C.N.); antonia.eilfort@balgrist.ch (A.M.E.)
3 Department of Health Sciences and Technology, ETH Zurich, 8093 Zurich, Switzerland
4 Spinal Cord Injury Center, Balgrist University Hospital, University of Zurich, 8008 Zurich, Switzerland
* Correspondence: linard.filli@balgrist.ch

Abstract: Slips are a leading cause of injury and hospitalization among at-risk individuals. Replicating real-world slips by experimental, mechanical perturbations is essential for characterizing reactive balance mechanisms activated during near-fall situations and for training these mechanisms in fall prevention programs. This study compared treadmill-based, slip-like perturbations targeting the early (early perturbations, EP) vs. late stance phase (late perturbations, LP) in 22 young and 21 older adults. Biomechanical and neuromuscular responses were assessed using full-body kinematics and surface electromyography (EMG). Additionally, participants provided subjective rating of perturbation intensity and inconvenience. EP elicited stronger reactive balance responses than LP, characterized by greater deviations in leg joint and trunk kinematics, as well as shorter EMG onset latencies and enhanced EMG peak amplitudes. Gait parameters required longer to recover to baseline following EP than LP. Subjectively, EP were rated as more intense and inconvenient, and were perceived to more closely mimic real-world slips. Older adults showed delayed and attenuated reactive balance responses compared to younger adults. These findings highlight the importance of targeting the vulnerable early stance phase to accurately simulate real-world slip events. Such perturbation paradigms may support the development of more effective, task-specific perturbation-based training programs aimed at reducing falls in at-risk populations.

Keywords: slip responses; mechanical perturbations; automatic postural responses; reactive balance; fall prevention; fall simulation; reactive balance training; slipping

1. Introduction

Falls are a major cause of injuries and hospitalization among older adults and individuals with musculoskeletal or neurological disorders [1,2]. More than one-third of older adults experience at least one fall per year [3]. A significant proportion of injury-related falls occur due to slips during walking that result in a sudden loss of balance [4].

Slips occur when the friction coefficient (available friction) is lower than the ratio of shear to normal foot forces (required friction). The initial stance phase, immediately after foot contact, is the most vulnerable period for slips in the real-world setting [5,6], causing the foot to slide forward. Previous studies have demonstrated that the timing of perturbation onset within the gait cycle significantly influences the magnitude of the reactive response [7,8]. Intriguingly, most treadmill-based slip paradigms trigger belt deceleration at foot contact, resulting in peak slip velocity occurring during mid-to-late stance [9–12]. In contrast, experimental slips peaking during the critical early stance phase remain rare, likely due to methodological challenges in initiating perturbations prior to foot contact.

Previous studies investigating the biomechanical aspects of slips have employed oily surfaces [13–15] and moveable platforms [8,16]. Whereas these methods effectively replicate the mechanical characteristics of slipping, they are limited in their ability to randomize the timing or location of the perturbation due to their fixed positioning. Consequently, participants often anticipate slip events (e.g., by adopting a more cautious gait), which substantially confounds the interpretation of stabilizing responses. In contrast, treadmill-based perturbations allow for fully unpredictable slip timing and enable the collection of a large number of steps and perturbation events. Treadmill-based systems also provide high reliability in delivering perturbations with consistent amplitude and precise timing within specific phases of the gait cycle [9,10,17]. Therefore, treadmill-based perturbations offer a valid and accurate approach for examining fast postural responses and locomotor recovery following slips. While the effects of perturbation intensity on slip-induced falls have been extensively investigated [18–20], the influence of perturbation timing on slipping remains poorly understood.

Locomotor adaptability typically declines with age, becoming more challenging and less effective [21]. This is largely attributed to age-related neuromuscular and sensory deterioration, decreased tendon stiffness, and reduced muscle strength, all of which impair motor control and balance [21,22]. However, the impact of aging on reactive balance remains inconclusive: while some studies report substantial differences between younger and older individuals [21–23], others show no significant age-related differences [12]. The most prominent age-related differences include attenuated EMG responses [22] and prolonged recovery times following perturbations in older adults [21,23].

This study aimed at developing a novel perturbation algorithm targeting the critical initial stance phase to more accurately replicate real-world slip conditions. Specifically, we compared the biomechanical effects of identical deceleration perturbations applied during either the early or late stance phase in younger and older adults using multimodal instrumented motion capture and EMG. We hypothesized that slip-like perturbations during early stance would induce stronger reactive responses and prolonged recovery phases than those applied during late stance. Furthermore, we expected older participants to exhibit more pronounced perturbation responses and delayed recovery than their younger counterparts.

The findings of this study advance our understanding of how perturbation timing and age influence reactive responses to slipping. By establishing an experimental paradigm that closely replicates key features of real-world slips, this work may inform the development of more effective, task-specific training protocols to improve reactive balance and reduce fall risk.

2. Materials and Methods

2.1. Participants

Twenty-two healthy young and 22 healthy older adults were included in this study. No *a priori* power analysis was conducted to determine the sample size. However, a population size of approximately 20 healthy participants is frequent in studies examining the effects of mechanical perturbations on biomechanical aspects [10]. Only participants able to walk at least 30 min without assistance or rest were included. Exclusion criteria included pregnancy, breastfeeding, and any neurological or orthopedic conditions potentially affecting walking function or balance. One participant from the older group discontinued the study due to a muscle injury sustained during testing. Therefore, 22 young and 21 older adults were included in the final data analysis.

2.2. Experimental Protocol

Gait perturbations were applied using the GRAIL system (Motek, Houten, The Netherlands) that consists of ten motion capture cameras (Vicon, Oxford, UK) operating at 200 Hz, a split-belt treadmill with two embedded force plates sampling at 1000 Hz, and a 180° immersive virtual screen. Throughout the experiment, participants walked within an immersive virtual environment depicting a New York City scene (Motek, Houten, The Netherlands). Handrails were removed and participants were secured by a safety harness to prevent falls. Full body kinematics were recorded using a modified version of the Plug-in Gait model containing 36 markers. Surface EMG was performed using a wireless system (Myon Aktos, Cometa Systems, Bareggio, Italy) to assess activity in the vastus medialis (VM), semitendinosus (SM), tibialis anterior (TA) and gastrocnemius medialis (GM) muscles with a sampling frequency of 1000 Hz. Electrodes were placed on muscles of the leg ipsilateral to the perturbation (VM, SM, TA, GM) and the corresponding contralateral muscles (c_VM, c_SM, c_TA, c_GM). Electrode placement was conducted according to surface electromyography for the non-invasive assessment of muscles (SENIAM) guidelines where applicable (http://seniam.org (accessed on 24 July 2024)). Skin impedance was optimized by shaving and carefully abrading (Nuprep gel, Waver and Company, Aurora, CO, USA) the skin overlying the muscles of interest. The skin was then cleaned with alcohol prior to electrode placement.

Prior to the perturbation trials, all participants filled out the Activities-Specific Balance Confidence (ABC) scale questionnaire to assess the self-perceived balance confidence in performing various activities of daily life [24]. Additionally, the functional gait assessment (FGA) was conducted to measure the participants' dynamic stability and balance [25]. Then, participants were familiarized with treadmill walking at different speeds for six minutes [26]. Thereafter, participants completed three perturbation blocks, each consisting of ten perturbations. They walked on the treadmill at a fixed speed of 1.2 m/s, while perturbations were induced through either deceleration or acceleration of the treadmill belt applied at different timepoints within the gait cycle. A fixed walking speed of 1.2 m/s was selected based on previous findings reporting it as a comfortable pace for both young and older adults [12]. Maintaining a constant walking speed across age groups ensured comparability of perturbation intensity and responses across participants.

For data analysis, we focused exclusively on the two deceleration perturbation types that mimic forward movements of the foot during slips. Importantly, both perturbations were identical in terms of their deceleration profile. Specifically, they were applied while participants walked at a fixed walking speed of 1.2 m/s. A deceleration of 5 m/s^2 was imposed for 0.33 s, resulting in a negative peak belt velocity of −0.45 m/s. There was an immediate re-acceleration of the treadmill belt at 5 m/s^2 for 0.33 s to return to the baseline speed of 1.2 m/s. However, the two slipping perturbations were applied at different timepoints within the gait cycle: the first deceleration algorithm was triggered upon foot contact, as defined by Zeni at al. [27], resulting in peak perturbation amplitude occurring during mid-to-late stance phase. The second deceleration algorithm was initiated during the swing phase, inducing the peak perturbation amplitude shortly after foot contact. Perturbations in which this peak velocity occurred before 5% of the gait cycle were excluded from analysis. For each perturbation, ten trials were assessed, with their order presented in a pseudo-randomized sequence to avoid anticipatory responses. At the end of the experiment, each perturbation type was individually evaluated by participants using self-reported ratings for perceived inconvenience and intensity (each reaching from 0 to 10), and their perceived similarity to a real-life situation causing instability.

2.3. Data Analysis

All data were analyzed using Vicon Nexus (version 2.10.3 Vicon Nexus, Oxford, UK) and custom-written Matlab scripts (version 2024a, The Mathworks, Natick, MA, USA). The marker data was filtered using a Woltring mean squared error (MSE) filter [28] and EMG data with a second order bandpass filter (10–500 Hz) followed by signal rectification. Gait events were identified by the algorithm developed by Zeni et al. [27] and manually corrected if needed. The following spatiotemporal parameters were analyzed: step length, step width, step duration and stance phase duration. Kinematic parameters were extracted from Plug-in-Gait. For each parameter, twenty gait cycles were analyzed prior to each perturbation to establish a baseline. Moreover, the perturbation step (Pert), as well as the ten steps post perturbation (P1 to P10) were examined to assess balance recovery. Cross-steps between treadmill belts were excluded from the analysis. Baseline EMG activity was determined over ten gait cycles without perturbations. Reaction time was defined as the point at which EMG activity exceeded the baseline mean + 2 standard deviations. EMG amplitude was evaluated by calculating the maximal change in the EMG signal between regular and perturbed walking conditions.

2.4. Statistical Analyses

Statistical analysis was performed using RStudio (version 4.4.2). The significance level was set at $\alpha = 0.05$ for all statistical tests. Normality of the data was investigated using the Shapiro–Wilk test [29]. Normally distributed data sets were analyzed using parametric statistical tests, while those with non-normal distribution were assessed using non-parametric tests. Demographic differences between the young and older age group were investigated using independent t-tests (body height and body weight) or non-parametric Mann–Whitney tests (age, FGA and ABC scale) [30]. Gender distribution was tested using a 2-tailed Fisher's Exact Test.

Peak velocity within the gait cycle was assessed using a paired t-test for LP, and a paired Wilcoxon test for EP, as the latter data set was not normally distributed. Subjective ratings of perturbation intensity and inconvenience, treated as ordinal data, were assessed using a Wilcoxon's sign rank test.

Linear mixed models (lmer function of the lme4 package) were used to assess EMG reaction times and amplitudes, with perturbation (EP, LP) and muscle (SM, VM, GM, TA, c_SM, c_VM, c_GM and c_TA) included as fixed factors, and subjects as a random effect. For assessing recovery of spatiotemporal gait parameters (step length, step width, step duration and stance phase duration) upon perturbations, models were fitted with perturbation (EP, LP) and step (base, P1-P10) as fixed factors, and subjects as a random effect. A type-I ANOVA was performed on the fitted model, followed by Tukey's honest significance difference (HSD) test for pairwise comparison.

Furthermore, one-dimensional continuous time series data, such as joint angles, were analyzed using MATLAB 2024a (The Mathworks, Natick, MA, USA) with the Statistical Parametric Mapping 1D approach (SPM 1D, www.spm1d.org) that is based on random field theory [25]. Data normality was assessed using the spm1d build in function (spm1d.stats.normality.anova1rm). Depending on the outcome of the data normality tests, either the statistical parametric mapping (spm1d.stats1d.anova1rm) or the statistical non-parametric mapping (spm1d.stats1d.nonparam.anova1rm) was applied. Post hoc analyses were conducted using the spm1d build in function (spm1d.stats1d.anova1_posthhoc) to compare the perturbations algorithms to normal walking. The null hypothesis was rejected if the SPM {t} exceeded the critical threshold t^* at alpha = 0.05.

3. Results

Twenty-two healthy young (11 females, 28.3 ± 4.8 years) and 21 older participants (10 females, 66.1 ± 3.9 years) were included in the analysis (Table 1). No significant group differences were observed in gender distribution ($p = 1.0$), body height ($p = 0.1841$; d = −0.411) and weight ($p = 0.6923$; d = −0.122). However, older participants showed reduced gait stability, as reflected by lower scores in the FGA (young vs. old: 29.8 ± 0.4 pts vs. 29.0 ± 0.9 pts; $p = 0.0007$; r = 0.520) and reduced balance confidence measured by the ABC scale (young vs. old: 97.6 ± 2.5% vs. 91.4 ± 10.4%; $p = 0.0143$; r = 0.375).

Table 1. Demographic characteristics of the young ($n = 22$) and older ($n = 21$) participant group. Values are presented as mean ± standard deviation. The Functional Gait Assessment (FGA) has a maximum score of 30 points, whereas the Activities-specific Balance Confidence (ABC) scale has a maximum score of 100%. Abbreviations: F: female; M: male.

	Young	Old	*p*-Value
Gender [M/F]	11/11	11/10	1.0
Age [years]	28.3 ± 4.8	66.1 ± 3.9	<0.0001
Height [m]	1.73 ± 0.08	1.70 ± 0.07	0.1841
Weight [kg]	69.3 ± 13.1	67.8 ± 11.0	0.6923
FGA [score]	29.8 ± 0.4	29.0 ± 0.9	0.0007
ABC scale [%]	97.6 ± 2.5	91.4 ± 10.4	0.0143

The timing of perturbation peak velocity within the gait cycle differed significantly between perturbation types in both age groups. In young adults, early perturbations (EP) occurred at 15.3 ± 2.8% and late perturbations (LP) at 47.5 ± 3.7% of the gait cycle (Z = 4.1069; $p < 0.0001$; rs = 0.6635). Similarly, in older adults, EP occurred at 15.9 ± 3.4% and LP occurred at 48.3 ± 5.2% of the gait cycle (Z = 4.0145; $p < 0.0001$; rs = 0.1143).

3.1. *Initial Response to Experimental Slips in Young Participants*

3.1.1. Kinematics

Overall, EP elicited greater initial kinematic responses than LP (Figure 1). Specifically, EP induced enhanced trunk flexion relative to normal walking from 28.1 to 100% of the gait cycle ($p < 0.0001$). This marked abdominal flexion likely serves to shift the center of pressure (CoP) anteriorly, thereby counteracting backward destabilization and preventing falls. In contrast, LP did not result in altered trunk kinematics relative to normal walking.

Both EP and LP led to significant alterations of hip and knee angle trajectories, mainly manifesting as enhanced flexion during stance, and modified movement patterns during the swing phase. For EP, significant deviations were observed at the hip from 14.4 to 67.0% of the gait cycle ($p < 0.0001$) and at the knee from 4.8 to 15.4% ($p = 0.0002$), 19.1–57.7% ($p < 0.0001$), 61.0–79.2% ($p < 0.0001$). For LP, significant changes occurred at the hip from 27.6 to 69.8% of the gait cycle ($p < 0.0001$), and at the knee from 16.9 to 21.8% ($p = 0.0073$), 31.7–57.9% ($p < 0.0001$), 61.5–82.2% ($p < 0.0001$). Additional deviations from normal joint angle trajectories were observed during the swing phase, likely as a consequence of the pronounced initial flexion. For EP, significant deviations were noted at the hip between 72.2 and 81.4% ($p = 0.0054$) and 88.6–99.8% ($p = 0.003$), and at the knee between 82.3 and 99.0% ($p < 0.0001$) and 99.3–100% ($p = 0.0166$). For LP, deviations were present at the hip from 90.2 to 95.4% ($p = 0.0113$), and at the knee from 84.9 to 100% ($p < 0.0001$). Overall, aberrant flexion movements at both the hip and knee were substantially more pronounced following EP compared to LP (Figure 1).

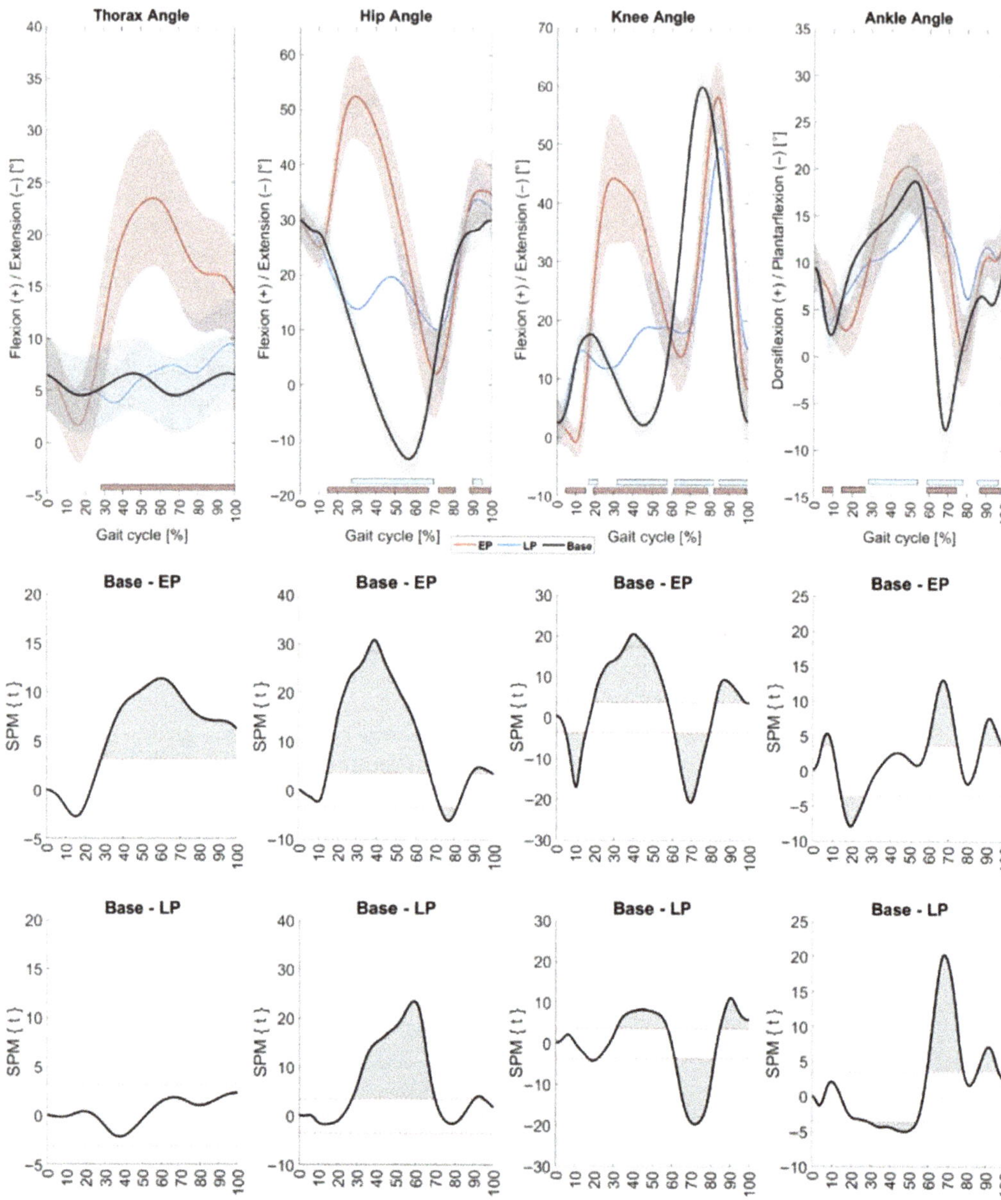

Figure 1. Initial kinematic responses to perturbations in young adults. (**Top row**) Mean sagittal plane kinematics of the thorax, hip, knee and ankle during regular walking (black lines; shaded areas represent ± 1 standard deviation), and in response to EP (red) and LP (blue). (**Middle row**) Statistical comparison between regular walking (base) and EP for thorax, hip, knee and ankle movements using Statistical Parametric Mapping (SPM). (**Bottom row**) SPM comparison between regular walking (base) and LP for all walking parameters. All data are time-normalized to the gait cycle. Joint angles for the hip, knee and ankle are shown for the leg ipsilateral to the perturbation. Significant differences between regular walking and EP are indicated by red bars at the lower part of the top figure row. Statistical differences between regular walking and LP are indicated by blue bars. Abbreviations: EP: early perturbations; LP: late perturbations.

Perturbation-induced deviations in ankle angle trajectories were generally comparable between EP and LP. EP elicited a delayed ankle plantarflexion after initial contact, with deviations emerging between 4.6 and 9.9% ($p = 0.0068$) and 14.5–27.0% ($p = 0.0001$)) of the gait cycle relative to normal walking. In contrast, LP induced a recued dorsiflexion during mid-stance, with significant alterations occurring between 28.5 and 54.2% ($p < 0.0001$) of the gait cycle. Later in the gait cycle, deviations were similar between EP and LP (EP vs. normal: 59.0–75.0% ($p < 0.0001$) and 87.0–98.5% ($p = 0.0003$): LP vs. normal: 59.2–78.4% ($p < 0.0001$) and 85.6–96.7% ($p = 0.0009$)).

3.1.2. EMG

Muscle activity profiles of the VM, SM, GM and TA on the perturbed side revealed substantial initial responses induced by both EP and LP (Figure 2). Across all muscles, EMG responses to EP appeared earlier within the gait cycle compared to LP, consistent with the earlier timing of EP application (Figure 2). Additionally, the magnitude of perturbation-induced EMG activity was greater in response to EP than LP.

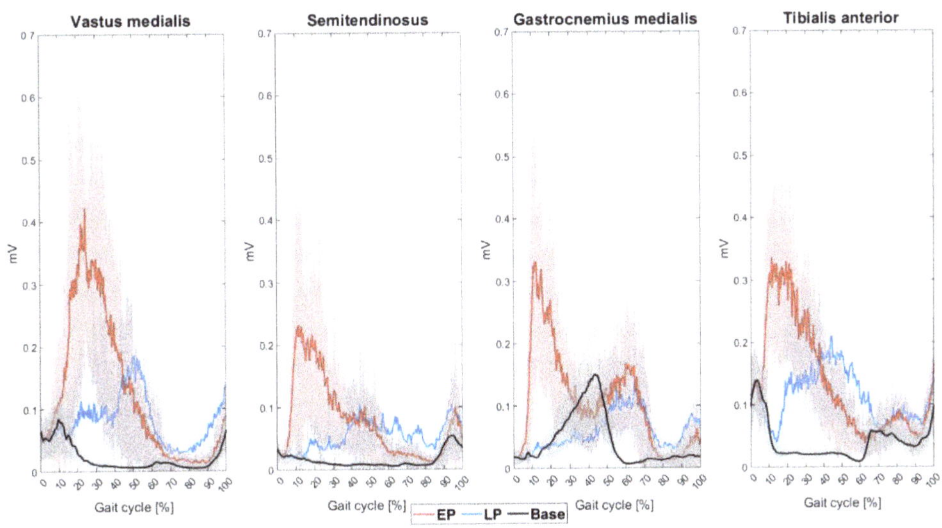

Figure 2. EMG responses to perturbations in various leg muscles of young adults. EMG activity of the vastus medialis, semitendinosus, gastrocnemius medialis and tibialis anterior muscles during regular walking (black curves), and in response to EP (red) and LP (blue). Shaded areas represent ±standard deviation for the respective conditions. All data are time-normalized to the gait cycle. Abbreviations: EP: early perturbations; LP: late perturbations.

EMG reaction times revealed significant main effects of *perturbation* ($F(1,315) = 113.31$, $p < 0.0001$), *muscle* ($F(7,315) = 45.80$, $p < 0.0001$), and their interaction (*perturbation*muscle:* $F(7,315) = 67.17$, $p < 0.0001$). Post hoc analysis demonstrated significantly shorter reaction times following EP vs. LP in the ipsilateral GM, as well as in the VM, TA and GM contralateral to the perturbation (Table 2). In contrast, reaction times in the ipsilateral VM were prolonged during EP, a phenomenon that might be attributed to the sudden passive extension of the ipsilateral hip and knee that potentially inhibits VM activity.

Maximal EMG amplitudes were significantly affected by the main factors *perturbation* ($F(1,315) = 136.52$, $p < 0.0001$) and *muscle* ($F(7,315) = 17.84$, $p < 0.0001$), as well as their interaction ($F(7,315) = 9.85$, $p < 0.0001$). Initial EMG responses showed enhanced amplitudes upon EP vs. LP across all muscles (Table 2). This effect reached statistical significance in all muscles, except the SM and GM on the contralateral side.

Table 2. Reaction times and peak amplitudes of initial EMG responses to EP and LP in various leg muscles of young participants. Values present the mean ± standard deviation. Statistics include effects sizes measures. (estimate (β) and t ratio (t)). Abbreviations: c_: contralateral; EP: early perturbations; GM: gastrocnemius medialis; LP: later perturbations; SM: semitendinosus; TA: tibialis anterior; VM: vastus medialis.

Muscle	Reaction Time [ms]				
	EP	**LP**	***p*-Value**	**B**	**t**
SM	88 ± 14	104 ± 33	0.2420	15.73	1.172
VM	166 ± 40	120 ± 18	0.0035	−39.45	−2.941
TA	101 ± 12	105 ± 18	0.9703	−0.50	−0.037
GM	100 ± 26	383 ± 127	<0.0001	315.09	23.485
c_SM	90 ± 11	105 ± 25	0.5050	8.95	0.667
c_VM	77 ± 13	103 ± 34	0.0362	28.23	2.104
c_TA	92 ± 13	121 ± 28	0.0374	28.05	2.090
c_GM	112 ± 14	157 ± 81	0.0004	47.86	3.567
Muscle	**Amplitude [mV]**				
	EP	**LP**	***p*-Value**	**B**	**t**
SM	0.37 ± 0.26	0.20 ± 0.16	0.0004	−0.1774	−3.558
VM	0.71 ± 0.25	0.35 ± 0.27	<0.0001	−0.3582	−7.182
TA	0.52 ± 0.15	0.39 ± 0.14	0.0078	−0.1336	−2.678
GM	0.58 ± 0.22	0.26 ± 0.10	<0.0001	−0.3253	−6.522
c_SM	0.36 ± 0.19	0.32 ± 0.19	0.5151	−0.0325	−0.652
c_VM	0.83 ± 0.39	0.38 ± 0.25	<0.0001	−0.4554	−9.131
c_TA	0.45 ± 0.14	0.31 ± 0.13	0.0073	−0.1347	−2.701
c_GM	0.37 ± 0.12	0.34 ± 0.13	0.5334	−0.0311	−0.624

3.2. Recovery Response in Young Participants

A significant main effect of *perturbation* was observed in step length ($F(1,441) = 4.64$, $p = 0.03174$), step duration ($F(1,441) = 21.57$, $p < 0.0001$) and stance phase ($F(1,441) = 31.61$, $p < 0.0001$). Moreover, the main factor *step after perturbation* significantly affected step length ($F(10,441) = 11.00$, $p < 0.0001$), step width ($F(10,441) = 9.58$, $p < 0.0001$), step duration ($F(10,441) = 133.10$, $p < 0.0001$) and stance phase ($F(10,441) = 149.13$, $p < 0.0001$). A significant interaction effect of *step after perturbation*perturbation* was observed in step length ($F(10,441) = 3.07$, $p = 0.0009$), step duration ($F(10,441) = 10.29$, $p < 0.0001$) and stance phase ($F(10,441) = 8.66$, $p < 0.0001$).

The time required for gait parameter recovery to baseline levels was slightly prolonged following EP compared to LP (Figure 3). After EP, step length returned to baseline by step P5, step width by P6, step duration and stance phase by P4. In contrast, following LP, step length was not significantly different from normal walking for two consecutive steps, and therefore no clear recovery phase was identified for this parameter. Step width recovered by P5, step duration and percentage of stance phase by P4 (Figure 3).

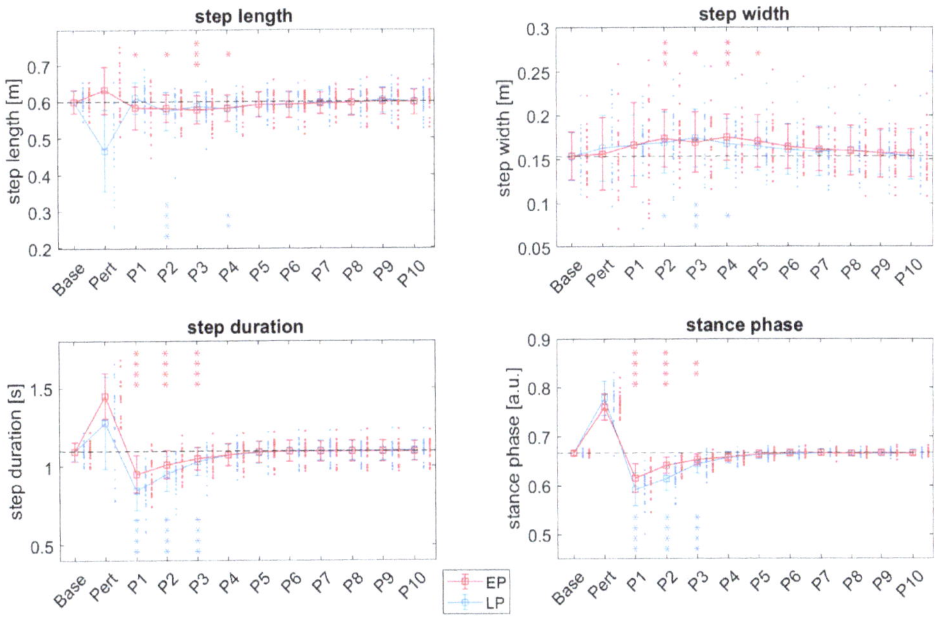

Figure 3. Recovery of spatiotemporal gait parameters following EP (red) and LP (blue) in young participants. The baseline (Base; dashed horizontal line) represents average values during regular walking, calculated from 20 unperturbed steps preceding the perturbation. Pert denotes the actually perturbed step, and P1-P10 indicate the ten subsequent recovery steps. Stance phase is reported as proportion of stance phase relative to step duration. Asterisks denote statistical significance: * $p < 0.05$, ** p-value < 0.01, *** p-value < 0.001, and **** $p < 0.0001$. Red asterisks indicate significant differences between EP and baseline; blue asterisks highlight differences between LP and baseline.

3.3. Subjective Perception of Perturbations in Young Participants

Participants rated the degree of perturbation inconvenience significantly higher for EP (median = 7.0, 95% CI, 6.0, 8.0) than LP (median = 3.0, 95% CI, 3.0, 5.0, Z = −3.9859; $p = 0.0002$; rs = 0.0831; Figure 4). Similarly, perceived perturbation intensity was greater for EP (median = 7.5, 95% CI, 7.0, 8.0) compared to LP (median = 3.0, 95% CI, 2.0, 5.0, Z = −3.9771; $p = 0.0002$; rs = 0.2652).

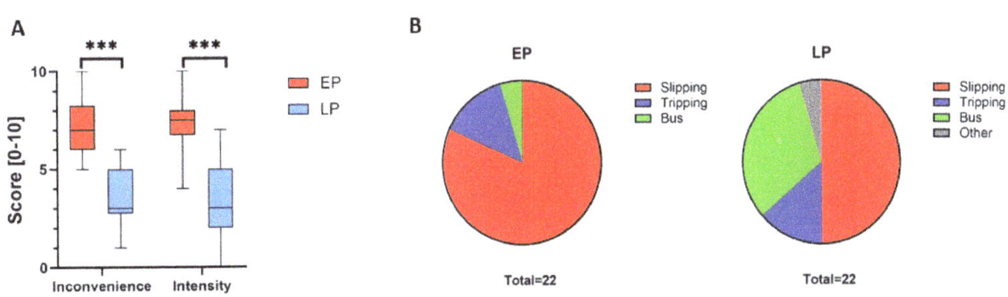

Figure 4. Subjective perception of the different perturbations in young adults. (**A**) Subjective ratings of EP (red) and LP (blue) with respect to perceived inconvenience and intensity. Rating ranged from 0 to 10, with 10 representing maximal inconvenience or intensity. (**B**) Comparison of EP and LP to real-life conditions including slipping, tripping, perturbations in bus and other conditions. *** represents p-value < 0.001.

When asked how they perceived the perturbations, young participants most commonly associated EP with slipping (81.8%), followed by tripping (13.6%) and a sudden bus stop (4.6%; Figure 4). LP was mostly perceived as slipping (50%) followed by a sudden bus stop (31.8%), tripping (13.6%) and other daily activities (4.6%). Interestingly, slipping was more frequently associated with EP than LP (81.8% vs. 50%), indicating that treadmill belt deceleration during early stance more closely mimics real-life slipping than perturbations applied during late stance.

3.4. *Age Differences*

3.4.1. Initial Response

Overall, kinematic responses to perturbations were largely similar between younger and older participants. Younger adults exhibited higher peak hip and knee flexion angles compared to older participants during both perturbations. In LP trials, significant knee angle differences were observed throughout both the stance and swing phase in the younger group. In contrast, older participants only showed significant alterations during the swing phase 61.6–84.0% ($p < 0.0001$) and 88.8–100% ($p = 0.0038$) (Figure S1).

A significant main effect of *age* was found for EMG reaction times ($F(1,41) = 22.56$, $p < 0.0001$). Additionally, significant *age* and *perturbation*age* effects were identified for the maximal amplitudes of initial EMG responses ($F(1,41) = 4.56$, $p = 0.0388$, $F(1,615) = 21.88$, $p < 0.0001$). Older adults exhibited prolonged reaction times and reduced EMG amplitudes compared to younger participants.

Both age groups demonstrated shorter EMG reaction times for EP vs. LP in the same set of muscles (ipsilateral VM and, contralateral VM, TA and GM). However, the increase in maximal amplitudes of EMG responses was attenuated in older participants (Table 3). In this group, enhanced maximal amplitudes were only observed in the SM ($p = 0.0195$), VM ($p < 0.0001$), GM ($p < 0.0001$) and c_VM ($p = 0.0012$; Table 3).

3.4.2. Recovery Response

In both age groups, comparable main effects of perturbation were observed for step length, step width, step duration and stance phase. However, subtle age-related differences emerged in the recovery time of spatiotemporal gait parameters. In older participants, step length recovered to normal walking at P4 following LP, whereas no significant deviation from normal walking was observed following EP, indicating no recovery steps were required (Figure S2). Step width recovered at P6 following EP and at P5 following LP, consistent with the recovery pattern observed in young participants. For step duration and stance phase duration, older adults required one additional step to return to baseline values compared to younger participants. Specifically, recovery occurred at step P5 in the older group versus P4 in the younger group for both perturbation types (Figures 3 and S2).

3.4.3. Subjective Perception of Perturbations

Analogous to their younger counterparts, older adults rated perturbation inconvenience higher for EP (median = 5.0, 95% CI, 3.0, 6.0) compared to LP (median = 3.0, 95% CI, 2.0, 3.0; $Z = -3.6031$; $p < 0.0001$; rs = 0.5025; Figure S3). Similarly, perceived perturbation intensity was significantly greater for EP (median = 5.0, 95% CI, 4.0, 7.0) than LP (median = 3.0, 95% CI, 2.0, 3.0; $Z = -3.8233$; $p < 0.0001$; rs = 0.1667). Overall, subjective ratings of both inconvenience and intensity were lower in older than younger participants (Figures 4 and S3).

In terms of perceived perturbation type, the majority of older participants associated EP with slipping (80.9%), followed by tripping (9.5%), a sudden bus stop (4.8%) and other daily activities (4.8%). For LP, slipping was also the most commonly mentioned perception (42.8%), followed by a sudden bus stop (28.6%) and tripping (28.6%; Figure S3).

Table 3. Reaction times and peak amplitudes (mean ± standard deviation) of initial EMG responses to EP and LP in various leg muscles of older participants. Statistics include effects sizes measures (estimate (β) and t ratio (t)). Abbreviations: c_: contralateral; EP: early perturbations; GM: gastrocnemius medialis; LP: later perturbations; SM: semitendinosus; TA: tibialis anterior; VM: vastus medialis.

Muscle	Reaction Time [ms]				
	EP	LP	*p*-Value	β	t
SM	108 ± 12	123 ± 48	0.2892	14.6	1.062
VM	216 ± 60	151 ± 33	<0.0001	−64.6	−4.705
TA	110 ± 12	128 ± 21	0.2002	17.6	1.284
GM	99 ± 45	415 ± 63	<0.0001	315.9	23.016
c_SM	109 ± 24	127 ± 43	0.2088	17.3	1.260
c_VM	103 ± 28	135 ± 56	0.0227	31.4	2.290
c_TA	116 ± 20	179 ± 119	<0.0001	63.4	4.618
c_GM	138 ± 30	168 ± 50	0.0271	30.5	2.221
Muscle	**Amplitude [mV]**				
	EP	**LP**	***p*-Value**	**β**	**t**
SM	0.30 ± 0.09	0.20 ± 0.11	0.0195	−0.0940	−2.348
VM	0.47 ± 0.22	0.25 ± 0.16	<0.0001	−0.2273	−5.674
TA	0.47 ± 0.21	0.41 ± 0.15	0.0940	−0.0673	−1.680
GM	0.41 ± 0.16	0.22 ± 0.13	<0.0001	−0.1829	−4.566
c_SM	0.27 ± 0.08	0.30 ± 0.17	0.3495	0.0375	0.937
c_VM	0.46 ± 0.20	0.33 ± 0.17	0.0012	−0.1310	−3.271
c_TA	0.42 ± 0.16	0.36 ± 0.16	0.0940	−0.0673	−1.680
c_GM	0.34 ± 0.12	0.28 ± 0.12	0.1070	−0.0648	−1.617

4. Discussion

Slips are a leading cause of injury among older adults and individuals with musculoskeletal or neurological disorders. Therefore, the development of experimental perturbation paradigms that closely mimic real-life slips is essential to better understand near-fall biomechanics and to exercise the reactive balance capacities critical for fall prevention. In this study, we applied treadmill-based, slip-like perturbations at different timepoints during the stance phase to examine differences in (1) kinematic gait patterns, (2) neuromuscular responses, and (3) subjective perception between perturbation types. Our findings highlight distinct, multimodal differences between perturbations with identical deceleration profiles applied during early stance (EP) vs. late stance (i.e., LP). Notably, initial responses to EP were more pronounced in both full-body kinematics and neuromuscular activity, reflecting enhanced reactive balance responses to perturbations targeting early stance. Specifically, EP elicited EMG responses with shorter onset latencies and higher peak amplitude compared to LP. Additionally, recovery of gait parameters to baseline levels was prolonged following EP, although this difference was marginal. Subjectively, EPs were more frequently perceived as real-time slips and EPs were rated as more intense and inconvenient than LPs. Overall, these findings indicate that EP elicits stronger reactive balance responses, and that precise perturbation timing is key for accurately replicating real-world slips.

Age-related differences were generally moderate. The most prominent differences were related to the initial EMG responses that revealed prolonged onset latencies and reduced peak amplitudes in older adults compared to younger ones across both perturbation types. Additionally, the phasic modulation of rapid muscle responses to EP compared to LP was attenuated in older participants. These findings indicate that reactive balance is diminished with aging, potentially contributing to the reduced ability of older individuals to respond and recover from unexpected perturbations in real-world scenarios.

4.1. Initial Responses to Perturbations

Immediate kinematic and neuromuscular responses were generally more pronounced following EP than LP. The initial biomechanical reactions to EP align with previously reported kinematic patterns in response to slip-like perturbations [31]: thorax and knee angles were initially extended for a short period, likely reflecting passive motion induced by the forward acceleration of the treadmill belt. Simultaneously, hip angles exhibited a pronounced flexion. These immediate biomechanical adaptations may reflect either passive, slip-induced mechanics or automated postural responses. Later during stance, both the thorax and knee transitioned into marked flexion, likely to stabilize the body and to reposition the center of mass (CoM) within the base of support [32,33]. Notably, adequate knee flexion has been identified as a critical factor in fall prevention [34]. Although similar patterns were observed in response to LP, the initial biomechanical adaptations were significantly attenuated, suggesting reduced balance demands during LP trials.

EMG reaction times and amplitudes in young participants were in line with previous findings [8,34]. Overall, EMG reaction times were substantially shorter following EP compared to LP. A single exception to this pattern was observed in the ipsilateral VM, which may have been initially suppressed due to the marked, passive hip flexion and knee extension induced by the perturbation. The more pronounced EMG responses following EP vs. LP align with a previous study applying slip-like over-ground perturbations [8], reinforcing the idea that the early stance phase—particularly initial foot contact—is a critical window for reactive balance responses. The phasic modulation of neuromuscular responses observed here is supported by observations that the central nervous system is dynamically modulated throughout the gait cycle. Notably, initial foot contact represents a particularly critical phase that is tightly controlled by descending motor systems and sensory afferents [35–37]. Enhanced neuromuscular control during initial foot contact likely facilitates rapid, reflexive responses essential for fall prevention and aligns with the assumption that reactive balance is a key mechanism to recover from near-fall situations [34,38].

Our findings of enhanced kinematic and neuromuscular responses to EP vs. LP indicate that experimental slips targeting the early stance phase induce a stronger gait distortion, underscoring the importance of precisely timed perturbations to accurately replicate the biomechanics of near-fall slips commonly encountered in daily life. Optimized slip simulations can enhance the effectiveness of perturbation-based training (PBT), providing a more task-specific stimulus to engage the reactive balance mechanisms critical for fall prevention. This, in turn, may improve the real-world transferability of PBT outcomes [39]. Interestingly, previous findings indicate that both young and older adults are able to improve their reactive balance performance through repeated exposure to unexpected gait perturbations [9,40,41], highlighting the adaptability of the neuromuscular system and the potential of PBT as a practical intervention for reducing fall risk.

4.2. Recovery from Perturbations

Beyond the immediate biomechanical and neuromuscular responses, both perturbation types also elicited longer-lasting responses. Specifically, step length, step duration and stance phase duration were reduced, while step width increased. Perturbation-induced reduction in step length aligns with previous studies [12,42] and is commonly interpreted as a shift towards a more cautious gait pattern [43]. Similarly, the increase in step width upon slip-like perturbations was reported previously [12,44] and represents a key compensatory strategy to enhance lateral stability during walking [43,44]. The observed stance phase shortening was previously identified as a critical component of recovery following slips [45].

Overall, recovery of gait parameters to baseline performance was slower following EP than LP, although these differences were modest. Importantly, all gait parameters normalized within the first five steps post perturbation, consistent with previous findings [12].

4.3. Subjective Perception

Participants rated early perturbations (EP) as significantly more intense and inconvenient than late perturbations (LP), suggesting that EP was perceived as a more disruptive and demanding gait disturbance. These subjective assessments align closely with the objective biomechanical data, reinforcing the conclusion that slip-like perturbations targeting the initial stance phase elicit stronger reactive balance responses and more accurately simulate near-fall situation in the real-world. Additionally, EP was associated more frequently with the sensation of slipping, further supporting its ecological validity in replicating authentic slip events. Collectively, these subjective evaluations strengthen the quantitative findings and underscore the relevance of early stance perturbations for realistic slip simulation and fall prevention research.

4.4. Age-Related Differences in Responses to Perturbations

Previous research on age-related differences in kinematic and neuromuscular responses to perturbations has yielded inconsistent results. Whereas some studies showed age-related variations in perturbation responses [21,46], others found no significant differences [12]. In our study, the most prominent age-related differences emerged in the initial neuromuscular responses. Specifically, older adults revealed significantly delayed EMG response onset latencies and markedly reduced response amplitudes for both perturbation types compared to younger adults. These findings align with previous results reporting diminished EMG amplitudes following tripping perturbations in older individuals [22]. The latency of neuromuscular responses to unexpected perturbations has been demonstrated to be a key factor whether a participant is able to recover or falls [34,38]. Additionally, our results revealed that the phasic modulation of EMG responses—i.e., the ability to scale responses based on the timing of the perturbation—is markedly attenuated in older adults, corroborating earlier findings [8]. Unlike younger participants, older adults showed a limited ability to enhance EMG amplitudes in response to early perturbations (EP), suggesting a reduced adaptability of the neuromuscular system. Summarized, these findings suggest that reactive balance capacity is diminished in older adults, potentially impairing their ability to recover from unexpected perturbations in real-world scenarios [8,39]. This impairment might result from age-related declines in supraspinal motor drive, reduced myelination of nerve fibers and decreased motoneuron excitability [47–50]. In addition, reduced sensitivity of muscle receptors and age-related changes in muscle fiber composition may further compromise balance responses [51,52]. Our findings suggest that reflexive muscle responses are a sensitive and valuable marker of reactive balance capacity. Incorporating such measures into future fall prevention research may enhance the identification of at-risk individuals and inform targeted intervention strategies.

Age-related differences in initial kinematic responses were moderate. However, younger participants showed higher peak flexion angles at the hip and knee, likely reflecting stronger reactive balance strategies aimed at repositioning the CoM to regain stability. Differences in recovery response between young and old participants were generally small and inconsistent. Whereas step duration and stance phase recovered slightly slower in the older age group, no age-related difference was observed in step width. Notably, only younger participants showed a reduction in step length following early perturbations (EP), indicating a more adaptive response to maintain stability.

The overall moderate age-related differences in perturbation responses may be attributed to the relatively high physical fitness and functional capacity of the older participants in our study, which likely enables them to tolerate the perturbations well. Nonetheless, the observed attenuation of neuromuscular responses in this group suggests the presence of impairments in reactive balance, even within a healthy aging population.

4.5. Limitations

This study has several limitations. First, perturbations were applied during treadmill walking, and the treadmill continued running after each perturbation. In contrast, real-life slips often result in an immediate cessation of walking. However, a treadmill-based setup was chosen for its advantages in triggering repetitive perturbations with high temporal accuracy, consistent amplitude and clearly defined timepoints that cannot be anticipated by participants. Second, we employed a fixed walking speed of 1.2 m/s for all participants. While previous studies identified this speed as close to comfortable walking speed for both young and older individuals [12], it may have been more demanding for some older participants. However, a fixed walking speed facilitated the comparability of perturbation intensity and responses across participants, thereby strengthening the consistency and interpretability of our findings. Third, the present study focused on the effects of perturbation timing on gait pattern changes. The influence of different perturbation intensity (i.e., acceleration and duration of perturbation) has not been explored here, although this factor is known to affect the response to perturbations [18–20].

5. Conclusions

Our findings underscore the critical role of perturbation timing in shaping reactive responses in both younger and older adults. Slip-like perturbations targeting the vulnerable, early stance phase elicited substantially greater responses compared to identical perturbations addressing the late stance phase. This was evident in amplified reactive balance responses and prolonged recovery phases to regain baseline gait patterns upon EP. Notably, EP were also subjectively rated as more intense and inconvenient, and were perceived to more closely replicate real-word slip events than LP.

Age-related differences were primarily observed in the initial neuromuscular responses, with older adults exhibiting prolonged muscle onset latencies, decreased response amplitudes and diminished modulation across perturbation types. These deficits reflect impaired reactive balance control, which may contribute to the elevated fall risk in older adults.

Our findings highlight that experimental, slip-like perturbations targeting the early stance phase provide a more ecologically valid simulation of real-world slip conditions. As such, they represent a valuable tool for task-specific, perturbation-based balance training interventions aimed at fall prevention in individuals at increased risk.

Supplementary Materials: The following supporting information can be downloaded at: https://www.mdpi.com/article/10.3390/bioengineering12121284/s1, The supplementary files (Figure S1, Figure S2 and Figure S3) have been uploaded separately. Figure S1. Initial kinematic responses to perturbations in older adults. Top row: Sagittal plane kinematics of the thorax, hip, knee and ankle during regular walking (black lines; shaded areas represent ±1 standard deviation), and in response to EP (red) and LP (blue). Middle row: Statistical comparison between regular walking (base) and EP for thorax, hip, knee and ankle movements using Statistical Parametric Mapping (SPM). Bottom row: SPM comparison between regular walking (base) and LP for all walking parameters. All data are time-normalized to the gait cycle. Joint angles for the hip, knee and ankle are shown for the leg ipsilateral to the perturbation. Significant differences between regular walking and EP are indicated by red bars at the lower part of the top figure row. Statistical differences between regular walking and LP are indicated by blue bars. Abbreviations: EP: early perturbations; LP: late perturbations. Figure S2. Recovery of spatiotemporal gait parameters following EP (red) and LP (blue) in older participants. The baseline (Base; dashed horizontal line) represents average values during regular walking, calculated from 20 unperturbed steps preceding the perturbation. Pert denotes the actually perturbed step, and P1-P10 indicate the ten subsequent recovery steps. Stance phase is reported as proportion of stance phase relative to step duration. Asterisks denote statistical significance: * $p < 0.05$, ** p-value < 0.01, *** p-value < 0.001, and **** $p < 0.0001$. Red asterisks indicate significant differences between EP and baseline; blue asterisks highlight differences between LP and baseline. Figure S3. Subjective perception of the different perturbations in older adults. (A) Subjective ratings of EP (red) and LP (blue) with respect to perceived inconvenience and intensity. Rating ranged from 0 to 10, with 10 representing maximal inconvenience or intensity. (B) Comparison of EP and LP to real-life conditions including slipping, tripping, perturbations in bus and other conditions. *** represents p-value < 0.001.

Author Contributions: Conceptualization, M.G. and L.F.; Methodology, M.G. and L.F. Validation, M.G. and L.F.; Formal Analysis, M.G.; Investigation, M.G., N.S.H., A.M.E., L.C.N. and L.F.; Resources, M.G., N.S.H., A.M.E., L.C.N. and L.F.; Data Curation, M.G.; Writing—Original Draft Preparation, M.G. and L.F.; Writing—Review and Editing, M.G., N.S.H., A.M.E., L.C.N. and L.F.; Visualization, M.G.; Supervision, L.F.; Project Administration, M.G. All authors have read and agreed to the published version of the manuscript.

Funding: This project was supported by the Balgrist Campus AG and the Balgrist Foundation.

Institutional Review Board Statement: The study was approved by the Ethics Committee of the Canton Zurich (Study-ID: 2023-00213; date of approval: 4 April 2023) and is registered online (clinicaltrials.gov; NCT05890755). The study was conducted according to the guidelines of the Declaration of Helsinki and Good Clinical Practice.

Informed Consent Statement: Written informed consent was obtained from all participants.

Data Availability Statement: The datasets generated and analyzed during the current study are available from the corresponding author upon reasonable request. All data of this study is included in the manuscript.

Acknowledgments: We thank all the volunteers who kindly participated in this study. We thank the Swiss Center for Movement Analysis (SCMA), Balgrist Campus AG, for supporting the conduction of this study. The authors would like to thank Beatrice Ottavia Kober and Sandra Mössner for their support.

Conflicts of Interest: Authors Marina Geissmann and Linard Filli are employed by the company Balgrist Campus AG. The authors declare that the research was conducted in the absence of any commercial or financial relationships that could be construed as a potential conflict of interest.

References

1. Ambrose, A.F.; Paul, G.; Hausdorff, J.M. Risk factors for falls among older adults: A review of the literature. *Maturitas* **2013**, *75*, 51–61. [CrossRef]
2. Berry, S.D.; Miller, R.R. Falls: Epidemiology, pathophysiology, and relationship to fracture. *Curr. Osteoporos. Rep.* **2008**, *6*, 149–154. [CrossRef]
3. Vieira, E.R.; Palmer, R.C.; Chaves, P.H. Prevention of falls in older people living in the community. *BMJ* **2016**, *353*, i1419. [CrossRef] [PubMed]
4. Pai, Y.-C.; Bhatt, T.; Wang, E.; Espy, D.; Pavol, M.J. Inoculation against falls: Rapid adaptation by young and older adults to slips during daily activities. *Arch. Phys. Med. Rehabil.* **2010**, *91*, 452–459. [CrossRef] [PubMed]
5. Perkins, P. *Measurement of Slip Between the Shoe and Ground During Walking*; ASTM International: West Conshohocken, PA, USA, 1978.
6. Redfern, M.S.; Cham, R.; Gielo-Perczak, K.; Grönqvist, R.; Hirvonen, M.; Lanshammar, H.; Marpet, M.; Pai, C.Y.; Powers, C. Biomechanics of slips. *Ergonomics* **2001**, *44*, 1138–1166. [CrossRef] [PubMed]

7. Golyski, P.R.; Vazquez, E.; Leestma, J.K.; Sawicki, G.S. Onset timing of treadmill belt perturbations influences stability during walking. *J. Biomech.* **2022**, *130*, 110800. [CrossRef]
8. Tang, P.-F.; Woollacott, M.H. Phase-dependent modulation of proximal and distal postural responses to slips in young and older adults. *J. Gerontol. Ser. A Biomed. Sci. Med. Sci.* **1999**, *54*, M89–M102. [CrossRef]
9. Rieger, M.M.; Papegaaij, S.; Pijnappels, M.; Steenbrink, F.; van Dieen, J.H. Transfer and retention effects of gait training with anterior-posterior perturbations to postural responses after medio-lateral gait perturbations in older adults. *Clin. Biomech.* **2020**, *75*, 104988. [CrossRef]
10. van den Bogaart, M.; Bruijn, S.M.; van Dieen, J.H.; Meyns, P. The effect of anteroposterior perturbations on the control of the center of mass during treadmill walking. *J. Biomech.* **2020**, *103*, 109660. [CrossRef]
11. Flux, E.; van der Krogt, M.M.; Harlaar, J.; Buizer, A.I.; Sloot, L.H. Functional assessment of stretch hyperreflexia in children with cerebral palsy using treadmill perturbations. *J. Neuroeng. Rehabil.* **2021**, *18*, 151. [CrossRef]
12. Roeles, S.; Rowe, P.J.; Bruijn, S.M.; Childs, C.R.; Tarfali, G.D.; Steenbrink, F.; Pijnappels, M. Gait stability in response to platform, belt, and sensory perturbations in young and older adults. *Med. Biol. Eng. Comput.* **2018**, *56*, 2325–2335. [CrossRef] [PubMed]
13. Lockhart, T.E.; Woldstad, J.C.; Smith, J.L. Effects of age-related gait changes on the biomechanics of slips and falls. *Ergonomics* **2003**, *46*, 1136–1160. [CrossRef] [PubMed]
14. Rakié, C.; Mark, S.R. Heel contact dynamics during slip events on level and inclined surfaces. *Saf. Sci.* **2002**, *40*, 559–576. [CrossRef]
15. Chambers, A.J.; Cham, R. Slip-related muscle activation patterns in the stance leg during walking. *Gait Posture* **2007**, *25*, 565–572. [CrossRef]
16. Bhatt, T.; Wening, J.D.; Pai, Y.C. Adaptive control of gait stability in reducing slip-related backward loss of balance. *Exp. Brain Res.* **2006**, *170*, 61–73. [CrossRef]
17. Sloot, L.H.; van den Noort, J.C.; van der Krogt, M.M.; Bruijn, S.M.; Harlaar, J. Can Treadmill Perturbations Evoke Stretch Reflexes in the Calf Muscles? *PLoS ONE* **2015**, *10*, e0144815. [CrossRef]
18. Brady, R.A.; Pavol, M.J.; Owings, T.M.; Grabiner, M.D. Foot displacement but not velocity predicts the outcome of a slip induced in young subjects while walking. *J. Biomech.* **2000**, *33*, 803–808. [CrossRef]
19. Lee, C.; Ahn, J.; Lee, B.C. The effects of perturbation intensities on backward slip-falls induced by a split-belt treadmill. *Sci. Rep.* **2025**, *15*, 5108. [CrossRef]
20. Troy, K.L.; Donovan, S.J.; Marone, J.R.; Bareither, M.L.; Grabiner, M.D. Modifiable performance domain risk-factors associated with slip-related falls. *Gait Posture* **2008**, *28*, 461–465. [CrossRef]
21. Suptitz, F.; Moreno Catala, M.; Bruggemann, G.P.; Karamanidis, K. Dynamic stability control during perturbed walking can be assessed by a reduced kinematic model across the adult female lifespan. *Hum. Mov. Sci.* **2013**, *32*, 1404–1414. [CrossRef]
22. Pijnappels, M.; Bobbert, M.F.; van Dieen, J.H. Control of support limb muscles in recovery after tripping in young and older subjects. *Exp. Brain Res.* **2005**, *160*, 326–333. [CrossRef] [PubMed]
23. McCrum, C.; Karamanidis, K.; Grevendonk, L.; Zijlstra, W.; Meijer, K. Older adults demonstrate interlimb transfer of reactive gait adaptations to repeated unpredictable gait perturbations. *Geroscience* **2020**, *42*, 39–49. [CrossRef] [PubMed]
24. Huang, T.T.; Wang, W.S. Comparison of three established measures of fear of falling in community-dwelling older adults: Psychometric testing. *Int. J. Nurs. Stud.* **2009**, *46*, 1313–1319. [CrossRef] [PubMed]
25. Wrisley, D.M.; Marchetti, G.F.; Kuharsky, D.K.; Whitney, S.L. Reliability, internal consistency, and validity of data obtained with the functional gait assessment. *Phys. Ther.* **2004**, *84*, 906–918. [CrossRef]
26. Meyer, C.; Killeen, T.; Easthope, C.S.; Curt, A.; Bolliger, M.; Linnebank, M.; Zorner, B.; Filli, L. Familiarization with treadmill walking: How much is enough? *Sci. Rep.* **2019**, *9*, 5232. [CrossRef]
27. Zeni, J.A., Jr.; Richards, J.G.; Higginson, J.S. Two simple methods for determining gait events during treadmill and overground walking using kinematic data. *Gait Posture* **2008**, *27*, 710–714. [CrossRef]
28. Woltring, H.J. A Fortran package for generalized, cross-validatory spline smoothing and differentiation. *Adv. Eng. Softw.* **1986**, *8*, 104–113. [CrossRef]
29. Habibzadeh, F. Data Distribution: Normal or Abnormal? *J. Korean Med. Sci.* **2024**, *39*, e35. [CrossRef]
30. Burkner, P.C.; Doebler, P.; Holling, H. Optimal design of the Wilcoxon-Mann-Whitney-test. *Biom. J.* **2017**, *59*, 25–40. [CrossRef]
31. Beschorner, K.E.; Redfern, M.S.; Cham, R. Earliest gait deviations during slips: Implications for recovery. *IIE Trans. Occup. Ergon. Hum. Factors* **2013**, *1*, 31–37. [CrossRef]
32. Cham, R.; Redfern, M.S. Lower extremity corrective reactions to slip events. *J. Biomech.* **2001**, *34*, 1439–1445. [CrossRef]
33. Ribeiro, N.F.; Armada, M.; Nunes, J.; Carvalho, Ó.; Santos, C.P. Unveiling human biomechanics: Insights into lower limb responses to disturbances that can trigger a fall. *Front. Robot. AI* **2024**, *11*, 1367474. [CrossRef] [PubMed]
34. Sawers, A.; Bhatt, T. Neuromuscular determinants of slip-induced falls and recoveries in older adults. *J. Neurophysiol.* **2018**, *120*, 1534–1546. [CrossRef] [PubMed]

35. Bent, L.R.; McFadyen, B.J.; Inglis, J.T. Vestibular contributions during human locomotor tasks. *Exerc. Sport. Sci. Rev.* **2005**, *33*, 107–113. [CrossRef] [PubMed]
36. Takahashi, M.; Uchida, N.; Yoshida, M.; Liang, N.; Nakazawa, K.; Sekikawa, K.; Inamizu, T.; Hamada, H. Phase-dependent modulation of corticospinal excitability during the observation of the initial phase of gait. *Somatosens. Mot. Res.* **2014**, *31*, 209–213. [CrossRef] [PubMed]
37. Filli, L.; Meyer, C.; Killeen, T.; Lörincz, L.; Göpfert, B.; Linnebank, M.; von Tscharner, V.; Curt, A.; Bolliger, M.; Zörner, B. Probing Corticospinal Control During Different Locomotor Tasks Using Detailed Time-Frequency Analysis of Electromyograms. *Front. Neurol.* **2019**, *10*, 17. [CrossRef]
38. Thelen, D.G.; Muriuki, M.; James, J.; Schultz, A.B.; Ashton-Miller, J.A.; Alexander, N.B. Muscle activities used by young and old adults when stepping to regain balance during a forward fall. *J. Electromyogr. Kinesiol.* **2000**, *10*, 93–101. [CrossRef]
39. McCrum, C.; Bhatt, T.S.; Gerards, M.H.G.; Karamanidis, K.; Rogers, M.W.; Lord, S.R.; Okubo, Y. Perturbation-based balance training: Principles, mechanisms and implementation in clinical practice. *Front. Sports Act. Living* **2022**, *4*, 1015394. [CrossRef]
40. Debelle, H.; Maganaris, C.N.; O'Brien, T.D. Biomechanical Mechanisms of Improved Balance Recovery to Repeated Backward Slips Simulated by Treadmill Belt Accelerations in Young and Older Adults. *Front. Sports Act. Living* **2021**, *3*, 708929. [CrossRef]
41. Epro, G.; McCrum, C.; Mierau, A.; Leyendecker, M.; Brüggemann, G.P.; Karamanidis, K. Effects of triceps surae muscle strength and tendon stiffness on the reactive dynamic stability and adaptability of older female adults during perturbed walking. *J. Appl. Physiol.* **2018**, *124*, 1541–1549. [CrossRef]
42. Madehkhaksar, F.; Klenk, J.; Sczuka, K.; Gordt, K.; Melzer, I.; Schwenk, M. The effects of unexpected mechanical perturbations during treadmill walking on spatiotemporal gait parameters, and the dynamic stability measures by which to quantify postural response. *PLoS ONE* **2018**, *13*, e0195902. [CrossRef]
43. McAndrew Young, P.M.; Dingwell, J.B. Voluntary changes in step width and step length during human walking affect dynamic margins of stability. *Gait Posture* **2012**, *36*, 219–224. [CrossRef]
44. Ren, X.; Lutter, C.; Kebbach, M.; Bruhn, S.; Bader, R.; Tischer, T. Lower extremity joint compensatory effects during the first recovery step following slipping and stumbling perturbations in young and older subjects. *BMC Geriatr.* **2022**, *22*, 656. [CrossRef]
45. Taborri, J.; Santuz, A.; Brüll, L.; Arampatzis, A.; Rossi, S. Measuring Kinematic Response to Perturbed Locomotion in Young Adults. *Sensors* **2022**, *22*, 672. [CrossRef]
46. Pijnappels, M.; Bobbert, M.F.; van Dieën, J.H. Push-off reactions in recovery after tripping discriminate young subjects, older non-fallers and older fallers. *Gait Posture* **2005**, *21*, 388–394. [CrossRef] [PubMed]
47. Dietz, V. Human neuronal control of automatic functional movements: Interaction between central programs and afferent input. *Physiol. Rev.* **1992**, *72*, 33–69. [CrossRef] [PubMed]
48. Mednikova, Y.S.; Kopytova, F. Some physiological characteristics of motor cortex neurons of aged rabbits. *Neuroscience* **1994**, *63*, 611–615. [CrossRef] [PubMed]
49. Sabbahi, M.A.; Sedgwick, E.M. Age-related changes in monosynaptic reflex excitability. *J. Gerontol.* **1982**, *37*, 24–32. [CrossRef]
50. Terao, S.-i.; Sobue, G.; Hashizume, Y.; Shimada, N.; Mitsuma, T. Age-related changes of the myelinated fibers in the human corticospinal tract: A quantitative analysis. *Acta Neuropathol.* **1994**, *88*, 137–142. [CrossRef]
51. Jakobsson, F.; Borg, K.; Edström, L.; Grimby, L. Use of motor units in relation to muscle fiber type and size in man. *Muscle Nerve* **1988**, *11*, 1211–1218. [CrossRef]
52. Lexell, J. Human aging, muscle mass, and fiber type composition. *J. Gerontol. A Biol. Sci. Med. Sci.* **1995**, *50*, 11–16. [CrossRef]

Disclaimer/Publisher's Note: The statements, opinions and data contained in all publications are solely those of the individual author(s) and contributor(s) and not of MDPI and/or the editor(s). MDPI and/or the editor(s) disclaim responsibility for any injury to people or property resulting from any ideas, methods, instructions or products referred to in the content.

bioengineering

MDPI

Article

Classification of Hemiplegic Gait and Mimicked Hemiplegic Gait: A Treadmill Gait Analysis Study in Stroke Patients and Healthy Individuals

Young-ung Lee [1], Seungwon Kwon [2], Cheol-Hyun Kim [1,3], Jeong-Woo Seo [4,5,*] and Sangkwan Lee [1,3,*]

1 Stroke Korean Medicine Research Center, Wonkwang University Gwangju Medical Center, Gwangju 61729, Republic of Korea; www8744@naver.com (Y.-u.L.); lambroskch@gmail.com (C.-H.K.)
2 Department of Cardiology and Neurology, Kyung Hee University College of Korean Medicine, Kyung Hee University Medical Center, Seoul 02447, Republic of Korea; kkokkottung@hanmail.net
3 Department of Internal Medicine and Neuroscience, College of Korean Medicine, Wonkwang University, Iksan 54538, Republic of Korea
4 Digital Health Research Division, Korea Institute of Oriental Medicine, Daejeon 34504, Republic of Korea
5 Korean Convergence Medical Science, University of Science and Technology, Daejeon 34113, Republic of Korea
* Correspondence: jwseo02@kiom.re.kr (J.-W.S.); sklee@wku.ac.kr (S.L.); Tel.: +82-42-868-9275 (J.-W.S.); +82-62-670-6700 (S.L.)

Abstract: Differentiating genuine hemiplegic gait (HG) in stroke survivors from hemiplegic-like gait voluntarily imitated by healthy adults (MHG) is essential for reliable assessment and intervention planning. Treadmill-based gait data were obtained from 79 participants—39 stroke patients (HG) and 40 healthy adults—instructed to mimic HG (MHG). Forty-eight spatiotemporal and force-related variables were extracted. Random Forest, support vector machine (SVM), and logistic regression classifiers were trained with (i) the full feature set and (ii) the 10 most important features selected via Random Forest Gini importance. Performance was assessed with 5-fold stratified cross-validation and an 80/20 hold-out test, using accuracy, F1-score, and the area under the receiver operating characteristic curve (AUC). All models achieved high discrimination (AUC > 0.93). The SVM attained perfect discrimination (AUC = 1.000, test set) with the full feature set and maintained excellent accuracy (AUC = 0.983) with only the top 10 features. Temporal asymmetries, delayed vertical ground reaction force peaks, and mediolateral spatial instability ranked highest in importance. Reduced-feature models showed negligible performance loss, highlighting their parsimony and interpretability. Supervised machine learning algorithms can accurately distinguish true hemiplegic gait from mimicked patterns using a compact subset of gait features. The findings support data-driven, time-efficient gait assessments for clinical neurorehabilitation and for validating experimental protocols that rely on gait imitation.

Keywords: stroke; hemiplegic gait; mimicked hemiplegic gait; machine learning; gait classification

1. Introduction

Stroke refers to neurological symptoms caused by damage to brain tissue due to either the blockage of blood vessels (ischemic stroke) or their rupture (hemorrhagic stroke) [1]. It is one of the leading causes of long-term disability, with more than 80% of survivors experiencing gait disturbances [2]. Even with continuous rehabilitation, approximately 18% of stroke patients are unable to walk, 11% require assistance, and only about half can regain independent walking ability [2]. The most common gait abnormality among stroke survivors is hemiplegic gait, which results from muscular weakness, impaired motor control, proprioceptive deficits, and increased muscle tone on the affected side [3]. This typically manifests as a flexor synergy in the upper limb and an extensor synergy in the lower limb, leading to joint patterns such as hip extension and internal rotation, knee extension, and ankle plantarflexion and inversion [1]. To achieve foot clearance during swing, patients often compensate through hip hiking or circumduction [4]. These compensatory strategies alter gait mechanics, causing increased energy expenditure and fatigue, and consequently elevate the risk of falls [5]. Therefore, the recovery of gait ability is a critical objective in stroke rehabilitation to promote independent daily functioning [6]. Recent studies have focused on quantifying gait impairments and identifying key variables for recovery using advanced analytical methods, including gait analysis systems, wearable sensors, and instrumented treadmills [7]. Given the distinguishable gait characteristics of stroke survivors, researchers have applied machine learning (ML) and deep learning techniques to develop automated algorithms capable of identifying gait deviations, predicting recovery outcomes, and classifying stroke severity [8]. These data-driven approaches have demonstrated promising performance; however, existing models primarily focus on distinguishing normal and pathological gait patterns under natural conditions. In real-world clinical and administrative settings, there are cases where patients may exaggerate or mimic hemiplegic gait, either consciously or due to external incentives such as insurance claims or return-to-work assessments. A previous study documented abnormal behaviors during rehabilitation by a stroke patient involved in a traffic accident [9], raising concerns about potential malingering or fraud. Other reports suggest that caregivers may also influence evaluations, as in Munchausen Syndrome by Proxy [10]. It is particularly challenging to detect mimicked hemiplegic gait visually because it is relatively easy to reproduce spatiotemporal patterns such as foot drop or pelvic tilting. Kinematic imitation involving joint angles can often be controlled voluntarily, making it difficult for clinicians to reliably differentiate between neurologically impaired and cognitively generated gait patterns. Despite growing interest in the objective quantification of gait impairments, there remains a lack of research specifically addressing the differentiation between genuine hemiplegic gait and its mimicked counterpart. Prior machine learning studies have not explored whether such models can detect intention-based imitation, a scenario with meaningful implications in clinical diagnostics, functional evaluations, and medico-legal contexts. Moreover, the interpretability, efficiency, and reproducibility of gait classification models remain underexplored, especially in settings where visual assessment may be subjective or inconsistent. The objective of this study was to determine whether machine learning techniques could accurately classify mimicked hemiplegic gait performed by healthy individuals and actual hemiplegic gait exhibited by stroke patients. Using treadmill-based spatiotemporal and force-related gait parameters, we developed and evaluated three supervised classifiers—Random Forest, Support Vector Machine (SVM), and Logistic Regression. We also investigated whether reduced-feature models using the top 10 most important gait parameters could maintain classification performance. Ultimately, this study aims to enhance the objectivity and reliability of clinical gait assessment, particularly in ambiguous or bias-prone scenarios, and to support functional evaluations for rehabilitation planning, insurance verification, and return-to-work decisions.

2. Materials and Methods

2.1. Data Sources and Participant Selection

This study retrospectively analyzed individuals who underwent gait analysis through a treadmill gait analysis system at Wonkwang University Korean Medicine Hospital in Gwangju (WKUGH). As this research only used simple measurement or observation equipment that does not lead to physical changes, it received review approval from the institutional review board of the hospital (WKIRB 2022-07, 29 June 2022). We selected data from subjects who visited WKUGH between November 1 2018 and June 30 2022, and who met the inclusion criteria for both the hemiplegic gait (HG) group and the mimicked hemiplegic gait (MHG) group and did not fall under the exclusion criteria (Table 1).

Table 1. Inclusion and exclusion criteria for the HG and MHG group.

	Inclusion Criteria	Exclusion Criteria
HG group	- Individuals diagnosed with stroke via CT or MRI and who have hemiparesis - Individuals capable of independent walking for more than 30 s on a treadmill (with Manual Muscle Testing (MMT) grades 3–5 for lower limbs, and Functional Ambulation Categories (FAC) 9 level 3–5).	- Individuals with clinical symptoms that could affect their walking ability (such as musculoskeletal diseases, acute sprain, etc.)
MHG group	- Individuals who have not been diagnosed with stroke - Individuals who can mimic hemiplegic gait following the instructions of the medical staff	

A total of 79 subjects were retrospectively analyzed in this study, consisting of 39 in the hemiplegic gait group (19 with left hemiparesis, 20 with right hemiparesis) and 40 in the mimicked hemiplegic gait group (20 mimicking left, 20 mimicking right hemiparesis) (Table 2).

Table 2. Demographic characteristics of subjects.

Characteristics		HG Group	MHG Group
Subjects (number)		39	40
Sex (number (%))	Male	20 (51.2%)	28 (70%)
	Female	19 (48.8%)	12 (30%)
Age (Mean (SD))		62.8 (6.44)	26.98 (2.27)
Affected side (number (%))	Left	19 (47.5%)	20 (50%)
	Right	21 (52.5%)	20 (50%)
MMT (median (IQR))	Upper limb	4 (1)	5 (0)
	Lower limb	4 (0)	5 (0)

HG, hemiplegic gait; MHG, mimicked hemiplegic gait; SD, standard deviation; IQR, interquartile range (at least 50% of the observations share the same value); MMT, manual muscle test.

2.2. Experiment and Equipment

We conducted a gait analysis using a treadmill equipped with a pressure plate (Figure 1). When the subject starts walking on the treadmill, the pressure exerted on the pressure plate is measured, and spatiotemporal features of gait are collected. The pressure applied to the treadmill (AP2010-2Si, Apsun Inc., Seoul, Republic of Korea) is transmitted to the Zebris FDM software (version 1.18.44, Zebris Medical GmbH, Isny/Allgäu, Germany) on the computer [11].

For the HG group, the subjects were asked to walk on the treadmill at their preferred speed for 30 s. For the MHG group, we conducted training on the flexor synergy pattern of the upper limbs and the extensor synergy pattern of the lower limbs, which are characteristic of post-stroke hemiparesis. They were instructed to mimic the characteristics of hemiplegic gait, including hip extension and internal rotation, knee extension, and plantar flexion and inversion of the ankle, while performing hip hike and circumduction during swing phase. Gait analysis was conducted when it was judged that they could sufficiently reproduce the hemiplegic gait after watching videos of actual hemiplegic gait of stroke patients and demonstrations by doctors of Korean Medicine. For the MHG group, the walking speed was limited to 0.7 km/h, which is the average walking speed of the HG group, as they tended to perform normal walking when the walking speed was set high.

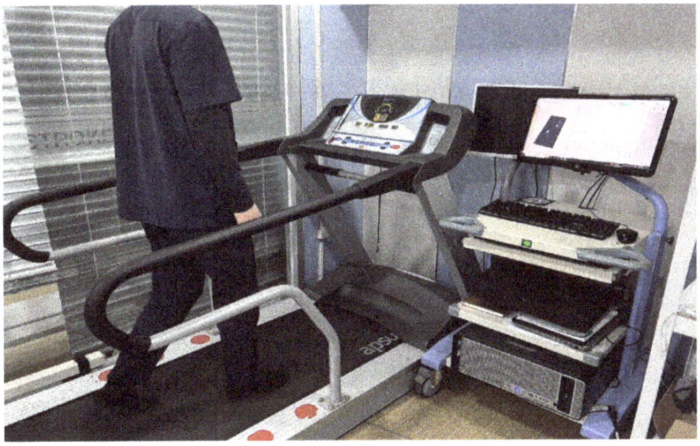

Figure 1. Gait analysis system using treadmill.

2.3. Gait Feature

The spatiotemporal features such as foot rotation degree, step length, stride length, velocity, cadence, and others, as well as the movement of the center of pressure (CoP) during gait, the ratio of the gait cycle of each lower limb, and the vertical ground reaction force (vGRF) generated during gait are calculated and obtained (Figure 2). These methods have been described previously [12].

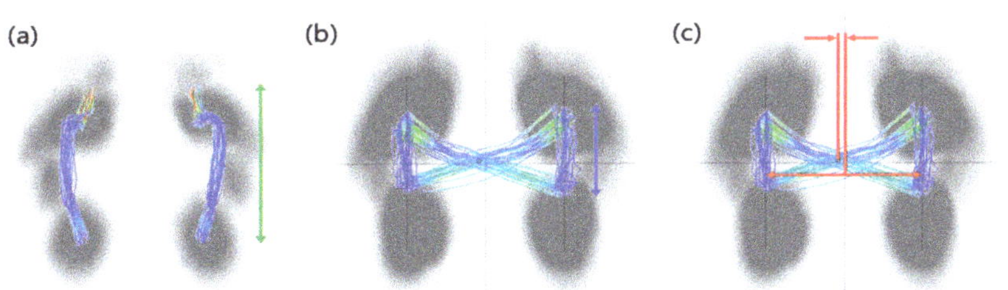

Figure 2. (**a**) Length of gait line (green), (**b**) single-limb support line (blue), and (**c**) lateral symmetry (red). The lines of single-limb support and lateral symmetry are derived from the butterfly-shaped diagram that illustrates the trajectory of the COP during walking.

The gait cycle is split into the stance and swing phases, which are determined by the toe off. The initial contact of the opposite side (left side in this case) happens when the right side reaches 50% of the cycle. There are two double limb support phases where both feet touch the ground: once at the start of the cycle (0–10%) and again midway (50–60%) (Table 3). Details of the gait cycle phases have been described previously [13].

Table 3. Gait features obtained by treadmill.

	Feature (Unit)	Description
Spatial feature	Foot rotation (degree) Step length (cm) Stride length (cm) Step width (cm)	positive: external rotation/negative: internal rotation from heel contact of one foot to the other foot initial contact of the same foot width between the feet
Temporal feature	Step time (sec) Stride time (sec) Cadence (steps/min) Velocity (km/h)	step time is the time taken between the heel contact of one foot and the heel contact of the other foot stride time is the elapsed time between the first contact of two consecutive footprints of the same foot steps per minute walking speed during gait analysis
CoP feature	Length of gait line (mm) Single-limb support line (mm) Lateral symmetry (mm)	CoP movement on one foot during the entire stance phase CoP movement during the single-leg support horizontal distance from the center point of the horizontal line
Gait event Feature	Stance phase (%) Load response (%) Single-limb support (%) Pre-swing (%) Swing phase (%) Double stance phase (%)	from heel strike to toe off begins with initial contact, the instant the foot contacts the ground the swing phase where only one limb in in contact with the ground final phase of stance, starting with initial contact of the opposite limb period during which the foot is in the air both feet are simultaneously in contact with the ground
Force feature	Time maximum force 1 (%)	first maximum vertical force, which occurs at the end of loading response

2.4. Statistical Analysis

All statistical analyses were performed using Python (version 3.10) and open source scientific libraries. Data preprocessing and management were conducted using Pandas, and group comparisons between the hemiplegic gait (HG) and mimicked hemiplegic gait (MHG) groups were performed using independent *t*-tests. The *t*-tests were implemented via the SciPy package [14].

To facilitate interpretation, since the direction of hemiparesis varies among the subjects, features that can be obtained from one side of the body (foot rotation, step length, stance phase, load response, single-limb support, pre-swing, swing phase, step time, length of gait line, single-limb support line, time maximum force 1) were uniformly converted to (+) for the unaffected side and (−) for the affected side, based on the study by Lee et al. [15].

For lateral symmetry, the unaffected direction was converted to (+) and the affected direction to (−). Additionally, to interpret time maximum force 1, the time maximum force ratio was calculated by dividing the unaffected side feature by the affected side feature, referencing Patterson's study method [16].

To assess between-group differences in gait features while controlling for the effect of age, an Analysis of Covariance (ANCOVA) was conducted for each dependent feature. The primary fixed factor was group type (hemiplegic gait [HG] vs. mimicked hemiplegic gait [MHG]), and age was treated as a covariate. The model also included the interaction term between age and group to test whether the relationship between age and the dependent feature differed across groups.

To examine group differences in gait features between the HG and MHG groups, appropriate statistical tests were selected based on normality assessments using the Shapiro–Wilk test. For features in which both groups satisfied the assumption of normality ($p > 0.05$), independent samples *t*-tests were employed. For non-normally distributed features, the non-parametric Mann–Whitney U test was applied.

2.5. Machine Learning Model

Since there is no established formula for calculating the required sample size in machine learning, we referred to the empirical rule-of-thumb for multiple regression proposed, which recommends a minimum sample size of $N \geq 50 + 8$ m, where m is the number of predictors [17]. For a maximum of 10 predictors, this criterion suggests that at least 130 participants are needed. However, our study included only 79 participants, falling short of this recommendation.

A post hoc sensitivity analysis was conducted as follows: for the full model test with m = 10 predictors and N = 79 participants, the numerator and denominator degrees of freedom were set to $df_1 = m = 10$ and $df_2 = N - m - 1 = 79 - 10 - 1 = 68$, respectively. At a significance level of $\alpha = 0.05$, the critical F-value was $F_{crit}(10,68) \approx 1.973$. The non-centrality parameter λ required to achieve 80% power was obtained from the noncentral F-distribution as $\lambda^* \approx 18.4875$. Based on this, the minimum detectable effect size was calculated as $f^2 = \frac{\lambda^*}{df_2} \approx 0.27$, $R^2 = \frac{f^2}{1+f^2} \approx 0.21$. This result indicates that while the study had adequate power to detect medium-to-large effects, it may have failed to detect smaller true effects. According to Cohen's conventional thresholds for multiple regression ($f^2 = 0.02$ for small, $f^2 = 0.15$ for medium, and $f^2 = 0.35$ for large effects), the calculated f^2 value of 0.2 corresponds to a medium-sized effect. This suggests that although the independent variables included in the model influence the dependent variable, the magnitude of this influence may not be substantial. Nevertheless, even very small effects can have considerable practical or clinical importance if they affect a large population.

A total of 79 observations were included in the data-set, consisting of two groups labeled as hemiplegic gait (HG) and mimicked hemiplegic gait (MHG) groups. Each observation included 26 spatiotemporal and force-related gait features, excluding age-sensitive features based on prior ANCOVA results.

To reduce model complexity and improve generalization due to the limited data-set size, feature selection was performed using the Gini impurity-based feature importance scores computed from a Random Forest classifier [18]. Specifically, a Random Forest model was trained on the entire standardized dataset using all available input features, and the importance of each feature was quantified by averaging the total reduction in Gini impurity that the feature contributed across all decision trees in the ensemble. Features that contributed more to reducing impurity were assigned higher importance scores. The features were then ranked in descending order based on their computed importance values, and the top 10 features were selected. These top-ranked features were consistently used in all subsequent modeling, hyperparameter tuning, and evaluation procedures to ensure comparability and to reduce the risk of overfitting [19].

To classify HG versus MHG by gait features, supervised machine learning models were developed using the top 10 features identified through feature selection. Three classification algorithms were employed: a Random Forest classifier, a Support Vector Machine (SVM) with a radial basis function (RBF) kernel [20], and a logistic regression model.

Random Forest is an ensemble method that constructs multiple decision trees and aggregates their outputs to improve prediction robustness. SVM identifies the optimal hyperplane to separate different classes, while Logistic Regression models the probability of class membership using a linear function. These models were chosen for their complementary strengths and their established use in biomedical data analysis

All models were implemented using scikit-learn (v1.3.0) with default hyperparameters initially, followed by hyperparameter tuning via grid search [21]. The Random Forest model leveraged ensemble decision trees to enhance robustness and interpretability, while the SVM model offered nonlinear boundary discrimination. Logistic regression was included for its simplicity and high interpretability in clinical contexts. All models were trained and evaluated on the same standardized feature set to ensure comparability across methods.

To mitigate the risk of overfitting due to the limited sample size, models were primarily evaluated using 5-fold stratified cross-validation, ensuring balanced representation of both gait groups within each fold [22]. In addition to cross-validation, an 80:20 holdout split was performed to further validate model performance on unseen data. Specifically, 80% of the data-set was randomly selected and used as a training-set for model fitting and hyperparameter tuning, while the remaining 20% was reserved as an independent test set for performance evaluation [23]. Model performance was assessed using accuracy, F1-score, and area under the Receiver Operating Characteristic—Area Under the Curve (ROC AUC), which reflect overall classification accuracy, robustness to class imbalance, and discriminative ability, respectively.

3. Results

3.1. Result of Age Effect

To examine the effect of age on gait features and to control for potential confounding, an analysis of covariance (ANCOVA) was performed with age as a covariate. The results indicated that age had a statistically significant effect on multiple features, including single-limb support line (+) (p = 0.003), foot rotation (+) (p = 0.007), velocity (p = 0.037), and step length (+) (p = 0.049) (Figure 3). No significant age-related effects were found in the remaining features. Additionally, no significant age × group interaction was found in any feature, suggesting that the effect of age was consistent across both groups.

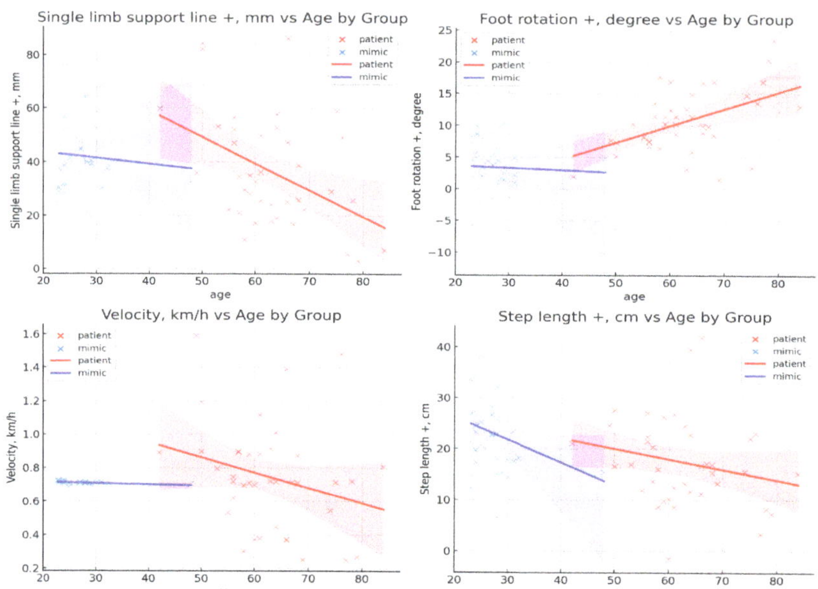

Figure 3. Distributional characteristics of features significantly influenced by age.

3.2. Result of Gait Feature

To examine group differences, independent samples t-tests were conducted for each variable, and Cohen's d was calculated as a measure of effect size. Furthermore, to assess the relative importance of the variables, a Random Forest classification model was employed, and the Gini importance for each variable was computed as the average decrease in Gini impurity contributed by that variable across the ensemble. The results revealed that several features showed statistically significant differences between the HG and MHG groups. Specifically, swing phase (−) ($p < 0.001$, Cohen's d = −2.103), stance phase (−) ($p < 0.001$, d = 2.103), and time maximum force1 (−) ($p < 0.001$, d = 1.556) showed large to very large effect sizes, indicating substantial biomechanical differences. Additionally, Time maximum force ratio ($p < 0.001$, d = −1.196) and step time (−) ($p < 0.001$, d = −0.615) also demonstrated meaningful group differences (Table 4).

Table 4. Comparison of features.

Features (Test Type)	HG Group	MHG Group	p-Value	Cohen's d	Gini
#Foot rotation (+) (b)	10.74 ± 4.97	3.43 ± 4.82	0.000 **	−1.492	0.051
Foot rotation (−) (b)	13.63 ± 8.14	3.96 ± 10.05	0.000 **	−1.056	0.037
#Step length (+) (b)	17.48 ± 8.73	23.19 ± 7.02	0.002 *	0.723	0.019
Step length (−) (b)	19.64 ± 8.48	20.32 ± 7.58	0.709	−0.084	0.004
Stride length (a)	37.12 ± 15.64	43.51 ± 6.34	0.022 *	−0.538	0.011
Step width (a)	15.27 ± 3.51	16.37 ± 4.49	0.230	−0.272	0.012
Stance phase (+) (a)	74.10 ± 5.54	78.32 ± 5.15	0.001 **	−0.791	0.018
Stance phase (−) (b)	72.74 ± 5.37	59.00 ± 7.50	0.000 **	2.103	0.138
Load Response (+) (b)	23.59 ± 5.11	19.48 ± 6.31	0.002 *	0.715	0.018
Load Response (−) (a)	23.72 ± 4.71	17.80 ± 4.71	0.000 **	1.256	0.038
Single-limb support (+) (b)	26.98 ± 5.61	41.06 ± 7.56	0.000 **	−2.110	0.144
Single-limb support (−) (b)	25.26 ± 6.31	21.67 ± 5.13	0.007 *	0.625	0.011
Pre-Swing (+) (a)	23.55 ± 4.93	17.79 ± 4.71	0.000 **	1.195	0.027
Pre-Swing (−) (b)	23.61 ± 5.29	19.50 ± 6.32	0.002 *	0.704	0.019
Swing phase (+) (a)	25.90 ± 5.54	21.68 ± 5.15	0.001 **	0.791	0.014
Swing phase (−) (b)	27.26 ± 5.37	41.00 ± 7.50	0.000 **	−2.103	0.155
Double stance phase (a)	47.10 ± 8.36	37.23 ± 8.09	0.000 **	1.200	0.037
Step time (+) (b)	0.98 ± 0.58	0.87 ± 0.22	0.274	0.252	0.008
Step time (−) (b)	1.02 ± 0.67	1.33 ± 0.22	0.010 *	−0.615	0.061
Stride time (b)	2.00 ± 1.24	2.20 ± 0.31	0.346	−0.217	0.016
Cadence (a)	72.66 ± 25.57	55.78 ± 8.37	0.000 **	0.892	0.017
#Velocity (a)	0.75 ± 0.32	0.71 ± 0.01	0.501	−0.155	0.025
Length of gait line (+) (a)	124.13 ± 22.62	134.88 ± 24.10	0.044 *	−0.460	0.007
Length of gait line (−) (a)	115.44 ± 27.07	101.73 ± 17.74	0.010 *	0.601	0.007
#Single-limb support line (+) (b)	36.55 ± 20.92	42.19 ± 14.65	0.171	0.313	0.005
Single-limb support line (−) (b)	22.26 ± 15.07	24.47 ± 8.32	0.424	−0.182	0.011
Lateral symmetry (a)	−14.51 ± 24.26	−21.60 ± 18.50	0.149	0.329	0.002
Time maximum force 1 (+) (b)	26.74 ± 5.44	28.50 ± 8.25	0.267	−0.251	0.013
Time maximum force 1 (−) (a)	28.67 ± 5.25	20.52 ± 5.22	0.000 **	1.556	0.042
Time maximum force ratio (b)	0.95 ± 0.19	1.46 ± 0.57	0.000 **	−1.196	0.035

Data are presented as mean ± standard deviation (SD). HG, hemiplegic gait; MHG, mimicked hemiplegic gait. (a): independent t-test; (b): Mann–Whitney U test. * p-value < 0.05; ** p value < 0.001; #: features excluded due to age. For HG and MHG groups, the values of the unaffected side and affected side were entered as (+) and (−), respectively. In case of the reference value, values corresponding to the right and left sides were entered in (+) and (−), respectively.

3.3. Result of Feature Importance Analysis

After excluding four features influenced by age (e.g., velocity, single-limb support line (+), foot rotation (+), step length (+)), the top 10 features with the highest importance scores were selected, and their relative contributions are visualized in Figure 4.

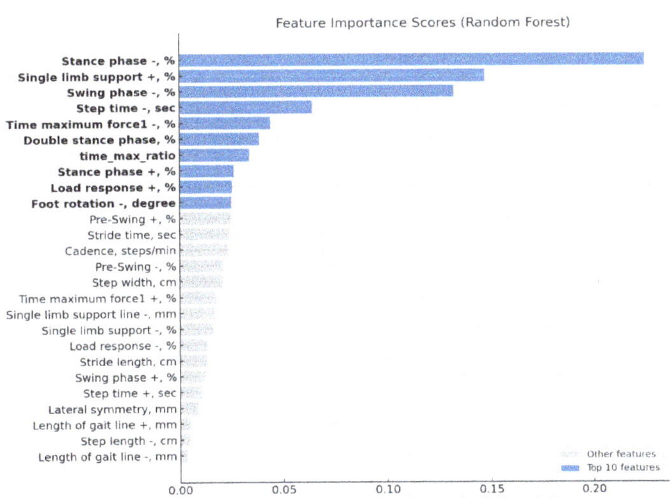

Figure 4. Feature importance scores by GINI Impurity of RF.

The most influential feature was stance phase (−) (Gini importance = 0.224), followed by single-limb support (+) (0.147), swing phase (−) (0.132), and step time (−) (0.064). Additional key features included time maximum force1 (−) (0.044), double stance phase (0.039), time_max_ratio (0.034), stance phase (+) (0.026), load response (+) (0.025), foot rotation (−), degree (0.025).

These top 10 features were subsequently used for feature-reduced model training, resulting in comparable or improved classification performance compared to models trained on the full feature set.

3.4. Result of Machine Learning Model

To evaluate classification performance, each model was trained and validated using both the full feature set (26 features) and a reduced feature set comprising the top 10 most important features selected via Random Forest. Table 5 summarizes the results of 5-fold stratified cross-validation across all models.

Table 5. The test results of classification models using top 10 features.

	Feature Set	Accuracy	F-1-Score	ROC AUC
Random Forest	All features	0.875	0.889	0.961
	Top 10 features	0.923	0.924	0.949
SVM (RBF Kernel)	All features	0.938	0.941	1.000
	Top 10 features	0.911	0.913	0.961
Logistic Regression	All features	0.911	0.901	0.932
	Top 10 features	0.911	0.907	0.941

When using the full feature set, the Support Vector Machine (SVM) with a radial basis function kernel demonstrated the highest classification performance, achieving an accuracy of 93.8%, F1-score of 0.941, and a perfect ROC AUC of 1.000. Logistic Regression also performed robustly on the full dataset, with an accuracy of 91.1% and ROC AUC of 0.932, while Random Forest yielded slightly lower accuracy (87.5%) but a comparably high AUC (0.961).

Upon restricting the input to the top 10 features, classification performance improved or remained stable across all models. Random Forest showed improved accuracy (92.3%) and F1-score (0.924), with a slight decrease in AUC to 0.949. The reduced-feature SVM achieved an accuracy of 91.1%, F1-score of 0.913, and maintained a high AUC of 0.961. Logistic Regression, using the same reduced features, also performed consistently well, with an accuracy of 91.1%, F1-score of 0.907, and AUC of 0.941 (Figure 5).

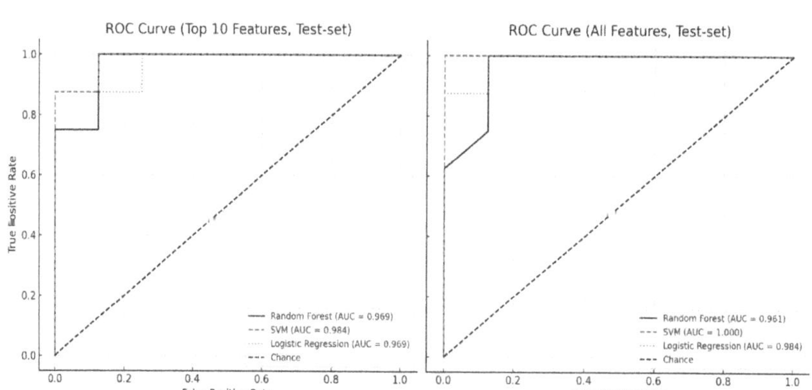

Figure 5. ROC curve comparison of three classifiers using top 10 and all features.

These results indicate that reducing the feature space to the most informative features not only maintained but, in some cases, enhanced model performance. Furthermore, while SVM demonstrated the highest discriminative capacity, both Random Forest and Logistic Regression achieved comparable results with the added benefit of interpretability and ease of integration in clinical settings.

3.5. Result of Machine Learning Model Using Non-Significant Variables

To examine whether the classification performance was solely driven by variables with significant group differences, we performed an additional analysis using only variables with $p > 0.05$ between the hemiplegic and mimicked hemiplegic gait groups. The variables included in this analysis were step length −, step width, step time +, stride time, velocity, single-limb support line +, single-limb support line −, lateral symmetry, and time maximum force1 +. Three classifiers—Random Forest, Support Vector Machine (SVM), and Logistic Regression classifiers—were trained on the training set (80%) and evaluated on the independent test set (20%) using Accuracy, F1-score, and ROC AUC metrics. The results are presented in Table 6 and Figure 6.

Table 6. The test results of classification models using non-significant features.

	Accuracy	F-1-Score	ROC AUC
Random Forest	0.875	0.875	0.969
SVM (RBF Kernel)	0.875	0.889	0.953
Logistic Regression	0.625	0.667	0.578

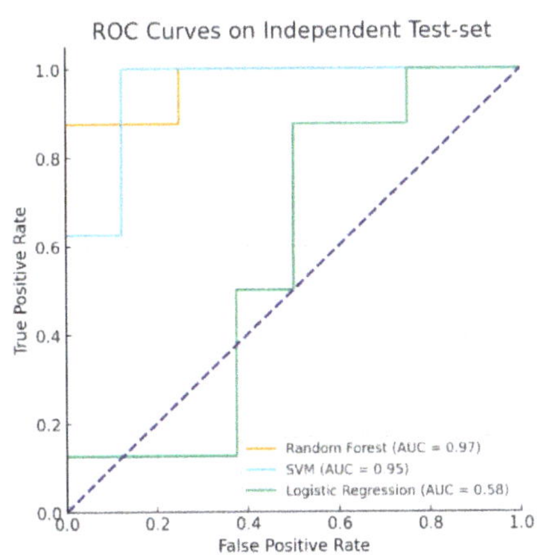

Figure 6. ROC curve comparison of three classifiers using non-significant (independent) features.

4. Discussion

This study aimed to identify key gait features and develop machine learning models to distinguish true hemiplegic gait (HG) from mimicked hemiplegic gait (MHG) using quantitative gait analysis data.

Gait features that can be collected through gait analysis include not only spatiotemporal features but also a wide variety of features related to the force, or movement of the center of pressure, making analysis difficult. In this study, machine learning was used to compare gait features obtained from numerous subjects in two groups to identify and classify the relationships between them. In this study, the collected gait analysis data were analyzed through machine learning, and the following results were obtained.

Firstly, In this study, ANCOVA revealed that four gait features—velocity, single-limb support line (+), foot rotation (+), and step length (+)—were significantly influenced by age. As a result, these features were excluded from intergroup statistical comparisons and machine learning modeling. Although each of these features represents clinically and biomechanically meaningful aspects of gait—including overall function, stability, joint control, and step efficiency—their strong association with age-related changes makes them less suitable for isolating pathological gait characteristics.

For example, velocity, a widely used marker of mobility and gait efficiency, is known to decrease with age due to reduced strength, balance, and neuromuscular coordination. Thus, differences in velocity may be attributed more to natural aging than to hemiparetic impairment [24,25]. Likewise, single-limb support line (+), derived from the trajectory of the center of pressure (COP), reflects the stability and duration of stance [26,27]. This feature is inherently sensitive to age-related decline in postural control, potentially confounding its interpretation as a group-specific gait deviation [28].

Foot rotation (+) indicates the degree of forefoot external rotation during gait. While such rotation is often seen in stroke-related compensatory movements, similar patterns can also emerge due to joint stiffness and muscular adaptations associated with aging, especially at the hip and ankle joints [29]. Step length (+), closely tied to stride mechanics, also decreases with age, as older adults typically exhibit reduced propulsion and joint range of motion. In this study, the absence of a significant difference in step length after adjusting for age supports this interpretation [30].

Importantly, all age-dependent gait variables identified in this study were derived from the unaffected side. While the unaffected side may exhibit more biomechanically stable patterns, it primarily reflects compensatory mechanisms rather than direct neurological impairments [31,32]. In contrast, the affected side provides richer pathological information, including asymmetry, altered timing, and deficits in force generation—features that are essential for distinguishing true hemiplegic gait from mimicked patterns [33]. Healthy individuals attempting to imitate hemiplegic gait are generally unable to replicate these subtle dysfunctions, making affected-side features especially valuable for classification. From a machine learning perspective, using predominantly affected-side parameters enhances discriminative power in differentiating neurologically impaired gait from cognitively generated imitation.

Secondly, a machine learning-based classification model was developed using unaffected-side gait features that were not significantly influenced by age. Feature importance analysis identified the top 10 features that most contributed to model performance. These features primarily comprised temporal gait features, phase-specific time ratios, and force timing characteristics, all of which captured essential distinctions between HG and MHG group.

Notably, features such as stance phase (−), single-limb support (+), swing phase (−), and step time (−) ranked among the most important. Among the top-ranked features identified in this study, stance phase (−), single-limb support (+), swing phase (−), and step time (−) reflect key spatiotemporal characteristics of hemiplegic gait. A reduced stance phase on the affected side indicates instability and diminished weight-bearing capacity, while increased single-limb support on the unaffected side reflects compensatory load-bearing strategies [31]. Shortened or delayed swing phase is commonly associated with impaired motor control and muscle weakness, and irregularities in step time reflect disrupted gait rhythm and temporal asymmetry [33]. These features capture pathological aspects of gait that are difficult for healthy individuals to replicate through mimicked hemiplegic gait, thus providing high discriminative power for classification. Although Rezgui et al. (2013) investigated the imitation of cerebral palsy gait rather than stroke-related hemiplegic gait, their findings support the notion that pathological gait patterns exhibit neuromechanical complexities that are difficult for healthy individuals to replicate accurately, thereby providing a relevant basis for our interpretation [34]. Their consistent emergence as important predictors in machine learning models highlights both their clinical relevance and their robustness in differentiating true hemiplegic gait from cognitively generated imitation. Furthermore, time-based kinetic features such as time_max_ratio and load response timing emerged as critical indicators. These features represent subtle shifts in the timing of ground reaction forces and suggest that temporal irregularities in neuromuscular response may serve as objective markers of pathological gait. Such micro-level deviations are unlikely to be perceived through visual inspection alone, underscoring the potential utility of data-driven metrics in clinical gait assessment.

Interestingly, the selected top features align well with those highlighted in previous clinical gait studies involving stroke patients. This convergence lends further support to their validity and highlights the importance of kinetic over kinematic features in distinguishing pathological gait. While kinematic features such as joint angles or step speed can be consciously manipulated by mimicry, kinetic features typically reflect involuntary motor output, offering greater diagnostic specificity.

In summary, the top 10 features identified in this study appear to capture fundamental biomechanical markers of true hemiplegic gait that are resistant to voluntary imitation. These findings suggest that carefully selected unaffected-side features—particularly those capturing temporal dynamics and weight transfer mechanisms—may serve as reliable components in objective gait classification systems. The results further support the use of explainable machine learning approaches to extract clinically relevant insights from quantitative gait analysis.

Thirdly, All three machine learning classification models developed in this study—Random Forest, Support Vector Machine (SVM), and Logistic Regression—demonstrated high performance in distinguishing hemiplegic gait (HG) from mimicked hemiplegic gait (MHG), supporting the feasibility of quantitative, data-driven gait classification. Among them, the SVM exhibited the highest discriminative power, achieving a perfect AUC (1.000) when trained on the full feature set and maintaining robust performance even when using only the top 10 features. This suggests that the SVM's ability to capture nonlinear decision boundaries may be particularly well-suited for modeling the complex patterns observed in hemiplegic gait.

The Random Forest model also achieved high accuracy and provided the added benefit of interpretability through feature importance scores. These importance scores were used to guide dimensionality reduction and contributed to maintaining model performance with fewer features. Logistic Regression, although slightly lower in AUC compared to the other models, offers advantages in transparency and clinical interpretability. In clinical settings where decision-making must be explainable, such simplicity is often valued despite minor performance trade-offs.

Importantly, models trained on only the top 10 most important features yielded comparable performance to models trained on the full feature set. This highlights the potential for efficient and lightweight gait assessment systems that minimize data collection burden without sacrificing diagnostic power. Such models may be more easily deployed in real-world settings, including wearable devices or bedside evaluation tools, and may support functional evaluations for rehabilitation planning, insurance verification, and return-to-work decisions. these models provide clinically meaningful insights into gait asymmetry and compensatory strategies. For example, the observed alterations in stance and swing phases correspond to well-known biomechanical consequences of muscle weakness and postural instability. Importantly, we found that models trained on only the top 10 most important features yielded comparable performance to those trained on the full feature set. This highlights the feasibility of developing efficient and lightweight gait assessment systems that minimize data collection burden without compromising diagnostic power. Such systems could be particularly advantageous for deployment in real-world clinical environments, including wearable devices or bedside evaluation tools, to support functional assessments for rehabilitation planning, insurance verification, and return-to-work decisions. Moreover, it should be acknowledged that the laterality of motor deficits may exert a significant influence on gait characteristics. Patients with left-sided hemiparesis often present with spatial neglect, which can exacerbate asymmetry and impair motor control, whereas right-sided hemiparesis may follow distinct compensatory mechanisms. Although our dataset did not allow for stratified analysis by side of involvement, future studies with larger cohorts should investigate laterality-specific gait alterations and their implications for personalized rehabilitation strategies. In addition, external validation using larger, multi-center datasets will be crucial to establish the robustness and generalizability of such lightweight models. Future research should also explore the integration of advanced algorithms, including deep learning and ensemble methods, to further enhance predictive performance while maintaining clinical interpretability.

Even when the analysis was restricted to variables showing no significant differences between groups ($p > 0.05$), Random Forest and SVM maintained high classification performance (ROC AUC = 0.97 and 0.95, respectively; Accuracy = 87.5%), demonstrating that the models learned complex multivariate patterns rather than exploiting obvious contrasts between groups. In contrast, Logistic Regression achieved substantially lower performance (ROC AUC = 0.58; Accuracy = 62.5%). This discrepancy can be attributed to the linear nature of Logistic Regression, which cannot adequately capture nonlinear relationships and higher-order interactions likely present in the selected variables. Moreover, potential multicollinearity among gait features and the limited sample size may have further reduced its performance. These findings collectively highlight the importance of nonlinear classification models in capturing complex gait patterns, particularly when apparent group differences are removed.

Several limitations of the present study should be acknowledged.

First, the training methodology for the MHG group poses concerns regarding ecological validity. Although participants were instructed using videos of actual stroke patients and demonstrations by doctors and were asked to reproduce characteristic hemiplegic gait patterns (hip extension and internal rotation, knee extension, ankle plantarflexion and inversion, hip hiking, and circumduction), no objective criteria or agreement scale was applied to confirm accurate imitation. Gait analysis was conducted only when physicians judged the mimicry to be sufficient, and treadmill speed was standardized at 0.7 km/h to minimize variability. Nevertheless, reliance on subjective assessment may have introduced uncontrolled variability, potentially compromising comparability with the HG group and leading to overestimation of the model's discriminatory capacity.

Second, the relatively small sample size (N = 79) limited the statistical power of the study. While sensitivity analysis confirmed that medium-to-large effects could be reliably detected, smaller effects might have been overlooked. According to Cohen's conventional thresholds for multiple regression ($f^2 = 0.02$ for small, $f^2 = 0.15$ for medium, and $f^2 = 0.35$ for large effects), our calculated $f^2 = 0.2$ corresponds to a medium-sized effect. This suggests that although the independent variables included in the model influence the dependent variable, the magnitude of this influence may not be substantial. Nevertheless, even very small effects can have considerable practical or clinical importance if they affect a large population.

Third, the machine learning models were trained and tested on a single-center dataset, raising concerns about external validity. To mitigate this, we applied cross-validation and developed a reduced model using only the top 10 key features identified through feature importance analysis, which showed comparable performance to the full model. However, such approaches cannot fundamentally resolve the limitation. We are therefore preparing additional patient recruitment and multi-center collaborative studies, and future work will focus on external validation with larger datasets to strengthen the generalizability of the model.

Fourth, although our models demonstrated high classification accuracy, it must be acknowledged that several gait features exhibited significant group differences between HG and MHG. This may have biased the classification results, favoring automatic discrimination and potentially inflating model performance beyond what might be expected in more ecologically valid conditions. Lastly, while we employed three widely used algorithms (Random Forest, SVM, Logistic Regression), future studies may benefit from exploring deep learning architectures, ensemble approaches, and refined threshold-tuning strategies to further enhance predictive accuracy and clinical applicability.

5. Conclusions

This study demonstrated that machine learning models can effectively distinguish hemiplegic gait from mimicked hemiplegic gait using quantitative gait features. By applying Random Forest, Support Vector Machine (SVM), and Logistic Regression classifiers, high classification performance was achieved even with a limited dataset, with SVM showing the highest AUC values. Feature importance analysis revealed that temporal asymmetries, such as altered stance and swing phases, along with force timing differences and spatial instability, were key discriminators. Notably, models trained using only the top 10 most informative features achieved comparable performance to those using the full feature set, suggesting that lightweight and interpretable models may be sufficient for clinical application. These findings support the potential of machine learning-based gait analysis as an objective tool for identifying pathological gait characteristics and contribute to the development of data-driven neurorehabilitation strategies. Further validation using external datasets and integration of additional physiological signals is recommended to enhance clinical utility and generalizability.

Author Contributions: Conceptualization, Y.-u.L.; methodology, Y.-u.L.; validation, S.L.; formal analysis, Y.-u.L.; investigation, C.-H.K.; data curation, J.-W.S. and S.K.; writing—original draft preparation, Y.-u.L.; writing—review and editing, J.-W.S. and S.K.; visualization, Y.-u.L.; supervision, S.L.; project administration, S.L.; funding acquisition, S.L. and C.-H.K. All authors have read and agreed to the published version of the manuscript.

Funding: This research was supported by a grant of the Korea Health Technology R&D Project through the Korea Health Industry Development Institute (KHIDI), funded by the Ministry of Health & Welfare, Republic of Korea (grant number: RS-2020-KH088006 & RS-2022-KH127675 & RS-2024-00442030).

Institutional Review Board Statement: The study was conducted in accordance with the Declaration of Helsinki and approved by the Institutional Review Board (IRB No., Wonkwang University Korean Medicine Hospital in Gwangju. WKIRB 2022-07, 29 June 2022).

Informed Consent Statement: Informed consent was obtained from all subjects involved in the study.

Data Availability Statement: The data presented in this study are available upon request from the corresponding author. These data are not publicly available because of privacy concerns.

Conflicts of Interest: The authors declare no conflicts of interest.

References

1. Li, S.; Francisco, G.E.; Zhou, P. Post-Stroke Hemiplegic Gait: New Perspective and Insights. *Front. Physiol.* **2018**, *9*, 1021. [CrossRef]
2. Balaban, B.; Tok, F. Gait Disturbances in Patients With Stroke. *PM&R* **2014**, *6*, 635–642. [CrossRef]
3. Murphy, S.J.X.; Werring, D.J. Stroke: Causes and Clinical Features. *Medicine* **2020**, *48*, 561–566. [CrossRef] [PubMed]
4. Eby, S.; Zhao, H.; Song, P.; Vareberg, B.J.; Kinnick, R.; Greenleaf, J.F.; An, K.-N.; Chen, S.; Brown, A.W. Quantitative Evaluation of Passive Muscle Stiffness in Chronic Stroke. *Am. J. Phys. Med. Rehabil.* **2016**, *95*, 899–910. [CrossRef] [PubMed]
5. Awad, L.N.; Palmer, J.A.; Pohlig, R.T.; Binder-Macleod, S.A.; Reisman, D.S. Walking Speed and Step Length Asymmetry Modify the Energy Cost of Walking After Stroke. *Neurorehabil. Neural Repair* **2015**, *29*, 416–423. [CrossRef] [PubMed]
6. Saunders, D.H.; Sanderson, M.; Hayes, S.; Kilrane, M.; Greig, C.A.; Brazzelli, M.; Mead, G.E. Physical fitness training for stroke patients. *Cochrane Database Syst. Rev.* **2020**, CD003316. [CrossRef]
7. Felius, R.A.W.; Geerars, M.; Bruijn, S.M.; Van Dieën, J.H.; Wouda, N.C.; Punt, M. Reliability of IMU-Based Gait Assessment in Clinical Stroke Rehabilitation. *Sensors* **2022**, *22*, 908. [CrossRef] [PubMed]
8. Kohnehshahri, F.S.; Merlo, A.; Mazzoli, D.; Bò, M.C.; Stagni, R. Machine Learning Applied to Gait Analysis Data in Cerebral Palsy and Stroke: A Systematic Review. *Gait Posture* **2024**, *114*, S39. [CrossRef]
9. Dolan, V.F. Narcotic-Seeking Behavior and Self-Injury: A Report of Three Cases. *J. Insur. Med.* **2025**, *52*, 23–30. [CrossRef]
10. Glaser, D. Fabricated or Induced Illness: From "Munchausen by Proxy" to Child and Family-Oriented Action. *Child Abuse Negl.* **2020**, *108*, 104649. [CrossRef]
11. M Patel, H.; M, B. Reliability, Agreement, and Validity of FDM Zebris Pressure Platform to Measure Lower Limb Weight Distribution during Quiet Standing. *Int. J. Curr. Res. Rev.* **2023**, *15*, 1–7. [CrossRef]
12. Esmaeilpour, F.; Letafatkar, A.; Karimi, M.T.; Khaleghi, M.; Rossettini, G.; Villafañe, J.H. Comparative Analysis of Ground Reaction Forces and Spatiotemporal Gait Parameters in Older Adults with Sway-Back Posture and Chronic Low Back Pain: A Cross-Sectional Study. *BMC Sports Sci. Med. Rehabil.* **2025**, *17*, 71. [CrossRef] [PubMed]
13. Kalron, A.; Achiron, A. The Relationship between Fear of Falling to Spatiotemporal Gait Parameters Measured by an Instrumented Treadmill in People with Multiple Sclerosis. *Gait Posture* **2014**, *39*, 739–744. [CrossRef] [PubMed]
14. Virtanen, P.; Gommers, R.; Oliphant, T.E.; Haberland, M.; Reddy, T.; Cournapeau, D.; Burovski, E.; Peterson, P.; Weckesser, W.; Bright, J.; et al. SciPy 1.0: Fundamental Algorithms for Scientific Computing in Python. *Nat. Methods* **2020**, *17*, 261–272. [CrossRef]
15. Lee, I.S.; Park, K.E.; Hong, H.J.; Sung, K.K.; Lee, S.K. The Change of Lateral Shift of Center of Pressure According to the Gait Improvement in Post-Stroke Hemiplegic Patients. *J. Intern. Korean Med.* **2014**, *35*, 448–454.
16. Patterson, K.K.; Gage, W.H.; Brooks, D.; Black, S.E.; McIlroy, W.E. Evaluation of Gait Symmetry after Stroke: A Comparison of Current Methods and Recommendations for Standardization. *Gait Posture* **2010**, *31*, 241–246. [CrossRef]
17. Green, S.B. How Many Subjects Does It Take to Do a Regression Analysis. *Multivar. Behav. Res.* **1991**, *26*, 499–510. [CrossRef]
18. Breiman, L. *Random Forests*; Springer Nature: Berlin/Heidelberg, Germany, 2001; Volume 45.
19. Guyon, I.; Elisseeff, A. An Introduction to Variable and Feature Selection. *J. Mach. Learn. Res.* **2003**, *3*, 1157–1182.
20. Chang, C.-C.; Lin, C.-J. LIBSVM: A Library for Support Vector Machines. *ACM Trans. Intell. Syst. Technol.* **2011**, *2*, 1–27. [CrossRef]
21. Pedregosa, F.; Pedregosa, F.; Varoquaux, G.; Varoquaux, G.; Org, N.; Gramfort, A.; Gramfort, A.; Michel, V.; Michel, V.; Fr, L.; et al. Scikit-Learn: Machine Learning in Python. *Mach. Learn. Python* **2011**, *12*, 2825–2830.
22. Kohavi, R. A Study of Cross-Validation and Bootstrap for Accuracy Estimation and Model Selection. *Int. Jt. Conf. Artif. Intell.* **1995**, *14*, 1137–1143.
23. Hastie, T.; Tibshirani, R.; Friedman, J. *The Elements of Statistical Learning: Data Mining, Inference, and Prediction*; Springer Series in Statistics; Springer: New York, NY, USA, 2009.
24. Bohannon, R.W. Comfortable and Maximum Walking Speed of Adults Aged 20–79 Years: Reference Values and Determinants. *Age Ageing* **1997**, *26*, 15–19. [CrossRef] [PubMed]
25. Studenski, S. Gait Speed and Survival in Older Adults. *JAMA* **2011**, *305*, 50. [CrossRef] [PubMed]
26. Ruhe, A.; Fejer, R.; Walker, B. Center of Pressure Excursion as a Measure of Balance Performance in Patients with Non-Specific Low Back Pain Compared to Healthy Controls: A Systematic Review of the Literature. *Eur. Spine J.* **2011**, *20*, 358–368. [CrossRef] [PubMed]
27. Lafond, D.; Corriveau, H.; Hébert, R.; Prince, F. Intrasession reliability of center of pressure measures of postural steadiness in healthy elderly people. *Arch. Phys. Med. Rehabil.* **2004**, *85*, 896–901. [CrossRef] [PubMed]
28. Maki, B.E. Gait Changes in Older Adults: Predictors of Falls or Indicators of Fear? *J. Am. Geriatr. Soc.* **1997**, *45*, 313–320. [CrossRef]
29. JudgeRoy, J.O.; Davis, B., III; Õunpuu, S. Step Length Reductions in Advanced Age: The Role of Ankle and Hip Kinetics. *J. Gerontol. Ser. A* **1996**, *51A*, M303–M312. [CrossRef]
30. Prince, F.; Corriveau, H.; Hébert, R.; Winter, D.A. Gait in the Elderly. *Gait Posture* **1997**, *5*, 128–135. [CrossRef]
31. Chen, G.; Patten, C.; Kothari, D.H.; Zajac, F.E. Gait Differences between Individuals with Post-Stroke Hemiparesis and Non-Disabled Controls at Matched Speeds. *Gait Posture* **2005**, *22*, 51–56. [CrossRef]

32. Olney, S.J.; Richards, C. Hemiparetic Gait Following Stroke. Part I: Characteristics. *Gait Posture* **1996**, *4*, 136–148. [CrossRef]
33. Patterson, K.K.; Parafianowicz, I.; Danells, C.J.; Closson, V.; Verrier, M.C.; Staines, W.R.; Black, S.E.; McIlroy, W.E. Gait Asymmetry in Community-Ambulating Stroke Survivors. *Arch. Phys. Med. Rehabil.* **2008**, *89*, 304–310. [CrossRef]
34. Rezgui, T.; Megrot, F.; Fradet, L.; Marin, F. On the Imitation of CP Gait Patterns by Healthy Subjects. *Gait Posture* **2013**, *38*, 576–581. [CrossRef]

Disclaimer/Publisher's Note: The statements, opinions and data contained in all publications are solely those of the individual author(s) and contributor(s) and not of MDPI and/or the editor(s). MDPI and/or the editor(s) disclaim responsibility for any injury to people or property resulting from any ideas, methods, instructions or products referred to in the content.

bioengineering

MDPI

Article

Feasibility and Preliminary Efficacy of Wearable Focal Vibration Therapy on Gait and Mobility in People with Multiple Sclerosis: A Pilot Study

Hongwu Wang [1,*], Yun Chan Shin [1], Nicole J. Tester [2] and Torge Rempe [3]

1 Department of Occupational Therapy, College of Public Health and Health Professions, University of Florida, Gainesville, FL 32611, USA; yunchan.shin@phhp.ufl.edu
2 University of Florida Health Rehabilitation at the Norman Fixel Institute for Neurological Disorders, University of Florida, Gainesville, FL 32628, USA; nicole.tester@ufhealth.org
3 Department of Neurology, College of Medicine, University of Florida, Gainesville, FL 32610, USA; torge.rempe@neurology.ufl.edu
* Correspondence: hongwu.wang@phhp.ufl.edu; Tel.: +1-(352)-2739934

Abstract: Multiple sclerosis (MS) is a chronic disease of the central nervous system that significantly impairs gait and mobility, contributing to a high risk of falls, reduced participation in daily activities, and diminished quality of life. Despite existing interventions such as exercise programs and pharmacological treatments, challenges such as fatigue, pain, and limited accessibility underscore the need for alternative therapies. Focal vibration therapy (FVT) has shown promise in improving gait, reducing spasticity, and enhancing mobility in people with MS (PwMS). However, further research is required to evaluate its long-term feasibility and optimize its parameters. This study examined the feasibility and preliminary efficacy of a home-based four-week wearable FVT device on gait and explored how FVT parameters impact gait and mobility outcomes. In this pilot double-blind randomized controlled trial, 22 PwMS were randomized into control and vibration groups (four FVT groups with varying vibration intensities/durations). Participants wore Myovolt® vibrators on distal quadricep muscles near the rectus femoris insertion (approximately 2 cm from the medial edge of the patella), gastrocnemius/soleus, and tibialis anterior muscles (10 min/muscle, 3 days/week, 4 weeks). Feasibility was evaluated via adherence and satisfaction (QUEST 2.0, interviews). Gait (3D motion analysis) and mobility (T25FW) were assessed at baseline and post-intervention. Data were analyzed using descriptive/inferential statistics and thematic analysis. Of 22 participants, 17 completed post-intervention (16 intervention, 1 control). Wearable FVT showed promising feasibility, with high satisfaction despite minor adjustability issues. Intervention groups improved gait speed (p = 0.014), stride length (p = 0.004), and ankle angle (p = 0.043), but T25FW was unchanged ($p > 0.05$). High-intensity FVT enhanced knee/hip moments. This study's results support the feasibility of wearable FVT for home-based management of mobility symptoms in MS with high participant satisfaction and acceptance. Notable gains in gait parameters suggest FVT's potential to enhance neuromuscular control and proprioception but may be insufficient to lead to mobility improvements. Subgroup analyses highlighted the impact of vibration intensity and duration on knee joint mechanics, emphasizing the need for personalized dosing strategies. Challenges included participant retention in the control group and burdensome biomechanical assessments, which will be addressed in future studies through improved sham devices and a larger sample size.

Keywords: focal vibration therapy; multiple sclerosis; motion capture analysis; gait biomechanics; feasibility; wearable

1. Introduction

Multiple sclerosis (MS) is a chronic autoimmune disease of the central nervous system (CNS) characterized by demyelination and axonal damage, leading to disrupted neural signal conduction and a range of neurological symptoms [1–3]. Among the most debilitating symptoms are gait and mobility impairments, driven by muscle weakness, spasticity, impaired coordination, sensory disturbances, and fatigue [4–6]. These challenges affect 50–70% of people with MS (PwMS), with 30% reporting multiple falls and related injuries within a few months [7,8], significantly reducing physical safety, daily activity participation, and quality of life [9,10].

Current interventions for MS-related mobility impairments, such as pharmacological treatments (e.g., dalfampridine) and exercise programs, face limitations, including side effects, limited efficacy, and accessibility barriers [11–14]. Fatigue and pain further hinder participation in exercise-based interventions, particularly for those with severe mobility limitations [15]. Consequently, there is a pressing need for safe, accessible, and cost-effective non-pharmacological therapies.

Focal vibration therapy (FVT), a non-invasive and portable intervention, stimulates sensory receptors in muscles and tendons to enhance proprioceptive input, neuromuscular control, and muscle activation [16,17]. FVT has shown potential benefits for gait and balance in various populations, including those with neurological conditions [18–20]. Four studies have investigated the use of FVT in PwMS. In people with secondary progressive MS who were non-responsive to common antispasmodic medication, repetitive FVT treatment (100 Hz, 0.2–0.5 mm amplitude) was associated with improved gait function by reducing spasticity and pain and improving quality of life [21]. In another study, walking also improved in PwMS (both those with and without spasticity) who received FVT (9000 Hz, < 0.8 N energy) compared with those who received sham vibration therapy [22]. The participants who received FVT improved gait velocity and cadence and took longer steps over a shorter time than the control group. The results reported by Paoloni et al. [23] (120 Hz) and Spina et al. [22] found that fatigue was significantly reduced in the FVT group, though there was no difference between the FVT and control groups. Ayvat et al. reported that FVT (50 Hz and 100 Hz, 1 mm amplitude) had a similar effect on spasticity, a better effect in increasing fascicle length with 50 Hz frequency, and improved stability in PwMS compared to an exercise program [24]. However, current research on FVT in MS is limited, and the optimal parameters, such as vibration frequency, amplitude, duration, and treatment intensity, have yet to be determined. Previous studies that have applied FVT to the lower extremities of people with MS have used different intensities and frequencies of FVT [21–24]. The measurements and equipment used to measure the effects also varied, making it difficult to assess the feasibility of their long-term usage [21–24].

This pilot study evaluated the feasibility and preliminary efficacy of a four-week home-based wearable FVT intervention on gait and mobility in PwMS. It aimed to assess the acceptability and feasibility of wearable FVT for home-based application in PwMS and explore how FVT parameters influence gait and mobility outcomes, with the long-term goal of optimizing treatment dosage to manage MS-related lower extremity symptoms effectively. We hypothesized that wearable FVT is feasible and would improve gait and mobility compared to baseline, with effects persisting at least four weeks post-intervention.

2. Materials and Methods

2.1. Study Design

This study was a pilot double-blind randomized controlled trial. Feasibility of the wearable FVT was assessed by participant acceptance, adherence, and satisfaction; while efficacy was evaluated using gait and functional mobility measures assessed at two timepoints: baseline evaluation before the start of the intervention, and post-intervention assessment immediately after the 4-week treatment period. As a pilot study, the target sample size was 30 participants (6 per group, including control), based on feasibility goals rather than a formal power calculation for efficacy, as is common in pilot trials (e.g., to assess recruitment, retention, and preliminary effect sizes). No a priori power calculation was performed for efficacy outcomes due to the exploratory nature.

2.2. Participants

Participants with clinically confirmed MS were recruited from the Oklahoma City area and surrounding clinics. The study was approved by the University of Oklahoma Health Sciences Center Institutional Review Board (IRB number 10785). Inclusion criteria were: (1) MS diagnosis defined by the 2017 revised McDonald criteria [25]; (2) age between 18 and 65 years; (3) subjects reporting impaired walking, assessed by clinical examination; (4) no clinical relapse in past 6 months; (5) ability to understand English instructions; (6) ability to sign an informed consent; and (7) normal or corrected vision. Participants with other symptoms or signs suggestive of peripheral neuropathy or other superimposed neurological or psychiatric conditions that could interfere with walking assessment, medical condition preventing the use of the vibration device, pregnancy, and a clinical diagnosis of moderate or severe dementia (defined as Montreal Cognitive Assessment [26] (MoCA) < 24 at screening) were excluded. Using a computer-generated randomization program, participants were randomized into five groups: a control group receiving non-functional sham vibration (showing the same vibration sounds but no actual vibration) and four intervention groups receiving different vibration dosages, as specified below. Allocation was concealed using sequentially numbered, opaque envelopes prepared by an independent researcher not involved in assessments. Envelopes were opened only after baseline consent. The sham vibration had an identical appearance to the experimental devices, with only auditory sounds, but no vibration. Participants were blinded via an identical device appearance (sham produced sound but no vibration). Outcome assessors (trained students) were blinded to allocation. Data analysts were blinded until the final analysis.

2.3. Intervention

Participants allocated to the FVT groups wore a portable vibration device (Myovolt®, Christchurch, New Zealand) placed bilaterally on three specific lower extremity muscle groups: the distal quadriceps muscle/tendon region near the rectus femoris insertion (approximately 2 cm from the medial edge of the patella), the gastrocnemius/soleus muscle/tendon region, and the tibialis anterior muscle belly (Figure 1). These muscles were selected because they are directly involved during walking, as supported by previous studies [21–24]. During each FVT session, participants sequentially received the prescribed focal vibration on the distal quadricep muscles, gastrocnemius, and tibialis anterior muscle groups. For the intervention groups, four vibration dosages were selected: Low-intensity short duration (LISD): 60 Hz frequency, 0.5 mm amplitude, 10 min per muscle (30 min/session); Low-intensity long duration (LILD): 60 Hz, 0.5 mm, two 10 min sessions per muscle with a 1-min break (60 min/session); High-intensity short duration (HISD): 120 Hz, 1 mm, 10 min per muscle (30 min/session); High-intensity long duration (HILD): 120 Hz, 1 mm, two 10-min sessions per muscle (60 min/session). These parameters were selected based on prior studies [21–24] and our pilot testing with people with strokes and diabetes and manufacturer (Myovolt®) recommendations for safe home use. All participants in the intervention groups performed three sessions per week over four consecutive weeks. The vibration intensity (frequency and amplitude) was predetermined for each intervention arm and remained constant throughout the intervention period. Participants in the control group wore the Myovolt device in the same locations using the sham vibrators.

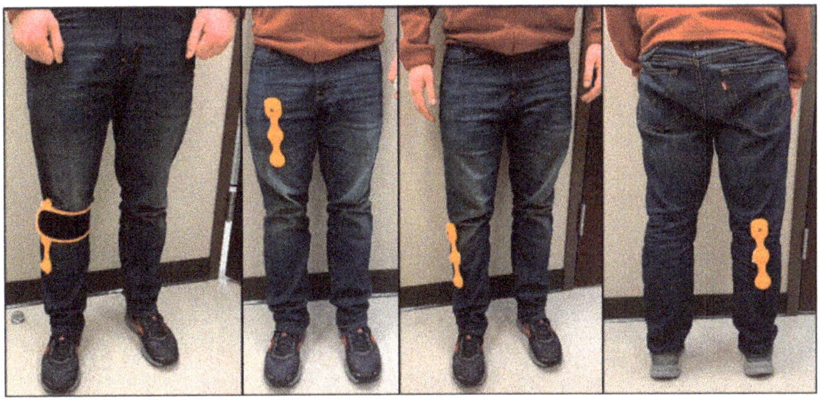

Figure 1. Myovolt wearable FVT device and application sites (left to right: vibration device with strap, quadriceps muscle/tendon region, gastrocnemius/soleus muscle/tendon region, and the tibialis anterior muscle belly).

At the initial visit, research staff trained all participants to don and doff the Myovolt device properly to avoid device slippage. All participants learned to switch the device on/off and charge the device. We provided each participant with a simple, intuitive user manual (as shown in the Supplementary Materials) to ensure the correct application at home. Participants were asked to note the date and time of the application of the FVT. Throughout the intervention, we maintained regular contact with participants to monitor adherence, troubleshoot device issues, and answer any questions.

2.4. Outcome Measurements

At each assessment, evaluators who did not know the intervention assignment recorded the outcomes. The evaluators were physical or occupational therapy students sufficiently trained by an experienced physical therapy researcher to ensure fidelity.

In the baseline assessment, participants' age, Body Mass Index (BMI), ethnicity, education level, duration of MS, Expanded Disability Status Scale (EDSS) score, ankle-foot orthosis/orthoses usage, walking aid (s) usage, MS medication, and self-reported physical limitation were collected via study personnel trained by a neurologist. The EDSS constitutes one of the oldest and probably most widely utilized assessment instruments in MS [27]. It has been used in virtually every major clinical trial conducted in MS during the last four decades and in numerous other clinical studies. The EDSS is an ordinal clinical rating scale ranging from 0 (normal neurologic examination) to 10 (death due to MS) in half-point increments. It has been shown to be a valid tool [28] for patients with multiple sclerosis with moderate intra-rater reliability [29].

The feasibility of the FVT intervention was assessed by the participants' adherence, acceptance, and satisfaction indicated by the Quebec User Evaluation of Satisfaction with Assistive Technology (QUEST 2.0) and semi-structured interviews. The Quebec User Evaluation of Satisfaction with QUEST is a standardized assessment tool designed to evaluate user satisfaction with assistive devices [30,31]. It has been shown with good test–retest reliability in people with MS [32]. Semi-structured interviews were conducted to collect qualitative data from participants about their acceptance, perceived usefulness, and experience of the FVT intervention.

Mobility was quantified using the Timed 25-Foot Walk Test (T25FW) at baseline and post-intervention. T25FW is a mobility test based on a timed 25-foot walk [33], with good test–retest reliability in people with MS [34]. The participant is directed to one end of a marked 25-foot course and is instructed to walk 25 feet as quickly as possible, but safely. The time is calculated from the initiation of the instruction to the start and ends when the participant has reached the 25-foot mark. The task is immediately administered again by having the participant walk back the same distance. Participants may use assistive devices when performing this task.

Quantitative gait parameters were collected using the Qualysis™ (Qualisys AB, Göteborg, Sweden) motion capture system and AMTI™ (Advanced Mechanical Technology, Inc., Watertown, MA, USA) force plates, placing reflective markers on 58 anatomical landmarks (Figure 2), using the Qualysis™ motion capture system's 12 cameras (sampling rate 120 Hz) and the AMTI™ force plates (sampling rate 1 kHz) to capture gait performance data. A physical therapist with over 15 years of experience in gait biomechanics and 8 years with the Qualisys motion capture system placed the markers. Each participant first performed a static trial to develop their individual skeletal model, which the investigators then exported to Visual3D© (C-Motion, Germantown, MD, USA) for data analysis. Participants then walked at a self-selected speed of 25 feet for three to five trials, using the normal pace they used for everyday life. From these trials, we analyzed and averaged data across all valid gait cycles captured, which typically ranged from 3 to 10 cycles per participant per assessment, depending on the quality of force plate contacts and the individual's stride length (ensuring clean, artifact-free data). Invalid cycles (e.g., those with partial force plate strikes or marker occlusions) were excluded. Gait cycles were primarily determined using force plate data, where heel strike (initial contact) and toe-off events were identified based on a vertical ground reaction force threshold of 20 N. When force plate data was unavailable or incomplete for a given step (e.g., due to the participant missing the plate), kinematic data from reflective markers (specifically, heel and toe marker trajectories and velocities) were used as a supplement to detect events via Visual3D's automated pipeline. This hybrid approach ensured accurate event detection while maximizing usable data. Investigators then calculated kinematic and kinetic data using Visual3D©. The following gait parameters were calculated: gait speed, stride length, stride width, stride time, left and right stance time, left and right swing time, cadence, duration of double support, left and right peak knee flexion, left and right peak dorsiflexion, left and right peak plantarflexion, left and right peak knee flexor moment, left and right peak plantar flexor moment, and left and right peak ankle joint power. Visual3D© defines the spatiotemporal measures as follows [35]: gait speed is the stride length divided by stride time, stride length is the distance from heel strike to heel strike on the same side, stride time is the duration of the gait cycle from heel strike to heel strike on the same side, left stance time is the time from left heel strike to left toe off, right stance time is the time from right heel strike to right toe off, left swing time is the time from left toe off to left heel strike, right swing time is the time from right toe off to right heel strike, mean cadence is the average number of steps taken per minute, and duration of double support is the amount of time spent with both feet in contact with the surface.

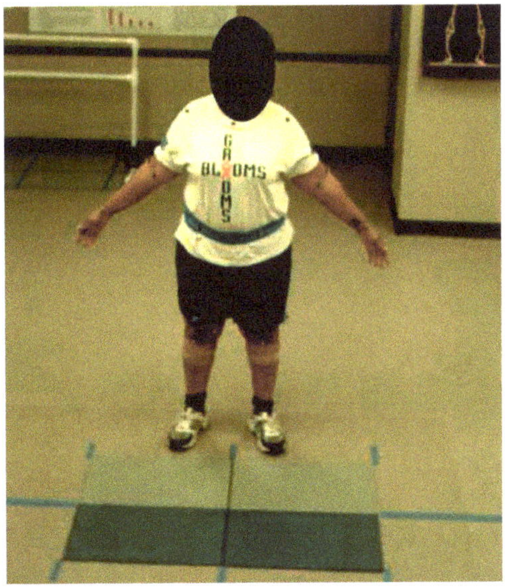

Figure 2. Reflective marker placement.

2.5. Statistical Analysis

All data were recorded on standardized case report forms and securely stored for subsequent analysis. All statistical analyses were conducted using IBM® SPSS Statistics for Windows, Version 26.0, and RStudio, Version 2022. Data were first screened for normality and homogeneity of variance before conducting inferential tests. Descriptive statistics were computed for participant demographics, feasibility data. Paired t-tests or Wilcoxon signed-rank tests were used to compare the gait variables and T25FW scores between baseline and post-intervention. Statistical significance was set at $p < 0.05$. Due to the exploratory nature of this pilot study, no adjustments were made for multiple comparisons in the analysis of gait parameters, which may increase the risk of false positives, as noted as a limitation. Effect sizes were calculated using Cohen's d for paired t-tests, where d = differences in the post and pre means / standard deviation of the difference (the standard deviation of the paired differences). For Wilcoxon signed-rank tests, the matched-pairs rank-biserial correlation (r) was computed and converted to d for consistency. Effect sizes were interpreted as small (d = 0.2–0.49), medium (d = 0.5–0.79), or large ($d \geq 0.8$) [36]. Qualitative data from semi-structured interviews were analyzed using thematic analysis to identify key themes related to participant satisfaction and usability.

3. Results

A total of 22 participants were recruited, with 19 completing the baseline assessment (17 intervention, 2 control) and 17 completing the post-intervention assessment (16 intervention, 1 control) (Figure 3). Three participants assigned to the control group withdrew from the study before the intervention started, and a baseline assessment due to the lack of perceived usefulness of the sham vibration. Two dropouts occurred, one from the HISD group and one from the control group. Consequently, only one participant from the control group completed the post-intervention assessment. The baseline characteristics of the total participants and each group are described in Tables 1 and 2. The mean age of the total experimental group, which completed the baseline evaluation, was 49.65 years (SD = 9.59), with 15 out of 17 participants (78.95%) being female. The control group had a mean age of 49.50 years (SD = 9.19), with 1 out of 2 participants being female. Therefore, due to the limited sample size, the initial plan to compare each of the four experimental groups with the control group was limited, and the analysis was conducted on the total experimental group and the data from the four individual experimental groups.

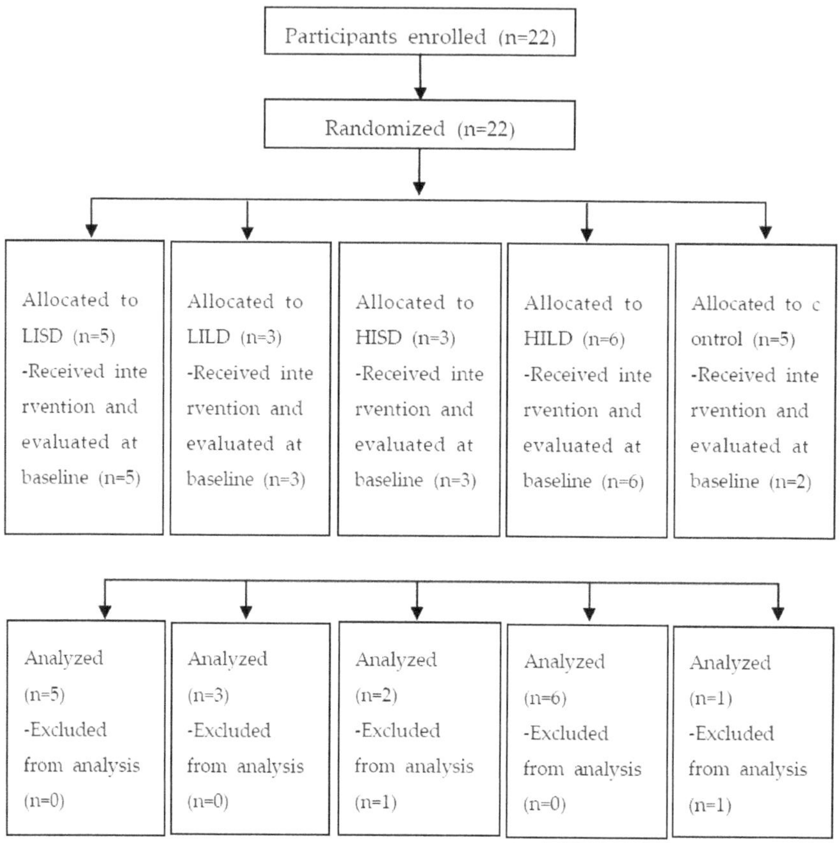

Figure 3. Flow of the trial selection process. Twenty-two participants were enrolled and randomized to different intervention and control groups. Nineteen participants completed the baseline assessment. Seventeen participants completed the post-intervention assessment. LISD: low intensity and short duration; LILD: low intensity and long duration; HISD: high intensity and short duration; HILD: high intensity and long duration.

Table 1. Participant Characteristics (n = 19).

	Experimental Group (n = 17)	Control Group (n = 2)
Age (mean, (SD))	49.65 (9.59)	49.50 (9.19)
Gender (n, (%))		
Male	3 (17.65%)	1 (50.00%)
Female	14 (82.35%)	1 (50.00%)
BMI (mean, (SD))	33.31 (7.86)	22.27 (0.97)

Table 1. *Cont.*

	Experimental Group (n = 17)	Control Group (n = 2)
Ethnicity (n, (%))		
African American	6 (35.29%)	1 (50.00%)
Caucasian	11 (64.71%)	1 (50.00%)
Education (n, (%))		
GED or High School Diploma	4 (23.53%)	1 (50.00%)
Some college	2 (11.76%)	0 (0.00%)
Bachelor's Degree	5 (29.41%)	0 (0.00%)
Master's Degree	3 (17.65%)	0 (0.00%)
Doctorate	1 (5.88%)	0 (0.00%)
Associate degree	1 (5.88%)	1 (50.00%)
Technical Certification	1 (5.88%)	0 (0.00%)
Years of MS (mean, (SD))	9.76 (7.53)	8 (9.90)
Baseline EDSS score (mean, (SD))	3.22 (0.93) ++	4.00 (0.00)
Ankle-foot orthoses usage (n, (%))		
Yes	1 (5.88%)	0 (0.00%)
No	16 (94.12%)	2 (100.00%)
Walking aids usage (n, (%))		
Yes	6 (35.29%)	1 (50.00%)
No	11 (64.71%)	1 (50.00%)
Using MS medication		
Yes	16 (94.12%)	2 (100.00%)
No	1 (5.88%)	0 (0.00%)
Perceived importance of medication use (mean, (SD))	9.82 (0.53)	9.00 (1.41)
Physical limitations affecting self-care (n, (%))		
Problems with hand	3 (17.65%)	0 (0.00%)
Problems with feet	8 (47.06%)	1 (50.00%)
Vision loss	1 (5.88%)	1 (50.00%)
Hearing loss	1 (5.88%)	0 (0.00%)

++: n = 16. Includes age, BMI, ethnicity, education level, MS duration, EDSS score, assistive devices usage, use of MS medication, and perceived importance of medication use (1–10 Likert scale: 1 = not important, 10 = very important).

Table 2. Baseline participants' demographics by intervention subgroups.

	Low-Intensity Vibration Group (n = 8)	High-Intensity Vibration Group (n = 9)	Short-Duration Vibration Group (n = 8)	Long-Duration Vibration Group (n = 9)
Age (mean, (SD))	50.00 (9.74)	49.33 (10.04)	50.88 (9.63)	48.56 (10.00)
Gender (n, (%))				
Male	2 (25.00%)	1 (11.11%)	2 (25.00%)	1 (11.11%)
Female	6 (75.00%)	8 (88.89%)	6 (75.00%)	8 (88.89%)
BMI (mean, (SD))	36.24 (7.28)	30.71 (7.82)	34.75 (7.94)	32.03 (8.03)
Ethnicity (n, (%))				
African American	2 (25.00%)	4 (44.44%)	2 (25.00%)	4 (44.44%)
Caucasian	6 (75.00%)	5 (55.56%)	6 (75.00%)	5 (55.56%)

Table 2. *Cont.*

	Low-Intensity Vibration Group (n = 8)	High-Intensity Vibration Group (n = 9)	Short-Duration Vibration Group (n = 8)	Long-Duration Vibration Group (n = 9)
Education (n, (%))				
GED or High School Diploma	1 (12.50%)	3 (33.33%)	1 (12.50%)	3 (33.33%)
Some college	2 (25.00%)	0 (0.00%)	1 (12.50%)	1 (11.11%)
Bachelor's Degree	3 (37.50%)	2 (22.22%)	3 (32.50%)	2 (22.22%)
Master's Degree	1 (12.50%)	2 (22.22%)	2 (25.00%)	1 (11.11%)
Doctorate	1 (12.50%)	0 (0.00%)	1 (12.50%)	0 (0.00%)
Associate degree	0 (0.00%)	1 (11.11%)	0 (0.00%)	1 (11.11%)
Technical Certification	0 (0.00%)	1 (11.11%)	0 (0.00%)	1 (11.11%)
Years of MS (mean, (SD))	7.75 (8.48)	11.56 (6.54)	8.13 (7.94)	11.22 (7.29)
Baseline EDSS score (mean, (SD))	2.79 (0.57) $^{+}$	3.56 (1.04)	3.36 (0.80) $^{+}$	3.11 (1.05)
Ankle-foot orthoses usage (n, (%))				
Yes	0 (0.00%)	1 (11.11%)	0 (0.00%)	1 (11.11%)
No	8 (100.00%)	8 (88.89%)	8 (100.00%)	8 (88.89%)
Walking aids usage (n, (%))				
Yes	1 (12.50%)	5 (55.56%)	3 (32.50%)	3 (33.33%)
No	7 (0.00%)	4 (44.44%)	5 (67.50%)	6 (66.67%)
Using MS medication				
Yes	8 (100.00%)	8 (88.89%)	8 (100.00%)	8 (88.89%)
No	0 (0.00%)	1 (11.11%)	0 (0.00%)	1 (11.11%)
Perceived importance of medication use (mean, (SD))	9.75 (0.71)	9.89 (0.33)	9.63 (0.74)	10.00 (0.00)
Physical limitations affecting the ability to perform self-care (n, (%))				
Problems with hand	2 (25.00%)	1 (11.11%)	1 (12.50%)	2 (22.22%)
Problems with feet	5 (62.50%)	3 (33.33%)	4 (50.00%)	4 (44.44%)
Vision loss	1 (12.50%)	0 (0.00%)	1 (12.50%)	0 (0.00%)
Hearing loss	1 (12.50%)	0 (0.00%)	0 (0.00%)	1 (11.11%)

$^{+}$: n = 7. Includes age, BMI, ethnicity, education level, MS duration, EDSS score, assistive devices usage, use of MS medication, and perceived importance of medication use (1–10 Likert scale: 1 = not important, 10 = very important).

3.1. Feasibility of the Wearable FVT Intervention

Seventeen participants completed the QUEST satisfaction survey regarding their experience with FVT (Table 3). Overall satisfaction was high. However, the lowest scores for "ease of adjusting" and "durability" were 2 points, with two participants expressing dissatisfaction with them. Additionally, one, one, and three participants scored "safe and secure," "comfort," and "how effective" as 3 points, respectively, reflecting a neutral level of satisfaction.

The feasibility measures are shown in Table 4. Sixteen participants, including one from the control group, completed the semi-structured interviews. Fifteen participants expressed acceptance of the FVT, except the one from the control group, who reported no perceived effect of the FVT. Of the 14 participants who responded that they would like to continue to use the focal vibration device, 9 expressed a desire to purchase it, and 3 indicated that they would consider purchasing it if certain improvements were made. Of the 16 participants, 13 did not experience any pain from using the device, with 2 reporting that the device may have caused muscle spasms or pain. The preference for the device included most participants stating that the device was "easy to use". Participant feedback (Table 4) indicated overall satisfaction with the FVT intervention but highlighted concerns regarding device adjustability (e.g., strap fit), durability (e.g., wear and tear), and comfort during prolonged use, as reported in semi-structured interviews. These findings suggest areas for device improvement in future iterations.

Table 3. QUEST results (n = 17).

Questions	Mean (SD)	Min Score
Satisfaction with the dimensions of the assistive device	4.76 (0.44)	4
Satisfaction with the weight	4.88 (0.33)	4
Satisfaction with the ease of adjusting the device	4.29 (1.05)	2
Satisfaction with how safe and secure of device is	4.71 (0.59)	3
Satisfaction with the durability	4.47 (1.07)	2
Satisfaction with ease of use	4.82 (0.39)	4
Satisfaction with the comfort of the device	4.71 (0.59)	3
Satisfaction with how effective the device is	4.53 (0.80)	3
Total satisfaction	37.18 (3.89)	27

Responses were collected via the Quebec User Evaluation of Satisfaction with Assistive Technology (QUEST 2.0) and semi-structured interviews, assessing satisfaction, perceived usefulness, and usability challenges (e.g., device adjustability, durability, comfort). Scores range from 1 (not satisfied) to 5 (very satisfied) for the QUEST items.

3.2. Gait Parameters

The experimental group demonstrated a significant gait speed increase ($p = 0.014$), along with stride length ($p = 0.004$) and the peak plantarflexion during the pre-swing phase of the more involved side ($p = 0.043$) after the FVT intervention (Tables 5 and 6). There were no significant changes in other spatiotemporal, kinematic, or kinetic variables (Tables 5–7). Trends toward significance were observed in the peak plantarflexion before heel strike ($p = 0.056$), peak hip flexion during stance ($p = 0.08$), peak ankle power in late stance ($p = 0.086$), peak ankle power in early stance ($p = 0.077$), peak knee flexor moment in early swing ($p = 0.076$), and peak knee power absorption in swing phase ($p = 0.065$) of the more involved side, respectively.

For the low intensity subgroup, the peak hip extension angle during the stance phase, the knee extension angle at the heel strike, and the peak knee flexion angle at the stance phase of the more involved side were significantly improved after the intervention. No significant changes were noted for other subgroups. We observed significantly improved peak knee flexion angle during the stance phase, peak knee flexion angle during the swing phase, and peak knee flexion moment during the stance phase in the more involved side in the participants receiving low-intensity FVT. For those who received high-intensity FVT, significantly improved peak hip extension power during the swing phase, peak knee flexion moment during the swing phase, and peak knee power during the stance phase were observed in the less involved side. The peak knee extension moment at the stance phase on the less involved side was the only gait parameter that showed a statistically significant difference when comparing the low-intensity and high-intensity groups.

3.3. Mobility

There were no statistically significant ($p = 0.54$) changes in the T25FW scores between the pre- (7.80 ± 3.50 s) and post-assessments (7.68 ± 3.09) for the experimental group. Minimal detectable clinical differences (20% change in the T25FW score [37]) were also not found in the total and each subgroup.

Table 4. Participants' feedback on feasibility (n = 16) based on post-intervention interviews.

	n
Willing to use FVT	15
Willing to purchase the device	9
Will not purchase the device	2
Willing to purchase the device after improvements (stronger intensity, clear evidence, appropriate cost)	3
Missed using the device	3
No pain during device use	13
Potential adverse events during device use (spasm or pain)	2
Device preference	
All the aspects	6
Ease of use	5
Flexibility	1
Easy to use	2
Simplicity	1
Fun to use	1
Lightweight	1

Table 5. Changes in spatiotemporal parameters (N = 16) for experimental participants.

Parameter: m = Meters; s = Second		All Participants Mean (Standard Deviation)	*p* Values	Estimated Effect Size
Gait speed (m/s)	pre	0.92 (0.30)	0.014	0.34
	post	0.98 (0.27)		
Stride length (m)	pre	1.05 (0.23)	0.004	0.44
	post	1.11 (0.19)		
Stride width (m)	pre	0.19 ± 0.04	0.613	0.02
	post	0.19 ± 0.03		
Stride time (s)	pre	1.20 (0.19)	0.76	0.01
	post	1.19 (0.23)		
More involved cadence (steps/min)	pre	101.01 (16.18)	0.53	0.03
	post	102.36 (18.26)		
Less involved cadence (steps/min)	pre	105.34 (15.53)	0.74	0.01
	post	105.83 (13.97)		
More involved stance (s)	pre	0.79 (0.15)	0.62	0.02
	post	0.78 (0.16)		
Less involved stance (s)	pre	0.81 (0.15)	0.63	0.02
	post	0.79 (0.18)		
More involved swing time (s) [a]	pre	0.40 (0.05)	0.57	0.02
	post	0.41 (0.07)		
Less involved swing time (s) [a]	pre	0.40 (0.06)	0.97	<0.01
	post	0.40 (0.05)		
Double limb support (s) [a]	pre	0.39 (0.11)	0.77	0.01
	post	0.39 (0.12)		

[a] N = 15 due to missed measures.

Table 6. Changes in kinematic parameters for experimental participants (N = 16).

Parameter: LI-Less Involved; MI-More Involved		All Participants Mean (Standard Deviation)	*p* Values	Estimated Effect Size
LI peak dorsiflexion at heel-off (°) [a]	pre	21.09 (2.41)	0.89	0.001
	post	21.24 (4.33)		
LI peak plantarflexion before heel strike (°) [a]	pre	−5.02 (6.26)	0.18	0.13
	post	−7.03 (6.36)		
LI peak dorsiflexion before heel-off (°) [a]	pre	11.55 (3.51)	0.97	<0.01
	post	11.52 (2.88)		
LI peak plantarflexion during pre-swing (°) [a]	pre	−6.48 (7.30)	0.28	0.08
	post	−8.42 (7.38)		
MI peak dorsiflexion at heel-off (°) [a]	pre	19.41 (2.96)	0.59	0.02
	post	19.79 (2.94)		
MI peak plantarflexion before heel strike (°) [a]	pre	−7.02 (8.38)	0.056	0.24
	post	−8.99 (8.07)		
MI peak dorsiflexion before heel-off (°) [a]	pre	10.60 (4.19)	0.62	0.02
	post	10.24 (4.97)		
MI peak plantarflexion during pre-swing (°) [a]	pre	−9.61 (9.87)	0.043	0.26
	post	−11.88 (9.69)		
LI knee flexion at heel stike (°)	pre	8.75 (9.93)	0.41	0.05
	post	10.10 (8.65)		
LI maximum knee flexion at stance (°)	pre	43.68 (8.91)	0.86	0.002
	post	43.26 (5.53)		
LI minum knee flexion at stance (°)	pre	4.58 (7.82)	0.51	0.03
	post	5.61 (7.23)		
LI maximum knee flexion at swing (°)	pre	54.36 (11.26)	0.53	0.03
	post	55.80 (6.44)		
LI minimum knee flexion at swing (°)	pre	6.44 (10.75)	0.50	0.03
	post	7.59 (9.83)		
MI knee flexion at heel stike (°)	pre	8.12 (9.59)	0.44	0.04
	post	9.52 (8.23)		
MI maximum knee flexion at stance (°)	pre	40.62 (7.73)	0.31	0.07
	post	42.82 (4.68)		
MI minimum knee flexion at stance (°)	pre	2.39 (7.02)	0.41	0.05
	post	3.67 (4.83)		
MI maximum knee flexion at swing (°)	pre	52.46 (10.78)	0.31	0.07
	post	54.70 (8.03)		
MI minimum knee flexion at swing (°)	pre	5.89 (10.53)	0.80	0.004
	post	6.32 (8.87)		
LI peak hip flexion at stance (°)	pre	23.63 (10.55)	0.18	0.12
	post	28.12 (8.51)		
LI peak hip extension at stance (°)	pre	−13.73 (11.94)	0.36	0.06
	post	−10.90 (10.11)		
LI peak hip flexion at swing (°)	pre	24.75 (11.03)	0.16	0.13
	post	29.64 (8.46)		

Table 6. *Cont.*

Parameter: LI-Less Involved; MI-More Involved		All Participants Mean (Standard Deviation)	*p* Values	Estimated Effect Size
LI peak hip extension at swing (°)	pre	−2.44 (12.86)	0.49	0.05
	post	−0.08 (10.02)		
MI peak hip flexion at stance (°)	pre	21.69 (12.09)	0.08	0.19
	post	27.41 (9.18)		
MI peak hip extension at stance (°)	pre	−14.86 (12.78)	0.29	0.07
	post	−11.66 (9.84)		
MI peak hip flexion at swing (°)	pre	23.20 (12.99)	0.11	0.16
	post	28.60 (8.91)		
MI peak hip extension at swing (°)	pre	−4.03 (13.97)	0.32	0.07
	post	−0.34 (10.64)		
LI minimum knee flexion at swing (°)	pre	6.44 (10.75)	0.50	0.03
	post	7.59 (9.83)		

[a] N = 15 due to missed ankle measurements.

Table 7. Changes in kinetic parameters for experimental participants (N = 13).

Parameter: LI-Less Involved; MI-More Involved		All Participants Mean (Standard Deviation)	*p* Values	Estimated Effect Size
LI peak plantar flexor moment (N · m/kg)	pre	1.10 (0.20)	0.15	0.16
	post	1.15 (0.16)		
LI peak ankle power in late stance (W/kg)	pre	1.89 (0.77)	0.058	0.27
	post	2.13 (0.82)		
LI peak ankle power in early stance (W/kg)	pre	−0.84 (0.41)	0.74	0.01
	post	−0.86 (0.31)		
MI peak plantar flexor moment (N · m/kg)	pre	1.10 (0.26)	0.37	0.07
	post	1.14 (0.22)		
MI peak ankle power in late stance (W/kg)	pre	1.81 (0.95)	0.086	0.23
	post	2.03 (1.11)		
MI peak ankle power in early stance (W/kg)	pre	−0.71 (0.27)	0.077	0.24
	post	−0.79 (0.32)		
LI peak knee extensor moment in early stance (N · m/kg)	pre	0.85 (0.29)	0.88	0.002
	post	0.85 (0.21)		
LI peak knee flexor moment in mid-stance (N · m/kg)	pre	−0.17 (0.08)	0.57	0.03
	post	−0.18 (0.06)		
LI peak knee flexor moment in early swing (N · m/kg)	pre	0.11 (0.06)	0.86	0.003
	post	0.11 (0.04)		
LI peak knee extensor moment in late swing (N · m/kg)	pre	−0.28 (0.09)	0.19	0.14
	post	−0.29 (0.08)		
LI peak knee power generation in stance (W/kg)	pre	0.55 (0.40)	0.13	0.18
	post	0.71 (0.47)		
LI peak knee power absorption in stance (W/kg)	pre	−1.38 (0.65)	0.69	0.01
	post	−1.43 (0.49)		

Table 7. Cont.

Parameter: LI-Less Involved; MI-More Involved		All Participants Mean (Standard Deviation)	p Values	Estimated Effect Size
LI peak knee power absorption in swing (W/kg)	pre	−0.97 (0.55)	0.55	0.03
	post	−1.01 (0.52)		
MI peak knee extensor moment in early stance (N · m/kg)	pre	0.74 (0.28)	0.19	0.14
	post	0.81 (0.27)		
MI peak knee flexor moment in mid-stance (N · m/kg)	pre	−0.18 (0.07)	0.67	0.02
	post	−0.19 (0.08)		
MI peak knee flexor moment in early swing (N · m/kg)	pre	0.08 (0.05)	0.076	0.24
	post	0.09 (0.06)		
MI peak knee extensor moment in late swing (N · m/kg)	pre	−0.26 (0.09)	0.27	0.10
	post	−0.28 (0.10)		
MI peak knee power generation in stance (W/kg)	pre	0.50 (0.29)	0.28	0.10
	post	0.57 (0.37)		
MI peak knee power absorption in stance (W/kg)	pre	−1.17 (0.58)	0.18	0.15
	post	−1.39 (0.61)		
MI peak knee power absorption in swing (W/kg)	pre	−0.87 (0.45)	0.065	0.26
	post	−1.03 (0.48)		
LI peak hip flexion moment in late stance (N · m/kg)	pre	1.19 (0.31)	0.31	0.09
	post	1.10 (0.33)		
LI peak hip extension moment in stance (N · m/kg)	pre	−0.33 (0.16)	0.26	0.10
	post	−0.37 (0.11)		
LI peak hip flexor moment in early swing (N · m/kg)	pre	0.21 (0.08)	0.25	0.11
	post	0.30 (0.25)		
LI peak hip power generation in terminal stance (W/kg)	pre	1.05 (0.36)	0.57	0.03
	post	1.09 (0.46)		
LI peak hip power absorption in stance (W/kg)	pre	−1.68 (0.78)	0.21	0.13
	post	−1.42 (0.56)		
LI peak hip power generation in swing (W/kg)	pre	0.61 (0.32)	0.61	0.02
	post	0.66 (0.30)		
MI peak hip flexion moment in late stance (N · m/kg)	pre	1.13 (0.38)	0.52	0.04
	post	1.07 (0.38)		
MI peak hip extension moment in stance (N · m/kg)	pre	−0.40 (0.17)	0.27	0.10
	post	−0.42 (0.16)		
MI peak hip flexor moment in early swing (N · m/kg)	pre	0.20 (0.09)	0.86	0.003
	post	0.20 (0.09)		
MI peak hip power generation in terminal stance (W/kg)	pre	1.00 (0.48)	0.67	0.02
	post	1.03 (0.38)		
MI peak hip power absorption in stance (W/kg)	pre	−1.54 (0.76)	0.33	0.08
	post	−1.36 (0.56)		
MI peak hip power generation in swing (W/kg)	pre	0.53 (0.30)	0.91	0.001
	post	0.54 (0.24)		

4. Discussion

This pilot study addressed a key gap in the literature: while focal vibration therapy (FVT) has shown preliminary benefits for gait and spasticity in people with multiple sclerosis (PwMS) in short-term, clinic-based settings [21–24], there is limited evidence on the feasibility and efficacy of wearable, home-based FVT over extended periods (e.g., 4 weeks), including optimal dosing parameters (intensity and duration) and their impact on detailed biomechanical gait outcomes. This research was needed because current interventions for MS-related mobility impairments, such as pharmacological treatments and exercise programs, often face limitations like side effects, accessibility barriers, and fatigue-related non-adherence [11,12,15], underscoring the importance of developing safe, portable, non-invasive alternatives to enhance neuromuscular control and daily function in PwMS. The primary purpose of this study was to evaluate the feasibility (adherence, satisfaction, acceptability) and preliminary efficacy of a 4-week home-based wearable FVT intervention on gait biomechanics and mobility in PwMS, while exploring dose–response effects to inform personalized protocols. Our hypothesis, that wearable FVT would be feasible and improve gait and mobility compared to baseline, with effects persisting at least four weeks post-intervention, was partially supported: feasibility was high with notable gait improvements (e.g., speed, stride length), but mobility (T25FW) remained unchanged, likely due to the short intervention duration and the test's limited sensitivity to subtle biomechanical changes; persistence could not be fully assessed as assessments were conducted immediately post-intervention, though gains were evident at that time-point.

Based on the QUEST satisfaction survey, most participants found the device acceptable and "easy to use." Semi-structured interviews further highlighted the general acceptance of FVT, with 15 out of 16 participants expressing positive attitudes toward its use. Notably, 14 participants indicated a willingness to continue using the device, with 9 expressing interest in purchasing it and 3 considering purchasing it if improvements were made, i.e., the strap. More than half of the participants expressed a desire for increased vibration. Two participants reported applying vibration to their wrists, noting improved hand function. Importantly, most participants did not report pain related to device use, though two individuals noted minor muscle spasms or pain. Areas for improvement were identified, particularly regarding "ease of adjusting" and "durability," which received the lowest satisfaction scores. Neutral feedback was also observed for "safety and security," "comfort," and "effectiveness." These concerns resonate with findings from other studies investigating wearable technology for MS and other central neurological disorders, emphasizing the importance of user-centered design to ensure that devices are not only effective but also practical and comfortable for everyday use [38–40]. This study supports the promising feasibility of wearable FVT for home-based management of mobility symptoms in MS, with generally positive participant satisfaction and acceptance. However, participant feedback highlighted challenges with device adjustability, durability, and comfort, which must be addressed to enhance usability and widespread adoption.

Improvements in gait parameters, such as increased gait speed, longer stride length, and alterations in ankle angle, aligned with previous studies demonstrating that FVT can positively influence neuromuscular control and proprioceptive feedback [41–43]. Similar patterns have been seen in other neurological populations, where kinematic and spatial-temporal gait parameter changes emerge even when mobility measures remain unchanged [44,45]. The lack of significant improvement in the T25FW may be attributed to its focus on short-distance walking, which may not fully capture subtle biomechanical improvements observed in gait parameters. Previous studies [22] suggest that short-distance tests like the T25FW may be less sensitive to neuromuscular changes compared to longer-distance measures, such as the Six-Minute Walk Test. Future studies will incorporate alternative functional mobility measures to better assess the translation of biomechanical gains into clinically meaningful outcomes. Interventions that improve underlying neuromuscular function often require additional time, training, or task-specific practice to translate into clinically meaningful outcomes in everyday mobility [46]. Since the wearable FVT could be self-applied at home, it could be used for a longer duration in future studies to lead to meaningful mobility improvements. This was reflected by the qualitative interview, which showed that more than half of the participants wanted more vibration. No standardized scales, such as the Multiple Sclerosis Impact Scale (MSIS-29), were collected alongside biomechanical measures in this study, as the pilot focused primarily on feasibility and biomechanical outcomes. However, during qualitative interviews, 5 to 6 participants spontaneously reported perceived increases in mobility and energy related to walking, suggesting potential subjective benefits that warrant further investigation. We plan to incorporate validated scales like the MSIS-29 in larger future trials to quantitatively assess these self-reported improvements.

The subgroup analyses indicated that vibration intensity and duration influenced only certain gait parameters, primarily related to knee joint mechanics. These results are consistent with prior research emphasizing the importance of selecting appropriate vibration parameters for different target symptoms [47,48]. The low- and high-intensity groups exhibited different patterns of knee moment changes on the less- and more involved side, which hints at the complexity of tailoring FVT doses and frequencies. These findings underscore the importance of personalized approaches in vibration therapy to optimize efficacy and minimize potential adverse effects. In future studies, we may need to apply different vibration intensities on different sides and adjust the vibration parameters as the rehabilitation progresses. Future studies with larger samples and standardized protocols are warranted to optimize dosing depending on the individual's baseline impairments, disease severity, and functional goals. We envision combining FVT with strength training (e.g., progressive resistance exercises) or balance training (e.g., Tai Chi), as vibration may enhance proprioception to amplify training effects. Dosing could interact by using lower intensities during acute training to avoid fatigue, or higher intensities for spasticity reduction pre-exercise. This is speculative and requires testing.

There were several limitations to this pilot study. Firstly, this study had a small sample size (n = 17 completing post-intervention assessments, with only one control group participant completing the study), which limited the statistical power and increased the risk of Type I and Type II errors. This study encountered significant challenges in participant recruitment and retention, largely due to the COVID-19 pandemic. Like other research [49], several participants were unable to continue participating in the study or were unable to enroll due to worsening health conditions, reduced clinical visits, and limited transportation. Secondly, only one of the five participants randomized to the control group completed the study, with three declining to participate in the study after trying the sham vibration device, as they did not feel the device would work for them, and one of the two control group participants who completed the baseline evaluation dropped out, making it impossible to compare data between the experimental and control groups. The high dropout rate in the control group, likely due to the lack of perceived benefit from the sham device, compromised the validity of comparisons between intervention and control groups. To address this, a new sham device generating both vibration sound and non-functional low-frequency vibration has been developed for future studies to improve participant retention. A larger follow-up study with an increased sample size and improved control group design is planned to enhance the robustness of findings. Another limitation of this study is that the gait biomechanical analysis was only conducted for the first two visits. One reason for the lack of assessments on the third visit was the assessment burden on the participants. The marker-based motion capture system requires around 40 min of preparation before the walking trail, which many participants felt was burdensome, as many MS participants reported fatigue at the end of the biomechanical test. In addition, participants using walkers or canes reported difficulty completing the biomechanical trail. We have established a new protocol using a markerless motion capture system to reduce the participants' burdens in future studies. Additionally, the analysis of multiple gait parameters without correction for multiple comparisons may have increased the risk of Type I errors, and these findings should be interpreted cautiously. Future studies will apply appropriate statistical corrections, such as Bonferroni adjustments, to account for multiple comparisons.

5. Conclusions

The present results highlight the potential of wearable FVT as a feasible and sustainable treatment for home-based mobility-associated symptoms management among people with MS. High participant satisfaction with wearable FVT supports its integration into MS rehabilitation protocols, promoting patient-centered care and functional independence. Preliminary improvements in gait speed, stride length, and ankle angle suggest FVT's potential to enhance neuromuscular control, reducing mobility-related disability and fall risk. While these subtle biomechanical improvements did not translate to significant improvements in a short-distance mobility test, they represent an encouraging step toward identifying how FVT can be optimally integrated into rehabilitation programs. Further research should focus on refining FVT parameters, combining vibration with other targeted therapies, and examining outcomes over longer distances and more ecologically valid scenarios to fully realize the potential of FVT in improving the mobility and quality of life of individuals with MS.

Supplementary Materials: The following supporting information can be downloaded at: https://www.mdpi.com/article/10.3390/bioengineering12090932/s1.

Author Contributions: Conceptualization, H.W.; methodology, H.W.; software, Y.C.S.; validation, H.W., N.J.T. and T.R.; formal analysis, H.W. and Y.C.S.; investigation, H.W.; resources, H.W. and T.R.; data curation, H.W. and Y.C.S.; writing—original draft preparation, H.W. and Y.C.S.; writing—review and editing, H.W., N.J.T. and T.R.; visualization, H.W. and Y.C.S.; supervision, H.W.; project administration, H.W.; funding acquisition, H.W. All authors have read and agreed to the published version of the manuscript.

Funding: This work was supported by the Presbyterian Health Foundation (PHF) Seed Grant, University of Oklahoma Health Sciences Center, 2019.

Institutional Review Board Statement: The study was conducted in accordance with the Declaration of Helsinki and approved by the Institutional Review Board (or Ethics Committee) of the University of Oklahoma Institutional Review Board (#10785, 15 July 2019).

Informed Consent Statement: Informed consent was obtained from the case participant involved in the study.

Data Availability Statement: The raw data supporting the conclusions of this article will be made available by the author upon request.

Acknowledgments: The investigators are grateful to the participants who gave their time and to the Department of Rehabilitation Sciences, Technology for Occupational Performance Laboratory for the use of their facilities. The investigators would like to thank Jenni Burzycki, Sarah Brown, Morgan Shuping, and Madeleine Foote for their assistance with patient testing and data collection. The investigators appreciate the technical support from Steve Leftly and Dianne Jones from Myovolt™.

The investigators would also like to acknowledge Carol Dionne (retired) and Nidhiben Anadani from the OUHSC for their support in participant recruitment.

Conflicts of Interest: The authors declare no conflicts of interest.

References

1. Filippi, M.; Bar-Or, A.; Piehl, F.; Preziosa, P.; Solari, A.; Vukusic, S.; Rocca, M.A. Multiple sclerosis. *Nat. Rev. Dis. Primers* **2018**, *4*, 43. [CrossRef]
2. Lassmann, H.; Brück, W.; Lucchinetti, C.F. The immunopathology of multiple sclerosis: An overview. *Brain Pathol.* **2007**, *17*, 210–218. [CrossRef]
3. Lubetzki, C.; Stankoff, B. Demyelination in multiple sclerosis. *Handb. Clin. Neurol.* **2014**, *122*, 89–99. [CrossRef] [PubMed]
4. Chee, J.N.; Sosnoff, J.J.; Sandroff, B.M.; Motl, R.W. Influence of multiple sclerosis on spatiotemporal gait parameters: A systematic review and meta-regression. *Arch. Phys. Med. Rehabil.* **2021**, *102*, 1801–1815. [CrossRef] [PubMed]
5. Braley, T.J.; Chervin, R.D. Fatigue in multiple sclerosis: Mechanisms, evaluation, and treatment. *Sleep* **2010**, *33*, 1061–1067. [CrossRef]
6. Comber, L.; Galvin, R.; Coote, S. Gait deficits in people with multiple sclerosis: A systematic review and meta-analysis. *Gait Posture* **2017**, *51*, 25–35. [CrossRef] [PubMed]
7. Cameron, M.H.; Nilsagard, Y. Balance, gait, and falls in multiple sclerosis. *Handb. Clin. Neurol.* **2018**, *159*, 237–250.
8. Matsuda, P.N.; Shumway-Cook, A.; Bamer, A.M.; Johnson, S.L.; Amtmann, D.; Kraft, G.H. Falls in multiple sclerosis. *PM R Phys. Med. Rehabil.* **2011**, *3*, 624–632. [CrossRef]
9. Finlayson, M.; Peterson, E.; Matsuda, P.N. Participation as an outcome in multiple sclerosis falls-prevention research: Consensus recommendation from the International MS Falls Prevention Research Network. *Int. J. MS Care* **2014**, *16*, 171–177. [CrossRef]
10. Van der Feen, F.E.; De Haan, G.A.; van der Lijn, I.; Heersema, D.J.; Meilof, J.F.; Heutink, J. Independent outdoor mobility of persons with multiple sclerosis—A systematic review. *Mult. Scler. Relat. Disord.* **2020**, *37*, 101463. [CrossRef]
11. Zhang, E.; Tian, X.; Li, R.; Chen, C.; Li, M.; Ma, L.; Wei, R.; Zhou, Y.; Cui, Y. Dalfampridine in the treatment of multiple sclerosis: A meta-analysis of randomised controlled trials. *Orphanet J. Rare Dis.* **2021**, *16*, 87. [CrossRef] [PubMed]
12. Dunn, J.; Blight, A. Dalfampridine: A brief review of its mechanism and efficacy in multiple sclerosis. *Drugs* **2011**, *71*, 471–480.
13. Du, L.; Xi, H.; Zhang, S.; Zhou, Y.; Tao, X.; Lv, Y.; Hou, X.; Yu, L. Effects of exercise in people with multiple sclerosis: A systematic review and meta-analysis. *Front. Public Health* **2024**, *12*, 1387658. [CrossRef]
14. Zou, L.; Wang, H.; Xiao, Z.; Fang, Q.; Zhang, M.; Li, T.; Du, G.; Liu, Y. Tai chi for health benefits in patients with multiple sclerosis: A systematic review. *PLoS ONE* **2017**, *12*, e0170212. [CrossRef]
15. Diaz-Quiroz, M.; Chicue-Cuervo, P.C.; Garcia-Moreno, L.; Gaviria-Carrillo, M.; Talero-Gutierrez, C.; Palacios-Espinosa, X. Fatigue in multiple sclerosis: A scoping review of pharmacological and nonpharmacological interventions. *Mult. Scler. J. Exp. Transl. Clin.* **2025**, *11*, 20552173241312527. [CrossRef]
16. Fattorini, L.; Pettorossi, V.E.; Marchetti, E.; Rodio, A.; Filippi, G.M. A review about muscle focal vibration contribution on spasticity recovery. *Front. Neurol.* **2025**, *16*, 1579118. [CrossRef]
17. Moggio, L.; de Sire, A.; Marotta, N.; Demeco, A.; Ammendolia, A. Vibration therapy role in neurological diseases rehabilitation: An umbrella review of systematic reviews. *Disabil. Rehabil.* **2022**, *44*, 5741–5749. [CrossRef] [PubMed]
18. Bessaguet, H.; Fernandez, B.; Malejac, V.; Nerriere, E.; Velarde, M.; Coiffet, A.; Rimaud, D.; Lapole, T. Effect of tibialis anterior focal muscle vibration for gait rehabilitation in hemiplegic individuals during the subacute phase after stroke: The NEUROVIB-AVC study protocol—A multicentric randomised controlled trial. *BMJ Open* **2025**, *15*, e102838. [CrossRef] [PubMed]
19. Alashram, A.R.; Padua, E.; Romagnoli, C.; Raju, M.; Annino, G. Clinical effectiveness of focal muscle vibration on gait and postural stability in individuals with neurological disorders: A systematic review. *Physiother. Res. Int.* **2022**, *27*, e1945. [CrossRef]
20. Ferrara, P.E.; Gatto, D.M.; Codazza, S.; Zordan, P.; Stefinlongo, G.; Coraci, D.; Lo Monaco, M.R.; Ricciardi, D.; Ronconi, G. Effects of focal muscle vibration on gait and balance in Parkinson patients: Preliminary results. *Appl. Sci.* **2022**, *12*, 10486. [CrossRef]
21. Camerota, F.; Celletti, C.; Di Sipio, E.; De Fino, C.; Simbolotti, C.; Germanotta, M.; Mirabella, M.; Padua, L.; Nociti, V. Focal muscle vibration, an effective rehabilitative approach in severe gait impairment due to multiple sclerosis. *J. Neurol. Sci.* **2017**, *372*, 33–39. [CrossRef]
22. Spina, E.; Carotenuto, A.; Aceto, M.G.; Cerillo, I.; Silvestre, F.; Arace, F.; Paone, P.; Orefice, G.; Iodice, R. The effects of mechanical focal vibration on walking impairment in multiple sclerosis patients: A randomized, double-blinded vs placebo study. *Restor. Neurol. Neurosci.* **2016**, *34*, 869–876. [CrossRef]
23. Paoloni, M.; Mangone, M.; Scettri, P.; Procaccianti, R.; Cometa, A.; Santilli, V. Segmental muscle vibration improves walking in chronic stroke patients with foot drop: A randomized controlled trial. *Neurorehabil. Neural Repair* **2010**, *24*, 254–262. [CrossRef]

24. Ayvat, F.; Özçakar, L.; Ayvat, E.; Aksu Yıldırım, S.; Kılınç, M. Effects of low vs. high frequency local vibration on mild-moderate muscle spasticity: Ultrasonographical and functional evaluation in patients with multiple sclerosis. *Mult. Scler. Relat. Disord.* **2021**, *51*, 102930. [CrossRef]
25. Thompson, A.J.; Banwell, B.L.; Barkhof, F.; Carroll, W.M.; Coetzee, T.; Comi, G.; Correale, J.; Fazekas, F.; Filippi, M.; Freedman, M.S.; et al. Diagnosis of multiple sclerosis: 2017 revisions of the McDonald criteria. *Lancet Neurol.* **2018**, *17*, 162–173. [CrossRef] [PubMed]
26. Tan, J.; Li, N.; Gao, J.; Wang, L.N.; Zhao, Y.M.; Yu, B.C.; Du, W.; Zhang, W.J.; Cui, L.Q.; Wang, Q.S.; et al. Optimal cutoff scores for dementia and mild cognitive impairment of the Montreal Cognitive Assessment among elderly and oldest-old Chinese population. *J. Alzheimers Dis.* **2015**, *43*, 1403–1412. [CrossRef] [PubMed]
27. Kurtzke, J.F. Rating neurologic impairment in multiple sclerosis: An expanded disability status scale (EDSS). *Neurology* **1983**, *33*, 1444–1452. [CrossRef]
28. Kuspinar, A.; Mayo, N.E. A review of the psychometric properties of generic utility measures in multiple sclerosis. *Pharmacoeconomics* **2014**, *32*, 759–773. [CrossRef] [PubMed]
29. Meyer-Moock, S.; Feng, Y.S.; Maeurer, M.; Dippel, F.W.; Kohlmann, T. Systematic literature review and validity evaluation of the Expanded Disability Status Scale (EDSS) and the Multiple Sclerosis Functional Composite (MSFC) in patients with multiple sclerosis. *BMC Neurol.* **2014**, *14*, 58. [CrossRef]
30. Demers, L.; Weiss-Lambrou, R.; Ska, B. Development of the Quebec User Evaluation of Satisfaction with assistive Technology (QUEST). *Assist. Technol.* **1996**, *8*, 3–13. [CrossRef]
31. Demers, L.; Weiss-Lambrou, R.; Ska, B. Item analysis of the Quebec User Evaluation of Satisfaction with Assistive Technology (QUEST). *Assist. Technol.* **2000**, *12*, 96–105. [CrossRef]
32. Demers, L.; Monette, M.; Lapierre, Y.; Arnold, D.L.; Wolfson, C. Reliability, validity, and applicability of the Quebec User Evaluation of Satisfaction with assistive Technology (QUEST 2.0) for adults with multiple sclerosis. *Disabil. Rehabil.* **2002**, *24*, 21–30. [CrossRef]
33. Goldman, M.D.; Motl, R.W.; Scagnelli, J.; Pula, J.H.; Sosnoff, J.J.; Cadavid, D. Clinically meaningful performance benchmarks in MS: Timed 25-foot walk and the real world. *Neurology* **2013**, *81*, 1856–1863. [CrossRef] [PubMed]
34. Oosterveer, D.M.; Wouda, N.C.; Volker, G.; van den Berg, C.; Terluin, B.; Hoitsma, E. Reliability parameters of the Timed 25-Foot-Walk (T25FW) in patients with Multiple Sclerosis: Lower walking speed is associated with greater Smallest Detectable Change. *Mult. Scler. Relat. Disord.* **2024**, *88*, 105731. [CrossRef] [PubMed]
35. C-Motion. Temporal Distance Calculations for Gait. Visual3D Wiki Documentation. Available online: https://c-motion.com/v3dwiki/index.php?title=Temporal_Distance_Calculations_for_Gait#Cadence (accessed on 6 October 2022).
36. Cohen, J. *Statistical Power Analysis for the Behavioral Sciences*, 2nd ed.; Lawrence Erlbaum Associates: Hillsdale, NJ, USA, 1988; pp. 19–27.
37. Coleman, C.I.; Sobieraj, D.M.; Marinucci, L.N. Minimally important clinical difference of the Timed 25-Foot Walk Test: Results from a randomized controlled trial in patients with multiple sclerosis. *Curr. Med. Res. Opin.* **2012**, *28*, 49–56. [CrossRef] [PubMed]
38. Horder, J.; Mrotek, L.A.; Casadio, M.; Bassindale, K.D.; McGuire, J.; Scheidt, R.A. Utility and usability of a wearable system and progressive-challenge cued exercise program for encouraging use of the more involved arm at-home after stroke—A feasibility study with case reports. *J. Neuroeng. Rehabil.* **2024**, *21*, 66. [CrossRef]
39. Martinez-Hernandez, U.; Metcalfe, B.; Assaf, T.; Jabban, L.; Male, J.; Zhang, D. Wearable assistive robotics: A perspective on current challenges and future trends. *Sensors* **2021**, *21*, 6751. [CrossRef]
40. Rodgers, M.M.; Alon, G.; Pai, V.M.; Conroy, R.S. Wearable technologies for active living and rehabilitation: Current research challenges and future opportunities. *J. Rehabil. Assist. Technol. Eng.* **2019**, *6*, 2055668319839607. [CrossRef]
41. Hebert, J.R.; Corboy, J.R. The association between multiple sclerosis-related fatigue and balance as a function of central sensory integration. *Gait Posture* **2013**, *38*, 37–42. [CrossRef]
42. Layne, C.S.; Malaya, C.A.; Levine, J.T. The effects of muscle vibration on gait control: A review. *Somatosens. Mot. Res.* **2019**, *36*, 212–222. [CrossRef]
43. Kerschan-Schindl, K.; Grampp, S.; Henk, C.; Resch, H.; Preisinger, E.; Fialka-Moser, V.; Imhof, H. Whole-body vibration exercise leads to alterations in muscle blood volume. *Clin. Physiol.* **2001**, *21*, 377–382. [CrossRef] [PubMed]
44. Lizrova Preiningerova, J.; Novotna, K.; Rusz, J.; Sucha, L.; Ruzicka, E.; Havrdova, E. Spatial and temporal characteristics of gait as outcome measures in multiple sclerosis. *J. Neuroeng. Rehabil.* **2015**, *12*, 14. [CrossRef]
45. Wonneberger, M.; Schmidt, H. Gait analysis in neurological diseases. *J. Neurol.* **2015**, *262*, 869–876.
46. Sokhangu, M.K.; Rahnama, N.; Etemadifar, M.; Rafeii, M.; Saberi, A. Effect of Neuromuscular Exercises on Strength, Proprioceptive Receptors, and Balance in Females with Multiple Sclerosis. *Int. J. Prev. Med.* **2021**, *12*, 5. [CrossRef] [PubMed]
47. Giorgi, F.; Donati, D.; Platano, D.; Tedeschi, R. Focal Vibration Therapy for Motor Deficits and Spasticity Management in Post-Stroke Rehabilitation. *Brain Sci.* **2024**, *14*, 1060. [CrossRef]

48. Lienhard, K.; Cabasson, A.; Meste, O.; Colson, S.S. Determination of the optimal parameters maximizing muscle activity of the lower limbs during vertical synchronous whole-body vibration. *Eur. J. Appl. Physiol.* **2014**, *114*, 1493–1501. [CrossRef]
49. Goyal, D.; Hunt, X.; Kuper, H.; Shakespeare, T.; Banks, L.M. Impact of the COVID-19 pandemic on people with disabilities and implications for health services research. *J. Health Serv. Res. Policy* **2023**, *28*, 77–79. [CrossRef] [PubMed]

Disclaimer/Publisher's Note: The statements, opinions and data contained in all publications are solely those of the individual author(s) and contributor(s) and not of MDPI and/or the editor(s). MDPI and/or the editor(s) disclaim responsibility for any injury to people or property resulting from any ideas, methods, instructions or products referred to in the content.

bioengineering

MDPI

Article

A Novel Protocol for Integrated Assessment of Upper Limbs Using the Optoelectronic Motion Analysis System: Validation and Usability in Healthy People

Luca Emanuele Molteni [1,*], Luigi Piccinini [1], Daniele Panzeri [1], Ettore Micheletti [1] and Giuseppe Andreoni [1,2]

1 Scientific Institute IRCCS "E.Medea", Bosisio Parini, 23842 Lecco, Italy; luigi.piccinini@lanostrafamiglia.it (L.P.); giuseppe.andreoni@polimi.it (G.A.)
2 Department of Design, Politecnico di Milano, 20133 Milano, Italy
* Correspondence: luca.molteni@lanostrafamiglia.it; Tel.: +39-031877695

Abstract: (1) Background: Upper limb (UL) function plays a central role in daily life, enabling essential tasks such as reaching, grasping, and eating. While numerous tools exist to evaluate UL kinematics, their application in pediatric populations is often limited by a lack of age-specific validation. This study presents a novel motion analysis protocol featuring a customized marker set, aimed at assessing UL movements in the three anatomical planes across different age groups, with a focus on pediatric applicability. (2) Materials and Methods: A SmartDX motion capture system was used, with 30 markers positioned on the upper body, referencing the trunk as the root of the kinematic chain. Ten healthy participants (mean age: 18.69 ± 12.45 years; range: 8.0–41.4) without UL impairments were recruited. The broad age range was intentionally selected to assess the protocol's transversal applicability. (3) Results: Results showed excellent intra-operator reliability for shoulder and wrist kinematics (ICC > 0.906) and good reliability for elbow movements (ICC > 0.755). Inter-operator reliability was good to excellent (shoulder ICC > 0.958; elbow ICC > 0.762; wrist ICC > 0.826) Usability, measured via the System Usability Scale, was rated as good (83.25). (4) Conclusions: The proposed protocol demonstrated strong reliability and practical usability, supporting its adoption in clinical and research settings. Its design allows for adaptability across motion capture platforms, promoting wider implementation in pediatric UL functional assessment.

Keywords: upper limb; functional assessment; kinematic analysis; shoulder kinematics; elbow kinematics; wrist kinematics

1. Introduction

Upper limb (UL) function is essential for performing everyday tasks such as pointing, grasping, handling, and eating. Accurate assessment of these movements is crucial in clinical medicine, rehabilitation, and ergonomics, particularly for tailoring therapeutic interventions in conditions like stroke and cerebral palsy (CP) [1,2]. Studies estimate that 50–85% of individuals with acute stroke and around 50% of those with chronic stroke exhibit UL impairments, which significantly affect independence and quality of life [3–5].

Various clinical tools are available to evaluate UL function [6], and guidelines emphasize the importance of using valid, reliable, and responsive outcome measures [7,8]. The literature proposes different methods like: The Melbourne Assessment of Unilateral Upper Limb Function (MUUL), Quality of Upper Extremity Skills Test (QUEST), and Shriners Hospital Upper Extremity Evaluation (SHUEE) [9–11]. These methods qualitatively assess motor performance of the upper extremity during different functional tasks [8]. However, these methods provide only general results, as they rely on weighted scores based on evaluator experience [12]. Distinguishing motor recovery from compensation can be difficult for these measures, which is crucial in therapies such as constraint-induced movement therapy (CIMT), trunk restraint therapy (TRT) and bilateral arm therapy (BAT) [5,13].

Combining clinical outcome measures with kinematic analysis is increasingly recognized as a valuable tool for assessing UL movement, with growing support from expert consensus and clinical research [14]. By providing objective, quantitative data on motor performance, kinematic analysis allows clinicians and researchers to better characterize recovery patterns, identify compensatory mechanisms, and improve prognostic accuracy. Kinematic assessments describe the biomechanical properties of movement with precision, offering accurate and reproducible information on motor control and coordination [15]. These metrics are critical for understanding dysfunction in specific anatomical regions and contribute to informed clinical decision-making regarding surgical intervention, pharmacological treatment, or rehabilitation planning [16]. For example, kinematic motion analysis is widely applied in conditions such as cerebral palsy (CP) to monitor motor performance during daily activities, support individualized rehabilitation strategies, and objectively evaluate treatment outcomes [17].

Kinematic metrics such as speed, smoothness, efficiency, accuracy, control strategy, and functional range of motion are often used in combination with clinical scales to evaluate UL function in patients with neurological conditions [18]. These tools allow for the assessment of reaching, gross, and fine motor abilities, as well as spatiotemporal movement characteristics. Jaspers et al. highlighted the importance of integrating kinematic data with qualitative scales to obtain a comprehensive picture of upper extremity function, which is essential for selecting the most appropriate treatment approach in pediatric patients with CP [17].

Despite these advantages, evidence regarding the responsiveness of kinematic measures in UL assessment remains limited [19]. Recent recommendations encourage standardization of kinematic analysis measurement protocols according to International Classification of Functioning (ICF) levels, tasks and conditions analyzed as well as psychometric properties [14,20]. Optoelectronic systems are considered the gold standard for UL kinematic analysis, offering high accuracy and temporal resolution [2]. However, standardized and validated protocols remain scarce. Implementing a standardized protocol to measure UL movement across three anatomical planes and to monitor the spatiotemporal characteristics of movement could serve as a valuable clinical tool. Combined with clinical scales, it can support the personalization and ongoing monitoring of rehabilitative interventions.

The aim of this study is to introduce and validate a novel motion analysis protocol for the UL, based on a dedicated marker set and an integrated biomechanical model. This protocol is designed for the global assessment of UL kinematics during functional movements, such as reach-to-target tasks, enabling a more detailed and objective evaluation of motor behavior and its potential abnormalities. Such detailed characterization is essential for improving the understanding of UL functionality in both healthy and clinical populations. Before clinical implementation, a newly developed protocol must undergo rigorous validation. Specifically, its repeatability—both intra- and inter-operator—must be established through testing on healthy participants. This study describes the methodological development of the protocol and presents the results of its validation in terms of accuracy, repeatability, and usability, considering both the experience of the operators and the feasibility for the subjects.

2. Materials and Methods

2.1. Subjects

To validate the protocol in both adults and children, ten healthy subjects (5 males, 5 females; mean age: 18.69, SD: 12.45; age range: 8.0–41.4) without any UL functional limitations voluntarily participated in the study. Informed consent was obtained from all adult participants and from the parents or legal guardians of the minors.

Inclusion criteria included the absence of functional impairments in the ULs. Exclusion criteria included behavioral, visual, or auditory disorders, as well as the presence of pain during UL movements. Baseline characteristics of the sample are presented in Table 1.

Table 1. Mean, standard deviation (SD), and range for baseline features of healthy subjects.

Baseline Features	
Age [y] (mean—SD; range)	18.69—SD 12.45; 8.0–41.4
Weight [Kg] (mean—SD; range)	44.5—SD 22.55; 24.00–90.00
Height [cm] (mean—SD; range)	144.5—SD 18.28; 124.0–167.0
BMI (mean—SD; range)	20.03—SD 5.65; 15.06–33.06

The study was approved by the Ethics Committee of the Institute (Approval Number: 55/23, Comitato Etico dell'Associazione "La Nostra Famiglia"—IRCCS "Eugenio Medea," 18 May 2023). The clinical trial has been registered on Clinical Trials.gov: NCT06400667.

2.2. Data Collections

Various protocols for UL kinematic assessment have been proposed in the literature; however, they often evaluate motion only in the sagittal plane and typically exclude trunk and head kinematics [21,22]. The present study aimed to develop a general-purpose protocol capable of capturing UL movement in all three anatomical planes—sagittal, frontal, and transverse—for the humerus, forearm, and hand. Additionally, trunk and head kinematics were included to capture the core contribution to motor behavior.

The protocol was designed to be applicable across the lifespan, including pediatric subjects. Therefore, special attention was paid to marker size, visibility, and placement to minimize occlusion and overlap. The anatomical coordinate system of each body segment was calculated by placing 28 reflective markers (10 mm diameter hemispherical spheres) [23]. Marker placement and the resulting biomechanical model are illustrated in Figure 1.

The model consists of 8 segments and allows the computation of 9 positional degrees of freedom (trunk position and fingertip position) and 22 joint angles. Segment reference frames were defined for the humerus, forearm, hand, thorax, and head following International Society of Biomechanics (ISB) guidelines [23,24]. Each segment, considering the relevant anatomical reference system, was calculated, as shown in Table 2. In particular, for the humerus, two distinct reference systems were used to calculate shoulder and elbow angles, respectively [25].

Obliquity, flexion-extension, and rotation angles of each segment were computed relative to adjacent segments or a global reference system, using Euler angles in the order: sagittal (flexion/extension), frontal (lateral bending), and transverse (axial rotation), following ISB recommendations [23].

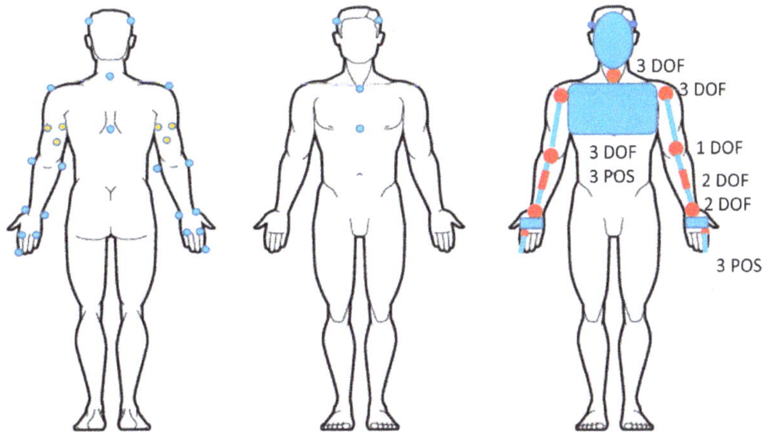

1	Right front side of the head	16	Right radial styloid
2	Left front side of the head	17	Right ulnar styloid
3	Right hind side of the head	18	Head second right metacarpal
4	L2ft hind side of the head	19	Head fourth second right metacarpal
5	Right Acromion	20	Right index nail
6	Left Acromion	21	Left lateral humeral condyle
7	Suprasternal notch	22	Left medial humeral condyle
8	Xiphoid process	23	Technical reference for thet arm
9	Spinous process last cervical vertebra	24	
10	Spinous process eighth thoracic vertebra	25	
11	Right lateral humeral condyle	26	Left radial styloid
12	Right medial humeral condyle	27	Left ulnar styloid
13	Technical reference for the right arm	28	Head second left metacarpal
14		29	Head fourth second left metacarpal
15		30	Left index nail

Figure 1. Positions of the markers on the subject and corresponding biomechanical model.

Table 2. Reference system of the different body segments.

Thorax coordinate system [23]	Origin:	The origin coincided with suprasternal notch (IJ)
	Y axis:	The line connecting the midpoint between xiphoid process (PX) and T8 and the midpoint between IJ and C7, pointing upward
	Z axis:	The line perpendicular to the plane formed by IJ, C7, and the midpoint between PX and T8, pointing to the right.
	X axis:	The common line perpendicular to the Z and Y axis, pointing forwards.
Proximal Humerus (note: This reference frame was used to calculate shoulder movement) [23]	Origin:	The origin coincident with GlenoHomeros (GH)
	Y axis:	The line connecting GH and the midpoint of lateral elbow (EL) and medial elbow (EM)), pointing to GH.
	Z axis:	The common line perpendicular to the Y and Z axis, pointing to the right
	X axis:	The line perpendicular to the plane formed by EL, EM, and GH, pointing forward.
Distal Humerus (note: This reference frame was used to calculate elbow movement) [25]	Origin:	coincides with midpoint of the elbow
	Y axis:	Forearm axis of rotation.
	Z axis:	The line perpendicular to the plane formed by Y and the Y axis of the proximal humerus reference frame
	X axis:	perpendicular to the plane formed by X and Y, POINTing forward

Table 2. *Cont.*

Forearm coordinate system [23]	Origin:	The origin coincided with ulnar styloid (US).
	Y axis:	the line connecting US and the midpoint between EL and EM, pointing proximally
	Z axis:	The common line perpendicular to the X and Y axis, pointing to the right.
	X axis:	The line perpendicular to the plane through US, radial styloid (RS), and the midpoint between EL and EM, pointing forward
Wrist coordinate system [23]	Origin:	The origin of the coordinate systems is located midway between the base and head of second metacarpal. In the transverse plane, it will be at the approximate center of the tubular bone.
	Y axis:	The line parallel to a line from the center of the distal head of the metacarpal to the midpoint of the base of the metacarpal.
	Z axis:	The common line perpendicular to the X and Y axis.
	X axis:	The X and Y axis will form a sagittal plane that splits the metacarpal into mirror images

Motion data were captured using an optoelectronic motion capture system (SMART DX, BTS Bioengineering, Milan, Italy) equipped with eight infrared cameras operating at 60 Hz. The cameras were positioned on the front and side walls of the room at approximately 2 m from the subject (Figure 2). Markers were placed directly on the subject's skin by trained physiotherapists experienced in anatomical landmark identification and motion analysis procedures.

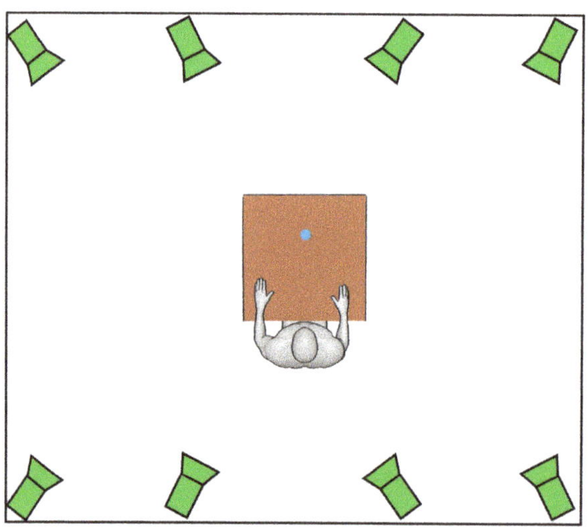

Figure 2. Laboratory setup and camera positions.

During acquisition, subjects were seated on a stool with their forearms resting on a table adjusted to navel height. During the test, the subject is required to reach a target on the table using the index finger. This ensures that all joints of the UL are engaged and that the movement is standardized. The target was placed at 80% of the subject's arm's length, over a cylinder with a height of about 8 cm, placed on the table. Each subject completed five "Hit-to-Target" (HtT) trials with the right arm, followed by five trials with the left arm. Each session was repeated twice by two different operators, resulting in a total of 20 trials per arm per subject.

The development of a new protocol of analysis requires the validation of its repeatability before its definitive and clinical application. The repeatability of the protocol was assessed by analyzing variability in outcome measures across sessions and between operators [26]. Specifically, both intra-operator (same operator, repeated sessions) and inter-operator (different operators) repeatability were evaluated. The experimental protocol for the intra- and inter-operator validation consisted of the following steps:

1. Preparation of the subject, positioning the markers (30) on the selected body landmarks.
2. The acquisition of 5 HtT trials with each arm;
3. Detachment of the markers from the subject.

For the analysis of intra and inter operative repeatability, the various steps were repeated 2 times by the same therapist, and 2 times by a different therapist. In total, each subject attended 4 sessions, so we analyzed 20 HtT trials for each arm in each subject. The repositioning of markers by both the same operator and the second operator was carried out in consecutive sessions, with about a three-minute break between each one. The total test time for this repeatability validation was about one hour and 30 min per session.

Usability evaluation is crucial for the successful clinical implementation of medical products [27]. According to ISO 9241–11 [28], usability encompasses effectiveness, efficiency, and user satisfaction. After each acquisition session, the participants were given the System Usability Scale (SUS) [29] 36 and an assessment to evaluate how challenging the different phases of the test were using a 5-point Likert-scale methodology (ranging from 1 to 5). The considered operations were as follows:

- Phase 1: instrument preparation and marker preparation (for the test subjects, the part of instrument preparation was excluded from the questionnaire because the subjects were not involved in this operation);
- Phase 2: marker positioning;
- Phase 3: recording the movements with the optoelectronic system;
- Phase 4: removing the markers.

Each phase was timed to assess the duration required.

2.3. Data Processing

Raw data were processed with Smart Analyzer software 1.10.0470 (BTS Bioengineering, Milano, Italy). First, the 3D data were filtered and eventually interpolated in cases of short periods of missing data. Subsequently, movement phases were segmented according to established criteria [30,31]:

- Going Phase: Begins when the velocity of the finger marker exceeds 50 mm/s and ends at the onset of the Adjusting Phase.
- Adjusting Phase: This phase was not defined by velocity thresholds, due to the fluctuating nature of speed during fine adjustments. Instead, it was identified based on the distance between the finger and the target, using a threshold set as the average distance plus three standard deviations across five movements. The end of this phase and the start of the Returning Phase were defined using the same criteria.
- Returning Phase: Starts at the conclusion of the Adjusting Phase and ends when the finger marker speed drops below 50 mm/s.

For each body segment, joint angle was normalized over the movement cycle. Range of motion (ROM) was calculated as the difference between the maximum and minimum angles across the entire movement. Mean angular velocity was computed for each joint and anatomical plane and segmented by movement phase. Additionally, we used other metrics from the literature, as follows:

- End-point (finger) metrics: Derived from finger kinematic data, these metrics assess movement speed, accuracy, efficiency, and smoothness.
- Trunk compensation metrics: Calculated from the marker placed on the sternum, these metrics quantified compensatory trunk movements during reaching tasks.

The metrics used are summarized in Table 3.

Table 3. Spatiotemporal metrics of movement.

	Metrics	
End-point (finger)	Time	This is calculated as the total time required for completing each task. In addition, the durations of the previous three phases were computed: the going phase, the adjusting phase, and the returning phase [31]
	Adjusting sway Index (ASI)	It is defined as the length of the 3D path described by the fingernail during the adjusting phase, which is a measure of the adjustments made to reach the final position. This represents an expression of the degree of precision [31].
	Mean Movement Velocity (MMV)	It is computed during the going phase and represents the mean velocity of the fingernail marker [31].
	Index of curvature (IC)	It is calculated as the ratio of the fingernail 3D path length to the linear distance between the initial and the final pointing position and is a representative of movement smoothness during the going phase [32].
	Number of Velocity Peaks (NVP)	It is a quality measure of movement smoothness computed from the speed profile of the finger during the entire movement [32].
Trunk compensation	Trunk compensation	It is defined as the length 3D path described by the marker placed on the sternum [33]
	Displacement along z-axis	Displacement of the marker placed on the sternum along the z-axis (towards the target) during the going phase. It quantifies trunk flexion [33].
	Displacement along x-axis	Displacement of the marker placed on the sternum along the x-axis during the going phase. It quantifies trunk lateral bending [33].

2.4. Statistical Analysis

For the technical and clinical validation phase, the protocol was tested on a sample of at least 10 participants and two clinical operators, with each procedure repeated five times per condition. This sample size is considered adequate to assess both the technical aspects of the protocol—such as intra- and inter-operator repeatability and measurement variability—and its procedural feasibility in a clinical setting, as reported in previous studies [26,34,35]. Intra- and inter-operator repeatability were evaluated by calculating the correlation coefficients of the average ROM across the five trials within corresponding sessions.

Usability was assessed through descriptive statistics (mean and standard deviation) for perceived usability and task difficulty, along with the average score obtained from the SUS questionnaire [36]. All statistical analyses were performed using SPSS 21 software (IBM Corp., Armonk, NY, USA).

3. Results

The proposed protocol is designed to quantify UL joint angles normalized over the movement cycle during a HtT task. Additionally, this study aimed to validate the kinematics of the UL and related spatiotemporal parameters. An example of the data output and automatically generated clinical report is shown in Figure 3.

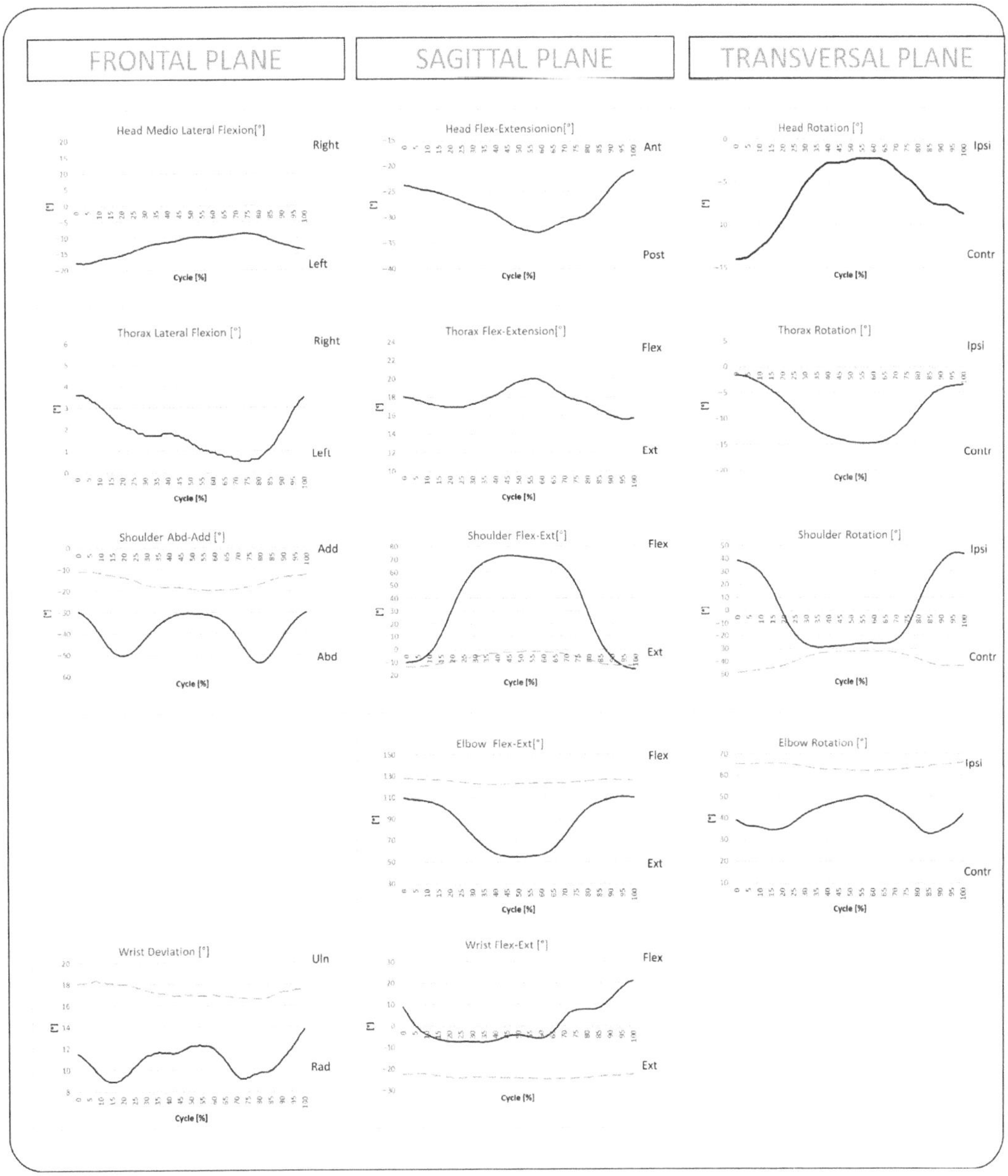

Figure 3. Example of UL angles in all three anatomical planes, normalized on the movement cycle. The black line represents the right UL; the gray dashed line represents the left UL.

To assess repeatability—both intra- and inter-operator—we computed the intraclass correlation coefficient (ICC) using a two-way mixed-effects model with absolute agreement and average measures. ICC values were calculated for the range of motion (ROM) of the UL joints and the extracted spatiotemporal parameters. The interpretation of ICC values followed established guidelines—values between 0.50 and 0.75 indicate moderate reliability, between 0.75 and 0.90 indicate good reliability, and values greater than 0.90 indicate excellent reliability [37].

3.1. Time Phases and End-Point Metrics

Regarding the repeatability analysis for intra-operator marking, Table 3 shows the results obtained. All the end-point indexes showed an ICC > 0.867, indicating good to excellent reliability. Only the Number of Velocity Peaks (NVP) parameters showed a lower ICC value of 0.739, indicating moderate reliability, although this value was close to the cutoff limit of 0.75. The time phases showed slightly worse results: reliability was moderate for the total time and for the adjustment phase (ICC > 0.785), while for the other phases, the reliability was also moderate (ICC > 0.725). Even in these cases, however, the ICC values were close to the cutoff limit of 0.75. Regarding the repeatability analysis for inter-operator reliability, the results are very close to the intra-operator reliability. Table 4 presents the obtained results. Similarly, the end-point metrics demonstrated good reliability (ICC > 0.793), except for the NVP, which showed moderate reliability (ICC = 0.721). Similarly to the intra-operator analysis, the time phases showed slightly worse results with moderate reliability.

Table 4. Intraclass correlation coefficient (ICC) and their levels about end-point metrics for intra and inter operator analysis (+++ = excellent, ++ = good, + = moderate, – poor) [37].

	Intra Operator		Inter Operator	
	ICC	ICC Level	ICC	ICC Level
T tot	0.785	++	0.715	+
T Going Phase	0.738	+	0.610	+
T Return Phase	0.725	+	0.552	+
T Adj Phase	0.839	++	0.816	++
Mean movement velocity (MMV)	0.896	++	0.953	+++
Curvature Index (CI)	0.898	++	0.898	++
Adjusting sway Index (ASI)	0.867	++	0.793	++
Number of Velocity Peaks (NVP)	0.739	+	0.721	+

3.2. Trunk Compensation Metrics

Regarding the intra-operator repeatability analysis for trunk compensation indices, Table 5 presents the results obtained for each movement phase. All indices demonstrated good to excellent reliability, with ICC values exceeding 0.79 and reaching a maximum of 0.956. In the inter-operator repeatability analysis, results were slightly lower but still acceptable, with trunk compensation indices showing moderate to good reliability (ICC > 0.696).

Table 5. Intraclass correlation coefficient (ICC) and their levels about trunk indexes for inter-operator analysis (+++ = excellent, ++ = good, + = moderate, – poor) [37].

	Intra Operator		Inter Operator	
	ICC	ICC Level	ICC	ICC Level
Thorax Length Going Phase	0.815	++	0.834	++
Antero-posterior Going Phase Displacement	0.818	++	0.890	++
Medio-lateral Going Phase Displacement	0.768	++	0.696	+
Thorax Length Adjusting Phase	0.926	+++	0.834	++
Antero-posterior Adjusting Phase Displacement	0.882	++	0.707	+
Medio-lateral Adjusting Phase Displacement	0.956	+++	0.854	++
Thorax Length Return Phase	0.870	++	0.870	++
Antero-posterior Return Phase Displacement	0.891	++	0.888	++
Medio-lateral Return Phase Displacement	0.815	++	0.825	++

3.3. Range of Motion

The repeatability analysis for the ROM showed consistent results between intra- and inter-operator assessments. Both the right and left ULs exhibited excellent reliability at the shoulder and wrist joints. Specifically, intra-operator reliability for these segments was ICC > 0.906, while inter-operator reliability was ICC > 0.941. The elbow joint demonstrated slightly lower reliability, showing good intra-operator repeatability and moderate to good inter-operator agreement. Reliability values for thorax and head segments ranged from moderate to good. Table 6 shows the results of ROM for different body segments.

Table 6. Intraclass correlation coefficient (ICC) and their levels about range of motion (ROM) for intra and inter operator analysis (+++ = excellent, ++ = good, + = moderate, − poor) [37].

	Intra Operator		Inter Operator	
	ICC	ICC Level	ICC	ICC Level
ROM Right Shoulder FE	0.983	+++	0.992	+++
ROM Left Shoulder FE	0.991	+++	0.992	+++
ROM Right Shoulder AA	0.906	+++	0.992	+++
ROM Left Shoulder AA	0.966	+++	0.958	+++
ROM Right Shoulder IE	0.917	+++	0.965	+++
ROM Left Shoulder IE	0.949	+++	0.954	+++
ROM Right Elbow FE	0.959	+++	0.950	+++
ROM Left Elbow FE	0.978	+++	0.953	+++
ROM Right Elbow PS	0.755	++	0.848	++
ROM Left Elbow PS	0.838	++	0.762	++
ROM Right Wrist FE	0.967	+++	0.826	++
ROM Left Wrist FE	0.949	+++	0.941	+++
ROM Right Wrist UR	0.934	+++	0.952	+++
ROM Left Wrist UR	0.949	+++	0.940	+++
ROM Right Thorax FE	0.869	++	0.952	+++
ROM Right Thorax ML	0.640	+	0.872	++
ROM Right Thorax IE	0.768	++	0.722	+
ROM Right Head FE	0.705	+	0.867	++
ROM Right Head ML	0.813	++	0.857	++
ROM Right Head IE	0.832	++	0.798	++

3.4. Usability Assessment

To evaluate the practical applicability of the proposed protocol in clinical settings, both operator and patient experiences were assessed. Perceived difficulty during the different phases of acquisition was rated by participants and clinicians, as summarized in Table 7.

Table 7. Assessment of the difficulty of the application of the protocol (1: very difficult–5: very easy).

	Operators				Patient		
Phase	1	2	3	4	1	2	3
Mean	4.83	4.68	4.95	4.98	4.88	4.90	4.70
Standard deviation	0.38	0.47	0.22	0.16	0.33	0.30	0.56
Max	5.00	5.00	5.00	5.00	5.00	5.00	5.00
Min	4.00	4.00	4.00	4.00	4.00	4.00	3.00

The phase1 correspond to the instrument preparation, phase 2 correspond to the subject preparation, phase 3 correspond to recording the movements with the optoelectronic system and the phase 4 correspond to the removing the markers.

The SUS was administered at the end of each session, resulting in an average score of 83.25, indicating a high level of usability. Furthermore, Table 8 presents the average time required for each procedural step, as well as the total duration of the entire acquisition process.

Table 8. Time required for the entire acquisition and for each phase. The phase1 correspond to the instrument preparation, phase 2 correspond to the marker positioning, phase 3 correspond to recording the movements with the optoelectronic system and the phase 4 correspond to the removing the markers.

	T [min]				
	1	2	3	4	TOT
Mean	2.00	6.05	10.13	1.80	19.97
Standar deviation	0.16	0.62	0.54	0.16	0.69
Max	2.32	7.22	11.73	2.10	21.50
Min	1.77	5.17	8.85	1.20	18.73

4. Discussion

The method presented in this study is a non-invasive and integrated approach for evaluating UL movement during functional tasks such as HtT movement. Its implementation requires a human motion analysis (MA) system, and its relative simplicity—developed in close collaboration with clinicians—makes it suitable for routine use in clinical practice. The proper balance between the need for a detailed motion description (requiring a high number of markers) and the limitation of the complexity (i.e., the number of markers to be prepared and placed onto the subject) not to affect the usability and acceptance in operators and subjects is respected. Indeed, the time needed for the participant for the examination is about 20 min for the entire process (Table 7). The relatively short completion time observed in this study was likely influenced by the characteristics of the recruited participants, who were all healthy and highly cooperative. In clinical populations, particularly in patients with neurological disorders or behavioral impairments, the time required for protocol execution may reasonably be longer. Furthermore, both clinicians and patients perceived the protocol as easy to perform. The usability evaluation, as measured by the SUS, yielded an average score of 83.25, indicating a high level of usability [38]. These results are particularly relevant for pediatric populations, where test duration and simplicity are critical due to reduced cooperation and limited attention spans in children. Short, engaging protocols like this one are likely to improve compliance and measurement accuracy in such groups. No major barriers were identified in this healthy adult cohort. Future clinical populations will be investigated to determine potential challenges, such as attention span, cooperation, or task comprehension, and any differences in perceived usability between children and adults.

In the intra- and inter-operator repeatability analyses, all endpoint indices demonstrated good to excellent reliability (ICC > 0.793), except for NVP, which showed moderate reliability. Trunk compensation indices also demonstrated good to excellent intra-operator reliability and moderate to good inter-operator reliability. Only two specific metrics—the medio-lateral displacement during the Going Phase and the antero-posterior displacement during the Adjusting Phase—showed ICC values close to the cut-off of 0.75. These lower values may be attributed to variability in the duration of movement phases. In fact, the temporal phase duration showed only moderate to good intra-operator reliability, indicating that time-dependent metrics are more sensitive to variability and potentially less robust. These findings confirm the consistency and robustness of the computed metrics in characterizing UL movement.

Regarding joint kinematics, intra-operator reliability showed excellent for shoulder and wrist kinematics (ICC > 0.906) and good reliability for elbow movements (ICC > 0.755). Inter-operator reliability was good to excellent (shoulder ICC > 0.958, elbow ICC > 0.762, wrist ICC > 0.826) Usability. Slightly lower reliability, ranging from moderate to good, was observed for the thorax and head segments. This is explained by the paravertebral muscles underneath the markers: during movement, their contractions modify the morphology of the back, thus adding an intrinsic 3D displacement to the corresponding markers and producing unavoidable, unremovable artifacts. The reliability values reported in our study are in line with previous findings in UL kinematic protocols [17,18], which report ICC values above 0.75 for most joint-level measures. Overall, these results support the conclusion that the proposed protocol is both reliable and repeatable. In particular, the kinematic data showed at least good repeatability, as well as some spatiotemporal parameters such as MMV, CI and ASI, which quantitatively describe the quality of movement. This set of outcomes, when combined with traditional clinical scales, could serve as a useful tool to support treatment personalization and to evaluate outcomes. Importantly, the protocol is simple to implement and adheres to ISB guidelines, which facilitates its adoption across a range of commercial optoelectronic systems beyond the specific system used in this study.

The proposed protocol provides a simple and efficient framework to calculate the main kinematic and spatiotemporal metrics of UL movement with a limited number of acquisitions. This approach is in line with previous studies on UL movement analysis, which emphasize the importance of balancing measurement accuracy with protocol simplicity and feasibility in clinical settings [17,18]. Furthermore, with respect to these studies, our protocol allows the evaluation of intra—and interoperative repeatability in healthy subjects, demonstrating reliability values higher than good.

The next step will be the clinical application of the protocol: together with clinical data, further validation will be obtained (through an intra and inter-operator reliability analyses) in subjects with UL altered movement patterns like cerebral palsy or acquired brain injury. The proposed protocol is subject to intrinsic limitations such as skin motion artifacts, although previous studies have demonstrated these to be negligible in terms of their impact on reliability [39]. The information related to the UL movement patterns during movement like hit to target is a fundamental outcome of this methodology it could be very useful for clinical diagnosis in several pathologies for an integrated functional assessment. The first one that will be investigated in the next months will be cerebral palsy and acquired brain injury in children.

Limitations

Despite the encouraging results, this study presents some limitations that should be acknowledged. First, the sample size was relatively small (n = 10), which is adequate for assessing technical reliability and repeatability [26,33], limits the generalizability of the findings to broader or more heterogeneous populations. Future studies including clinical populations and a larger number of participants are necessary to confirm the applicability and robustness of the protocol in real-world clinical scenarios. Lastly, although the protocol was designed to be general-purpose and pediatric-friendly, its performance in specific clinical populations—such as children with neuromotor impairments—has yet to be evaluated. These populations may present additional challenges, such as involuntary movements, limited range of motion, or attention deficits, which could impact marker placement accuracy and task execution.

5. Conclusions

This study presents the development and validation of a protocol for the integrated assessment of UL movements, providing a comprehensive analysis of the upper-quarter body kinematics in both pediatric and adult populations. The reliability of the protocol was validated on a sample of 10 healthy subjects, yielding satisfactory and reliable results. Usability assessments from both operators and patients were also positive, supporting the protocol's practicality in clinical settings. The demonstrated intra- and inter-operator repeatability suggests that this protocol can be confidently introduced into clinical practice for the diagnosis and monitoring of rehabilitative treatments. Furthermore, thanks to its simple implementation following ISB guidelines, the methodology is adaptable to various commercial optoelectronic systems, facilitating its adoption across different clinical environments. Although clinical scales remain the standard for evaluating UL functionality in diagnosis and rehabilitation, this optoelectronic-based protocol provides a reliable, non-invasive method to quantify detailed kinematic parameters relevant for clinical assessment and treatment planning. The collected dataset establishes preliminary normative values, which will be expanded in future studies to develop a comprehensive clinical database for specific pathologies.

Author Contributions: Conceptualization: L.P. and G.A.; Methodology: G.A., L.P. and L.E.M.; software: L.E.M.; data curation: L.E.M., D.P. and E.M.; writing—original draft preparation: L.E.M.; paper revision: G.A.; paper supervision: L.P. and G.A.; project administration: G.A. All authors have read and agreed to the published version of the manuscript.

Funding: This study was supported by "5 per mille" funds for biomedical research, in particular for the project "5x000/2023—Sviluppo di nuovi protocolli di valutazione funzionale multifattoriale e relativi indici per l'età pediatrica".

Institutional Review Board Statement: The study was approved by the Ethics Committee of the Institute (Approval Number: 55/23, Comitato Etico dell'Associ-azione "La Nostra Famiglia"—IRCCS "Eugenio Medea," 18 May 2023). The clinical trial has been registered on Clinical Trials.gov: NCT06400667.

Informed Consent Statement: Informed consent was obtained from all adult participants and from the parents or legal guardians of the minors.

Data Availability Statement: Data presented in this study are available on request to the corresponding author in anonymous form due to GDPR and informed consent.

Acknowledgments: The authors would like to thank the "5 per mille" program for biomedical research for supporting this study through the project "5x1000/2023—Development of new multifactorial functional assessment protocols and related indices for the pediatric age," awarded to Giuseppe Andreoni. We also thank the support provided by the Italian Ministry of Health (Ricerca Corrente 2024–2025, granted to Eng. E. Biffi).

Conflicts of Interest: No conflict of interest exists. The authors wish to confirm that there are no known conflicts of interest associated with this publication and there has been no financial support for this work that could have influenced its outcome.

Abbreviations

The following abbreviations are used in this manuscript:

UL	Upper Limb
CP	Cerebral Palsy
MUUL	The Melbourne Assessment of Unilateral Upper Limb Function
QUEST	Quality of Upper Extremity Skills Test
SHUEE	Shriners Hospital Upper Extremity Evaluation
CIMT	Constraint-Induced Movement Therapy
TRT	Trunk Restraint Therapy
BAT	Bilateral Arm Therapy
ICF	International Classification of Functioning
ISB	International Society of Biomechanics

HtT	Hit-to-Target
SUS	System Usability Scale
ROM	Range of motion
ICC	intraclass correlation coefficient
MMV	Mean Movement Velocity
IC	Index of curvature
NVP	Number of Velocity Peaks
MA	motion analysis

References

1. Langhorne, P.; Bernhardt, J.; Kwakkel, G. Stroke rehabilitation. *Lancet* **2011**, *377*, 1693–1702. [CrossRef] [PubMed]
2. Francisco-Martínez, C.; Prado-Olivarez, J.; Padilla-Medina, J.A.; Díaz-Carmona, J.; Pérez-Pinal, F.J.; Barranco-Gutiérrez, A.I.; Martínez-Nolasco, J.J. Upper limb movement measurement systems for cerebral palsy: A systematic literature review. *Sensors* **2021**, *21*, 7884. [CrossRef]
3. Santisteban, L.; Térémetz, M.; Bleton, J.P.; Baron, J.C.; Maier, M.A.; Lindberg, P.G. Upper limb outcome measures used in stroke rehabilitation studies: A systematic literature review. *PLoS ONE* **2016**, *11*, e0154792. [CrossRef]
4. Lemmens, R.J.M.; Timmermans, A.A.A.; Janssen-Potten, Y.J.M.; Smeets, R.J.E.M.; Seelen, H.A.M. Valid and reliable instruments for arm-hand assessment at ICF activity level in persons with hemiplegia: A systematic review. *BMC Neurol.* **2012**, *12*, 21. [CrossRef]
5. Demers, M.; Levin, M.F. Do Activity Level Outcome Measures Commonly Used in Neurological Practice Assess Upper-Limb Movement Quality? *Neurorehabil. Neural Repair* **2017**, *31*, 623–637. [CrossRef]
6. Ashford, S.; Slade, M.; Malaprade, F.; Turner-Stokes, L. Evaluation of functional outcome measures for the hemiparetic upper limb: A systematic review. *J. Rehabil. Med.* **2008**, *40*, 787–795. [CrossRef]
7. Murphy, M.A.; Resteghini, C.; Feys, P.; Lamers, I. An overview of systematic reviews on upper extremity outcome measures after stroke. *BMC Neurol.* **2015**, *15*, 29. [CrossRef]
8. Koman, L.A.; Smith, B.P.; Shilt, J.S. Cerebral palsy. *Lancet* **2004**, *363*, 1619–1631. [CrossRef]
9. Bourke-Taylor, H. Melbourne Assessment of Unilateral Upper Limb Function: Construct validity and correlation with the Pediatric Evaluation of Disability Inventory. *Dev. Med. Child Neurol.* **2003**, *45*, 92–96. [CrossRef] [PubMed]
10. Haga, N.; van der Heijden-Maessen, H.C.; van Hoorn, J.F.; Boonstra, A.M.; Hadders-Algra, M. Test-Retest and Inter- and Intrareliability of the Quality of the Upper-Extremity Skills Test in Preschool-Age Children With Cerebral Palsy. *Arch. Phys. Med. Rehabil.* **2007**, *88*, 1686–1689. [CrossRef]
11. Davids, J.R.; Peace, L.C.; Wagner, L.V.; Gidewall, M.A.; Blackhurst, D.W.; Roberson, W.M. Validation of the Shriners Hospital for Children Upper Extremity Evaluation (SHUEE) for children with hemiplegic cerebral palsy. *J. Bone Jt. Surg.* **2006**, *88*, 326–333. [CrossRef]
12. Bard, R.; Chaléat-Valayer, E.; Combey, A.; Bleu, P.E.; Perretant, I.; Bernard, J.C. Upper limb assessment in children with cerebral palsy: Translation and reliability of the French version for the Melbourne unilateral upper limb assessment (test de Melbourne). *Ann. Phys. Rehabil. Med.* **2009**, *52*, 297–310. [CrossRef]
13. Rohafza M, Fluet GG, Qiu Q, Adamovich S. Correlation of reaching and grasping kinematics and clinical measures of upper extremity function in persons with stroke related hemiplegi. *Physiol. Behav.* **2017**, *176*, 139–148. [CrossRef]
14. Kwakkel, G.; Lannin, N.A.; Borschmann, K.; English, C.; Ali, M.; Churilov, L.; Saposnik, G.; Winstein, C.; Van Wegen, E.E.H.; Wolf, S.L.; et al. Standardized Measurement of Sensorimotor Recovery in Stroke Trials: Consensus-Based Core Recommendations from the Stroke Recovery and Rehabilitation Roundtable. *Neurorehabil. Neural Repair* **2017**, *31*, 784–792. [CrossRef] [PubMed]
15. Mesquita, I.A.; Fonseca, P.F.P.d.; Borgonovo-Santos, M.; Ribeiro, E.; Pinheiro, A.R.V.; Correia, M.V.; Silva, C. Comparison of upper limb kinematics in two activities of daily living with different handling requirements. *Hum. Mov. Sci.* **2020**, *72*, 102632. [CrossRef] [PubMed]
16. Karakostas, T.; Watters, K.; King, E.C. Assessment of the Spastic Upper Limb with Computational Motion Analysis. *Hand Clin.* **2018**, *34*, 445–454. [CrossRef]
17. Jaspers, E.; Desloovere, K.; Bruyninckx, H.; Molenaers, G.; Klingels, K.; Feys, H. Review of quantitative measurements of upper limb movements in hemiplegic cerebral palsy. *Gait Posture* **2009**, *30*, 395–404. [CrossRef]
18. De Los Reyes-Guzmán, A.; Dimbwadyo-Terrer, I.; Trincado-Alonso, F.; Monasterio-Huelin, F.; Torricelli, D.; Gil-Agudo, A. Quantitative assessment based on kinematic measures of functional impairments during upper extremity movements: A review. *Clin. Biomech.* **2014**, *29*, 719–727. [CrossRef]
19. Alt Murphy, M.; Häger, C.K. Kinematic analysis of the upper extremity after stroke–how far have we reached and what have we grasped? *Phys. Ther. Rev.* **2015**, *20*, 137–155. [CrossRef]

20. Salter, K.; Jutai, J.W.; Teasell, R.; Foley, N.C.; Bitensky, J.; Bayley, M. Issues for selection of outcome measures in stroke rehabilitation: ICF activity. *Disabil. Rehabil.* **2005**, *27*, 315–340. [CrossRef]
21. Butler, E.E.; Ladd, A.L.; Louie, S.A.; LaMont, L.E.; Wong, W.; Rose, J. Three-dimensional kinematics of the upper limb during a Reach and Grasp Cycle for children. *Gait Posture* **2010**, *32*, 72–77. [CrossRef]
22. Artilheiro, M.C.; Corrêa, J.C.F.; Cimolin, V.; Lima, M.O.; Galli, M.; de Godoy, W.; Lucareli, P.R.G. Three-dimensional analysis of performance of an upper limb functional task among adults with dyskinetic cerebral palsy. *Gait Posture* **2014**, *39*, 875–881. [CrossRef]
23. Wu, G.; Van Der Helm, F.C.T.; Veeger, H.E.J.; Makhsous, M.; Van Roy, P.; Anglin, C.; Nagels, J.; Karduna, A.R.; McQuade, K.; Wang, X.; et al. ISB recommendation on definitions of joint coordinate systems of various joints for the reporting of human joint motion—Part II: Shoulder, elbow, wrist and hand. *J. Biomech.* **2005**, *38*, 981–992. [CrossRef]
24. Milanese, C.; Cavedon, V.; Corte, S.; Agostini, T. The effects of two different correction strategies on the snatch technique in weightlifting. *J. Sports Sci.* **2017**, *35*, 476–483. [CrossRef]
25. Kontaxis, A.; Cutti, A.G.; Johnson, G.R.; Veeger, H.E.J. A framework for the definition of standardized protocols for measuring upper-extremity kinematics. *Clin. Biomech.* **2009**, *24*, 246–253. [CrossRef] [PubMed]
26. Andreoni, G.; Negrini, S.; Ciavarro, G.L.; Santambrogio, G.C. ZooMS: A non invasive analysis of global and metameric movement of the lumbar spine. *Eura Medicophys* **2005**, *41*, 7–16.
27. Zapata, B.C.; Fernández-Alemán, J.L.; Idri, A.; Toval, A. Empirical Studies on Usability of mHealth Apps: A Systematic Literature Review. *J. Med. Syst.* **2015**, *39*, 1. [CrossRef] [PubMed]
28. *ISO 9241-11*; 2018 Ergonomics of Human-System Interactionpart 11: Usability: Definitions and Concepts. ISO/IEC: Geneva, Switzerland, 2018.
29. Friesen, E.L. Measuring at Usability with the Modified System Usability Scale (SUS). *Stud. Health Technol. Inform.* **2017**, *242*, 137–143. [CrossRef] [PubMed]
30. Menegoni, F.; Milano, E.; Trotti, C.; Galli, M.; Bigoni, M.; Baudo, S.; Mauro, A. Quantitative evaluation of functional limitation of upper limb movements in subjects affected by ataxia. *Eur. J. Neurol.* **2009**, *16*, 232–239. [CrossRef]
31. Cimolin, V.; Beretta, E.; Piccinini, L.; Turconi, A.C.; Locatelli, F.; Galli, M.; Strazzer, S. Constraint-induced movement therapy for children with hemiplegia after traumatic brain injury: A quantitative study. *J. Head Trauma Rehabil.* **2012**, *27*, 177–187. [CrossRef]
32. Butler, E.E.; Rose, J. The Pediatric Upper Limb Motion Index and a Temporal-Spatial Logistic Regression: Quantitative Analysis of Upper Limb Movement Disorders during the Reach & Grasp Cycle. *Physiol. Behav.* **2018**, *176*, 139–148. [CrossRef]
33. Beretta, E.; Cesareo, A.; Biffi, E.; Schafer, C.; Galbiati, S.; Strazzer, S. Rehabilitation of upper limb in children with acquired brain injury: A preliminary comparative study. *J. Healthc. Eng.* **2018**, *2018*, 4208492. [CrossRef] [PubMed]
34. Ciavarro, G.L.; Andreoni, G.; Negrini, S.; Santambrogio, G.C. Functional assessment of the lumbar spine through the optoelectronic ZooMS system. *Clin. Appl.* **2006**, *42*, 135–143.
35. Piccinini, L.; Molteni, L.E.; Panzeri, D.; Micheletti, E.; Pintabona, G.; Andreoni, G. Integrated Assessment of Gait and Spinal Kinematics Using Optoelectronic Motion Analysis Systems: Validation and Usability Assessment of a Novel Protocol. *Biomechanics* **2025**, *5*, 24. [CrossRef]
36. Brooke, J. SUS: A "Quick and Dirty" Usability Scale. *Usability Eval. Ind.* **1995**, *189*, 207–212. [CrossRef]
37. Koo, T.K.; Li, M.Y. A Guideline of Selecting and Reporting Intraclass Correlation Coefficients for Reliability Research. *J. Chiropr. Med.* **2016**, *15*, 155–163. [CrossRef]
38. Bangor, A.; Kortum, P.; Miller, J. Determining what individual SUS scores mean: Adding an adjective rating scale. *J. Usability Stud.* **2009**, *4*, 114–123.
39. Ciavarro, G.L.; Tramonte, A.; Fusca, M.; Santambrogio, G.C.; Andreoni, G. Evaluation of 3D kinematic model of the spine for ergonomic analysis. *SAE Tech. Pap.* **2004**, *113*, 2004. [CrossRef]

Disclaimer/Publisher's Note: The statements, opinions and data contained in all publications are solely those of the individual author(s) and contributor(s) and not of MDPI and/or the editor(s). MDPI and/or the editor(s) disclaim responsibility for any injury to people or property resulting from any ideas, methods, instructions or products referred to in the content.

bioengineering

Article

A High-Fidelity mmWave Radar Dataset for Privacy-Sensitive Human Pose Estimation

Yuanzhi Su [1], Huiying (Cynthia) Hou [1,*], Haifeng Lan [1] and Christina Zong-Hao Ma [2,3,4]

1 Department of Building Environment and Energy Engineering, The Hong Kong Polytechnic University, Hong Kong SAR, China; yuanzhi.su@connect.polyu.hk (Y.S.); haifeng.lan@connect.polyu.hk (H.L.)
2 Department of Biomedical Engineering, The Hong Kong Polytechnic University, Hong Kong SAR, China; czh.ma@polyu.edu.hk
3 Research Institute for Sports Science and Technology, The Hong Kong Polytechnic University, Hong Kong SAR, China
4 Research Institute for Smart Ageing, The Hong Kong Polytechnic University, Hong Kong SAR, China
* Correspondence: cynthia.hou@polyu.edu.hk

Abstract: Human pose estimation (HPE) in privacy-sensitive environments such as healthcare facilities and smart homes demands non-visual sensing solutions. Millimeter-wave (mmWave) radar emerges as a promising alternative, yet its development is hindered by the scarcity of high-fidelity datasets with accurate annotations. This paper introduces mmFree-Pose, the first dedicated mmWave radar dataset specifically designed for privacy-preserving HPE. Collected through a novel visual-free framework that synchronizes mmWave radar with VDSuit-Full motion-capture sensors, our dataset covers 10+ actions, from basic gestures to complex falls. Each sample provides (i) raw 3D point clouds with Doppler velocity and intensity, (ii) precise 23-joint skeletal annotations, and (iii) full-body motion sequences in privacy-critical scenarios. Crucially, all data is captured without the use of visual sensors, ensuring fundamental privacy protection by design. Unlike conventional approaches that rely on RGB or depth cameras, our framework eliminates the risk of visual data leakage while maintaining high annotation fidelity. The dataset also incorporates scenarios involving occlusions, different viewing angles, and multiple subject variations to enhance generalization in real-world applications. By providing a high-quality and privacy-compliant dataset, mmFree-Pose bridges the gap between RF sensing and home monitoring applications, where safeguarding personal identity and behavior remains a critical concern.

Keywords: mmWave radar; privacy-preserving sensing; human pose estimation

1. Introduction

Human pose estimation (HPE) has emerged as a foundational technology enabling transformative applications across healthcare monitoring [1–3], human–computer interaction [4–6], and smart environment systems [7–9]. In clinical contexts, continuous pose tracking facilitates early detection of critical events such as falls in elderly populations [10,11], while in residential settings, it supports intuitive gesture-based control of domestic appliances [5,12]. However, the predominant reliance on visual sensing modalities—particularly RGB cameras [13,14]—introduces significant limitations in privacy-sensitive environments. These systems inherently capture personally identifiable information, raising serious ethical and regulatory concerns in contexts like patient rooms, bathrooms, or private residences, where confidentiality is paramount. Moreover, their performance degrades substantially under suboptimal lighting conditions, limiting reliability in nocturnal care scenarios.

Millimeter-wave (mmWave) radar technology [15,16] presents a promising alternative, operating through radio frequency signals rather than optical capture. This modality offers two distinct advantages: immunity to lighting variations and inherent privacy preservation through non-visual data acquisition. By generating sparse 3D point clouds representing spatial coordinates without capturing biometric identifiers, mmWave systems fundamentally avoid the privacy violations associated with visual sensors. Despite these benefits, advancement in mmWave-based HPE has been constrained by the absence of high-fidelity datasets that simultaneously satisfy two critical requirements: precise annotations and coverage of wide daily movements.

Existing datasets exhibit notable limitations in this domain. The HuPR benchmark [17] leverages synchronized RGB cameras to generate pseudo-labels via pre-trained vision models, inheriting annotation inaccuracies while compromising privacy through visual data capture. Similarly, the dataset introduced by Sengupta et al. [18] relies on Microsoft Kinect for ground truth, introducing depth-sensing errors estimated at >50 mm positional deviation. More fundamentally, current resources lack comprehensive coverage of medically critical scenarios such as falls—events that demand high detection reliability but occur predominantly in privacy-sensitive contexts. This gap between technological potential and available training resources has impeded the development of robust mmWave HPE systems for real-world applications where privacy and accuracy are significant.

To address these challenges, we present mmFree-Pose, a novel dataset specifically designed for privacy-sensitive human pose estimation using mmWave radar. The specific comparison is shown in Figure 1. Our acquisition framework employs synchronized mmWave radar and inertial motion-capture sensors, eliminating optical sensors entirely from the data collection pipeline. This approach ensures fundamental privacy protection while achieving medical-grade annotation precision. The dataset comprises 4534 temporally aligned samples capturing 10+ actions performed by three subjects, encompassing both basic movements (e.g., arm waving and leg lifts) and complex scenarios (e.g., forward/backward falls) in multiple orientations relative to the radar. Each sample provides five-dimensional point cloud data (x, y, z, velocity, and intensity) paired with precise 23-joint skeletal annotations.

The primary contributions of this work are threefold:

- We establish a privacy-by-design data acquisition paradigm, enabling high-fidelity pose estimation in privacy-sensitive environment.
- We establish the first mmWave radar dataset with high-fidelity full-body pose annotations generated without any optical or visual data.
- Experimental validation demonstrates executive performance on complex poses, with testing on several benchmark models, achieving a significant performance.

Collectively, this resource bridges a critical gap in sensing infrastructure for applications where privacy constraints preclude visual monitoring, such as healthcare facilities or smart homes.

The remainder of this paper is structured as follows: Section 2 examines related work on privacy-preserving human pose estimation, mmWave-based pose estimation, and identifies specific limitations in existing datasets and inertial motion capture for annotation. Section 3 details the sensor synchronization methodology and data collection protocol. Section 4 presents benchmark evaluations and comparative analysis. Section 5 discusses practical applications, limitations, and future research directions. Concluding remarks are provided in Section 6.

Dataset	Number	Dimension	Type	Movement	Keypoint	Device
MS COCO	Over 20k	3	Full-visual	-	17	Camera
UCH-Thermal-pose	904	1	Semi-visual	-	17	Thermal Imager
HuPR	141k	4	Semi-visual	3	14	mmWave Radar
Ours	4534	5	Non-visual	11	23	mmWave Radar

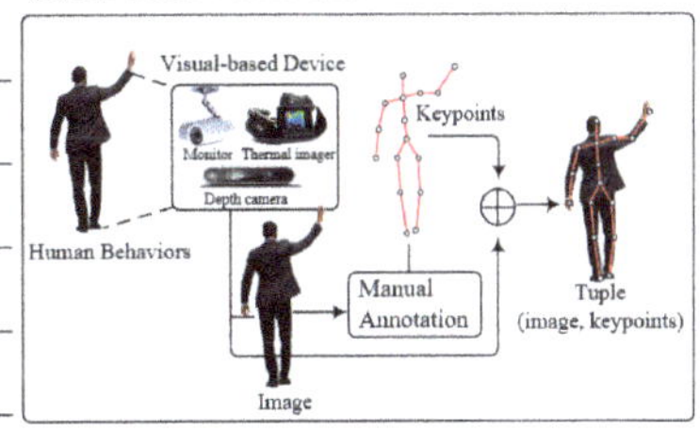

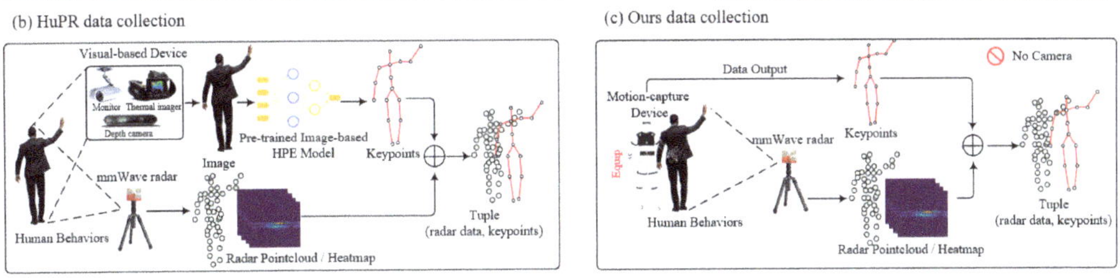

Figure 1. Comparative framework of human pose dataset acquisition: visual vs. non-visual paradigms. (**a**) Traditional visual/semi-visual methods (MS COCO and UCH-Thermal-Pose). (**b**) Semi-visual pseudo-labeling (HuPR). (**c**) Proposed privacy-centric framework with visual-free annotation.

2. Related Work

2.1. Privacy-Preserving Human Pose Estimation

Traditional vision-based human pose estimation (HPE) [4,6,19–27] methodologies face fundamental limitations in privacy-sensitive contexts. RGB-D systems [26] like Microsoft Kinect capture detailed body silhouettes, risking biometric identifier exposure that violates relevant regulations in healthcare settings. Infrared alternatives [28,29] offer partial mitigation by eliminating texture and color information, but thermal imagery still retains spatial heat distributions that, when combined with shape priors, can be reverse-engineered to approximate human identity or body type. Recent RF-based approaches [30,31] using Wi-Fi or ultrawideband radar provide anonymity through signal-scattering patterns, yet suffer from low spatial resolution (>20 cm error), making them unsuitable for fine-grained tasks, particularly in applications requiring higher localization accuracy. In this landscape, millimeter-wave (mmWave) radar emerges as a balanced solution, offering centimeter-level spatial resolution through short-wavelength signal propagation, while preserving subject anonymity by avoiding any visual or thermal representation. Its non-invasive nature aligns well with privacy-by-design frameworks, making it particularly suitable for sensitive environments like bathrooms, bedrooms, or eldercare facilities. Yet paradoxically, many existing mmWave HPE implementations still rely on optical sensors (RGB cameras and depth sensors) [17,18,32,33] to generate annotated ground truth, introducing privacy compromise at the training phase even if inference is performed using radar alone. This reliance not only undermines privacy claims but also restricts the deployment of such models in privacy-critical applications due to regulatory scrutiny.

Our work directly addresses this conflict by proposing a fully visual-free data acquisition pipeline, thereby eliminating the need for camera-based annotation while maintaining high fidelity via inertial motion capture. This resolves the long-standing trade-off between privacy preservation and annotation accuracy, a crucial step toward enabling ethically compliant, real-world human monitoring solutions.

2.2. Fundamentals of mmWave Radar Sensing

Millimeter-wave (mmWave) radar [15,16] operates by emitting high-frequency radio waves (typically 60–80 GHz) and analyzing reflections from objects [20]. Unlike cameras, it captures motion through radio signals rather than light. The fundamental operating principle of mmWave radar involves transmitting electromagnetic waves in the millimeter-wave range and analyzing the signals reflected from objects within the radar's field of view. The radar system transmits a millimeter-wave signal through an antenna array. This signal is modulated to increase linearly over a defined time interval as it propagates through the environment and interacts with objects in its path. Depending on the material properties and surface geometry of these objects, a portion of the signal is reflected back toward the radar. The receiving antenna captures these reflected signals and combines them with a segment of the transmitted signal, producing an intermediate frequency (IF) signal.

These IF signals are digitized and processed through a series of Fast Fourier Transforms (FFTs) to resolve range, Doppler velocity, and angle information. Specifically, a 3D radar point is formed using range FFT (distance resolution), Doppler FFT (velocity measurement), and angle FFT (azimuth/elevation angles). Then Constant False Alarm Rate (CFAR) detection isolates valid human targets from noise, followed by coordinate conversion to Cartesian space. Hence, each point is represented as $p = \{x, y, z, \text{velocity}, \text{intensity}\}$, where the coordinates (x, y, z) define the object's location, and the additional attributes indicate the object's velocity and signal intensity within the radar's field of view. By repeating this process, a series of signals received by mmwave radar can be converted into a point set, which can be represented as point cloud $P = \left\{p_i \middle| p_i = \{x_i, y_i, z_i, \text{velocity}_i, \text{intensity}_i\} \in R^5, i = 1, 2, \ldots, N\right\}$, where N indicates the number of points.

For generating 3D point clouds where each point represents a detected surface location, velocity, and reflectivity, this technology leverages two key physical properties:

(1) High-frequency waves provide fine spatial resolution (centimeter-level), enabling detection of small body movements like joint rotations.
(2) Signal time-of-flight measurements calculate object distance, while Doppler shifts in reflected waves reveal limb velocity.

For human pose estimation, mmWave radar offers inherent privacy advantages: its output contains only geometric coordinates without visual details (e.g., facial features or skin texture), making it compliant for sensitive settings. Additionally, it functions reliably in darkness and through light obstructions (e.g., clothing or curtains), addressing critical limitations of optical sensors. While challenges like sparse data points remain, these characteristics position mmWave as a unique enabler for ethical human monitoring where cameras cannot be deployed.

2.3. mmWave Radar Datasets for HPE

Existing mmWave HPE datasets exhibit critical limitations in privacy compliance and annotation quality. The emergence of mmWave radar technology has opened new avenues for HPE and provides a robust alternative to visual sensors. At present, several datasets have been developed to explore this potential. For instance, Sengupta et al. [18] proposed an HPE dataset using mmWave radar, which consists of radar reflection data encoded as RGB images, with pixel values representing 3D coordinates and reflection intensity, along with ground-truth skeletal joint data captured via Microsoft Kinect. Xue et al. provided a detailed dataset for 3D mesh reconstructions from radar data, offering a valuable resource for developing and benchmarking 3D HPE algorithms. Another notable dataset, HuPR [17], incorporates the synchronized vision and radar components for cross-modality training. HuPR leverages pre-trained 2D pose estimation networks on RGB images to generate pseudo-label annotations for radar data, thereby avoiding manual labeling efforts and enhancing training efficiency.

Despite these valuable contributions, existing radar datasets suffer from several drawbacks, such as limited diversity in human poses and inaccurate data annotations, all of which hinder broader experimentation and development in the field. In contrast, this paper presents a comprehensive dataset that includes a wide range of human poses, from simple to complex, and features high-fidelity annotations obtained via motion-capture technology. This approach ensures accurate ground-truth data, free from the limitations of model-generated annotations, and provides a richer, more diverse dataset for training robust mmWave radar-based HPE models. By directly addressing the shortcomings of existing datasets, our work advances the capabilities of RF-based HPE technologies, paving the way for real-world applications.

2.4. Inertial Motion Capture for Annotation

Inertial measurement unit (IMU)-based systems [34] offer privacy-compliant alternatives for motion capture. The VDSuit-Full system deployed in this work utilizes 23 wireless IMUs to reconstruct skeletal poses without optical inputs. Comparable systems like Xsens MVN [35] provide medical-grade kinematics but require proprietary software that impedes annotation extraction. Recent work [36–38] demonstrates IMU-based operating-room monitoring, validating inertial systems' clinical reliability. However, IMUs are susceptible to integration drift, quadrature errors, and cross-axis sensitivity over time, particularly during dynamic sequences. Existing works have attempted to model and mitigate such effects via compensation schemes [39].

Despite limitations such as potential drift over long sequences and reliance on initial calibration, IMUs remain particularly well-suited for annotating mmWave radar data. Their high temporal resolution compensates for radar's lower frame rate and point cloud sparsity, while their numerical output avoids any form of biometric reconstruction. This synergy allows for accurate spatial–temporal alignment and robust pose labeling without compromising privacy. Our approach represents one of the first to harness this complementary relationship, enabling precise, scalable annotation of mmWave point clouds without invoking visual sensing at any stage—effectively resolving the longstanding trade-off between privacy and annotation fidelity that constrains prior mmWave HPE datasets.

3. Privacy-First Data Construction

3.1. Privacy-by-Design Framework

The core architecture of our data collection framework implements a strict privacy-by-design paradigm through the complete exclusion of optical sensors. Millimeter-wave radar captures motion data exclusively as sparse 3D point clouds, $P = \{p_i | p_i = (x, y, z, v, I)\} \in R^5$, inherently incapable of reconstructing visual identifiers such as facial features or body morphology. Simultaneously, the VDSuit-Full motion-capture system employs several inertial measurement units (IMUs), directly generating joint coordinates without recording any visual representations. Additionally, the point cloud representation provides information-theoretic anonymity through dimensionality reduction. Crucially, the system operates without supplemental RGB, infrared, or depth cameras that could compromise privacy, establishing a new standard for ethically compliant human sensing.

3.2. Action Design

Action sequences in the dataset were carefully curated to address critical gaps in privacy-sensitive monitoring scenarios, particularly those relevant to healthcare, eldercare, and smart home environments. A total of 11 representative human actions were selected, spanning a spectrum from low-dynamic daily tasks to high-risk emergency motions. These actions were classified into three functional categories:

- Basic gestures, such as single-hand waving and shoulder touching, reflect common interactive movements that may be used in gesture-controlled interfaces or passive monitoring of user activity.
- Activities of daily living (ADLs), including sitting-to-standing transitions and simulated dressing motions, are essential for assessing autonomy and physical function—especially in bathroom or bedroom settings, where visual sensors are categorically prohibited due to privacy regulations.
- Critical fall scenarios, including forward, backward, and lateral falls, were deliberately designed and validated by referencing the established fall-detection literature. These sequences simulate the most frequent and injurious fall patterns observed in elderly care environments.

Additional movements, such as controlled leg raises, static balancing poses, and transitional weight shifts, were incorporated to increase diversity in joint kinematics and center-of-mass dynamics. Importantly, to model viewpoint and orientation variance, each action was performed at three different yaw angles relative to the radar's boresight (0°, 90°, and 180°), ensuring robustness of the dataset against rotation-dependent occlusion and sensor placement biases.

Each sequence spans approximately 5 to 15 s, capturing the complete temporal evolution of the motion from initiation to resolution. This full-trajectory coverage is crucial for downstream learning tasks such as sequence-based pose estimation, activity classification, and time-series fall prediction. The design ensures that mmFree-Pose reflects realistic movement complexity under privacy-preserving conditions, providing a benchmark that is both ethically compliant and technically challenging.

3.3. Data Preprocessing Pipeline

Using the IWR6843 ISK radar sensor from Texas Instruments, raw data underwent rigorous preprocessing to enhance quality while preserving privacy attributes. Radar point clouds were filtered to remove non-human points and environmental noise, retaining only clusters corresponding to body segments. Moreover, precise alignment between radar and motion-capture systems was achieved through temporal signal. Additionally, spatial calibration employed a hip-centered coordinate system where $J_{\text{hip}} = (0,0,0)$, with Kabsch algorithm optimization minimizing residual error between radar centroids and mocap joint positions. Skeletal data was normalized to the hip joint origin through affine transformation, $\hat{J}_k = J_k - J_{hip}$, ensuring consistent coordinate frames despite participant movement. To compensate for radar sparsity, we applied a simple temporal fusion technique by averaging five consecutive frames to enhance point density. While this approach helps reduce transient noise and improve annotation alignment with IMU data, it may also introduce temporal smoothing effects that can blur rapid motions. In future work, we aim to adopt more advanced temporal denoising methods, such as Kalman filtering or learned temporal smoothers, to better preserve dynamic motion characteristics. Final anonymization scrubbed all metadata, including timestamps, locations, and anthropometric records, assigning de-identified participant codes (P01–P03). The resulting dataset comprises 4534 samples with matched point clouds and 23-joint annotations, partitioned into training (80%), validation (10%), and test sets (10%) while maintaining temporal continuity within sequences. A data exemplar is provided in Figure 2a.

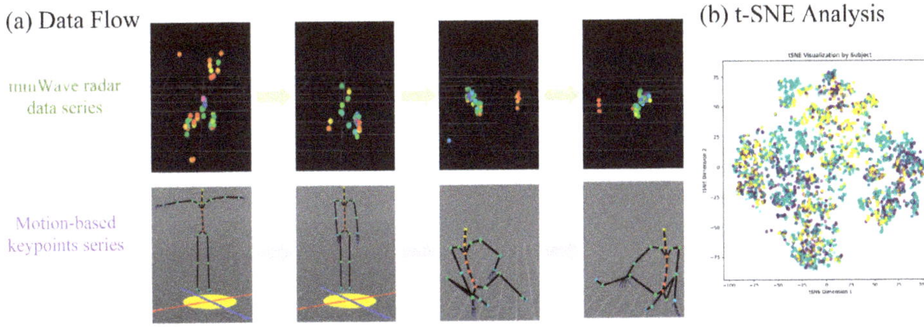

Figure 2. Temporal synchronization and feature Analysis of mmFree-Pose data: (**a**) time-aligned data flow—synchronized mmWave radar point clouds (**top**) and motion-capture keypoints (**bottom**); and (**b**) t-SNE visualization of pose feature embeddings (colored by participant).

Furthermore, to visually observe the impact of subjects on data distribution and action categories, we performed t-SNE visualization on the data samples, as shown in Figure 2b. The visualization results revealed that the inter-subject variability in point cloud distributions is relatively small compared to the variability introduced by different poses and actions. This suggests that the model's performance is more influenced by pose diversity than by individual anthropometric differences.

4. Data Value Validation

4.1. Experimental Protocol

The validation framework employed standardized evaluation metrics and baseline models to objectively quantify dataset efficacy. Point Transformer [40], PointNet [41], and DGCNN [42] architectures served as reference models, representing fundamental point cloud processing approaches widely adopted in mmWave HPE research. The models are evaluated under three different settings—11, 16, and 23 joints—representing varying levels of model complexity and granularity in estimating human poses; more details are illustrated in Figure 3.

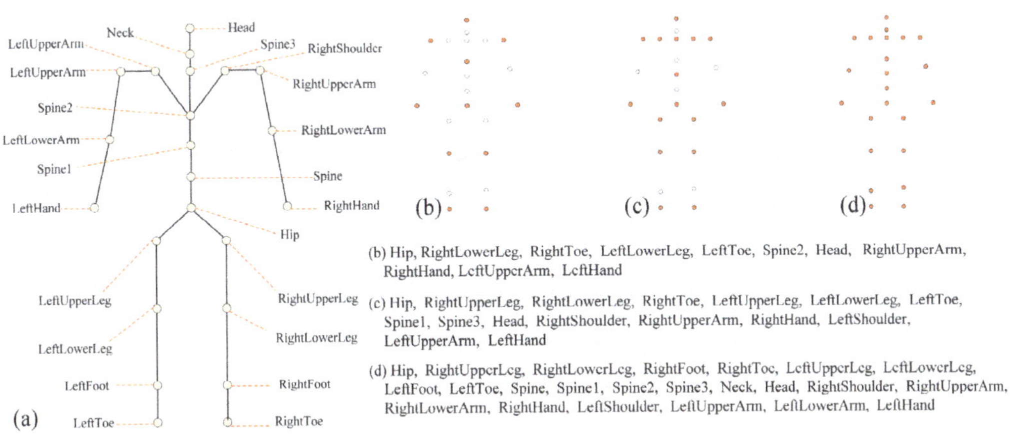

Figure 3. Three different joint settings are used in our experiments to assess the model's robustness under varying joint counts. (**a**) displays a full human body skeleton with 23 labeled joint points. (**b–d**) show point sets of body joints with 11, 16, and 23 joints, respectively. The incremental number of joints allows us to evaluate the model's performance across different levels of complexity.

Performance was assessed through three complementary metrics: Percentage of Correct Keypoints within a 10 cm threshold (PCK@5 cm), Mean per Joint Position Error (MPJPE), and Average Precision across Object Keypoint Similarity thresholds from 0.5 to 0.95 (AP). Statistical significance against existing datasets was established via Wilcoxon signed-rank tests with $\alpha = 0.01$ confidence level. The experiment setup is illustrated in Figure 4.

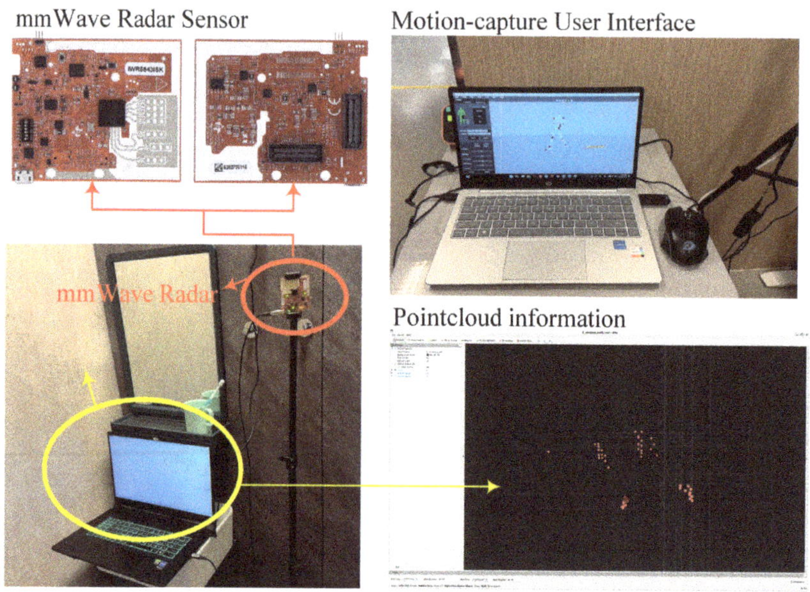

Figure 4. (**Left**) Hardware setup: mmWave radar sensor and laptop terminal for real-time data processing. (**Right**) Motion-capture interface displaying synchronized point cloud visualization.

4.2. Benchmark Performance

As shown in Table 1, PointNet demonstrates superior performance across all joint configurations and metrics, achieving State-of-the-Art results on the mmFree-Pose dataset. For the critical 23-joint evaluation, PointNet reaches the lowest Mean Localization Error (12.39 cm vs. DGCNN's 13.01 cm) while improving PCK (47.18% vs. Point Transformer's 40.89%) and AP (95% vs. DGCNN's 89%). Notably, its advantage widens with simpler skeletons (16 joints: 44.17% PCK higher than DGCNN), suggesting exceptional efficiency in core joint tracking. Surprisingly, the attention-based Point Transformer underperforms despite its theoretical capacity, indicating sparse mmWave point clouds (~50 points/frame) may hinder complex architectural learning. These results establish PointNet as the optimal baseline for privacy-sensitive HPE applications requiring balance between accuracy and computational efficiency. Visualization results, provided in Figure 5, further emphasize the robustness of deep learning approaches in accurately estimating human poses across different keypoint configurations, regardless of complexity.

Table 1. Quantitative comparison of 3D deep HPE methods on curated datasets. Arrows show optimization directions: ↑ for higher-better (PCK, AP); ↓ for lower-better (MLE).

Approach	11 Joints			16 Joints			23 Joints		
	MLE↓	PCK↑	AP↑	MLE↓	PCK↑	AP↑	MLE↓	PCK↑	AP↑
Point Transformer	16.37	37.93	84	14.22	40.21	90	14.31	40.89	91
PointNet	14.39	42.19	91	10.61	44.17	94	12.39	47.18	95
DGCNN	14.86	38.49	85	13.06	41.13	90	13.01	42.01	89

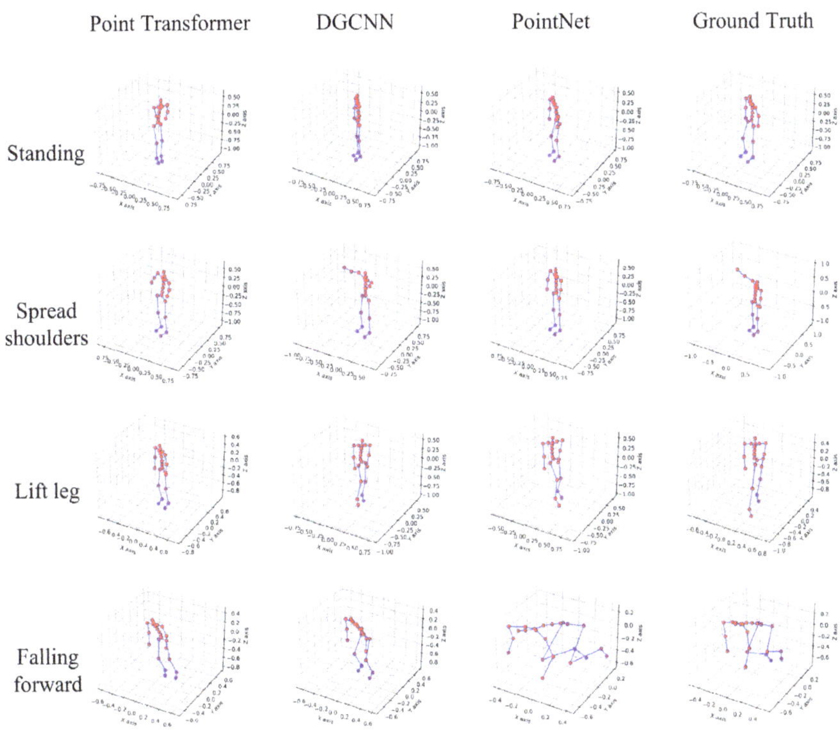

Figure 5. Qualitative comparison of pose estimation models on privacy-sensitive actions.

Error distribution: As detailed in Table 2, joint-wise error analysis reveals a consistent hierarchy in prediction accuracy across all evaluated models. Core joints—notably the hip and spine—demonstrate substantially lower MPJPEs compared to peripheral joints. For example, hip localization errors range from 0.001 cm (DGCNN) to 0.202 cm (Point Transformer), while spine-related joints maintain sub-2 cm accuracy. In contrast, extremities such as hands and feet exhibit much higher error rates, ranging from ~18 cm to over 27 cm, with the left hand reaching 26.27 cm error in Point Transformer and 23.24 cm in PointNet.

Table 2. Mean per Joint Position Error (MPJPE) is used to measure the average Euclidean distance between the predicted keypoints and the ground truth for each joint, where a lower MPJPE indicates higher accuracy. The comparison of several benchmarks is conducted on the full dataset, using a setting of 23 joints for evaluation.

Keypoint \ Approach	Point Transformer	PointNet	DGCNN
Hip	0.202	0.093	0.001
Right upper leg	6.088	4.118	4.054
Right lower leg	16.259	14.449	15.854
Right foot	21.383	18.981	20.893
Right toe	24.712	20.836	23.029
Left upper leg	6.403	4.250	4.229
Left lower leg	15.873	14.495	14.296
Left foot	20.323	18.303	17.995
Left toe	23.127	19.719	19.505
Spine	1.954	1.833	1.884
Spine 1	3.966	3.880	3.911
Spine 2	6.384	6.240	6.308
Spine 3	8.891	8.746	8.707
Neck	11.719	11.397	11.275
Head	13.786	13.276	13.061
Right shoulder	10.992	9.912	9.954
Right upper arm	17.584	13.608	13.538
Right lower arm	20.406	15.961	17.114
Right hand	27.221	21.990	25.288
Left shoulder	9.884	9.854	9.832
Left upper arm	16.090	13.235	13.112
Left lower arm	19.670	16.519	18.219
Left hand	26.269	23.236	27.215

This disparity is primarily attributable to point cloud sparsity and radar reflectivity variance: the torso typically generates denser and more stable radar returns due to its larger surface area and proximity to the radar boresight, whereas smaller appendages, like wrists, toes, and fingers, contribute weaker, noisier returns that may intermittently disappear from the radar's field of view during rapid motion or occlusion. Moreover, limb extremities exhibit greater range of motion, increasing prediction difficulty under non-uniform sampling.

Efficiency trade-offs: The further comparison for real-world deployment feasibility is summarized in Table 3. Computational benchmarks reveal that PointNet achieves an optimal trade-off between efficiency and accuracy, making it well-suited for latency-sensitive and resource-constrained environments such as smart home hubs, mobile health monitors, or embedded fall detection units.

Specifically, PointNet requires only 11.45 million floating-point operations (FLOPs)—largely fewer than DGCNN (54.69 M)—while maintaining a low inference latency of 2 milliseconds per frame. This low computational footprint ensures high responsiveness even on non-GPU devices or low-power processors, which are common in medical wearables or IoT edge systems. While Point Transformer exhibits superior parameter efficiency (298.18 K parameters vs. PointNet's 349.12 K), its higher FLOPs (24.48 M) indicate more intensive real-time processing demands, which—combined with its significantly lower fall detection PCK—limit its viability in clinical applications, where both accuracy and reaction time are essential.

Table 3. The computational comparison of model components at FLOPs, parameters, and inference time per frame.

Approach	23 Joints		
	FLOPs (M)	Parameter (K)	Inference Time (ms)
Point Transformer	24.48	298.18	2
PointNet	11.45	349.12	2
DGCNN	54.69	594.88	3

Collectively, these findings establish PointNet as the most deployable architecture under practical constraints. Its balance of accuracy, low latency, and moderate complexity makes it ideal for real-world HPE systems deployed in privacy-sensitive, real-time, and resource-limited environments.

4.3. Performance on Complex Motions

In challenging fall scenarios—one of critical but technically demanding tasks for human pose estimation—PointNet demonstrates superior robustness compared to competing architectures (Table 4). Specifically, it achieves an MLE of 16.73 cm, representing a 16.2% improvement over DGCNN (18.99 cm) and a 24.4% improvement over Point Transformer (22.13 cm). Furthermore, it records the highest AP of 90%, indicating a reliable capacity to localize joints even under rapid, chaotic movement conditions common in falls.

Table 4. Quantitative comparison of 3D deep HPE methods on curated datasets in complicated fall patterns. Arrows show optimization directions: ↑ for higher-better (PCK, AP); ↓ for lower-better (MLE).

Approach	23 Joints		
	MLE↓	PCK↑	AP↑
Point Transformer	22.13	33.34	60
PointNet	16.73	43.93	90
DGCNN	18.99	43.66	70

This performance is particularly significant given the inherent difficulties in radar-based estimation of high-velocity limb trajectories. Fall events typically involve sudden, multi-joint rotations and ground contact within a short time span, often accompanied by partial occlusion or transient disappearance of extremity reflections in the radar signal. Such dynamics challenge model inference due to sparse and noisy point clouds, and degrade spatial coherence across frames.

Despite these constraints, PointNet achieves a Peak Correct Keypoint (PCK) of 43.93%, narrowly outperforming DGCNN (43.66%) and clearly surpassing Point Transformer (33.34%). The margin suggests that simpler architectural designs may generalize better to data-sparse, high-variance scenarios than transformer-based networks, which tend to rely on dense attention patterns ill-suited for radar sparsity (typically <200 points/frame). The reliability of PointNet in fall detection extends its potential for real-time applications.

5. Reproducibility and Applications

The mmFree-Pose dataset enables transformative applications in privacy-sensitive domains where visual monitoring is ethically or legally prohibited. In clinical settings, its high-fidelity fall sequences support developing non-invasive emergency alert systems for elderly care facilities, operating reliably in darkness without compromising patient dignity. For smart homes, gesture recognition during activities like sitting-to-standing control of bathroom appliances, while low-latency inference (e.g., PointNet at 2 ms) facilitates deployment on resource-constrained edge devices. Indus-trial safety monitoring further benefits from the inherent anonymity of point clouds, enabling worker activity tracking in hazardous zones.

Despite these advances, three limitations warrant consideration. First, peripheral joint localization remains challenged during dynamic motions, with high hand errors (Table 4) due to radar shortcomings—a fundamental constraint of mmWave sparsity. Second, demographic coverage is currently limited to three subjects (age 25–32, BMI 18.5–24.9), restricting generalizability to diverse populations such as pediatric or obese individuals. Third, while the dataset includes multiple orientations, it lacks arbitrary view angles and continuous transitions between poses. This discrete setup limits the ecological realism of natural human behavior, where orientation and pose evolve fluidly. Finally, data collection occurred in controlled lab environments, omitting real-world interference like moving furniture or pets, potentially inflating performance metrics versus field deployments.

Future work will address these constraints through targeted innovations. Demographic diversity will be expanded via recruiting more representative subjects without additional privacy-sensitive captures. Finally, we will initiate real-world validation in assisted living facilities, incorporating environmental clutter to bridge the lab-to-field gap. These efforts will solidify mmFree-Pose as a foundational resource for privacy-centric human sensing, advancing technologies that harmonize safety with uncompromising ethical standards.

6. Conclusions

This paper presents mmFree-Pose, the first dedicated mmWave radar dataset explicitly designed to address the critical challenge of privacy preservation in human pose estimation (HPE). By establishing a novel visual-free acquisition framework, we eliminate the ethical and technical risks associated with optical sensors while achieving medical-grade annotation accuracy through synchronized inertial motion capture. The dataset covers 11 safety-critical and socially relevant actions—from basic gestures to high-risk falls—captured under multiple orientations relative to the radar. Each sample provides raw 3D point clouds (with Doppler velocity and intensity) paired with precise 23-joint skeletal annotations, enabling robust model training without compromising subject anonymity.

Our experimental validation demonstrates that mmFree-Pose bridges the gap between RF sensing and privacy-critical applications. Benchmark evaluations reveal that PointNet achieves a State-of-the-Art performance on complex motions, outperforming transformer-based and graph convolutional counterparts. This underscores its suitability for latency-sensitive deployments in eldercare monitoring or smart home systems, where low computational overhead (11.45 M FLOPs, 2 ms inference time) is essential. Crucially, the dataset's design directly resolves the longstanding trade-off between annotation fidelity and privacy compliance, setting a new standard for ethically grounded human sensing.

Despite its contributions, limitations remain: peripheral joint localization errors persist due to radar sparsity, demographic diversity is currently limited, and real-world environmental interference was not modeled. Future work will expand subject diversity (e.g., age and BMI), integrate multi-radar configurations to mitigate occlusion, and validate the framework in operational settings such as assisted-living facilities. We aim to catalyze advancements in privacy-preserving HPE, ultimately enabling technologies that safeguard dignity while enhancing safety in sensitive environments.

Author Contributions: Y.S. contributed to data collection and analysis, data interpretation, draft of the manuscript, and editing; H.H. contributed to concept development, draft of the manuscript, project management, student supervision, and funding acquisition; H.L. contributed to concept development and data collection; C.Z.-H.M. contributed to draft of the manuscript and editing. All authors have read and agreed to the published version of the manuscript.

Funding: This study was supported by grants from the Hong Kong Polytechnic University: Start-Up Fund for New Recruits (Project ID: P0040305) and departmental fund by the Department of Building Environment and Energy Engineering (Project ID: P0052446).

Institutional Review Board Statement: The ethics of this study was approved by the Hong Kong Polytechnic University (reference number: HSEARS20240926009, 7 October 2024).

Informed Consent Statement: Informed consent was obtained from all subjects involved in the study.

Data Availability Statement: The original contributions presented in this study are included in the article. Further inquiries can be directed to the corresponding authors.

Acknowledgments: All the authors would like to thank the anonymous participants who volunteered to participate in this study.

Conflicts of Interest: The authors declare no conflicts of interest.

References

1. Stenum, J.; Cherry-Allen, K.M.; Pyles, C.O.; Reetzke, R.D.; Vignos, M.F.; Roemmich, R.T. Applications of Pose Estimation in Human Health and Performance across the Lifespan. *Sensors* **2021**, *21*, 7315. [CrossRef]
2. Zhu, Y.; Xiao, M.; Xie, Y.; Xiao, Z.; Jin, G.; Shuai, L. In-Bed Human Pose Estimation Using Multi-Source Information Fusion for Health Monitoring in Real-World Scenarios. *Inf. Fusion* **2024**, *105*, 102209. [CrossRef]
3. Chen, K.; Gabriel, P.; Alasfour, A.; Gong, C.; Doyle, W.K.; Devinsky, O.; Friedman, D.; Dugan, P.; Melloni, L.; Thesen, T. Patient-Specific Pose Estimation in Clinical Environments. *IEEE J. Transl. Eng. Health Med.* **2018**, *6*, 1–11. [CrossRef]
4. Huo, R.; Gao, Q.; Qi, J.; Ju, Z. 3d Human Pose Estimation in Video for Human-Computer/Robot Interaction. In Proceedings of the International Conference on Intelligent Robotics and Applications, Hangzhou, China, 5–7 July 2023; Springer: Singapore, 2023; pp. 176–187.
5. Neto, P.; Simão, M.; Mendes, N.; Safeea, M. Gesture-Based Human-Robot Interaction for Human Assistance in Manufacturing. *Int. J. Adv. Manuf. Technol.* **2019**, *101*, 119–135. [CrossRef]
6. Liu, H.; Nie, H.; Zhang, Z.; Li, Y.-F. Anisotropic Angle Distribution Learning for Head Pose Estimation and Attention Understanding in Human-Computer Interaction. *Neurocomputing* **2021**, *433*, 310–322. [CrossRef]
7. Cosma, A.; Radoi, I.E.; Radu, V. Camloc: Pedestrian Location Estimation through Body Pose Estimation on Smart Cameras. In Proceedings of the 2019 International Conference on Indoor Positioning and Indoor Navigation (IPIN), Pisa, Italy, 30 September–3 October 2019; IEEE: Piscataway, NJ, USA, 2019; pp. 1–8.
8. Palermo, M.; Moccia, S.; Migliorelli, L.; Frontoni, E.; Santos, C.P. Real-Time Human Pose Estimation on a Smart Walker Using Convolutional Neural Networks. *Expert Syst. Appl.* **2021**, *184*, 115498. [CrossRef]
9. Wu, C.; Aghajan, H. Real-Time Human Pose Estimation: A Case Study in Algorithm Design for Smart Camera Networks. *Proc. IEEE* **2008**, *96*, 1715–1732. [CrossRef]
10. Beddiar, D.R.; Oussalah, M.; Nini, B. Fall Detection Using Body Geometry and Human Pose Estimation in Video Sequences. *J. Vis. Commun. Image Represent.* **2022**, *82*, 103407. [CrossRef]
11. Juraev, S.; Ghimire, A.; Alikhanov, J.; Kakani, V.; Kim, H. Exploring Human Pose Estimation and the Usage of Synthetic Data for Elderly Fall Detection in Real-World Surveillance. *IEEE Access* **2022**, *10*, 94249–94261. [CrossRef]
12. Coronado, E.; Villalobos, J.; Bruno, B.; Mastrogiovanni, F. Gesture-Based Robot Control: Design Challenges and Evaluation with Humans. In Proceedings of the 2017 IEEE international conference on robotics and automation (ICRA), Singapore, 29 May–3 June 2017; IEEE: Piscataway, NJ, USA, 2017; pp. 2761–2767.
13. Mehta, D.; Sridhar, S.; Sotnychenko, O.; Rhodin, H.; Shafiei, M.; Seidel, H.-P.; Xu, W.; Casas, D.; Theobalt, C. Vnect: Real-Time 3d Human Pose Estimation with a Single Rgb Camera. *ACM Trans. Graph. (TOG)* **2017**, *36*, 1–14. [CrossRef]
14. Zheng, C.; Wu, W.; Chen, C.; Yang, T.; Zhu, S.; Shen, J.; Kehtarnavaz, N.; Shah, M. Deep Learning-Based Human Pose Estimation: A Survey. *ACM Comput. Surv.* **2023**, *56*, 1–37. [CrossRef]
15. Rao, S.; Texas Instruments. *Introduction to Mmwave Sensing: FMCW Radars*; Texas Instruments: Dallas, TX, USA, 2017.

16. Bi, X.; Bi, X. Millimeter Wave Radar Technology. In *Environmental Perception Technology for Unmanned Systems*; Springer: Berlin/Heidelberg, Germany, 2021; pp. 17–65.
17. Lee, S.P.; Kini, N.P.; Peng, W.H.; Ma, C.W.; Hwang, J.N. HuPR: A Benchmark for Human Pose Estimation Using Millimeter Wave Radar. In Proceedings of the Proceedings—2023 IEEE Winter Conference on Applications of Computer Vision, WACV 2023, Waikoloa, HI, USA, 2–7 January 2023.
18. Sengupta, A.; Jin, F.; Zhang, R.; Cao, S. Mm-Pose: Real-Time Human Skeletal Posture Estimation Using MmWave Radars and CNNs. *IEEE Sens. J.* **2020**, *20*, 10032–10044. [CrossRef]
19. Liu, H.; Liu, T.; Zhang, Z.; Sangaiah, A.K.; Yang, B.; Li, Y. ARHPE: Asymmetric Relation-Aware Representation Learning for Head Pose Estimation in Industrial Human–Computer Interaction. *IEEE Trans. Ind. Inf.* **2022**, *18*, 7107–7117. [CrossRef]
20. Newell, A.; Yang, K.; Deng, J. Stacked Hourglass Networks for Human Pose Estimation. In Proceedings of the Computer Vision–ECCV 2016: 14th European Conference, Amsterdam, The Netherlands, 11–14 October 2016; Proceedings, Part VIII 14; Springer: Cham, Switzerland, 2016; pp. 483–499.
21. Sharma, A.M.; Venkatesh, K.S.; Mukerjee, A. Human Pose Estimation in Surveillance Videos Using Temporal Continuity on Static Pose. In Proceedings of the 2011 International Conference on Image Information Processing, Shimla, India, 3–5 November 2011; IEEE: Piscataway, NJ, USA, 2011; pp. 1–6.
22. Li, M.; Hu, H.; Xiong, J.; Zhao, X.; Yan, H. TSwinPose: Enhanced Monocular 3D Human Pose Estimation with JointFlow. *Expert Syst. Appl.* **2024**, *249*, 123545. [CrossRef]
23. Zhao, M.; Li, T.; Abu Alsheikh, M.; Tian, Y.; Zhao, H.; Torralba, A.; Katabi, D. Through-Wall Human Pose Estimation Using Radio Signals. In Proceedings of the IEEE Conference on Computer Vision and Pattern Recognition, Salt Lake City, UT, USA, 18–23 June 2018; pp. 7356–7365.
24. Li, J.; Bian, S.; Zeng, A.; Wang, C.; Pang, B.; Liu, W.; Lu, C. Human Pose Regression with Residual Log-Likelihood Estimation. In Proceedings of the IEEE/CVF International Conference on Computer Vision, Montreal, QC, Canada, 10–17 October 2021; pp. 11025–11034.
25. Manzo, G.; Serratosa, F.; Vento, M. Online Human Assisted and Cooperative Pose Estimation of 2D Cameras. *Expert Syst. Appl.* **2016**, *60*, 258–268. [CrossRef]
26. Zimmermann, C.; Welschehold, T.; Dornhege, C.; Burgard, W.; Brox, T. 3d Human Pose Estimation in Rgbd Images for Robotic Task Learning. In Proceedings of the 2018 IEEE International Conference on Robotics and Automation (ICRA), Brisbane, QLD, Australia, 21–25 May 2018; IEEE: Piscataway, NJ, USA, 2018; pp. 1986–1992.
27. Chen, S.; Xu, Y.; Zou, B. Prior-Knowledge-Based Self-Attention Network for 3D Human Pose Estimation. *Expert Syst. Appl.* **2023**, *225*, 120213. [CrossRef]
28. Guo, Y.; Chen, Y.; Deng, J.; Li, S.; Zhou, H. Identity-Preserved Human Posture Detection in Infrared Thermal Images: A Benchmark. *Sensors* **2022**, *23*, 92. [CrossRef]
29. Smith, J.; Loncomilla, P.; Ruiz-Del-Solar, J. Human Pose Estimation Using Thermal Images. *IEEE Access* **2023**, *11*, 35352–35370. [CrossRef]
30. Xie, C.; Zhang, D.; Wu, Z.; Yu, C.; Hu, Y.; Sun, Q.; Chen, Y. Accurate Human Pose Estimation Using RF Signals. In Proceedings of the 2022 IEEE 24th International Workshop on Multimedia Signal Processing (MMSP), Shanghai, China, 26–28 September 2022; IEEE: Piscataway, NJ, USA, 2022; pp. 1–6.
31. Yu, C.; Zhang, D.; Wu, Z.; Xie, C.; Lu, Z.; Hu, Y.; Chen, Y. Fast 3D Human Pose Estimation Using RF Signals. In Proceedings of the ICASSP 2023—2023 IEEE International Conference on Acoustics, Speech and Signal Processing (ICASSP), Rhodes Island, Greece, 4–10 June 2023; IEEE: Piscataway, NJ, USA, 2023; pp. 1–5.
32. Li, G.; Zhang, Z.; Yang, H.; Pan, J.; Chen, D.; Zhang, J. Capturing Human Pose Using MmWave Radar. In Proceedings of the 2020 IEEE International Conference on Pervasive Computing and Communications Workshops (PerCom Workshops), Austin, TX, USA, 23–27 March 2020; IEEE: Piscataway, NJ, USA, 2020; pp. 1–6.
33. Cui, H.; Zhong, S.; Wu, J.; Shen, Z.; Dahnoun, N.; Zhao, Y. Milipoint: A Point Cloud Dataset for Mmwave Radar. *Adv. Neural Inf. Process. Syst.* **2023**, *36*, 62713–62726.
34. Ahmad, N.; Ghazilla, R.A.R.; Khairi, N.M.; Kasi, V. Reviews on Various Inertial Measurement Unit (IMU) Sensor Applications. *Int. J. Signal Process. Syst.* **2013**, *1*, 256–262. [CrossRef]
35. Roetenberg, D.; Luinge, H.; Slycke, P. Xsens MVN: Full 6DOF Human Motion Tracking Using Miniature Inertial Sensors. *Xsens Motion Technol. BV Tech. Rep.* **2009**, *1*, 1–7.
36. Felius, R.A.W.; Geerars, M.; Bruijn, S.M.; van Dieën, J.H.; Wouda, N.C.; Punt, M. Reliability of IMU-Based Gait Assessment in Clinical Stroke Rehabilitation. *Sensors* **2022**, *22*, 908. [CrossRef] [PubMed]
37. Felius, R.A.W.; Geerars, M.; Bruijn, S.M.; Wouda, N.C.; Van Dieën, J.H.; Punt, M. Reliability of IMU-Based Balance Assessment in Clinical Stroke Rehabilitation. *Gait Posture* **2022**, *98*, 62–68. [CrossRef] [PubMed]

38. Kobsar, D.; Charlton, J.M.; Tse, C.T.F.; Esculier, J.-F.; Graffos, A.; Krowchuk, N.M.; Thatcher, D.; Hunt, M.A. Validity and Reliability of Wearable Inertial Sensors in Healthy Adult Walking: A Systematic Review and Meta-Analysis. *J. Neuroeng. Rehabil.* **2020**, *17*, 62. [CrossRef] [PubMed]
39. Marano, D.; Cammarata, A.; Fichera, G.; Sinatra, R.; Prati, D. Modeling of a Three-Axes MEMS Gyroscope with Feedforward PI Quadrature Compensation. In Proceedings of the Advances on Mechanics, Design Engineering and Manufacturing: Proceedings of the International Joint Conference on Mechanics, Design Engineering & Advanced Manufacturing (JCM 2016), Catania, Italy, 14–16 September 2016; Springer: Cham, Switzerland, 2016; pp. 71–80.
40. Zhao, H.; Jiang, L.; Jia, J.; Torr, P.H.S.; Koltun, V. Point Transformer. In Proceedings of the IEEE/CVF International Conference on Computer Vision, Montreal, QC, Canada, 10–17 October 2021; pp. 16259–16268.
41. Qi, C.R.; Su, H.; Mo, K.; Guibas, L.J. Pointnet: Deep Learning on Point Sets for 3d Classification and Segmentation. In Proceedings of the IEEE Conference on Computer Vision and Pattern Recognition, Honolulu, HI, USA, 21–26 July 2017; pp. 652–660.
42. Wang, Y.; Sun, Y.; Liu, Z.; Sarma, S.E.; Bronstein, M.M.; Solomon, J.M. Dynamic Graph Cnn for Learning on Point Clouds. *ACM Trans. Graph. (TOG)* **2019**, *38*, 1–12. [CrossRef]

Disclaimer/Publisher's Note: The statements, opinions and data contained in all publications are solely those of the individual author(s) and contributor(s) and not of MDPI and/or the editor(s). MDPI and/or the editor(s) disclaim responsibility for any injury to people or property resulting from any ideas, methods, instructions or products referred to in the content.

bioengineering

MDPI

Article

Lower Limb Inter-Joint Coordination and End-Point Control During Gait in Adolescents with Early Treated Unilateral Developmental Dysplasia of the Hip

Chu-Fen Chang [1,2], Tung-Wu Lu [1,3,4,*], Chia-Han Hu [1], Kuan-Wen Wu [3,4,5], Chien-Chung Kuo [6] and Ting-Ming Wang [3,4,5,*]

1 Department of Biomedical Engineering, National Taiwan University, Taipei 10617, Taiwan; cfchang711@mail.tcu.edu.tw (C.-F.C.); d12528026@ntu.edu.tw (C.-H.H.)
2 Department of Physical Therapy, Tzu Chi University, Hualien 970374, Taiwan
3 Health Science and Wellness Research Center, National Taiwan University, Taipei 10617, Taiwan; wukuanwen@gmail.com
4 Department of Orthopaedic Surgery, School of Medicine, National Taiwan University, Taipei 10617, Taiwan
5 Department of Orthopaedic Surgery, National Taiwan University Hospital, Taipei 10002, Taiwan
6 Department of Orthopaedics, China Medical University Hospital, Taichung 40447, Taiwan; d4306kcc@gmail.com
* Correspondence: twlu@ntu.edu.tw (T.-W.L.); tingmingwang@ntu.edu.tw (T.-M.W.)

Abstract: Background: Residual deficits after early treatment of developmental dysplasia of the hip (DDH) using osteotomy often led to asymmetrical gait deviations with increased repetitive rates of ground reaction force (GRF) in both hips, resulting in a higher risk of early osteoarthritis. This study investigated lower limb inter-joint coordination and swing foot control during level walking in adolescents with early-treated unilateral DDH. **Methods**: Eleven female adolescents treated early for DDH using Pemberton osteotomy were compared with 11 age-matched healthy controls. The joint angles and angular velocities of the hip, knee, and ankle were measured, and the corresponding phase angles and continuous relative phase (CRP) for hip–knee and knee–ankle coordination were obtained. The variability of inter-joint coordination was quantified using the deviation phase values obtained as the time-averaged standard deviations of the CRP curves over multiple trials. **Results**: The DDH group exhibited a flexed posture with increased variability in knee–ankle coordination of the affected limb throughout the gait cycle compared to the control group. In contrast, the unaffected limb compensated for the kinematic alterations of the affected limb with reduced peak angular velocities but increased knee–ankle CRP over double-limb support and trajectory variability over the swing phase. **Conclusions**: The identified changes in inter-joint coordination in adolescents with early treated DDH provide a plausible explanation for the previously reported increased GRF loading rates in the unaffected limb, a risk factor of premature OA.

Keywords: developmental dysplasia of the hip (DDH); Pemberton's osteotomy; gait analysis; coordination; continuous relative phase; phase plot; variability

1. Introduction

Developmental dysplasia of the hip (DDH) is characterized by a poorly developed acetabulum and displaced femoral head, often leading to hip joint instability and subluxation [1]. Undetected or untreated DDH can result in limb-length discrepancies, snapping sensation, and limited hip motion [2]. The hip incongruence and deformity also increase the joint contact pressures during walking [3], raising the risk of hip osteoarthritis (OA) [4]. In children with DDH, these changes in biomechanics lead to alterations in gait and movement control.

Early surgical correction for DDH is essential to achieve optimal functional outcomes and prevent the development of associated sequelae [5–7]. However, adolescents who underwent corrective surgery in infancy were reported to sustain repetitive loads of greater-than-normal rates on both hips around heel strike, increasing their risks of developing premature hip OA [8]. Similar findings have been observed in juveniles treated for unilateral DDH during toddlerhood, and the magnitudes of the loading rates in the lower limb joints during gait correlated with the morphology of the unaffected hip [8]. Thus, monitoring through gait analysis for changes in loading rates post-surgery is essential in identifying the residual sequelae of hip OA until growth maturity.

Human locomotion is a complex task that requires highly coordinated movements of body segments and continuous precise end-point motion control while negotiating environmental constraints to meet task demands. As a multi-segment system, the joint angles determine the position of the end-point of the lower limbs (i.e., foot segments) [9,10]; therefore, smooth and stable inter-joint coordination is essential for achieving precise control and maintaining dynamic stability during level walking [11,12]. During walking, a rapid increase in the ground reaction force (GRF) around the heel strike is linked to the impact of the foot when its velocity suddenly becomes zero [13]. Such high loading rates may initiate joint OA and accelerate damaged cartilage fibrillation, as has been observed in advanced OA [14]. Smooth endpoint contact with the ground around the heel strike can reduce the GRF loading rates, which can be achieved by proper control of the joint velocities of the lower limbs [15]. In contrast, compromised inter-joint coordination in limb control may lead to inaccurate endpoint contact, with a subsequent increase in GRF loading rates [16]. Residual deficits in the operated hip have been shown to lead to angular deviations or active compensatory changes in the lower-limb joints with high repetitive GRF loading rates during gait in children with DDH [17]. Our previous study also showed that adolescents with early-treated unilateral DDH exhibited asymmetrical gait patterns, characterized by anterior pelvic tilt, pelvic hiking on the affected side, pelvic rotation toward the unaffected side, and increased knee flexion and ankle dorsiflexion in the affected limb [13]. Thus, quantifying the coordinated movements between the lower limb joints in such patients may provide useful information to gain more insight into the effects of residual deficits on gait patterns in treated DDH hips.

The relationship between the angular positions and velocities of one joint relative to another is a common representation of inter-joint coordination involving the interplay between efferent motor control and afferent joint receptors [18]. Information on inter-joint coordination helps investigate how redundant degrees of freedom of the joints in the neuromusculoskeletal system are organized to achieve smooth, accurate, and efficient functional movement [19]. With the relative phase analysis method incorporating joint position and velocity information, the patterns and variabilities of inter-joint coordination during functional movement in various populations have been studied, including healthy young adults, older adults, and patients with diseases or injuries [11,20]. The variability observed in the relative phase plots from repeated trials served as an indicator of the stability of inter-joint coordination [20]. Generally, reduced variability is considered a lack of flexibility, while excessive variability may be associated with injury, injury risks, or conditions changing motor control patterns [18]. Considering the residual gait deviations in patients with an early reduction in unilateral DDH [13], different inter-joint coordination patterns with greater variability during level walking may be expected. More insight into lower limb inter-joint coordination may help explain the harmful loading rates around heel strike observed in patients with early reduction for unilateral DDH [17].

The current study aimed to determine the patterns and variability of inter-joint coordination in the lower extremities during gait in children treated for unilateral DDH during infancy, and to compare them with their typically developing peers. It was hypothesized that the DDH group would demonstrate altered bilateral hip–knee and knee–ankle coordination patterns during gait with greater variability than typically developing controls.

2. Materials and Methods

2.1. Participants

Eleven female adolescents with unilateral DDH treated using Pemberton osteotomy during infancy participated in the study (DDH group: age = 10.55 ± 0.99 years; age at surgery = 1.63 ± 0.47 years; postoperative duration = 8.64 ± 1.19 years; mass = 33.6 ± 8.3 kg; height = 140.82 ± 7.98 cm; leg length (LL) = affected limb = 73.27 ± 6.35 cm and unaffected limb = 72.27 ± 6.68 cm). A control group of eleven age-matched healthy peers was included for comparison (Control group: age = 10.99 ± 1.48 years; mass = 35.75 ± 7.74 kg; height = 143.52 ± 9.83 cm; LL = 76.12 ± 6.08 cm). Written consent was obtained from the participants after the Institutional Review Board approved the study and their parents or legal guardians provided informed consent. The DDH group was community ambulatory with no history of hip pain, infection, or other musculoskeletal disorders, and had not undergone any operation other than Pemberton's osteotomy. According to the X-ray data, the frontal-plane acetabular coverage increased to within the normal range six months after surgery. The sample size in each group was determined through an a priori power analysis for a two-group independent *t*-test using G*POWER [21], based on pilot data of the deviation phase (DP) values for the hip–knee and knee–ankle continuous relative phase (CRP) curves, obtained from four participants in each group. The analysis indicated that a minimum of nine participants per group would be required to achieve a statistical power of 0.8 with a large effect size (Cohen's d = 0.6) at a significance level of 0.05. Based on this estimation, 11 participants per group were considered appropriate for the current study.

2.2. Experimental Protocol

In the gait laboratory of a university hospital, every participant walked on an 8 m walkway at their preferred speed. The segmental motions of the pelvis–leg apparatus were measured using 28 retroreflective markers placed on standard anatomical landmark points commonly used in gait analysis [22,23]. Three-dimensional marker trajectories were measured using a motion capture system with seven infrared cameras (Vicon 512, Oxford Metrics Group, Oxford, UK) at 120 Hz and low-pass filtered using a fourth-order Butterworth filter with a cutoff frequency of 5 Hz before subsequent analysis, and the ground reaction forces (GRF) were measured using two force plates (AMTI, Advanced Mechanical Technology, Watertown, MA, USA) at 1080 Hz [13,24,25]. Each participant completed at least six successful trials, containing complete data for the entire gait cycle.

2.3. Data Analysis

Each segment of the pelvis–leg apparatus is represented as a rigid body. Each segment was fixed with an orthogonal coordinate system, with the positive x-axis directed anteriorly, positive y-axis superiorly, and positive z-axis directed right, following recommendations of the International Society of Biomechanics [26]. The angular displacement of a joint (joint angle) was calculated as the rotational movement of the distal segment relative to the proximal segment following a Cardanic rotation sequence of z-x-y. The angular velocities were calculated by fitting cubic splines to the time series of the angle and obtaining the first derivatives using the generalized cross-validation spline (GCVSPL) method [27]. Sign conventions of the angles and angular velocities follow the coordinate and Cardan angle definitions and are indicated in Figure 3 To reduce the negative effects of marker-skin movement artifacts, a global optimization method with joint constraints was used, which minimized the weighted sum of the squared distances of the model-experiment marker positions [17]. The peak values of the joint angles and angular velocities over the gait cycle, the values at ipsilateral and contralateral heel strike and toe off, and the subsequent ipsilateral heel strike were obtained for the statistical analysis. Standard temporospatial gait parameters, including speed, stride length, cadence, step length, and step width, were obtained. To assess the between-trial variability of the end-point trajectories, the standard deviations of the vertical and anterior–posterior components of the ensemble trajectories for the toe and heel markers were averaged over the swing phase. The stance phase was defined as the period from heel strike to toe off over the gait cycle.

To generate the phase plots of the joints, the joint angular displacements were normalized to a range between -1 and 1, centered at zero. The angular velocity values were normalized based on the maximum absolute velocity over the gait cycle [11]. These normalization procedures are helpful in reducing the influence of different movement amplitudes and frequencies [28]. For each joint, a phase plot was generated by plotting the normalized angular velocities (x') against the normalized angular displacements (x), and the angle from the positive x-axis to the ray from the origin to the point (x, x') calculated using the 2-argument arctangent function yielded the phase angle (φ) [29]. Any phase angle discontinuity with magnitudes of π or greater was corrected to less than π by adding multiples of $\pm 2\pi$ [20] (Figure 1).

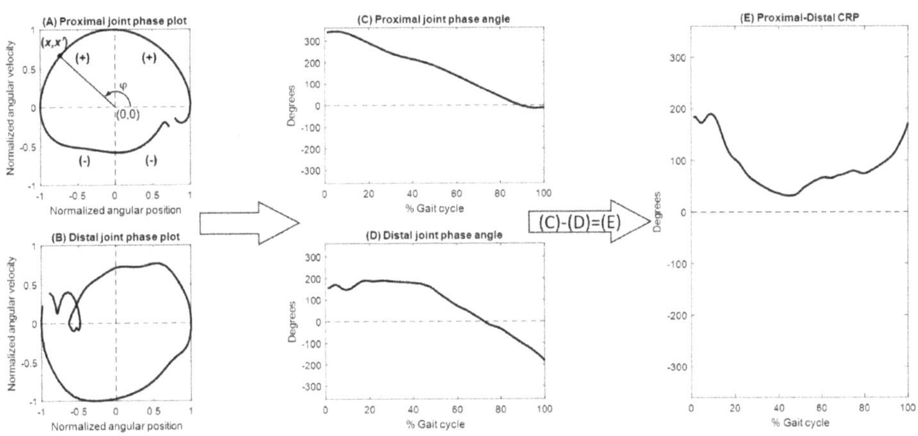

Figure 1. Schematic illustration of the analytical process for computing continuous relative phase (CRP). (**A**,**B**) depict the phase plots of the proximal and distal joints, respectively. (**C**,**D**) present the corresponding phase angles of the proximal and distal joints across the gait cycle, respectively. (**E**) shows the CRP profile obtained as the difference between the proximal and distal joint phase angles (**C**,**D**).

The coordination between two adjacent joints was described by the CRP, which was calculated by subtracting the phase angle of the distal joint from that of the proximal joint [30]. In the current study, the coordination between the hip and knee was described by the hip–knee CRP ($\varphi_{hip-knee}$) and that between the knee and ankle by the knee–ankle CRP ($\varphi_{knee-ankle}$) (Figure 2). When the CRP was close to 0° or 360°, the two adjacent joints moved in a similar pattern or in-phase, whereas the CRP was close to 180°, representing an opposite or out-of-phase fashion. When the proximal joint leads the distal joint, the CRP value is positive, whereas a negative value indicates an opposite. The CRP curves of both limbs from the six walking trials were ensemble-averaged across all participants in each subject group to obtain general inter-joint coordination patterns. For each of the initial and terminal double-leg stance (DLS), single-limb support (SLS), and swing phases, phase-averaged CRP values for each inter-joint relationship were obtained. Another parameter, the coefficient of multiple correlations (CMC) [20] was used to quantify the similarity of CRP patterns between the Control and DDH groups. A CMC value approaching unity indicates that the patterns were congruent. Root-mean-squared differences (RMSD) were used to quantify between-group differences in the ensemble-averaged CRP curves for each phase. While CMC identified temporal differences in phase shifts, RMSD characterized deviations in the relative phase pattern magnitudes and fluctuations. Therefore, a high CMC with a low RMSD denotes a similar pattern and magnitude between the two given curves. The CMC values were interpreted as follows: 0.65–0.75, moderate, 0.75–0.85 indicates good, 0.85–0.95 is very good, and 0.95–1 is excellence level [31]. The variability of inter-joint coordination was quantified by the DP values obtained as the time-averaged standard deviations of the CRP curves for each gait phase over multiple trials [28] (Figure 2). A low DP value indicates a less variable and more stable inter-joint coordination relationship.

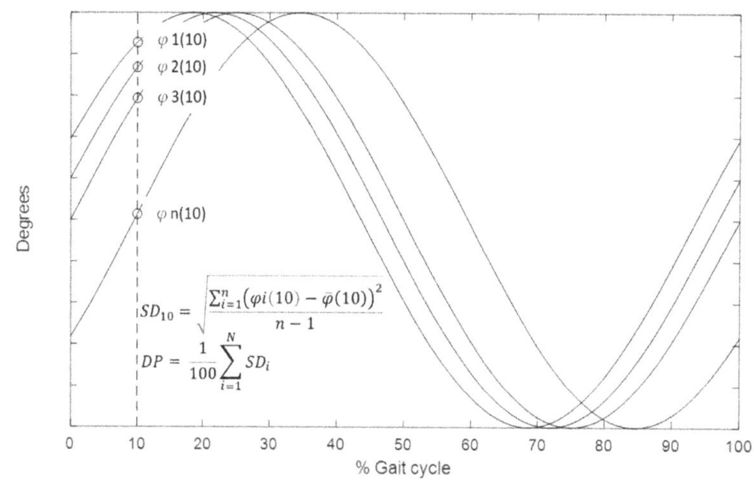

Figure 2. Schematic illustration of the computation of deviation phase (DP) values. At each time point of the gait cycle, the standard deviation (SDi) of continuous relative phase (CRP) values across multiple trials is calculated. The DP value is then obtained as the time-averaged standard deviation over the entire gait cycle, representing the variability of the CRP profiles.

2.4. Statistical Analysis

The Shapiro–Wilk test was used to determine the normality of all calculated variables. Independent *t*-tests were used to compare differences between the groups for normally distributed data, whereas paired *t*-tests were used to identify differences between the affected and unaffected limbs in the DDH group. For non-normally distributed variables, between-group differences were assessed using the Mann–Whitney U-test, whereas differences between the affected and unaffected limbs of the DDH group were detected using the Wilcoxon signed-rank test. A significance level of 0.05 was set for all tests.

3. Results

Compared with the control group, individuals with DDH showed a significant increase in step width, but without significant differences in the other spatiotemporal parameters

(Table 1). The DDH group also demonstrated a significant increase in deviation values for the end-point trajectories (both toe and heel) over the swing phase in the unaffected limb compared to the control group (Table 1). Significant differences in the joint angles were found between the affected limb and control, and between the affected and unaffected limbs, while differences in the joint angular velocities were found between the unaffected limb and control (Figure 3 and Supplementary Table S1). Over the entire gait cycle, the DDH group exhibited a more flexed posture in the affected limb with greater knee flexion and ankle dorsiflexion than the control group but without significant differences in joint angular velocities. In contrast, the unaffected limb showed significantly higher hip flexion peak velocity and ankle plantarflexion peak velocity, but lower knee joint angular velocities around toe off, without significant differences in the joint angles. The affected limb showed greater knee flexion and ankle dorsiflexion but a smaller hip extension than the unaffected limb during the entire gait cycle. No significant differences between the limbs were found in the angular velocities of any joint.

Table 1. Means (standard deviations) of the spatiotemporal parameters and the deviation values of the heel/toe end-point trajectories in the DDH and Control groups.

	Control Group	DDH Group		Pg		Ps
		Affected	Unaffected	Affected	Unaffected	
Gait speed (m/s)	1.22 (0.24)	1.13 (0.13)	1.10 (0.23)	0.306	0.314	0.819
Stride length (mm)	112.31 (9.93)	110.91 (8.52)	111.02 (7.00)	0.730	0.741	0.904
Cadence (1/s)	118.72 (12.82)	111.10 (10.94)	113.63 (12.40)	0.162	0.365	0.353
Step length (mm)	579.93 (49.23)	579.5 (39.75)	560.6 (31.01)	0.983	0.300	0.054
Step width (mm)	832.52 (268.51)	1070.30 (389.52)		0.001 *		
End-points (during the swing phase): Heel						
Anterior-posterior component (mm)	22.69 (9.12)	35.83 (24.37)	36.31 (17.71)	0.110	0.035 *	0.959
Vertical component (mm)	11.99 (5.88)	19.98 (15.19)	20.65 (10.78)	0.119	0.030 *	0.906
End-points (during the swing phase): Toe						
Anterior-posterior component (mm)	28.07 (10.65)	40.65 (31.97)	39.38 (15.68)	0.230	0.042 *	0.907
Vertical component (mm)	5.35 (0.85)	8.47 (5.05)	9.80 (2.74)	0.069	0.001 *	0.451

Pg: *p*-values for between-group comparisons using U-test; Ps: *p*-values for between-limb comparisons in the DDH group using Wilcoxon signed ranks test; *: Significant difference ($p < 0.05$).

Both groups showed nearly closed limit circles for the phase trajectories of the hip, knee, and ankle; however, the phase plots for the ankle exhibited different trajectories (Figure 4). The differences between the groups in each phase trajectory were visible during DLS (Figure 5).

Both groups displayed similar patterns of inter-joint coordination in the hip–knee and knee–ankle CRP curves (Figure 5). For the hip–knee CRP patterns over the gait phases, good to excellent correlations (CMC: 0.79 to 0.94) with the control group were found for both the affected and unaffected limbs of the DDH group (Table 2). No significant between-group or between-limb differences in the phase-averaged CRP values for the DDH group were found in the hip–knee CRP curves ($p > 0.05$; Table 2), with between-group RMSD values ranging from 2.52° to 13.53° for both the affected and unaffected limbs (Table 2). No significant between-group differences were found in DP values for any gait phase, regardless of the affected or unaffected limb ($p > 0.05$; Table 3).

For the knee–ankle CRP patterns over the gait phases, the affected limb showed good to excellent correlation with the control group (CMC: 0.75 to 0.85), while the unaffected limb showed almost no correlation with the control (Table 2). No significant between-group or between-limb differences were found in the phase-averaged CRP values for most gait phases ($p > 0.05$), except for the initial and terminal DLS of the unaffected limb, which showed significantly greater phase-averaged CRP values than the control ($p < 0.05$; Table 2).

The RMSD values for the affected and unaffected limbs ranged from 5.46° to 15.69° over most gait phases, except for the initial and terminal DLS of the unaffected limb, which had RMSD values of 20.94° and 40.93°, respectively (Table 3). For inter-joint coordination variabilities, significantly greater DP values of the knee–ankle CRP in the affected limb were found during the stance phase of the DDH group (i.e., DLS and SLS) than in the controls (Table 3).

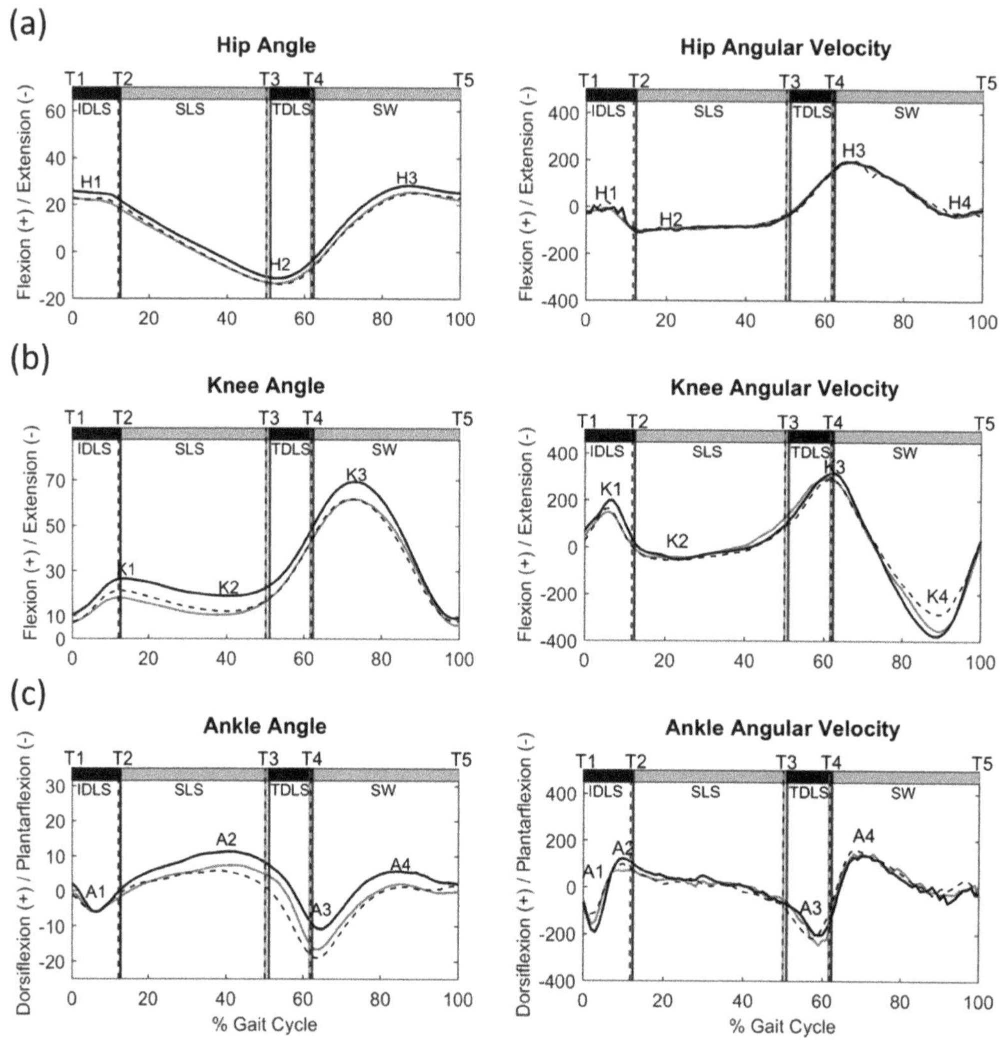

Figure 3. Ensemble–averaged angles (°) and angular velocities (°/s) of (**a**) the hip, (**b**) knee and (**c**) ankle of the affected limb (black, solid line) and unaffected limb (black, dotted line) in the DDH group and Control group (grey, solid line) during level walking. T1: Heel strike; T2: Contralateral toe off; T3: Contralateral heel strike; T4: Toe off; T5: Subsequent heel strike; H1–H4: Peaks and troughs in the hip curves; K1–K4: Peaks and troughs in the knee curves; A1–A4: peaks and troughs in the ankle curve.

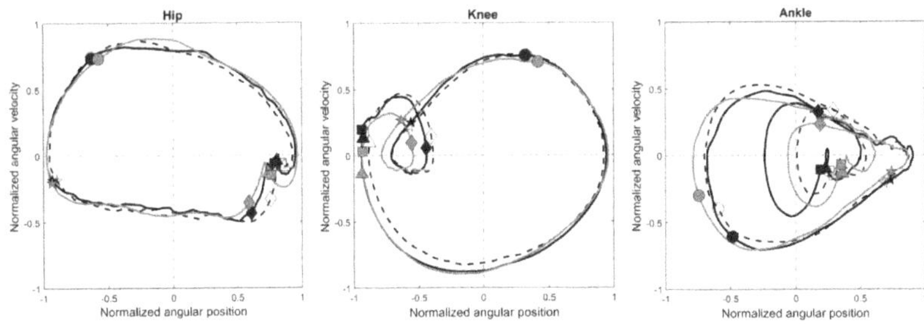

Figure 4. Ensemble−averaged phase plots of the hip, the knee and the ankle of the affected limb (black, solid line) and unaffected limb (black, dotted line) in the DDH group and the Control group (grey, solid line) during level walking. Square markers: Heel strike; Diamond markers: Contralateral toe off; Pentagram markers: Contralateral heel strike; Circular markers: Toe off; Triangular markers: Subsequent heel strike.

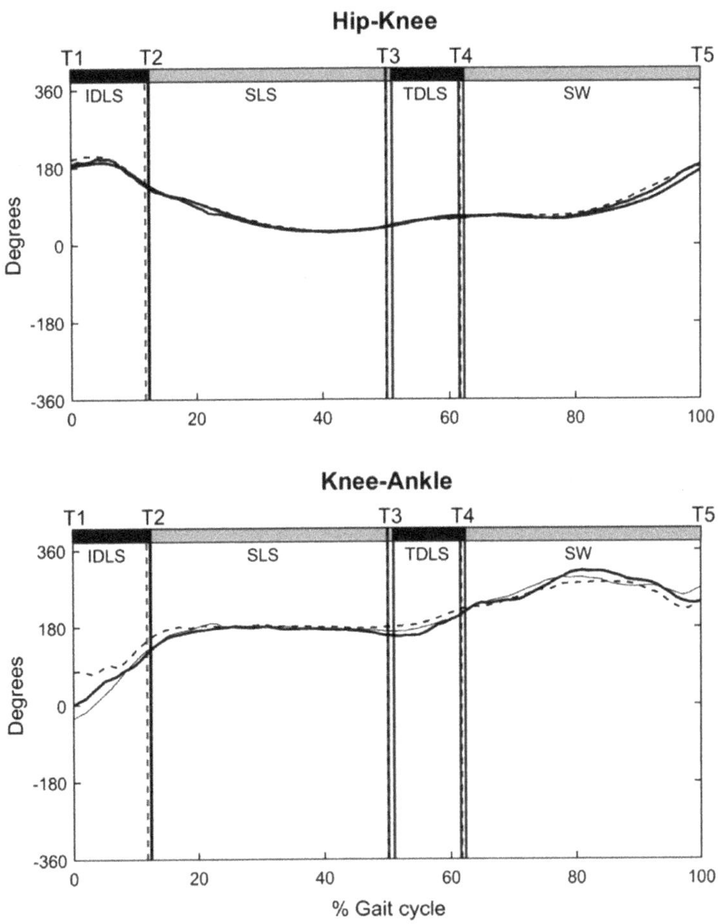

Figure 5. Ensemble−averaged CRP curves of the hip−knee and knee−ankle coordination of the affected limb (black, solid line) and unaffected limb (black, dotted line) in the DDH group and the Control group (grey, solid line) during gait.

Table 2. Means (standard deviations) of phase-averaged CRP of the hip–knee and knee–ankle coordination and coefficient of multiple correlation (CMC) values and the RMS differences (RMSD) of the CRP curves between DDH and Control groups.

Phase	CRP	Control Group	DDH Group		Pg		Ps	CMC		RMSD	
			Affected	Unaffected	Affected	Unaffected		Affected	Unaffected	Affected	Unaffected
Initial DLS	Hip–Knee	177.99 (13.08)	180.75 (16.62)	187.01 (11.07)	0.670	0.096	0.311	0.94	0.83	6.05	11.57
	Knee–Ankle	62.21 (77.97)	43.62 (42.29)	97.66 (57.41)	0.495	0.023 *	0.210	0.85	0.31	15.32	40.93
SLS	Hip–Knee	63.45 (9.87)	59.67 (9.04)	63.48 (8.88)	0.360	0.994	0.330	0.97	0.99	4.97	2.52
	Knee–Ankle	172.30 (9.77)	174.12 (7.44)	179.69 (8.27)	0.629	0.700	0.112	0.75	0.02	5.46	9.46
Terminal DLS	Hip–Knee	56.75 (11.72)	55.18 (10.54)	52.68 (8.69)	0.743	0.366	0.552	0.91	0.79	2.74	4.26
	Knee–Ankle	178.24 (18.43)	184.52 (21.92)	196.39 (16.97)	0.475	0.026 *	0.171	0.76	0.09	10.01	20.94
Swing	Hip–Knee	89.18 (9.03)	91.93 (6.54)	96.38 (13.86)	0.424	0.164	0.346	0.94	0.86	8.99	13.53
	Knee–Ankle	277.99 (35.92)	268.57 (20.11)	257.21 (22.49)	0.456	0.119	0.226	0.75	0.71	14.19	15.69

SLS: Single limb support; DLS: Double limb support; Pg: *p*-values for between-group comparisons using U-test; Ps: *p*-values for between-limb comparisons in the DDH group using Wilcoxon signed ranks test; *: Significant difference ($p < 0.05$).

Table 3. Means (standard deviation) of the DP values for CRP curves of the DDH and Control groups.

Phase	CRP	Control Group	DDH Group		Pg		Ps
			Affected	Unaffected	Affected	Unaffected	
Initial DLS	Hip–Knee	16.80 (8.33)	26.00 (9.92)	22.22 (8.42)	0.360	0.163	0.369
	Knee–Ankle	8.81 (2.92)	11.72 (5.51)	10.31 (3.78)	0.040 *	0.156	0.514
SLS	Hip–Knee	8.49 (4.02)	6.59 (3.19)	6.63 (3.04)	0.254	0.256	0.976
	Knee–Ankle	7.86 (2.87)	11.69 (4.41)	8.97 (4.30)	0.032 *	0.507	0.176
Terminal DLS	Hip–Knee	66.44 (34.64)	62.77 (27.48)	55.21 (27.93)	0.796	0.434	0.549
	Knee–Ankle	12.49 (4.06)	15.49 (10.08)	14.44 (5.97)	0.039 *	0.404	0.777
Swing	Hip–Knee	13.77 (6.04)	16.02 (7.54)	18.05 (6.37)	0.469	0.138	0.522
	Knee–Ankle	22.46 (9.74)	29.02 (14.79)	26.31 (15.43)	0.255	0.513	0.692

SLS: Single limb support; DLS: Double limb support; Pg: *p*-values for between-group comparisons using U-test; Ps: *p*-values for between-limb comparisons in the DDH group using Wilcoxon signed ranks test; *: Significant difference ($p < 0.05$).

4. Discussion

The DDH group adopted a more flexed posture in the affected limb throughout the gait cycle with significantly increased knee flexion and ankle dorsiflexion compared to the Control, but with no significant differences in joint angular velocities (Table 2). The observed more flexed posture of the affected limb may be related to residual deficits in muscle strength, such as hip flexors and abductors, and knee extensors in the affected limb, which are often observed in patients treated with DDH [13]. While the observed angular displacement and velocity changes corresponded with altered phase trajectories of the knee and ankle (Figure 5), the inter-joint coordination patterns in the affected limb remained comparable to those of healthy controls, as suggested by the good to excellent correlations and low RMSD of the CRP curves (Table 3). In contrast, although the unaffected limb showed similar joint angles to the controls, differences in joint angular velocities around initial and terminal DLS were observed (Table 2), which were associated with variations in the phase trajectories of the knee and ankle (Figure 5) and lower correlations with the knee–ankle inter-joint coordination patterns of the healthy controls. From the current results, it appears that the unaffected limb compensated for the changes in the affected limb by altering the joint angular velocities, which are more likely controlled by normal muscle strength, and thus knee–ankle coordination to maintain close to normal inter-joint coordination patterns in the affected limb.

While the affected limb showed inter-joint coordination patterns similar to those of the healthy control, the knee–ankle coordination during the stance phase was less stable than that of the control group, with DP values greater than those of the control. Excessive variability may indicate a less stable movement pattern [11,18]. The greater variability of the knee–ankle coordination in the affected limb during stance corresponded to the greater variability of the swing foot and toe trajectories of the unaffected limb during the swing phase and shortly before heel strike. Precision control of the endpoint of the lower limb throughout the swing phase is essential for smooth heel contact to reduce GRF loading rates [9,16,32]. Previous studies have found that adolescents treated for DDH show significantly increased loading rates in both the affected and unaffected limbs [8]. It has been suggested that impaired control over the swing limb after osteotomy may increase the loading rates of the GRF, extending to the lower limb joints [33]. The current findings provide a possible explanation for increased GRF loading rates observed in the unaffected limb. That is, the less stable control of the knee–ankle inter-joint coordination in the affected limb during stance led to greater variability in the trajectories of the swing foot and endpoints and the subsequent impact on the ground, and thus increased GRF loading rates, a factor closely related to the development of OA [8].

Only female adolescents with early treated unilateral DDH were included in the current study because females are 5–9 times more likely to be affected than males [34], making it feasible to recruit a clinically homogeneous sample. Although sex differences in motor control strategies have been reported, particularly in adults, this study focused on a typical adolescent female cohort without aiming to examine sex-related differences in movement control. Further research may be needed to determine whether male patients have comparable inter-joint control strategies. Future investigations may also include patients with bilateral DDH. Functional tasks that demand more joint motion, such as stair walking and sit-to-stand movements, may be needed to provide deeper insights into the mechanical functions of DDH. Future investigations may benefit from comparing patient-specific joint angles with the established normative range of motion data to better characterize active compensatory strategies in both the affected and unaffected limbs. Including the trunk segment in inter-joint coordination in other planes may be necessary for pathological conditions that involve whole-body movement beyond the sagittal plane.

5. Conclusions

In addition to significant changes in the individual joint kinematics, the adolescents with early treated DDH also changed the way the motions of the lower limb joints are coordinated during level walking and displayed asymmetrical inter-joint coordination patterns between limbs. Compared to the Control, the DDH group showed a more flexed posture with increased variability in knee–ankle CRP curves in the affected limb throughout the gait cycle. It appears that the unaffected limb compensated for the kinematic alterations of the affected limb with decreased peak joint angular velocities but increased the knee–ankle CRP mean values over double-limb support and trajectory variability over the swing phase. The observed greater variability in the knee–ankle inter-joint coordination of the affected limb during stance and the trajectories of the end-points of the unaffected swing foot provide a possible explanation for the increased GRF loading rates in the unaffected limb, a risk factor for the initiation of OA at the lower limb joints.

Supplementary Materials: The following supporting information can be downloaded at: https://www.mdpi.com/article/10.3390/bioengineering12080836/s1, Table S1: Means (standard deviations) of the angles and angular velocities at the hip, knee and ankle joints in the DDH and Control groups.

Author Contributions: C.-F.C.: data curation, resources, and writing—original draft; T.-W.L.: conceptualization, methodology, supervision, writing—original draft, and writing—review and editing; C.-H.H.: formal analysis, and writing—original draft; K.-W.W.: data curation and writing—original draft; C.-C.K.: data curation and writing—original draft; T.-M.W.: conceptualization, resources, supervision and writing—review and editing. All authors have read and agreed to the published version of the manuscript.

Funding: The authors are grateful for the financial support from the National Science Council of Taiwan (Grant Number: NSC 90-2314-B-002-223).

Institutional Review Board Statement: The study was conducted in accordance with the Declaration of Helsinki, and approved by the Institutional Review Board of National Taiwan Hospital University.

Informed Consent Statement: Informed consent was obtained from all subjects involved in the study.

Data Availability Statement: The datasets used and/or analyzed during the current study are available from the corresponding author upon reasonable request.

Acknowledgments: We sincerely thank all the participants who generously volunteered their time and contributed to this study.

Conflicts of Interest: The authors declare no conflicts of interest with any financial organization regarding the materials discussed in this manuscript.

References

1. Nandhagopal, T.; De Cicco, F.L. *Developmental Dysplasia of the Hip*; StatPearls Publishing LLC.: Treasure Island, FL, USA, 2024.
2. Han, J.; Li, Y. Progress in screening strategies for neonatal developmental dysplasia of the hip. *Front. Surg.* **2022**, *9*, 995949. [CrossRef] [PubMed]
3. Constantinou, M.; Loureiro, A.; Carty, C.; Mills, P.; Barrett, R. Hip joint mechanics during walking in individuals with mild-to-moderate hip osteoarthritis. *Gait Posture* **2017**, *53*, 162–167. [CrossRef]
4. Scott, E.J.; Dolan, L.A.; Weinstein, S.L. Closed Vs. Open Reduction/Salter Innominate Osteotomy for Developmental Hip Dislocation After Age 18 Months: Comparative Survival at 45-Year Follow-up. *J. Bone Jt. Surg. Am.* **2020**, *102*, 1351–1357. [CrossRef] [PubMed]
5. Pemberton, P.A. Pericapsular osteotomy of the ilium for the treatment of congenitally dislocated hips. *Clin. Orthop. Relat. Res.* **1974**, *98*, 41–54. [CrossRef] [PubMed]
6. Young, J.R.; Anderson, M.J.; O'Connor, C.M.; Kazley, J.M.; Mantica, A.L.; Dutt, V. Team approach: Developmental dysplasia of the hip. *JBJS Rev.* **2020**, *8*, e20. [CrossRef]
7. Çiçekli, Ö.; Doğan, M. Evaluation of surgical outcome in advanced age patients with developmental hip dysplasia. *Int. J. Surg.* **2018**, *52*, 44–49. [CrossRef]

8. Chang, C.F.; Wang, T.M.; Wang, J.H.; Huang, S.C.; Lu, T.W. Adolescents After Pemberton's Osteotomy for Developmental Dysplasia of the Hip Displayed Greater Joint Loading than Healthy Controls in Affected and Unaffected Limbs during Gait. *J. Orthop. Res.* **2011**, *29*, 1034–1041. [CrossRef]
9. Ivanenko, Y.P.; Cappellini, G.; Dominici, N.; Poppele, R.E.; Lacquaniti, F. Modular control of limb movements during human locomotion. *J. Neurosci.* **2007**, *27*, 11149–11161. [CrossRef]
10. Hicheur, H.; Terekhov, A.V.; Berthoz, A. Intersegmental coordination during human locomotion: Does planar covariation of elevation angles reflect central constraints? *J. Neurophysiol.* **2006**, *96*, 1406–1419. [CrossRef]
11. Chiu, S.L.; Lu, T.W.; Chou, L.S. Altered Inter-joint Coordination during Walking in Patients with Total Hip Arthroplasty. *Gait Posture* **2010**, *32*, 656–660. [CrossRef]
12. Winter, D.A. Foot trajectory in human gait: A precise and multifactorial motor control task. *Phys. Ther.* **1992**, *72*, 45–53. [CrossRef]
13. Chang, C.-F.; Wang, T.-M.; Wang, J.-H.; Huang, S.-C.; Lu, T.-W. Residual gait deviations in adolescents treated during infancy for unilateral developmental dysplasia of the hip using Pemberton's osteotomy. *Gait Posture* **2012**, *35*, 561–566. [CrossRef]
14. Jørgensen, A.E.M.; Kjær, M.; Heinemeier, K.M. The effect of aging and mechanical loading on the metabolism of articular cartilage. *J. Rheumatol.* **2017**, *44*, 410–417. [CrossRef] [PubMed]
15. Tajima, T.; Tateuchi, H.; Koyama, Y.; Ikezoe, T.; Ichihashi, N. Gait strategies to reduce the dynamic joint load in the lower limbs during a loading response in young healthy adults. *Human. Mov. Sci.* **2018**, *58*, 260–267. [CrossRef] [PubMed]
16. Shih, Y.; Teng, H.-L.; Powers, C.M. Lower extremity stiffness predicts ground reaction force loading rate in heel strike runners. *Med. Sci. Sports Exerc.* **2019**, *51*, 1692–1697. [CrossRef]
17. Lee, W.C.; Chen, T.Y.; Hung, L.W.; Wang, T.M.; Chang, C.H.; Lu, T.W. Increased Loading Rates During Gait Correlate With Morphology of Unaffected Hip in Juveniles With Treated Developmental Hip Dysplasia. *Front. Bioeng. Biotechnol.* **2021**, *9*, 704266. [CrossRef] [PubMed]
18. Bars, S.L.; Bourgeois-Gironde, S.; Wyart, V.; Sari, I.; Pacherie, E.; Chambon, V. Motor Coordination and Strategic Cooperation in Joint Action. *Psychol. Sci.* **2022**, *33*, 736–751. [CrossRef]
19. St-Onge, N.; Feldman, A.G. Interjoint coordination in lower limbs during different movements in humans. *Exp. Brain Res.* **2003**, *148*, 139–149. [CrossRef]
20. Kuo, C.C.; Chen, S.C.; Wang, J.Y.; Ho, T.J.; Lin, J.G.; Lu, T.W. Effects of Tai-Chi Chuan Practice on Patterns and Stability of Lower Limb Inter-Joint Coordination During Obstructed Gait in the Elderly. *Front. Bioeng. Biotechnol.* **2021**, *9*, 739722. [CrossRef]
21. Erdfelder, E.; Faul, F.; Buchner, A. GPOWER: A general power analysis program. *Behav. Res. Methods Instrum. Comput.* **1996**, *28*, 1–11. [CrossRef]
22. Wu, G.; Van der Helm, F.C.; Veeger, H.D.; Makhsous, M.; Van Roy, P.; Anglin, C.; Nagels, J.; Karduna, A.R.; McQuade, K.; Wang, X. ISB recommendation on definitions of joint coordinate systems of various joints for the reporting of human joint motion—Part II: Shoulder, elbow, wrist and hand. *J. Biomech.* **2005**, *38*, 981–992. [CrossRef] [PubMed]
23. Wu, G.; Siegler, S.; Allard, P.; Kirtley, C.; Leardini, A.; Rosenbaum, D.; Whittle, M.; D D'Lima, D.; Cristofolini, L.; Witte, H. ISB recommendation on definitions of joint coordinate system of various joints for the reporting of human joint motion—Part I: Ankle, hip, and spine. *J. Biomech.* **2002**, *35*, 543–548. [CrossRef]
24. Kim, H.K.; Dai, X.; Lu, S.-H.; Lu, T.-W.; Chou, L.-S. Discriminating features of ground reaction forces in overweight old and young adults during walking using functional principal component analysis. *Gait Posture* **2022**, *94*, 166–172. [CrossRef]
25. Kim, H.K.; Lu, S.-H.; Lu, T.-W.; Chou, L.-S. Contribution of lower extremity muscles to center of mass acceleration during walking: Effect of body weight. *J. Biomech.* **2023**, *146*, 111398. [CrossRef]
26. Grood, E.S.; Suntay, W.J. A joint coordinate system for the clinical description of three-dimensional motions: Application to the knee. *J. Biomech. Eng.* **1983**, *136*, 144. [CrossRef]
27. Woltring, H.J. A Fortran package for generalized, cross-validatory spline smoothing and differentiation. *Adv. Eng. Softw.* **1986**, *8*, 104–113. [CrossRef]
28. Stergiou, N.; Scholten, S.D.; Jensen, J.L.; Blanke, D. Intralimb coordination following obstacle clearance during running: The effect of obstacle height. *Gait Posture* **2001**, *13*, 210–220. [CrossRef]
29. Kurz, M.J.; Stergiou, N. Effect of Normalization and Phase Angle Calculations on Continuous Relative Phase. *J. Biomech.* **2002**, *35*, 369–374. [CrossRef]
30. Burgess-Limerick, R.; Abernethy, B.; Neal, R.J. Relative Phase Quantifies Interjoint Coordination. *J. Biomech.* **1993**, *26*, 91–94. [CrossRef] [PubMed]
31. Ferrari, A.; Cutti, A.G.; Garofalo, P.; Raggi, M.; Heijboer, M.; Cappello, A.; Davalli, A. First in Vivo Assessment of "Outwalk": A Novel Protocol for Clinical Gait Analysis Based on Inertial and Magnetic Sensors. *Med. Biol. Eng. Comput.* **2010**, *48*, 1–15. [CrossRef] [PubMed]
32. Schmitz, A.; Pohl, M.B.; Woods, K.; Noehren, B. Variables during swing associated with decreased impact peak and loading rate in running. *J. Biomech.* **2014**, *47*, 32–38. [CrossRef] [PubMed]

33. Silverman, A.K.; Fey, N.P.; Portillo, A.; Walden, J.G.; Bosker, G.; Neptune, R.R. Compensatory mechanisms in below-knee amputee gait in response to increasing steady-state walking speeds. *Gait Posture* **2008**, *28*, 602–609. [CrossRef] [PubMed]
34. Woodacre, T.; Ball, T.; Cox, P. Epidemiology of developmental dysplasia of the hip within the UK: Refining the risk factors. *J. Child. Orthop.* **2016**, *10*, 633–642. [CrossRef] [PubMed]

Disclaimer/Publisher's Note: The statements, opinions and data contained in all publications are solely those of the individual author(s) and contributor(s) and not of MDPI and/or the editor(s). MDPI and/or the editor(s) disclaim responsibility for any injury to people or property resulting from any ideas, methods, instructions or products referred to in the content.

bioengineering

MDPI

Article

In Vitro Biomechanical Experiment on the Effect of Unilateral Partial Facetectomy Performed by Percutaneous Endoscopy on the Stability of Lumbar Spine

Tao Ma [1,2,†], Xiaoshuang Tu [1,2,†], Junyang Li [1,2,†], Jingwei Wu [1,2] and Luming Nong [1,3,4,*]

1 Orthopedics Department, The Third Affiliated Hospital of Nanjing Medical University, Changzhou 213164, China; matao@stu.njmu.edu.cn (T.M.); 13330732948@163.com (X.T.); 2024122109@stu.njmu.edu.cn (J.L.); wujingwei1999@outlook.com (J.W.)
2 Orthopaedics Department, Nanjing Medical University, Nanjing 211103, China
3 Changzhou Medical Center, Nanjing Medical University, Changzhou 213164, China
4 The Affiliated Changzhou No.2 People's Hospital of Nanjing Medical University, No.29 Xinglong Lane, Tianning District, Changzhou 213000, China
* Correspondence: tessys2008@163.com; Tel.: +86-138-6115-7520
† These authors are co-first authors of the article.

Abstract: Objectives: This study's purpose is to investigate the lumbar biomechanical effects of unilateral partial facetectomy (UPF) of different facet joint (FJ) portions under percutaneous endoscopy. Methods: Forty fresh calf spine models were used to simulate UPF under a physiological load performed through three commonly used needle insertion points (IPs): (1) The apex of the superior FJ (as the first IP); (2) The midpoint of the ventral side of the superior FJ (as the second IP); (3) The lowest point of the ventral side of the superior FJ (as the third IP). The range of motion (ROM) and the L4/5 intradiscal maximum pressure (IMP) were measured and analyzed under a physiological load in all models during flexion, extension, left–right lateral flexion, and left–right axial rotation. Results: When UPF was performed through the second IP, the ROM of the lumbar spine and the L4/5 IMP in the calf spine models were not statistically different from the intact calf spine model. Conclusions: UPF through the second IP resulted in a minimal impact on the biomechanics of the lumbar spine. Thus, it might be considered the most appropriate IP for UPF.

Keywords: biomechanics; bioengineering; preclinical studies; therapeutics; unilateral partial facetectomy

1. Introduction

Lumbar hypermobility following traditional open spinal surgery is a major cause of chronic low back pain, affecting long-term patient outcomes [1,2]. This instability often results from the disruption of spinal anatomical structures during surgical interventions. To address these limitations, percutaneous endoscopic transforaminal discectomy (PETD) has emerged as a minimally invasive alternative, offering reduced tissue damage and faster recovery [3,4]. However, a critical challenge in PETD is the unavoidable partial resection of the facet joint (FJ) to access the spinal canal [5–8]. Clinical studies indicate that such resection may lead to postoperative hypermobility [9,10], underscoring the need to balance decompression with biomechanical preservation. The facet joints are pivotal in maintaining spinal stability by resisting compression, shear, and rotational forces [11,12]. Disruption of their integrity redistributes stress to adjacent structures, accelerating degeneration [13,14].

Prior biomechanical studies primarily focused on facetectomy volume [15], yet neglected the impact of resection location—a critical factor in clinical practice where surgeons select specific insertion points (IPs). This study aims to systematically evaluate the biomechanical effects of unilateral partial facetectomy (UPF) performed through three clinically relevant IPs. By measuring intradiscal pressure (IMP) and range of motion (ROM), we identify the optimal IP that minimizes biomechanical disruption.

2. Materials and Methods

2.1. Calf Spine Specimen Preparation

Fifty fresh calf lumbar segments (L3–L6) were collected from 15-month-old calves with uniform weight and spinal status, and all specimens were X-rulated for structural integrity, excluding fractures, tumors, and severe osteoporosis, and 40 were used in follow-up experiments. All specimens were wrapped in gauze soaked in saline, sealed in a double-layer plastic bag, and stored at −20 °C. Before testing, specimens were first thawed at 4 °C for 12 h to minimize structural damage [16], followed by an additional 8 h thawing period at room temperature. During this period, ice cubes were placed around the specimens to maintain a low temperature and prevent tissue degeneration. Subsequently, muscle and adipose tissue were carefully removed, preserving the integrity of the bony structures, intervertebral discs, facet joints, and ligaments. The integrity of the bony structure, lumbar intervertebral disc, FJ, and ligament tissue should be maintained by paying attention during the handling of the specimen, which was then covered with gauze soaked in saline to keep it moist. Since the calf specimens possessed a long transverse process, all calf specimens were partially cut (retaining approximately 7 cm in length) in order to facilitate the experimental operation. The two ends of the L3 and L6 segments of the specimen were fixed in a special test mold using Kirschner wires, embedded in self-curing denture powder (dental polymethyl methacrylate), and kept horizontal to facilitate the installation of the specimen on the loading device.

2.2. Insertion Point (IP) Determination

According to the actual clinical surgery method, facetectomy was performed by removing the ventral side of the superior FJ up to the dorsal side. Thus, three commonly used clinical needle IPs were selected: (1) The apex of the superior FJ (as the first IP); (2) The midpoint of the ventral side of the superior FJ (as the second IP); (3) The lowest point of the ventral side of the superior FJ (as the third IP). In this experiment, a trephine with a diameter of 7.5 mm commonly used in clinical surgery was used to simulate the UPF.

2.3. Facetectomy Simulation and Grouping

Calf Spine Model

Figure 1 shows the percutaneous lumbar facetectomy instrument used in the experiment. First, the tip of the duckbill protective sleeve was pushed from the lateral posterior approach through the lower half of the left intervertebral foramen of the specimen to the level of the upper endplate of the L5. The oblique opening of the sleeve faced the back side of the lumbar spine and the sleeve pressed against the IP on the L5 superior FJ. The sleeve formed an angle of 20° with the coronal surface of the lumbar spine specimen and was parallel to the plane of the intervertebral disc. The intervertebral foramen was formed and enlarged by the matching trephine through the inner cavity of the protective sleeve. The inner diameter of the enlarged protective sleeve was 8.0 mm, and the outer diameter of the trephine was 7.5 mm. Forty fresh calf spine specimens were randomly divided into 4 groups with 10 specimens in each group. The control group was represented by the intact calf spine. Group A was represented by the calf spine model in which UPF was performed through the first IP. Group B was represented by the calf spine model in which UPF was performed through the second IP. Group C was represented by the calf spine model in which UPF was performed through the third IP. Figure 2 shows the calf spine models after UPF.

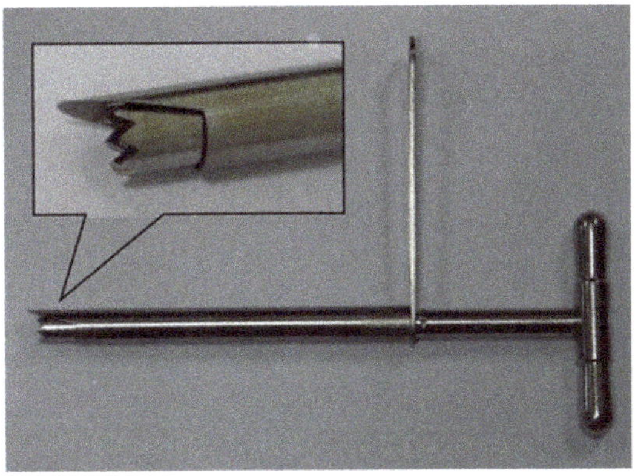

Figure 1. The trephine used in the biomechanical experiment of calf spine specimens.

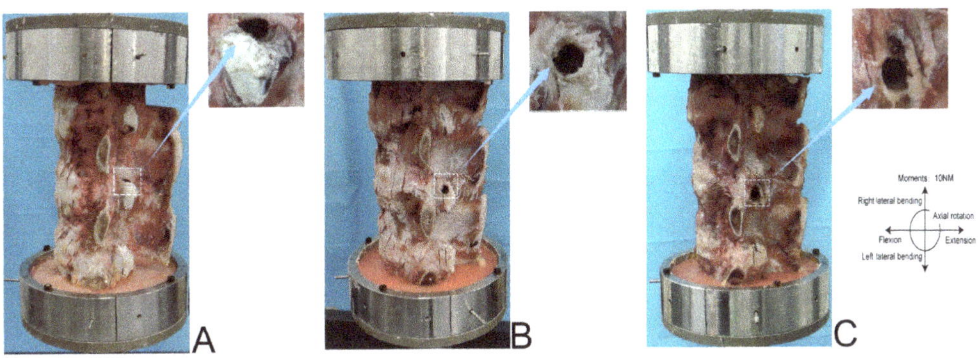

Figure 2. The schematic diagram of L5 left superior facet joint resection in the calf spine specimens: (**A**) Group A. (**B**) Group B. (**C**) Group C.

2.4. Model Boundaries and Load Conditions

Calf Spine Model

IMP and ROM were chosen as the core parameters because they reflect intervertebral disc load distribution (IMP) and spinal range of motion (ROM), respectively, which are the gold standards for evaluating postoperative stability. A scalpel was used to perform a horizontal incision of 1 cm parallel to the endplate of the vertebral body in the center of the L4/5 intervertebral disc, the needle to test the pressure (approximately 1 mm in diameter) was inserted parallel to the endplate of the vertebral body into the posterior edge of the intervertebral disc, and the Gaeltec pressure sensor was connected to measure the IMP. Before the test, the calf spine specimens were fixed on the Intron E10000 tension and torsion biaxial universal material biomechanical testing machine using a special fixture for testing calf spine mechanics. An electronic digital level for a spine biomechanical test installed above the special fixture was present to measure lumbar spine ROM (Figure 3). According to the standards of the calf spine specimen test proposed by Wilke et al. [17], the torque was set to 10 N·m and the constant axial force was set to 400 N. The specimens were loaded and unloaded twice to remove their viscoelasticity before measuring the ROM of the calf spine flexion, extension, lateral bending, axial rotation, and the L4/5 IMP, in order to ensure the accuracy of the data, and the results were recorded on the third round of measurements, so that relatively stable kinematic test data could be obtained. The specimens were continuously sprayed with saline during the entire test to keep them moist and minimize tissue degeneration.

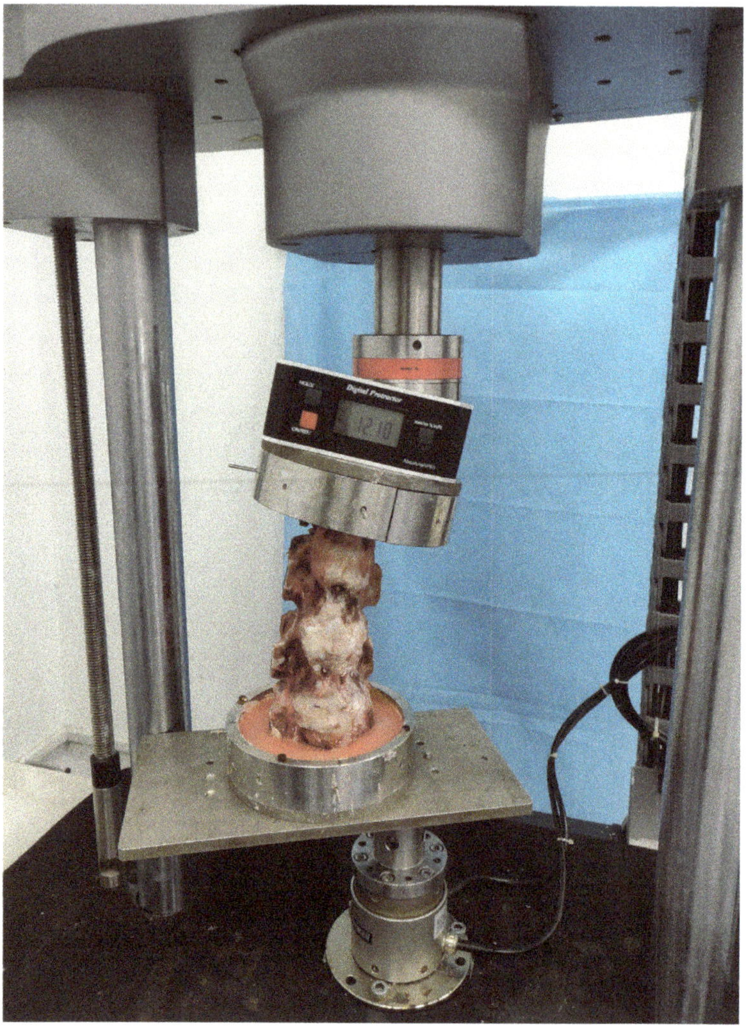

Figure 3. The Intron E10000 tension and torsion biaxial universal material biomechanical testing machine and electronic digital level for calf spine specimens biomechanical test.

2.5. Statistical Analysis

Statistical analysis was performed using SPSS (version 22.0; IBM Corp., Armonk, NY, USA). The mean and standard deviation (SD) of IMP and ROM were calculated using one-way ANOVA and the measured data were expressed as "x ± s". All reported *p* values were two-tailed, and *p* values less than 0.05 were considered statistically significant.

3. Results

3.1. Calf Spine Models

3.1.1. L4/5 IMP

The data of the pressure sensor in the L4/5 intervertebral disc of the calf spine specimen were recorded and analyzed. The L4/5 IMP showed a significant increase among Groups A, B, C, and the control group in flexion, extension, left–right lateral flexion, and left–right axial rotation. The L4/5 IMP significantly increased under extension in Group A compared with the control group ($p < 0.05$). The L4/5 IMP slightly increased in Group B compared with its value in the control group during extension and left–right axial rotation, but the difference was not statistically significant. The difference in flexion and left–right lateral flexion was also not statistically significant compared with the control group. Compared to the control group, in flexion, extension, left–right lateral flexion, and left–right axial rotation, the L4/5 IMP (intervertebral disc space) in Group C showed a significant increase. ($p < 0.05$). The detailed data are listed in Table 1.

Table 1. The L4/5 intradiscal maximum pressure of calf spine specimens after facetectomy (Kpa).

Grouping	Control	A	B	C	*F* Value	*p* Value
Flexion	572.48 ± 23.38	694.91 ± 29.65	654.64 ± 15.99	729.48 ± 24.22 [a]	54.926	$p < 0.001$
Extension	627.53 ± 41.22	941.51 ± 39.62 [a]	714.05 ± 41.35	1000.23 ± 52.32 [a]	66.921	$p < 0.001$
Left lateral flexion	556.37 ± 43.42	682.89 ± 51.74	638.08 ± 33.68	715.79 ± 46.29 [a]	78.891	$p < 0.001$
Right lateral flexion	578.47 ± 52.12	705.20 ± 55.48	664.88 ± 43.15	738.40 ± 46.53 [a]	68.212	$p < 0.001$
Left axial rotation	685.28 ± 37.42	794.08 ± 48.26	742.27 ± 33.82	1123.47 ± 33.58 [a]	88.651	$p < 0.001$
Right axial rotation	663.78 ± 46.96	786.45 ± 45.92	725.11 ± 47.15	1047.60 ± 51.62 [a]	85.621	$p < 0.001$

Note: Compared to the control group, [a] $p < 0.05$.

3.1.2. ROM

The ROM of the calf spine specimens was obtained by recording the electronic digital level on the upper end of the specimen fixture (Table 2). There was a significant increase in ROM between Group A, B, C and the control group in left–right axial rotation, with no significant differences in flexion, extension, and left–right lateral flexion. No significant difference in ROM was found under the six motions of flexion and extension, left–right lateral flexion, and left–right axial rotation in Group A and Group B compared with the control group. No significant difference in ROM was found under the four motions of flexion and extension, left–right lateral flexion and left–right axial rotation in Group C compared with the control group. However, the ROM was significantly increased under left–right axial rotation in Group C compared with its value in the control group ($p < 0.05$).

Table 2. The range of motion of calf spine specimens after facetectomy (°).

Grouping	Control	A	B	C	*F* Value	*p* Value
Flexion	10.23 ± 2.09	11.44 ± 3.29	11.55 ± 2.12	12.68 ± 3.11	2.052	$p > 0.05$
Extension	7.20 ± 1.77	7.85 ± 1.64	7.65 ± 0.84	8.15 ± 1.14	1.986	$p > 0.05$
Left lateral flexion	8.33 ± 1.27	8.95 ± 1.19	8.90 ± 1.11	10.45 ± 1.53	1.999	$p > 0.05$
Right lateral flexion	8.85 ± 1.25	9.47 ± 1.34	8.95 ± 1.18	10.15 ± 1.20	1.879	$p > 0.05$
Left axial rotation	4.80 ± 0.75	5.35 ± 0.68	5.20 ± 0.76	9.23 ± 1.50 [a]	10.598	$p < 0.001$
Right axial rotation	5.85 ± 0.84	6.35 ± 0.67	6.55 ± 0.75	10.15 ± 1.44 [a]	12.368	$p < 0.001$

Note: Compared to the control group, [a] $p < 0.05$.

4. Discussion

This study evaluated the biomechanical effects of three facet excision approach points using a bovine lumbar spine model. The results showed that the second approach (ventral midpoint) performed best in preserving spinal stability, while the first and third approaches resulted in increased disc pressure and abnormal range of motion, respectively. These findings provide a key biomechanical basis for optimizing percutaneous endoscopic surgery (PETD).

Our findings demonstrate that the choice of insertion point (IP) during unilateral partial facetectomy (UPF) critically impacts lumbar spine stability [18–21]. While previous studies focused on facetectomy volume thresholds, our work uniquely evaluates the biomechanical effects of UPF performed through different IPs, aligning with clinical surgical practices [1,22,23]. At present, lumbar hypermobility is diagnosed by the relative displacement or angle of the vertebral body in the flexion and extension positions. Hasegawa K. et al. also believed that the increase in the FJ space is the strongest predictor of lumbar hypermobility [24]. Therefore, the integrity and health of the FJs are essential in the stability of the lumbar spine. The best choice for testing the biomechanics of lumbar spine is the use of specimens from a fresh human cadaver. However, it is difficult to obtain a sufficient number of cadavers of the same age and gender. Calf vertebral bodies are similar in size to the human ones and have a wide variety of sources. Therefore, the experiments in this work were performed using 40 calf spine specimens to perform UPF.

During the PETD surgery, an insertion operation is performed under local anesthesia in the posterior aspect of the vertebral body to allow direct entry into the spinal canal to perform the discectomy. The surgery is performed far from the outlet and dorsal root ganglia, avoiding as much as possible the muscles and ligaments adjacent to the vertebral body, but a partial destruction of the FJ is inevitable. Some biomechanical studies showed that the destruction of FJs increases the risk of spinal hypermobility and spinal degeneration [25–27].

However, recent advances in finite element (FE) research on facetectomy have been made. In 2014, Erbulut [28] performed an FE analysis and found that the FE model of the lumbar spine is severely affected in extension and axial rotation after the complete removal of one FJ side. Thus, lumbar fusion or pedicle screw fixation is required after the removal of the bilateral FJs of the lumbar spine. However, in 2017, Zeng et al. [7] simulated the resection of the 50% of one FJ side on a lumbar FE model and they realized that the intradiscal pressure and intervertebral ROM were not significantly different from their value in the intact model. Thus, these patients do not need lumbar fusion or lumbar fixation. On the other hand, in 2019, Li et al. [29] simulated the graded resection of the lumbar FJs through FE analysis and discovered that the removal of 50% of the unilateral lumbar FJ increased the risk of biomechanical degeneration of the lumbar spine and the occurrence of failed back surgery syndrome. In 2020, S. Ahuja et al. [15] performed an FE analysis and discovered that the lumbar spine ROM, the pressure in the FJs, and the pressure in the intervertebral disc significantly increase when more than 30% of a unilateral facet joint is removed. The conclusions of the above studies on the biomechanics of facetectomy are different, because none of these studies established a unified standard in the resection of the lumbar FJs. The experiments performed in previous works were mostly resection of the superior FJ from the dorsal side to the ventral side, which is not in agreement with what is performed in clinical practice, and the cutting method was a longitudinal cut of the artificial division [8,15,28–31]. Indeed, a trephine is used in clinical practice to perform a cut from the ventral side of the superior FJ to the dorsal side, and from the head to the tail end [32–34]. The resected superior FJ is left with an arc-shaped gap. Therefore, the previous studies are not applicable in clinical surgery, thus having less significance.

The three IPs selected in our experiments were needle IPs currently used in clinical surgery, with the first IP (the apex of the superior FJ) as the most commonly used IP. The percutaneous endoscopic discectomy was invented in 1993 by the German spine surgeon Hoogland Thomas [35] who chose the apex of the superior FJ as the needle IP [4,36]. Therefore, this IP was selected also in this work as one of the IPs to perform the experiments. In our experiment, the height of the L5 superior FJ of the lumbar FE model was 13.4 mm, the average height of the L5 superior FJ of the calf spine models was greater than 13 mm, and the radius of the trephine was 3.75 mm, thus, the height of the superior FJ was sufficient to divide the three IPs, all placed at the edge of the superior FJ. Facetectomy performed through the ventral edge of the superior FJ can maximize the expansion of the intervertebral foramen. In addition, the test data on these three IPs could be compared with each other to evaluate the impact of facetectomy of the different FJ portions on the biomechanics of the lumbar spine.

The bilateral FJs and the intervertebral disc form a spine unit that shares the pressure of the trunk on the vertebral body [37–39]. Since the top of the superior FJ is triangular, a stress concentration may easily occur at the tip of the superior FJ under physiological conditions, meaning that the stress sustained in this point is relatively large. The facetectomy performed through the first IP resulted in the destruction of the integrity of the superior FJ, leading to stress redistribution, and the larger stress sustained by the apex of the superior FJ was distributed to the adjacent intervertebral disc and the contralateral FJ. The first IP (the apex of the superior FJ) was the most commonly used IP. The in vitro biomechanics test revealed no significant difference in the ROM of the lumbar spine after facetectomy of the calf spine models between Group A compared with the control group. However, compared with the control group, the L4/5 IMP under extension in Group A was significantly increased. This might be related to the protection of the joint capsule of the FJs. Indeed, some studies showed that the joint capsule of the FJs not only protects and nourishes the FJs, but also shares the physiological load, thus limiting the excessive movement of the lumbar spine [9,40,41]. The second IP was located on the outer edge of the intervertebral foramen. In the in vitro biomechanics test, no statistically significant difference was found in the L4/5 IMP and ROM of the lumbar spine in Group B compared with the control group. The third IP was performed in the thickest part of the superior FJ, where the stress was the largest. The in vitro biomechanics test revealed a statistically significant difference in the L4/5 IMP and ROM of the lumbar spine in Group C compared with the control group.

This work has a limitation. No specimens from cadavers were used to perform the in vitro biomechanical studies, thus, calf spine specimens were preferred since calf vertebral bodies are similar in size to the human ones, and because calf spine specimens represent the best replacement for cadaver spine specimens to perform biomechanical research. However, in the present experiments, the FJs of the calf spine specimens possessed thicker joint capsules and greater bone density, which increased the difficulty in the removal of the excess muscle and soft tissues from the specimens. The outer diameter of the trephine used in the experiment was 7.5 mm, therefore, the biomechanical effect of other size trephine or tools used for facetectomy on the lumbar spine needs further study and additional clinical research.

5. Conclusions

This study systematically evaluated the biomechanical effects of unilateral partial facetectomy (UPF) performed through three insertion points (IPs) in calf spine models. Key findings include: Firstly, UPF through the second IP (midpoint of the ventral superior facet joint) minimized biomechanical disruption, with no significant differences in ROM or L4/5 IMP compared to intact specimens. Secondly, UPF through the first IP (apex of the superior facet joint) increased L4/5 IMP during extension, suggesting potential risks for postoperative instability. Finally, the third IP (lowest ventral point) induced significant biomechanical degradation, validating its unsuitability for clinical application.

These results emphasize the importance of IP selection in UPF procedures. UPF performed through the midpoint of the ventral side of the superior FJ resulted in a minimal impact on the biomechanics of the lumbar spine, suggesting that it might be the most appropriate IP for UPF.

Author Contributions: Conceptualization, T.M. and L.N.; methodology, L.N.; software, T.M.; validation, T.M., X.T. and J.L.; formal analysis, T.M.; investigation, J.W.; resources, L.N.; data curation, J.W.; writing—original draft preparation, T.M., X.T. and J.L.; writing—review and editing, L.N.; visualization, J.W.; supervision, L.N.; project administration, L.N.; funding acquisition, L.N. All authors have read and agreed to the published version of the manuscript.

Funding: "Changzhou High-level Medical Talents Training Project (2022CZLJ016)", "Changzhou Science and Technology Bureau Project (CJ20245030)", "Clinical project of Changzhou Medical Center of Nanjing Medical University: CMCC202404".

Institutional Review Board Statement: This study was approved by the Ethics Committee of The Affiliated Changzhou No.2 People's Hospital of Nanjing Medical University [2021]KY113-01. This study was approved by the Ethics Committee of The Affiliated Changzhou No.2 People's Hospital of Nanjing Medical University [2021]KY113-01.

Informed Consent Statement: Informed consent was obtained from all subjects involved in the study.

Data Availability Statement: The data that support the findings of this study are available from the corresponding author upon reasonable request.

Acknowledgments: We would like to express our sincere gratitude to the patients who participated in this study, as well as to our colleagues who contributed to its completion.

Conflicts of Interest: The authors declared no potential conflicts of interest with respect to the research, authorship, and/or publication of this article.

References

1. Hlaing, S.S.; Puntumetakul, R.; Wanpen, S.; Boucaut, R. Balance Control in Patients with Subacute Non-Specific Low Back Pain, with and without Lumbar Instability: A Cross-Sectional Study. *J. Pain Res.* **2020**, *13*, 795–803. [CrossRef] [PubMed]
2. Sun, C.; Tian, W.J.; Liu, H.X.; Guan, P.G. Outcomes of multisegmental transforaminal enlarged decompression plus posterior pedicle screw fixation for multilevel lumbar spinal canal stenosis associated with lumbar instability. *Int. J. Surg.* **2018**, *50*, 72–78. [CrossRef]
3. Gu, G.; Wang, C.; Gu, X.; Zhang, H.; Zhao, Y.; He, S. Percutaneous Transforaminal Endoscopic Discectomy for Adjacent Segment Disease After Lumbar Fusion in Elderly Patients Over 65 Years Old. *World Neurosurg.* **2018**, *112*, e830–e836. [CrossRef] [PubMed]
4. Hoogland, T.; van den Brekel-Dijkstra, K.; Schubert, M.; Miklitz, B. Endoscopic transforaminal discectomy for recurrent lumbar disc herniation: A prospective, cohort evaluation of 262 consecutive cases. *Spine* **2008**, *33*, 973–978. [CrossRef]
5. Li, X.R.; Yu, J.; Zhang, W.; Gao, G.M.; Han, L.; Chen, L.; Nong, L.M. Biomechanical Model Study of the Effect of Partial Facetectomy on Lumbar Stability Under Percutaneous Endoscopy. *World Neurosurg.* **2020**, *139*, e255–e264. [CrossRef]
6. Liu, X.; Huang, Z.; Zhou, R.; Zhu, Q.; Ji, W.; Long, Y.; Wang, J. The Effects of Orientation of Lumbar Facet Joints on the Facet Joint Contact Forces: An In Vitro Biomechanical Study. *Spine* **2018**, *43*, E216–E220. [CrossRef]
7. Zeng, Z.L.; Zhu, R.; Wu, Y.C.; Zuo, W.; Yu, Y.; Wang, J.J.; Cheng, L.M. Effect of Graded Facetectomy on Lumbar Biomechanics. *J. Healthc. Eng.* **2017**, *2017*, 7981513. [CrossRef] [PubMed]
8. Kiapour, A.; Ambati, D.; Hoy, R.W.; Goel, V.K. Effect of graded facetectomy on biomechanics of Dynesys dynamic stabilization system. *Spine* **2012**, *37*, E581–E589. [CrossRef]
9. Bermel, E.A.; Barocas, V.H.; Ellingson, A.M. The role of the facet capsular ligament in providing spinal stability. *Comput. Methods Biomech. Biomed. Eng.* **2018**, *21*, 712–721. [CrossRef]
10. Haher, T.R.; O'Brien, M.; Dryer, J.W.; Nucci, R.; Zipnick, R.; Leone, D.J. The role of the lumbar facet joints in spinal stability. Identification of alternative paths of loading. *Spine* **1994**, *19*, 2667–2670; discussion 2671. [CrossRef]
11. Campos, W.K.; Linhares, M.N.; Sarda, J.; Santos, A.R.S.; Lin, K.; Latini, A.; Walz, R. Predictors of Pain Recurrence After Lumbar Facet Joint Injections. *Front. Neurosci.* **2019**, *13*, 958. [CrossRef]
12. Schmidt, H.; Galbusera, F.; Rohlmann, A.; Zander, T.; Wilke, H.J. Effect of multilevel lumbar disc arthroplasty on spine kinematics and facet joint loads in flexion and extension: A finite element analysis. *Eur. Spine J.* **2012**, *21* (Suppl. S5), 663–674. [CrossRef]

13. Ebenbichler, G.R.; Leitgeb, J.; Amtmann, G.; Konig, F.; Schernthaner, M.; Resch, K.L.; Kainberger, F. Degeneration and Instability and the Relation to Patients' Function Late After Lumbar Disc Surgery: Data from a 12-Year Follow-Up. *Am. J. Phys. Med. Rehabil.* **2016**, *95*, 871–879. [CrossRef] [PubMed]
14. Yee, T.J.; Terman, S.W.; La Marca, F.; Park, P. Comparison of adjacent segment disease after minimally invasive or open transforaminal lumbar interbody fusion. *J. Clin. Neurosci.* **2014**, *21*, 1796–1801. [CrossRef]
15. Ahuja, S.; Moideen, A.N.; Dudhniwala, A.G.; Karatsis, E.; Papadakis, L.; Varitis, E. Lumbar stability following graded unilateral and bilateral facetectomy: A finite element model study. *Clin. Biomech.* **2020**, *75*, 105011. [CrossRef] [PubMed]
16. Park, S.W.; Lim, T.J.; Park, J. A biomechanical study of the instrumented and adjacent lumbar levels after In-Space interspinous spacer insertion. *J. Neurosurg. Spine* **2010**, *12*, 560–569. [CrossRef] [PubMed]
17. Wilke, H.J.; Mathes, B.; Midderhoff, S.; Graf, N. Development of a scoliotic spine model for biomechanical in vitro studies. *Clin. Biomech.* **2015**, *30*, 182–187. [CrossRef]
18. Mas, Y.; Gracia, L.; Ibarz, E.; Gabarre, S.; Pena, D.; Herrera, A. Finite element simulation and clinical follow-up of lumbar spine biomechanics with dynamic fixations. *PLoS ONE* **2017**, *12*, e0188328. [CrossRef]
19. Hsieh, Y.Y.; Chen, C.H.; Tsuang, F.Y.; Wu, L.C.; Lin, S.C.; Chiang, C.J. Removal of fixation construct could mitigate adjacent segment stress after lumbosacral fusion: A finite element analysis. *Clin. Biomech.* **2017**, *43*, 115–120. [CrossRef]
20. Tang, S.; Rebholz, B.J. Does lumbar microdiscectomy affect adjacent segmental disc degeneration? A finite element study. *J. Surg. Res.* **2013**, *182*, 62–67. [CrossRef]
21. Adams, M.A.; Freeman, B.J.; Morrison, H.P.; Nelson, I.W.; Dolan, P. Mechanical initiation of intervertebral disc degeneration. *Spine* **2000**, *25*, 1625–1636. [CrossRef]
22. Denteneer, L.; Stassijns, G.; De Hertogh, W.; Truijen, S.; Van Daele, U. Inter- and Intrarater Reliability of Clinical Tests Associated With Functional Lumbar Segmental Instability and Motor Control Impairment in Patients With Low Back Pain: A Systematic Review. *Arch. Phys. Med. Rehabil.* **2017**, *98*, 151–164. [CrossRef] [PubMed]
23. Ferrari, S.; Manni, T.; Bonetti, F.; Villafane, J.H.; Vanti, C. A literature review of clinical tests for lumbar instability in low back pain: Validity and applicability in clinical practice. *Chiropr. Man. Therap* **2015**, *23*, 14. [CrossRef]
24. Hasegawa, K.; Shimoda, H.; Kitahara, K.; Sasaki, K.; Homma, T. What are the reliable radiological indicators of lumbar segmental instability? *J. Bone Joint Surg. Br.* **2011**, *93*, 650–657. [CrossRef] [PubMed]
25. Sairyo, K.; Chikawa, T.; Nagamachi, A. State-of-the-art transforaminal percutaneous endoscopic lumbar surgery under local anesthesia: Discectomy, foraminoplasty, and ventral facetectomy. *J. Orthop. Sci.* **2018**, *23*, 229–236. [CrossRef] [PubMed]
26. Phillips, F.M.; Tzermiadianos, M.N.; Voronov, L.I.; Havey, R.M.; Carandang, G.; Renner, S.M.; Rosler, D.M.; Ochoa, J.A.; Patwardhan, A.G. Effect of the Total Facet Arthroplasty System after complete laminectomy-facetectomy on the biomechanics of implanted and adjacent segments. *Spine J.* **2009**, *9*, 96–102. [CrossRef]
27. Okuda, S.; Miyauchi, A.; Oda, T.; Haku, T.; Yamamoto, T.; Iwasaki, M. Surgical complications of posterior lumbar interbody fusion with total facetectomy in 251 patients. *J. Neurosurg. Spine* **2006**, *4*, 304–309. [CrossRef]
28. Erbulut, D.U. Biomechanical effect of graded facetectomy on asymmetrical finite element model of the lumbar spin. *Turk. Neurosurg.* **2014**, *24*, 923–928. [CrossRef]
29. Qian, J.; Yu, S.S.; Liu, J.J.; Chen, L.; Jing, J.H. Biomechanics changes of lumbar spine caused by foraminotomy via percutaneous transforaminal endoscopic lumbar discectomy. *Zhonghua Yi Xue Za Zhi* **2018**, *98*, 1013–1018. [CrossRef]
30. Li, J.; Zhang, X.; Xu, W.; Xi, Z.; Xie, L. Reducing the extent of facetectomy may decrease morbidity in failed back surgery syndrome. *BMC Musculoskelet. Disord.* **2019**, *20*, 369. [CrossRef]
31. Lee, K.K.; Teo, E.C.; Qiu, T.X.; Yang, K. Effect of facetectomy on lumbar spinal stability under sagittal plane loadings. *Spine* **2004**, *29*, 1624–1631. [CrossRef] [PubMed]
32. Xie, P.; Feng, F.; Chen, Z.; He, L.; Yang, B.; Chen, R.; Wu, W.; Liu, B.; Dong, J.; Shu, T.; et al. Percutaneous transforaminal full endoscopic decompression for the treatment of lumbar spinal stenosis. *BMC Musculoskelet. Disord.* **2020**, *21*, 546. [CrossRef]
33. Wang, Y.B.; Chen, S.L.; Cao, C.; Zhang, K.; Liu, L.M.; Gao, Y.Z. Percutaneous Transforaminal Endoscopic Discectomy and Fenestration Discectomy to Treat Posterior Ring Apophyseal Fractures: A Retrospective Cohort Study. *Orthop. Surg.* **2020**, *12*, 1092–1099. [CrossRef]
34. Chen, Z.; Zhang, L.; Dong, J.; Xie, P.; Liu, B.; Wang, Q.; Chen, R.; Feng, F.; Yang, B.; Shu, T.; et al. Percutaneous transforaminal endoscopic discectomy compared with microendoscopic discectomy for lumbar disc herniation: 1-year results of an ongoing randomized controlled trial. *J. Neurosurg. Spine* **2018**, *28*, 300–310. [CrossRef] [PubMed]
35. Hoogland, T. Percutaneous endoscopic discectomy. *J. Neurosurg.* **1993**, *79*, 967–968.
36. Schubert, M.; Hoogland, T. Endoscopic transforaminal nucleotomy with foraminoplasty for lumbar disk herniation. *Oper. Orthop. Traumatol.* **2005**, *17*, 641–661. [CrossRef]
37. Szkoda-Poliszuk, K.; Zak, M.; Pezowicz, C. Finite element analysis of the influence of three-joint spinal complex on the change of the intervertebral disc bulge and height. *Int. J. Numer. Method. Biomed. Eng.* **2018**, *34*, e3107. [CrossRef]

38. Abbas, J.; Slon, V.; Stein, D.; Peled, N.; Hershkovitz, I.; Hamoud, K. In the quest for degenerative lumbar spinal stenosis etiology: The Schmorl's nodes model. *BMC Musculoskelet. Disord.* **2017**, *18*, 164. [CrossRef]
39. Li, Z.; Liu, F.; Liu, S.; Chen, Z.; Jiang, C.; Feng, Z.; Jiang, X. Miniopen Transforaminal Lumbar Interbody Fusion with Unilateral Fixation: A Comparison between Ipsilateral and Contralateral Reherniation. *Biomed. Res. Int.* **2016**, *2016*, 7261027. [CrossRef]
40. Zehr, J.D.; Barrett, J.M.; Fewster, K.M.; Laing, A.C.; Callaghan, J.P. Strain of the facet joint capsule during rotation and translation range-of-motion tests: An in vitro porcine model as a human surrogate. *Spine J.* **2020**, *20*, 475–487. [CrossRef] [PubMed]
41. Widmer, J.; Cornaz, F.; Scheibler, G.; Spirig, J.M.; Snedeker, J.G.; Farshad, M. Biomechanical contribution of spinal structures to stability of the lumbar spine-novel biomechanical insights. *Spine J.* **2020**, *20*, 1705–1716. [CrossRef] [PubMed]

Disclaimer/Publisher's Note: The statements, opinions and data contained in all publications are solely those of the individual author(s) and contributor(s) and not of MDPI and/or the editor(s). MDPI and/or the editor(s) disclaim responsibility for any injury to people or property resulting from any ideas, methods, instructions or products referred to in the content.

bioengineering

MDPI

Article

The Utah Manipulation and Locomotion of Large Objects (MeLLO) Data Library

Nathaniel G. Luttmer *, Nathan I. Baum, Josue Flores-Gonzalez, John M. Hollerbach and Mark A. Minor *

University of Utah Robotics Center, John and Marcia Price College of Engineering, University of Utah, Salt Lake City, UT 84112, USA
* Correspondence: nluttmer1@gmail.com (N.G.L.); mark.minor@utah.edu (M.A.M.)

Abstract: The purpose of this paper is to provide researchers with a description of a data library representing human interaction with medium- to large-sized objects in everyday life. The library includes motion capture data characterizing human and object motion, as well as data for characterizing haptic interaction with the object via force and torque measurements via a load cell and inertial measurement unit (IMU) readings of the object accelerations. Objects include a box, luggage, briefcase, walker, shopping cart, wheelbarrow, and door. The data collected includes multiple types of interactions with each object, such as manipulating the object and walking while interacting with the object (e.g., pulling, pushing, carrying, operating, etc.). Data processing techniques for synchronizing data, deriving human biomechanics, and segmenting trials are presented. Examples of how the data in the library can be manipulated and processed further are provided. This includes combining ten wheelbarrow lifts of one subject together and analyzing the knee motion, object acceleration, and load cell readings (force and torque) with mean trajectories and standard deviations of the trajectories. From there, the range of motion can be extracted, such as for the hip, knee, and ankle joint minimum angles, maximum angles, and range of motion. A comparison of walking with and without a wheelbarrow is presented using spatiotemporal parameters and cyclograms to demonstrate their differences. The database is available on AddBiomechanics, SimTK, and GitHub.

Keywords: databases; kinematics; kinetics; dynamics; human–object interaction; haptics; legged locomotion; data models

1. Introduction

Humans interact with many different objects throughout their daily activities. Some examples include carrying a briefcase to work, pushing a cart while shopping for groceries, working in the garden with a wheelbarrow, and lifting and moving boxes. Likewise, humans who have trouble walking use assistive devices to help them walk to places they need to go. The way humans interact with these different objects varies in many ways. Some objects can be interacted with using only one hand, and some need to be interacted with using both hands due to the size and shape of the object. The area where humans place their hands to interact with the object is also different given the shape and size of different objects. Humans approach and interact with these objects differently, and the biomechanics moving these objects also varies. This paper presents a library of data characterizing humans interacting with several objects from daily life, which will be used to develop a better understanding of human motion, object motion, and haptic interaction between humans and objects in future work.

2. Motivation

Libraries of data characterizing human manipulation and interaction help scientists and engineers characterize how humans interact with those objects. Such data provide a foundation for ergonomists, biomechanicians, roboticists, and virtual reality and gaming engineers seeking to characterize human biomechanics and develop new devices and technology to simulate those interactions. Understanding the forces, torques, and dynamics produced on objects when a human interacts with them is crucial [1]. The motion of a human walking up to the object and interacting with the object, i.e., grabbing, lifting, pushing, etc., is also important to characterize the typical ways humans interact with these objects. This research produces a library of data representing user biomechanics while interacting with those objects. The library will be used in future work to evaluate interaction with the objects and to design haptic manipulators that will mimic the objects in virtual reality. The haptic devices and virtual objects will then be used in user studies comparing virtual and real objects using the data from this library.

Our motivation for creating the library is somewhat unique. Many libraries, such as the KIT database [2], are used to create a database representing human–object interactions with multiple objects, but they usually focus on motion alone, and often strive to mimic that motion in related applications. Motion capture data from the KIT library, for example, is used to control robotic humanoids in a simulation [3] using a reference kinematics and a dynamics model of the human body called the master motor map (MMM). The KIT database is also used to segment bimanual manipulation from household tasks based upon human demonstration [4], which is also used to control humanoid robots. Other researchers have also used the KIT database to create motions for humanoid robots [5] based upon motions of humans.

While these research endeavors characterize human kinematics while interacting with an object, we also aim to characterize haptic interactions with objects. While the KIT database has been applied to create a taxonomy differentiating coordination patterns in human bimanual manipulation [6], our motivation is to eventually characterize human interactions with objects from both a biomechanics and haptics perspective, which will be used as a baseline for evaluating the haptic manipulators that we are developing. While the data from our library might be used to create a taxonomy like in [6], this is not a specific motivation for our research.

To characterize human kinematics and haptic interaction, our library comprises a combination of motion capture data, load cell data of the interaction between humans and different objects, and IMU (inertial measurement unit) readings of the object when it is being manipulated.

3. Related Work

3.1. Haptics

Haptics is the study of touch and motion. For us specifically, we are researching how subjects touch and move different objects from everyday life. The field of haptics is an ongoing research topic [7,8]. There are four main subareas in haptics: human haptics, machine haptics, computer haptics, and multimedia haptics [9]. Human haptics is more focused on physiological response, such skin stretching in response to forces, which is not related to this work. Machine haptics is more focused on design and control of a device to mimic haptic interactions, which will be more a focus in our future work designing and evaluating haptic manipulators based upon the library in this paper. In this study, we focus on the forces, torques, and manipulation of objects by humans and the way humans orient themselves to interact with these objects. Motion capture, load cells on the objects, and an IMU on the object track the human subject and provide haptic measurements when the subjects interact with the objects. Computer graphics haptics is more focused on the visual display of objects moving due to haptic interaction, which will be the focus of future work citing this library. Multimedia haptics is more focused on the ability of multimedia display to mimic haptic interaction, such as the work in [10], where environmental displays such as wind and mist were used to create haptic sensations, which is quite different from this work.

Adding load cells to objects that humans are interacting with has been performed before. Russo et al. studied humans balanced on a wooden beam while holding two canes with load cells in the base and motion capture to track the forces and human orientations used to balance themselves on the beam [11]. McClain et al. conducted a similar experiment of a human using a walker for load support, but used strain gauges on the tubes supporting the handles to measure interaction forces [12]. The data were used to design a new walker and its control systems to support similar forces. In this study, we use a 6-DoF load cell to obtain interaction forces, and evaluate how a user interacts with haptic manipulators mimicking a walker. We believe that the work presented here is unique, since the goal is to create a library of such biomechanical and haptic interactions with objects while standing and walking.

3.2. Similar Databases

There are many openly available human motion databases that include a wide range of information. These databases are essential for many different fields, such as computer vision, computer graphics, multimedia, robotics, human–computer interaction, and machine learning. Zhu et al. [13] provide an extensive survey of human motion databases, characterizing them by measurement techniques, types of motion and manipulation used to generate the data, and the types of data contained in the studies. Common data sources include marker-based motion capture, ground reaction force data, inertial measurements, video, and imagery. A wide variety of motions are studied, such as walking, lifting, kicking, dancing, and interaction with different objects. Some tasks require single-handed manipulation, and others require two-handed manipulation. Objects range from small household items, such as bottles, caps, and utensils, to hand-held tools, and large items, such as furniture, boxes, and doors.

Of the many databases described in [13], the work presented here is most similar to those focusing on manipulation of medium-to-large objects from daily life combined with locomotion, specifically where one- and two-handed manipulation is required. Human motion and kinematics, object motion, and kinetic interactions with the object are characterized. A brief review of the most related datasets is provided below and summarized in Table 1, which highlights the different types of data presented, the types of motion used to collect data, and the objects that are manipulated.

In [14], Bassani et al. provide a dataset characterizing human motion and muscular activity in manual material handling tasks, which is typical in the biomechanics and ergonomics fields. Users lifted and moved a small barbell weight with one arm and a medium-sized box using bimanual manipulation, amongst other tasks. Data were collected using an Xsens MVN suit (Movella, Henderson, NV, USA) composed of seventeen 9-axis IMU sensors and 8 sEMG sensor readings containing data from 14 subjects. Subjects stood in the N-pose in front of a table, lifted the object from the floor, kept it lifted with the elbow flexed at 90 degrees, and placed it on a table. Subjects then lifted the object from the table, carried it to another position, and placed it on the floor. Their box manipulation task is like the box manipulation task in our library, but our study uses the box as an instrument to measure interaction wrenches and uses motion capture to measure kinematics, which is unique, since our database provides a baseline for characterizing haptic interaction.

Table 1. Comparison of our dataset library and existing ones.

Database	Human Sensing	Haptic Sensing	Object Sensing	Object Size (S, M, L)	Similar Objects	Locomotion with Objects	Number of Subjects
Dataset of Human Motion and Muscular Activities [14]	IMU, sEMG	None	None	M	B	Yes	14
Dataset of Unscripted Human Motion [15]	IMU	None	None	S, M, L	B, D, SC	Yes	13
HBOD [16]	MoCap, IMU	None	MoCap	S, M	None	No	5
An Industry-Oriented Dataset [17]	IMU, MoCap	Pressure Sensor	None	S, M, L	None	Yes	13
BEHAVE [18]	RGBD Images	None	RGBD Images	S, M, L	B, L	No	8
KIT [2]	MoCap	None	MoCap	S, M, L	B	Yes	43
Our Database	MoCap	Load Cell	MocCap, IMU	M, L	B, D, BC, L, W, WB, SC	Yes	6

Box (B), door (D), briefcase (BC), luggage (L), walker (W), wheelbarrow (WB), shopping cart (SC).

Geissinger et al. [15] used an XSens MVN with sparse IMUs to measure human kinematics during activities of daily life on a university campus, driving, going to a variety of different stores, working in a machine shop and laboratory, exercising, and at home. This generated a large dataset across 13 subjects, which was then used to train deep learning networks to predict upper body motion and full body motion. While some of the activities, such as walking up to a door and opening it, pushing a cart, or lifting a box, are like those in our study, they only focus on the kinematics of the human, whereas the database presented here also characterizes kinetic interaction with the object and its resulting motion.

The hand–body–object dataset (HBOD) includes data of subjects moving and interacting with a screwdriver, hammer, spanner, electrical drill, and rectangular workpiece with one hand [16]. Data are derived from 12 IMUs placed on body segments and a Cyberglove 2, which together measure body and hand kinematics. In this case, motion capture markers were used to measure the posture of the objects being manipulated. Five subjects then lifted and placed objects at high positions and performed tool manipulation. While the measurement of human and object kinematics are similar to our database, ref. [16] focuses more on dexterous kinematics, and kinetics are not measured. Likewise, the objects being manipulated are quite different than those presented in this paper.

The industry-oriented dataset for collaborative robotics includes data of human postures and actions that are common in industry [17]. Like HBOD, [17] measures whole body kinematics using both IMUs and a glove with flexion sensors to measure hand kinematics. Similarly to our work, they also use marker-based motion capture to measure human kinematics. Their gloves use pressure sensors to detect contact with the objects, but this does not provide kinetic information about interaction forces as we do in this paper. The study emphasizes tasks typical of assembly lines, which are mainly focused on picking up small parts, carrying them, and then assembling them with other objects. They do, however, evaluate lifting larger loads and moving them to a shelf, which is like the box lift task in our study. Unlike HBOD and this paper, the object motions in [17] are not measured. Measurements from 13 subjects are reported in [17], in which two cameras are used for video recording tasks, but data are not derived from them.

The BEHAVE dataset [18] includes a large set of images of eight subjects interacting with objects in natural environments. This dataset contains multiview RGBD frames with accurate pseudo-ground-truth SMPL (skinned multi-person linear model). The objects manipulated include various boxes, chairs, and tables, as well as a crate, backpack, trash-can, monitor, keyboard, suitcase, basketball, exercise ball, yoga mat, stool, and toolbox. Interactions include lifting, carrying, sitting, pushing, and pulling, as well as unstructured free movement combined with object interactions. One- and two-handed manipulations are provided with hands, as well as manipulations using feet. Imagery data does not measure kinematics and kinetic interaction directly, but the authors do provide computer vision code to demonstrate a basic reconstruction of kinematics using the data. It is not clear if such information is sufficient for characterizing haptic interaction.

The KIT database includes a dataset of full-body human and object motion capture using one- and two-hand manipulation [2]. This database has 43 different subjects and 41 different objects with raw data and post-processed motions. This dataset includes a full body motion capture marker setup with 56 markers and markers placed on each of the objects to analyze object movement. The objects and interactions include tasks such as opening a door, manipulating a box, walking up and down stairs, and interaction between subjects. This is a very extensive database and includes a plethora of other objects, but it is mainly focused on kinematics. Kinetic interaction is not measured.

While these studies have provided detailed insight into how people interact with specific objects, our end goal focuses on haptic interaction with a series of everyday objects combined with locomotion. The database described in this paper includes full body motion capture and object motion capture data, which is only present in a few studies, such as [2]. Unique to our database is object instrumentation using IMU measurements of the object's motion when a human is moving the object and measurements of interaction wrenches using 6-DOF load cells. This allows the detailed measurement of forces and torques exerted on the object combined with the object's accelerations and position, which should be sufficient to characterize haptic interaction with the object. This new information can be used to characterize the different object models for future applications, such as haptics and virtual reality (VR). Further unique to this study is that this haptic interaction is combined with measuring human motion during that interaction, which allows for the simultaneous characterization of human gait and kinematics during haptic interaction. This knowledge will be helpful for validating interactions with future haptic devices mimicking these objects in a virtual world.

4. Tasks

Several activities of daily life have been identified as motivating tasks for this research based on coordination of locomotion and manipulation. The first task uses two-handed oppositional grasp and is shown in Figure 1a, where a user is grasping and lifting a box on a virtual table. The next task uses a piece of luggage, also known as a roller-board, where the user supports the luggage by the handle and pulls it behind them as they walk, Figure 1b. This task is proposed as an example of a person walking through an airport. A task using a briefcase, Figure 1c, is shown in the user's right hand, which is carried like a person walking to work. A walker usage task is presented, Figure 1d, which is motivated by our prior work with subjects with Parkinson's disease [19] and spinal cord injury [20] where the walker is used to help support the user while they walk. Walker usage usually requires the user to lift the handles slightly and push it to locomote. The shopping cart task, shown in Figure 1e, requires the user to push the cart using different levels of force in each hand to control the cart direction. Figure 1f illustrates a task where the user operates a wheelbarrow, which is common for yard work around the home. This requires the user to lift the back of the wheelbarrow with the handles and then push it forward while walking. They may slightly tip side to side to control steering. Depending on the load in the wheelbarrow (e.g., dirt or concrete versus wood chips or leaves), this can be incredibly demanding, requiring both strength, coordination, and balance. Hence, we will use wheelbarrow operation to display more physically challenging tasks to the user. The door opening task is proposed, as shown in Figure 1g, which was selected since this is consistently repeated in everyday life. The door is configured to open inward and pivot on its right side, such that the user pushes the door open with their right hand and steps through.

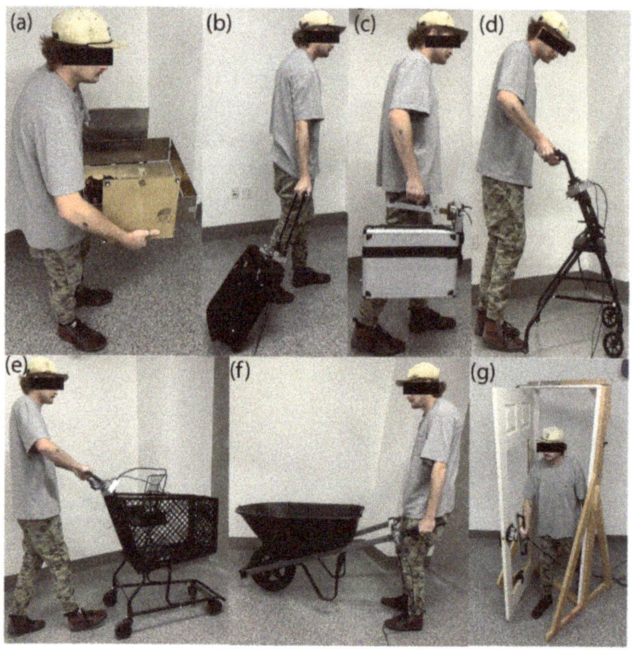

Figure 1. Tasks performed in everyday life: (**a**) manipulating a box, (**b**) walking with luggage, (**c**) carrying a briefcase, (**d**) using a walker, (**e**) pushing a cart, (**f**) manipulating a wheelbarrow, and (**g**) opening a door.

5. Methods and Procedures

This paper presents methods and procedures used to create a database describing how humans interact with the objects which were presented in Section 4. The human walked up to these objects, grabbed the handles, lifted/lowered, pushed, or walked with a steady gait while grasping/manipulating the object. During the study, information such as forces, torques, object motion, human kinematics, and human gait were collected. Furthermore, 6-DOF load cells were incorporated into the object's interaction areas, such as handles, record forces, and torques applied to the object by the human. Body and object kinematics and dynamics were studied using full body motion capture and IMU readings of the object motion when a human interacts with the object.

5.1. Motion Capture Volume

The motion capture system consisted of a 10-camera VICON motion capture system with a mixture of MXF20 and MXF40 cameras (Oxford, UK). The capture volume was designed to capture full body motion in an 8.2 by 4.5 by 2 m sized space. This ensured that we captured full body data for a subject who is 1.9 m tall, locomoting for multiple gait cycles and interacting with the objects naturally. The room was sufficiently large so that users could begin walking and establish a gait pattern.

5.2. Marker Set

The full body marker setup is shown in Figure 2. Reflective markers were placed on all main segments and on rotational joints [21,22]. A minimum of three markers were placed on each of the segments to fully define the segment and record its movement. The motion capture setup was found to be sufficient enough to obtain full body motions for all sizes of participants in the study. These data were exported in CSV and C3D files to be viewed in the database.

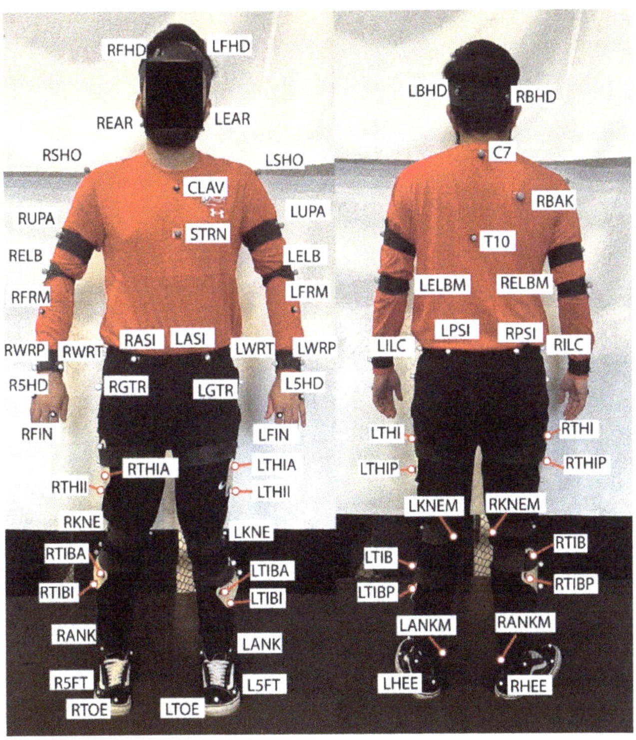

Figure 2. Motion capture marker setup [21,22].

5.3. Instrumentation and Syncronization

Each object was instrumented with force/torque sensors, an IMU, and motion capture markers. The force/torque sensors were 6-DOF sensors from ATI Industrial Automation (9105-TIF-OMEGA85), (Apex, NC, USA). The IMU was a Parker Lord Microstrain IMU, (3DMGX5-AR), (Williston, VT, USA) which can capture a wide variety of different readings. We are mainly interested in the acceleration of the object when it is manipulated by the user. One of the load cells and the IMU were encased inside the IMU/load cell casing to keep the IMU safe and have the respective coordinate frames stay consistent between the load cell and the IMU (Figure 3). The load cell/IMU casing had a marker extension with VICON markers on it designed to produce an unobstructed coordinate frame when connected to the different objects. The second load cell case was similar, but did not have an IMU inside of it.

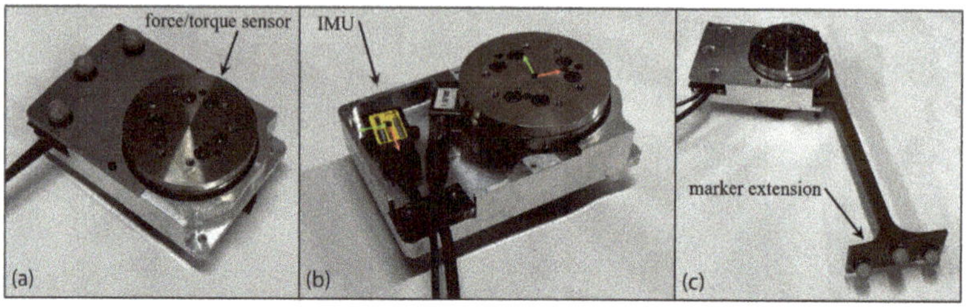

Figure 3. The load cell and IMU case (**a**) with the cover on, (**b**) with the cover off, (**c**) with the marker extension.

Loads were applied to the objects via handles that were attached to the force/torque sensor, as indicated in Figure 3a–c, which is the output of the load cell. As a result, most of the mass of the load cell and the case supporting it were included in the mass of the object being manipulated, as indicated in the next section. Since the handles were attached to the output of the load cell, the load cell could not measure the forces/torques due to the handle's motion, but they were small compared to the forces/torques required to manipulate the objects. For example, as indicated in the next section, the handles and output plate had a mass of 0.24 kg to 1.2 kg, whereas the masses of the objects were ~8 kg to ~40 kg. The case, IMU, and load cell had a mass of 1.5 kg and measured 15.24 by 10.16 by 4.62 cm.

Each sensor was logged on a separate computer, which required a method of data synchronization. The dSpace system sent a chain of impulses to the VICON DAQ (Oxford, UK) to line up the data between the load cell and the motion capture data. To synchronize all of these data, the object was given 10 short impulses by the subject, resulting in accelerations in the IMU, and force measurement in the force/torque sensor. Displacements in the motion capture data, which are synchronized in time, can be used to check the synchronization between all the different datasets. Synchronization between the different sensors/computers is essential to keeping the data consistent.

5.4. Object Instrumentation

5.4.1. Box

The box used in this study was heavy and large, so this was more challenging than other tasks. The box object was constructed to model a 50.5 × 45.7 × 45.7 cm cardboard box with moderate rigidity. The box weighed 8 kg and had an additional 1.4 kg weight placed inside. Figure 4 shows the box object, which comprised three parts: the main body of the box, and then two separate sides. The main body was constructed of thin, aluminum plates with small brackets for added rigidity. The sides were made of large aluminum brackets with cardboard mounted externally, allowing the user to feel the texture of cardboard during manipulation. The two force/torque sensors were mounted between the main body and each of the sides. The IMU was encased inside the IMU/load cell casing, and was between the main body and the left side, as shown in Figure 4.

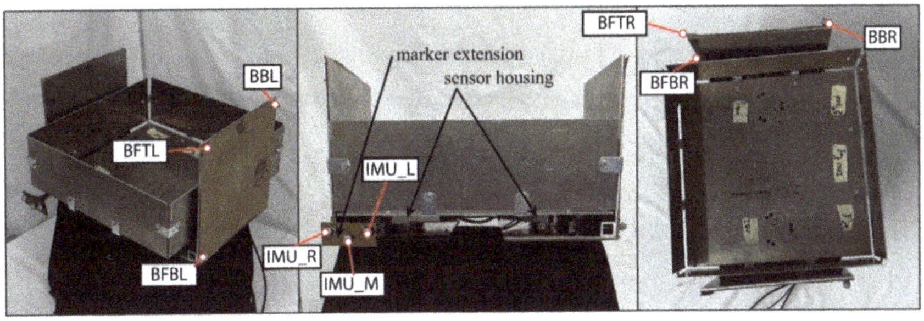

Figure 4. The box apparatus.

5.4.2. Luggage

The luggage object was a 48.3 by 33 by 17.8 cm roller luggage compartment with an instrumented handle, as shown in Figure 5. There was a 4.5 kg weight added inside the luggage compartment to simulate a packed piece of luggage. The luggage itself weighed about 2.3 kg. The sensor housing containing the load cell and IMU was between the luggage compartment and the handle. It was positioned here to measure the forces exerted by the human when holding the handle and walking with the object. Motion capture markers surrounded the compartment and were on either side of the handle. There were also markers placed on the sensor housing to know the location of the load cell and IMU.

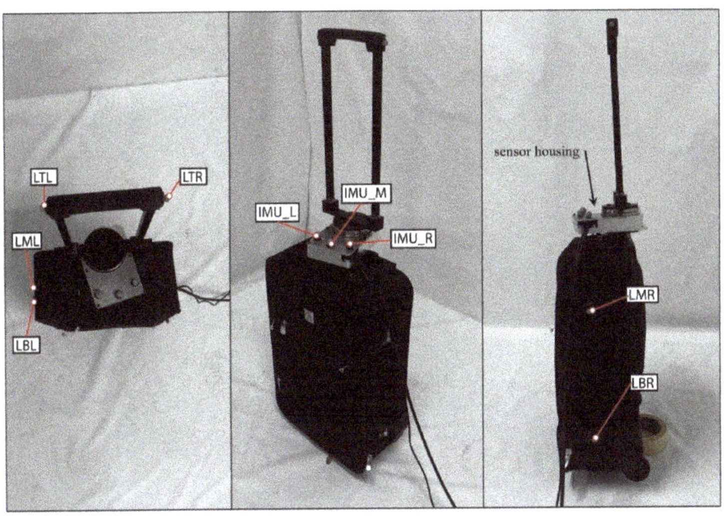

Figure 5. The luggage/roller board apparatus.

5.4.3. Briefcase

The briefcase was a 48.3 by 12.7 by 45.7 cm briefcase with an articulating handle, as shown in Figure 6. The briefcase had weight added inside of it to simulate a full briefcase weighing 8 kg. The briefcase handle was prepared by detaching it from the briefcase and putting it on a fixture consisting of aluminum and 3D-printed parts. This fixture was connected to the load cell, which was connected to the sensor which also housed the IMU. The handle was able to rotate exactly the same as the original briefcase design. An aluminum plate was bolted to the side of the hard case of the briefcase to be able to mount the handle and the sensor housing. The handle was in the relative location, as it was when connected to the briefcase, but elevated slightly to accommodate the sensor housing. Motion capture markers were placed around the briefcase and on the sensor housing.

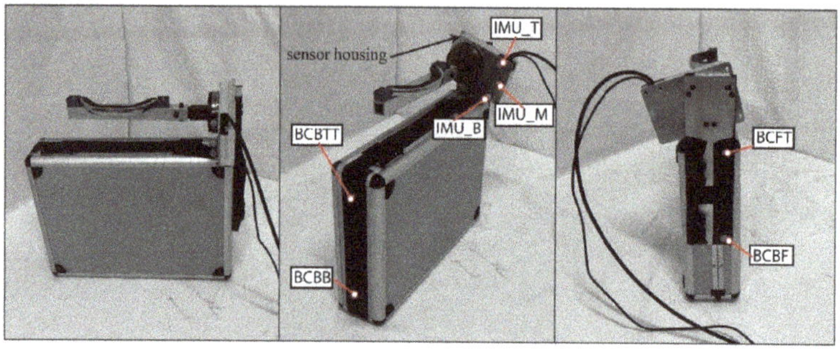

Figure 6. The briefcase apparatus.

5.4.4. Walker

The walker object was a modified assistive walker, with the handle height being 94 cm high and the handles being 61 cm apart with a weight of about 7.5 kg, as shown in Figure 7. The load cells/IMU casings were located between the handles and the adjustable height bars. The height was adjustable, but set to a position that an average person can comfortably use. Motion capture markers were placed around the lower frame of the walker and the load cell/IMU casings.

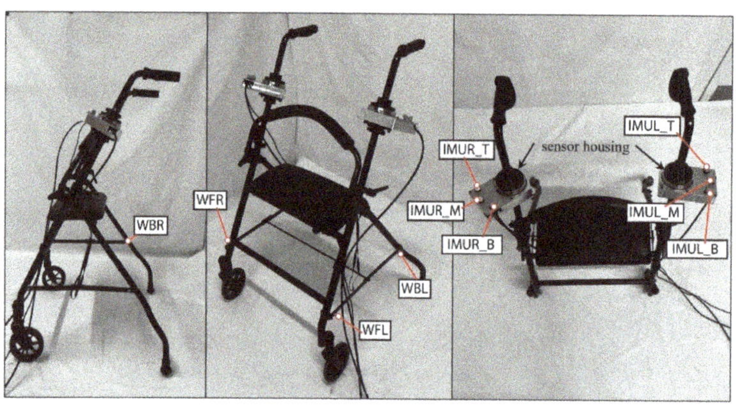

Figure 7. The walker apparatus.

5.4.5. Shopping Cart

The shopping cart was a standard shopping cart typical of a US grocery store, as shown in Figure 8. The shopping cart was 91.5 by 61 by 112 cm, with the handles located 112 cm above the ground. The shopping cart weight was 19.5 kg, and there was also a 22.7 kg plate fixed inside the shopping cart to simulate the cart carrying groceries. The cart was painted matte black so it did not affect the motion capture cameras when capturing datasets. The load cells and IMU were located between the handles, which were split, and the shopping cart body. The frame of the handles was cut so that they sat at the same location as a normal shopping cart. There were motion capture markers placed around the lower frame, near the wheels, and around the top of the cart basket.

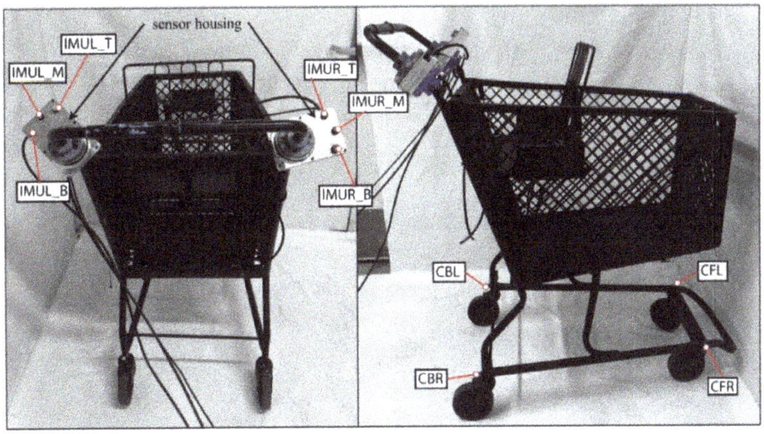

Figure 8. Shopping cart apparatus.

5.4.6. Wheelbarrow

The wheelbarrow was a standard steel wheelbarrow purchased from Home Depot, as shown in Figure 9. The wheelbarrow was a 68.58 by 67.8 by 115 cm fixed wheelbarrow which weighed 16.3 kg. The wheelbarrow also had a 22.7 kg plate in it to simulate the wheelbarrow carrying a load, such as dirt. The load cell and IMU cases were located between the chassis of the wheelbarrow and the handles. The end of the handles were in the same position as they were originally, so as to not change the overall design. There were motion capture markers located around the bucket of the wheelbarrow and on the load cell/IMU casings. The wheelbarrow was painted matte black to prevent interference with the motion capture system.

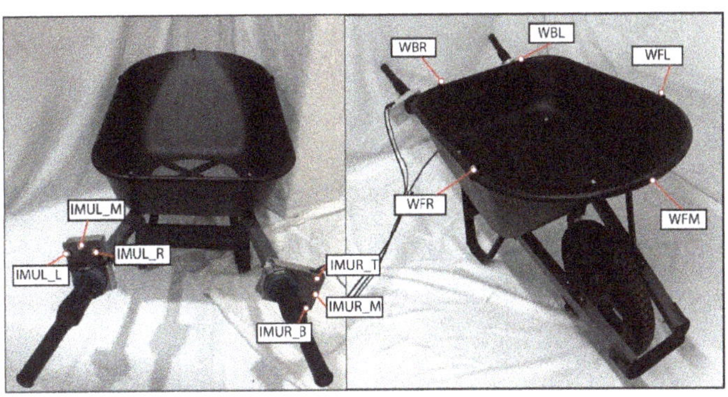

Figure 9. Wheelbarrow apparatus.

5.4.7. Door

The door was a standard solid core-molded composite interior door, purchased from Home Depot (Item No. THDQC225400566). The door was 76.2 cm wide by 203.2 cm high, and weighed 25.4 kg. The door was cut out in the middle to allow the motion capture cameras to see through the door and view the motion capture markers on the front of the subject (Figure 10). Due to cutting out a large portion of the door, added weights were placed on the door to simulate a heavy door weighing 15.87 kg. The door had a door closer, so there was added tension on the door, and the door closed by itself. The door handle was a standard long door handle, which was affixed to the load cell and IMU case, and then attached to the door where a standard door handle would be. The load cell and IMU case had the extension on it to put the motion capture markers in an area where they can be seen by the motion capture cameras. There were also motion capture markers placed on both sides of the door and around the frame of the door so the door angle could be found when opening it.

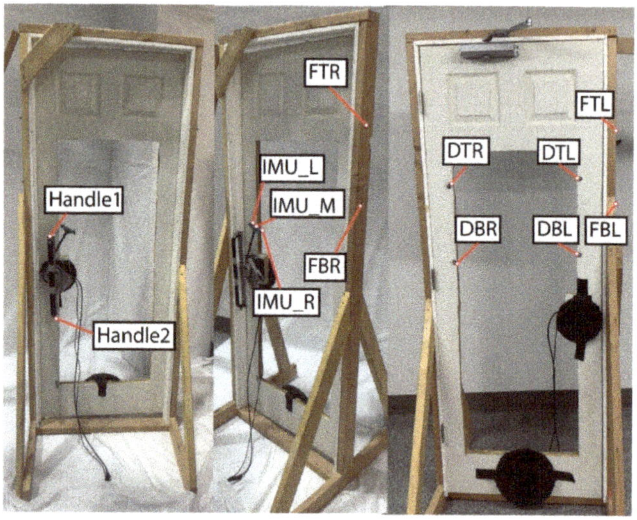

Figure 10. The door apparatus.

5.5. Transformations

The information provided in the library from the sensors (IMU and load cell) was in the respected coordinate frame of the sensor. To move that information from the sensor to the handle where the interaction took place, the information needed to be manipulated through a transform to calculate the forces and torques at the handle. This provided the haptic information between the subject and the handle of the object. The calculation was performed by taking the sum of forces and moments at the load cell. The top diagram in Figure 11 shows a wheelbarrow handle diagram of the world origin, IMU, VICON marker, load cell, and subject hands coordinate frames with the transformation between them. The lower image in Figure 11 shows the forces and moments acting on the wheelbarrow handle.

An example of how to perform this calculation is provided. Consider that F_H is the force vector at the handle exerted by the subject's hand and F_{LC} is the force vector measured at the load cell. Summing the forces provides,

$$\sum F = F_H - F_{LC} = 0 \tag{1}$$

Which can be solved to show that the load cell forces are equal and opposite to the handle forces, such that $F_H = F_{LC}$. Summing moments about the load cell then results in,

$$\sum M = -M_H + M_{LC} - F_H \times T = 0 \tag{2}$$

where M_H is the moment exerted on the handle by the subject, and M_{LC} is moment acting on the load cell. T is the homogeneous transformation matrix from the load cell to the handle of the object

$$T = \begin{bmatrix} R & d \\ 0 & 1 \end{bmatrix} \tag{3}$$

which is constructed from the rotation matrix, R,

$$R = \begin{bmatrix} r_{11} & r_{12} & r_{13} \\ r_{21} & r_{22} & r_{23} \\ r_{31} & r_{32} & r_{33} \end{bmatrix} \tag{4}$$

from the load cell to the handle, and d is the displacement from the load cell to the handle,

$$d = \begin{bmatrix} d_1 \\ d_2 \\ d_3 \end{bmatrix}$$

The moment equation can then be solved to calculate the moment at the handle, N_H, as follows:

$$M_H = M_{LC} - F_{LC} \times T \tag{5}$$

Combined, F_H and M_H indicate the forces and moments supported by the user.

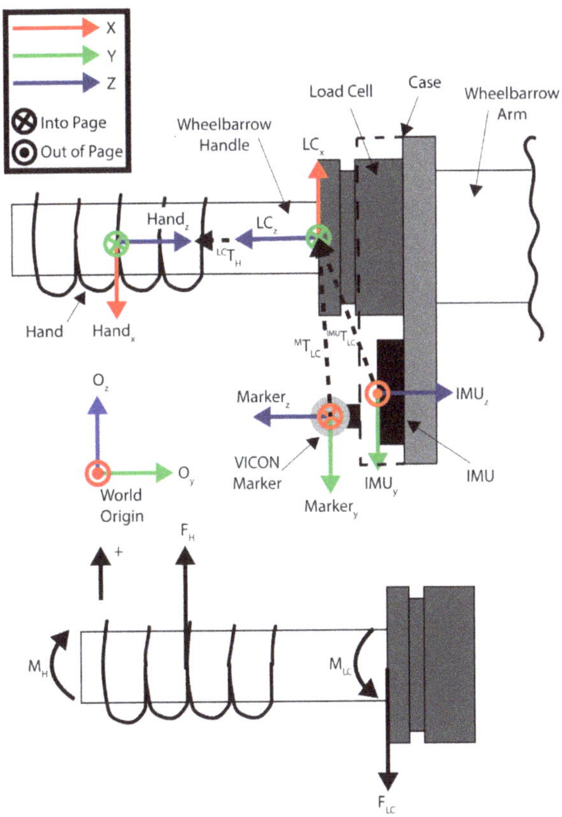

Figure 11. Diagram of the wheelbarrow handle, load cell, and IMU case with VICON markers, and the wheelbarrow arm. The top diagram shows the coordinate frames of the VICON markers relative to the motion capture origin, the marker, IMU, load cell, and the subject's hand. The transformations, T, are shown between the marker and load cell, IMU and load cell, and the load cell and subject's hand. The coordinate frames (blue, red, and green vectors correlating to x, y, and z, respectively) show the orientations of each of the sensors relative to the world coordinate frame. The lower image shows the forces at the hand and how they relate to the load cell forces.

The transformation, T, for each object handle is provided in the data library, which allows load cell data to be transformed to calculate forces and moments exerted by the user for each object. Transformations between the marker to the load cell, IMU to the load cell, and the transformation between the load cells are also included in the data library. This can be used to calculate the position, velocity, and acceleration of the object being manipulated using standard coordinate transformation techniques [23].

5.6. Object Interaction Protocols

The database included a variety of human motion capture files, object motion capture files, and sensor files specific to interactions with the objects mentioned in Section 3. Separate protocols for each object were used to provide similar interactions amongst the subjects. While all interactions involved walking and manipulation of the object, they were all slightly different due to the unique ways humans interacted with each of them. We generally evaluated multiple interactions with each object, such that lifting an object was considered separately from walking with the object. This allowed us to decouple the two types of interactions for evaluation in future studies. Likewise, tasks involving walking while manipulating the object initiated the gait with the left foot, allowing a common gait pattern to be established in all the trials. All interactions were designed to mimic natural interactions with the objects, although interactions were segmented, as indicated above.

(1) Box: The box had two types of interactions. The first was lifting. The box was sitting on a stand. The subject started standing straight up, then bent down and grabbed the sides of the box with an oppositional two-handed grasp and then lifted the box. They then lowered the box back down to the stand, let go, and stood back up. In the second interaction, the subject carried the box while walking. The subject started at one end of the capture volume holding the box with a two-handed oppositional grasp, and then walked through the volume. They started with their left foot and walked to the other side of the volume with a steady gait while holding the box.
(2) Luggage: The subject started at one end of the capture value holding the handle of the luggage. They then walked through the capture volume, pulling the roller luggage behind them. They began walking with their left foot first, while keeping a steady gait until they reached the other side of the capture volume.
(3) Briefcase: The briefcase had two different types of interactions. The first was lifting. At the start, the subject was standing straight up, then bent down and grabbed the handle, and then lifted the briefcase. They then lowered the briefcase to the ground, let go, and stood back up. In the second interaction, the subject carried the briefcase while walking. They started at one end of the capture volume while holding the briefcase in their right hand. They then walked, starting with their left foot, through the volume to the other side, with a steady gait, while holding the briefcase.
(4) Walker: In this interaction, the subject walked through the motion capture volume using the walker for support. They started at one end of the volume with their hands grasping the walker handles. The subject then lifted the handles slightly and pushed the roller walker forward while extending their arms. They set the handles down and then applied downward force on the handles to support their weight while stepping towards the walker. The process was repeated until the subject traversed the capture volume.
(5) Shopping cart: The subject approached the shopping cart and then pushed it through the motion capture volume. The subject started in a standing position a step back from the shopping cart. They stepped towards the cart and placed their hands on its handles; both of their arms were lifted up and grasped the shopping cart. They then pushed the shopping cart through the volume while walking.

(6) Wheelbarrow: The wheelbarrow had two types of interactions. The first was lifting the handles. The subject started in a standing position between the handles. They then bent down, grabbed the handles, and lifted the wheelbarrow handles. The handles were then lowered until the back of the wheelbarrow again contacted the ground. The subject then released the handles and stood back up. In the second task, the subject pushed the wheelbarrow through the volume while walking. The subject started at one end of the capture volume while holding the wheelbarrow handles, meaning that the back of the wheelbarrow was lifted and the front was balanced on its wheel. They then walked through the volume while pushing the wheelbarrow. They started walking with their left foot, developed a steady gait, and pushed the wheelbarrow through the capture volume.

(7) Door: The subject walked up to the door, opened it, stepped through, and released the door handle. They began standing a few steps away from the door. Unlike the other walking trials, the subject first took a step with their right foot due to the location of the door so they could more naturally open the door and step through it. After the right step, they stepped with their left foot towards the door while also reaching with their right hand to grasp the door handle. They then pushed the door open with their right hand and walked through, with their left foot leading. This is due to the fact that it was a right-handed door, meaning that the hinge was on the right side of the door and the handle and opening were on the left side. They then finished stepping through the door with their right foot and released the handle, allowing it to start closing. They then took a half step with their left foot, such that it evened up with their right foot. The subject was then standing straight up, and the door had closed behind them.

(8) Gait: Natural gait was also measured, since so many of the tasks involved walking with objects. This allowed a baseline comparison in future studies so that the effect of handling the objects could be considered. The subject stood at one end of the capture volume and started walking with their left foot. They walked across the capture volume and their gait was recorded.

6. Data Processing

6.1. VICON

Processing started with the data collected via our VICON motion capture system. Marker registration was verified first to ensure that all markers were continuously registered through the motion sequence, since markers may be lost occasionally. VICON Nexus data gap-filling (i.e., spline, cyclic, and pattern filling) was applied to resolve unregistered markers. For small gaps, a mixture of cyclic and spline gap-filling was applied. Cyclic filling used information from the whole trial. Since we were repeating gaits, cyclic was a great option due to the repetitive nature of the study. Spline filling used cubic spline interpolation of the points around the marker gap. Pattern filling was used for large gaps where cyclic and spline filling failed. Pattern filling referenced other markers that experience the same trajectory characteristics (rigid bodies) on the same segment.

After marker filling, VICON data were then exported. Exporting was the same for all studies, no matter the object or trial. For each full trial, trajectory data were exported in CSV data files and C3D motion files while the trigger data were exported in CSV files. Trigger data were generated by the dSpace system, as indicated later in this section. Trajectory data included motion capture data from both the subject and object.

Full trial data were also segmented in Nexus to create short segments for repeated tasks. For example, a subject may have lifted an object multiple times in a full trial, or may have pushed an object multiple times in a full trial. The segmented trajectory data were trimmed to windows where only the whole human and object marker sets were visible. Segmented trajectory data are provided in CSV data file and C3D motion file formats in the database.

6.2. AddBiomechanics

AddBiomechanics is an open-source motion capture pipeline developed at Stanford University that uses optimization to process uploaded motion capture data faster and more efficiently [24]. The C3D files from the previous subsection were uploaded to AddBiomechanics along with subject demographic, height, and weight information. The C3D data were combined with a musculoskeletal model of the subject. The OpenSim musculoskeletal model by Rajagopal et al. [25] was adapted to use our marker set, which was included in the library. The single markers used by Rajagopal at the thigh and shank were replaced by the marker rigid marker plates that we used at these locations. The four markers used by Rajagopal at the shoulder were replaced by our single marker. Our marker set also included an additional marker on the hand and three extra markers on the trunk, which were added to the model. The modified musculoskeletal model is provided in the database and is stored in AddBiomechanics with the data.

AddBiomechanics was then used to process the data. AddBiomechanics first estimated the functional joint centers and then created an initial guess for body segment scales and marker registrations [24]. Bilevel optimization was applied to fit the model geometry and kinematics to the marker data. AddBiomechanics was then used to produce exportable files that include joint and segment rotational angles. The files produced byAddBiomechanics were marker error (CSV), the joint and segment angles (MOT), and PDF previews of the data. All of these data are available in AddBiomechanics and in our database.

6.3. dSpace/Load Cells

The dSpace file was presented as a MAT file type, and contained the information from both of the load cells (force and torque). This file included time syncing data (i.e., trigger data) and force and torque measurements. Both raw and filtered data were included. Filtered data were also included by using a low pass filter with a 20 Hz cutoff frequency.

6.4. IMU

The IMU data were presented as a CSV file, and included data reported by the IMU located on the object. Data were transmitted by serial communications to the dSpace computer using the SensorConnect 15.6.4 software. The information in this file included the acceleration readings of the object when it was interacted with, and the gyroscopic readings when the object was manipulated.

6.5. Final Data Synchronization and Export

Once the data processing, described in the previous subsections, was complete, final synchronization and file generation was performed, as shown in Figure 12. Data were synchronized and exported for each subject, object, and interaction separately. A MATLAB 2024b script first loaded the data:

- VICON trajectory CSV,
- VICON trigger data CSV,
- Cut VICON trajectory CSV,
- AddBiomechanics MOT motion file,
- Load cell MAT file,
- IMU CSV file.

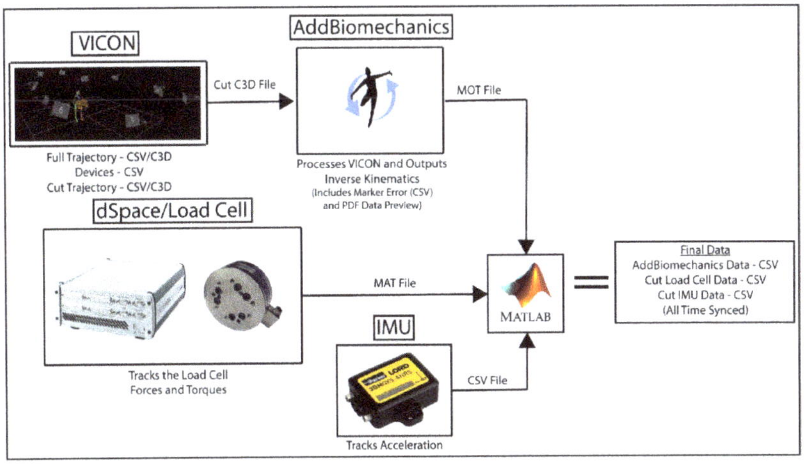

Figure 12. Data processing flowchart.

This MATLAB script then synchronized the different datasets. The VICON trigger data CSV contained analog measurements of the trigger signal which was produced by dSpace when the measurements started. The same trigger signal was recorded in the load cell MAT file, and was used to align the timestamps of the two datasets. The load cell MAT file and IMU CSV file timestamps were then synchronized by detecting the 10 taps, as indicated in Section 5.3. The cut VICON trajectory CSV timestamps were the same as those in the VICON trajectory CSV, so the timestamps in the Cut VICON data are then used segment the Load Cell and IMU data correspondingly for each trial. This allows the cut data to represent both the kinematics and kinetics for each trial separately. AddBiomechanics shifts the start time for each trial to zero to represent the start of each trial uniformly. The segmented Load Cell data and IMU data for each trial are likewise shifted to zero to correlate to the AddBiomechanics data. MATLAB exports the synchronized Final Data (AddBiomechanics, Load Cell, and IMU) in CSV format.

7. Results

7.1. Subjects

The dataset currently contains data from six subjects, which will be expanded as this project continues. The subjects are all healthy males ranging from 18 to 30 years old. They range from 1.6 to 1.9 m in height and 56.6 to 133 kg in weight. Data were collected according to University of Utah IRB #00123921.

7.2. Datasets

Our dataset includes a few different datasets from the different stages of processing, as shown in Figure 12.

(1) The main dataset is located on GitHub and SimTK and contains all the files described in Section 6 and shown in Figure 13. Data are arranged by subject, object, and task. The AddBiomechanics folder contains the data generated from the AddBiomechanics which is the marker error (CSV), motion files (MOT), and PDFs that show a preview of the data in the motion files. The cut VICON data folder contains the windowed marker data from VICON (CSV/C3D). The dSpace data contains an MAT file of each load cell and additional data needed for time syncing. The full VICON data folder contains the whole marker trajectory file for each task (CSV/C3D) and the trigger data file for syncing (CSV). The IMU data folder contains the IMU sensor data (CSV). The

final data folder contains the synced AddBiomechanics full body joint and segment angles (CSV), the force and torque from the load cells (CSV), and the IMU data (CSV) of the windows of the VICON data. The entire library of data is available on GitHub and SimTK.

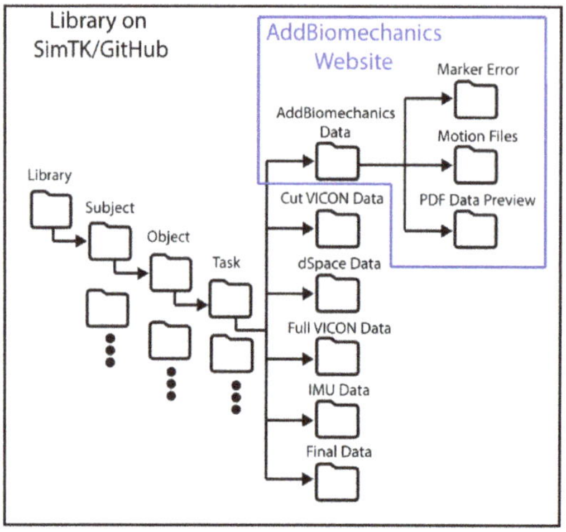

Figure 13. Database file organization.

(2) The AddBiomechanics data are also available on the AddBiomechanics website and contain everything that is processed through AddBiomechanics, as shown in Figure 13. It also contains the uploaded files used to generate the AddBiomechanics data. It contains the PDF, the marker errors, and the motion files described above. It contains the marker data in a (TRC) file and the OpenSim models used to obtain this information. AddBiomechanics is provided so that other researchers can evaluate the data processing, and have ready access to raw and processed data.

(3) The main dataset is also available on GitHub and SimTK, and contains everything that is in the main database file described above. There is also the OpenSim model used for AddBiomechanics (OSIM), example processing code (MATLAB), and the homogeneous transformations (CSV) described in Section 5.5, which are available in the library.

7.3. Data Sample

There is a large amount of data in the library, and many different actions/objects. An example of the data is shown in Figure 14. Using the cut dataset from VICON, the AddBiomechanics dataset was generated. An example of the motion data included in the AddBiomechanics output is shown in Figure 14. The data shown are the right and left knee angles of a subject picking up a briefcase and then setting it back down ten times. These are only a subset of the kinematic angles available in the dataset. The dataset contains joint angles and segment angles of the whole body in the MOT files in the AddBiomechanics folder. As seen from the knee data, the angles of both knees increase as the subject bends down and reaches a position to grab the briefcase, and then it decreases back to ~zero in a standing position. The subject then bends back down to place the briefcase on the ground and releases the handle.

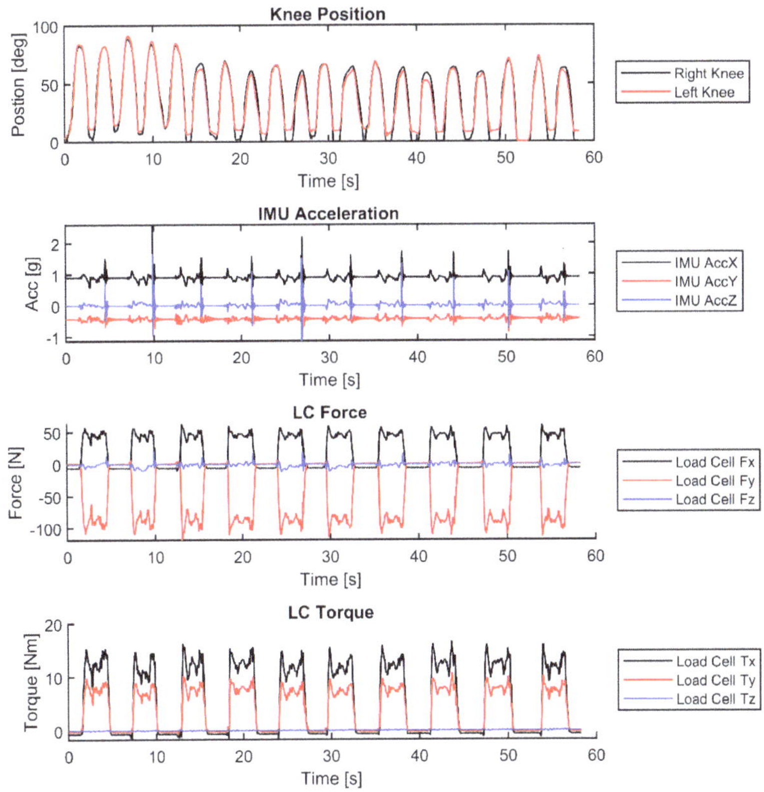

Figure 14. Example of typical data showing knee rotation from AddBiomechanics, IMU acceleration of the object when it is being manipulated, and force and torque from the load cell of the subject lifting and manipulating a briefcase.

Example data from the load cell and the IMU are also presented in Figure 14. These data are aligned with respect to the time of the cut VICON and AddBiomechanics data. When the object is interacted with, the load cell and IMU signals vary. An example of the accelerometer data is shown in Figure 14. Spikes correlate to when the briefcase is picked up and when it is set back down. Non-zero forces and torques between the spikes correlate to the load cell data measured while the subject lifts and lowers the briefcase. The load cell data then returns to ~zero when the briefcase is set on the ground and released.

7.4. Data Analysis Example: Wheelbarrow

Data from the library are intended to be used to characterize how subjects interact with large objects using one- and two-handed manipulation while locomoting. Such information is beneficial to the biomechanics and robotics communities, where gait, interaction forces, and object motion can be studied. The biomechanics community, for example, may be interested in gait changes between normal walking and walking while carrying an object. Data are commonly analyzed to provide data such as spatiotemporal gait characteristics (e.g., stride length or cadence, etc.) [19,26,27], biomechanical characteristics (e.g., knee range of motion), joint trajectories (e.g., knee joint angle vs. gait cycle) [26,28] and cyclograms (e.g., comparing joint angles, such as knee vs. hip angle for one leg [28,29] or left vs. right angles for the knee joint [27]). Data from the library can provide such information, but require additional data processing, as described below. In the first example, we characterize a user lifting the wheelbarrow. In the second example, we characterize a person walking with and without the wheelbarrow.

7.4.1. Time Series Data: Wheelbarrow Lift

Data can be analyzed to characterize typical results during an interaction. In this case, we show how data from lifting and lowering the wheelbarrow repeatedly can be processed to identify mean values and confidence intervals during the lifting motion. These data are cut using the AddBiomechanics right knee data. In this case, we show how the data can be analyzed to determine when a user is lifting the wheelbarrow. Data cutting analyzes 25 knee angle points moving along the signal. As the user crouches down to reach the handle, the knee angle increases, which produces positive slope between measurements. The user will eventually stand up with the wheelbarrow handle, which causes the knee angle to decrease. The transition from crouching to lifting is determined by when a positive slope has been detected 24 times and then a negative slope occurs at the next point. As the user lifts the wheelbarrow, knee angle measurements continue to decrease, producing negative slopes. When a negative slope has been detected 24 times and the knee angle starts to increase, a positive slope is determined, which indicates that the user is beginning to crouch down with the wheelbarrow, marking the end of the lifting.

Once the lift cycles are found, the sensor readings from the IMU and load cell are cut and processed based upon the start and end of the lifting cycle to show mean values and confidence intervals during the lifting cycle. The data in Figure 15 show this process applied to knee angle, IMU acceleration, and load cell torque and force. The data shows ten lift cycles of a wheelbarrow from one of the subjects, shown as gray lines in the plot. The larger black signal is the mean value of those signals. The bold red signals represent the ±95% confidence intervals from the data. This analysis shows how this subject typically lifts the wheelbarrow. Future work could then combine data from multiple subjects to show broader trends of how users lift wheelbarrows. The trajectories from different subjects can also be compared using cross-correlation [30] to characterize their similarity.

Once the data are cut up into the ten lifts, the data can be analyzed further. Using the AddBiomechanics data, the angles of the right hip, knee, and ankle are analyzed. The mean and standard deviation of the minimum angle, maximum angle, and the range of motion of the hip, knee, and ankle angles from the 10 lifts are shown in Table 2. This information is useful to understand the amount of movement these joints undergo while lifting a wheelbarrow. These data could be used to compare how different users lift a wheelbarrow in future work.

Table 2. The mean and standard deviation of the minimum, maximum, and range of motion of the knee during a wheelbarrow lift.

Joint	Minimum Angle (Degrees)	Maximum Angle (Degrees)	Range of Motion (Degrees)
Hip	12.5 ± 8.2	75.3 ± 7.4	62.8 ± 7.3
Knee	15.5 ± 3.6	76.6 ± 6.8	61.1 ± 8.2
Ankle	−14.1 ± 1.6	4.3 ± 5.0	18.4 ± 4.2

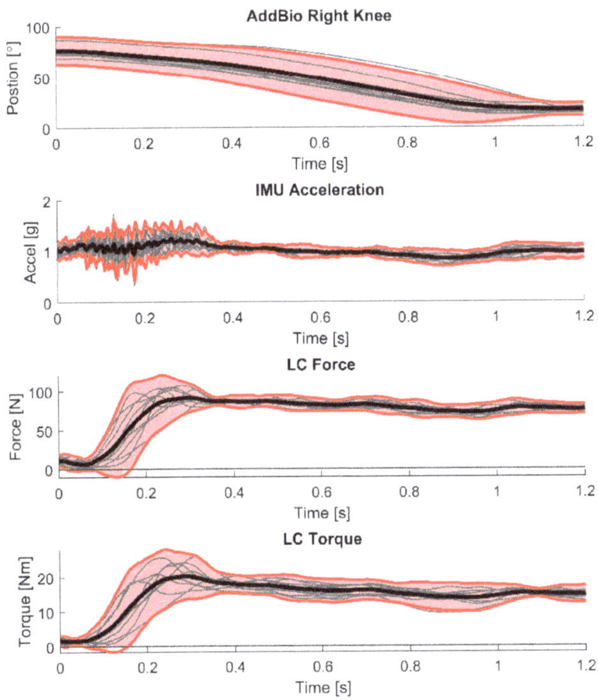

Figure 15. Example of 10 lift cycles of a wheelbarrow from one subject and the sensor readings during lift (IMU, load cell). The gray signals are the 10 trials, the bold red signals are the ±95% confidence intervals, and the black signal is the mean of the signals.

7.4.2. Gait Characterization: Regular Gait vs. Wheelbarrow Gait

Data can also be analyzed to provide information about gait characteristics. In this case, we show how one subject's gait varies while pushing the wheelbarrow compared to their regular gait. In the future, spatiotemporal parameters and kinematics data will be examined, and kinetics data will be examined to show nominal parameters during, gait as well as cyclograms, to indicate variations during gait.

Data characterization requires segmenting data based upon the cyclic nature of the data and comparing data between cycles. Data are segmented based upon right heal strike, which is estimated based upon when the right heal marker (i.e., RHEE, Figure 2) z position reaches a minimum. These data are segmented by heel strikes, but midstance and toe off can be used instead following Luttmer et al. midstance and toe-off algorithms in our prior work [31]. Each data segment is then analyzed to estimate spatiotemporal gait parameters for each gait cycle, which then provide mean and standard deviations of the parameters across multiple cycles.

The data library contains six subjects and is growing. An example of spatiotemporal parameters from one subject with ten gait trajectories is shown in Table 3. The table shows the differences in spatiotemporal parameters between the subject's regular gait and when the subject is manipulating a wheelbarrow while walking. From the table, regular gait step length, stride length, walking speed, cadence, and stride frequency are all larger than that of the subject walking with the wheelbarrow. The step time and stride time is also slower when the subject is manipulating the wheelbarrow, which correlates to the user being more careful while carrying a load. From this analysis, there is a difference in the gait of a subject with and without manipulating an object. Future work will combine all the subjects' data in the library and perform statistical analysis.

Table 3. Spatiotemporal parameters of a regular gait and gait while manipulating a wheelbarrow.

Parameters	Regular Gait	Wheelbarrow Carry Gait
Step Length [m]	0.66 ± 0.22	0.63 ± 0.03
Step Time [s]	0.58 ± 0.08	0.63 ± 0.04
Stride Length [m]	1.45 ± 0.04	1.24 ± 0.06
Stride Time [s]	1.21 ± 0.03	1.25 ± 0.05
Walking Speed [m/s]	1.20 ± 0.04	0.99 ± 0.06
Cadence [steps/m]	49.7 ± 1.15	48.0 ± 2.00
Stride Frequency [strides/m]	24.9 ± 0.56	24.0 ± 1.00

Cyclograms are also used for characterizing gait. Cyclograms plot one joint angle versus another joint angle during a gait cycle [29]. Changes in gait are denoted by changes in the shape of the plots [29]. Comparing knee and hip angle from one leg allows comparison of changes in gait [28,29], while comparing similar joints (e.g., hip or ankle) from the left and right legs can highlight asymmetry in gait [27]. Data provided in this database can provide either type of cyclogram, since the motion of legs was captured.

This data library contains the regular gait of the subjects and the gait of the subject while walking and interacting with each of the objects. Figure 16 shows the regular gait of a subject compared to the gait of a subject while manipulating a wheelbarrow. The gait is from heel strike to heel strike. The plots on the left side show the knee–knee cyclograms comparing the subject's regular walking gait and walking gait when pushing a wheelbarrow. The shapes of the plots are similar, but they are offset. When pushing the wheelbarrow, the left leg produces a larger range of motion and the right leg shows a shorter range of motion. The envelopes enclosed by the curves while pushing the wheelbarrow are larger in some regions and smaller in other regions compared to the regular gait, also indicating that there is variation in relative knee angles when pushing the wheelbarrow.

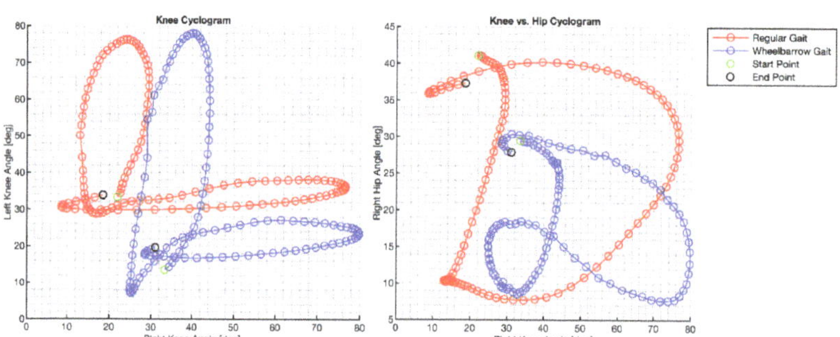

Figure 16. Example cyclogram of a subject's regular gait versus the subject's gait while manipulating a wheelbarrow.

The right subfigure in Figure 16 examines the same walking gaits, but plots the cyclograms comparing the right hip and right knee angle. There is a significant difference between regular walking gait and walking with the wheelbarrow. The range of motion of both the hip and knee have both decreased and shifted. The right knee angle is nominally larger but has less variation. The right hip angle is nominally smaller and shows less variation. As a result, the envelope enclosed by the curve while manipulating the wheelbarrow is significantly smaller compared to the envelope from the regular gait. There is also a small cusp at the bottom left corner of the envelope with regular gait where angles are at their minimum values, whereas the cusp encloses a much larger volume when pushing the wheelbarrow. This indicates that the regular gait joint angles both reach their minimum values simultaneously, whereas the gait with the wheelbarrow results in the joints reaching their minimum in a more staggered behavior. These cyclograms highlight that the gait is very different when the subject is manipulating the object while walking.

8. Conclusions

We have presented a database characterizing human interaction with medium-to-large-sized objects from daily living. Unique to this database is its focus on characterizing data important for representing haptic interaction with objects, such as interaction forces, inertial measurements, and object motion, in addition to normal human biomechanical data. Such information should be useful for researchers working in ergonomics, biomechanics, robotics, virtual reality, and gaming.

Methods for collecting the data were presented. The various sensors used to create this database were described. Motion capture marker locations on the human subjects and objects were indicated. The transformations between the sensors, markers, and the human hand were described and included in the library. Data processing through VICON, AddBiomechanics, and MATLAB were presented to produce data that is useful for future applications. An example subset of data was presented to show the output of one of our trials for one object interaction trial. Examples of how these data can be used for different types of processing it were also described. This included looking at ten signals of wheelbarrow lift with means and 95% confidence intervals of the knee joint and sensor signals, accompanied by joint range of motion means and standard deviation of the hip, knee, and ankle. The dataset has gait trials which can be compared, such as the differences between spatiotemporal parameters of a regular gait and when the subject is manipulating a wheelbarrow. Cyclograms of regular gait and gait with a wheelbarrow are shown, which is another way these data can be used. The library is posted on AddBiomechanics, GitHub, and SimTK, with their URLs listed in the Data Availability Statement.

Future work will include continuing to grow the database, identifying object properties, and characterizing human interaction with those objects. Object characteristics will then be programmed into haptic manipulators. Similar studies to those presented here will evaluate human subjects interacting with the manipulators and will be added to this database.

Author Contributions: Conceptualization, N.G.L., N.I.B., J.M.H. and M.A.M.; methodology, N.G.L., N.I.B., J.F.-G., J.M.H. and M.A.M.; software, N.G.L., N.I.B. and J.F.-G.; validation, N.G.L., N.I.B. and J.F.-G.; formal analysis, N.G.L. and J.F.-G.; investigation, N.G.L., N.I.B., J.M.H. and M.A.M.; resources, N.G.L. and M.A.M.; data curation, N.G.L. and M.A.M.; writing—original draft preparation, N.G.L., N.I.B. and M.A.M.; writing—review and editing, N.G.L. and M.A.M.; visualization, N.G.L., J.M.H. and M.A.M.; supervision, N.G.L., J.M.H. and M.A.M.; project administration, M.A.M.; funding acquisition, N.G.L., J.M.H. and M.A.M. All authors have read and agreed to the published version of the manuscript.

Funding: This research was funded by the US National Science Foundation, grant number 1911194.

Institutional Review Board Statement: The study was conducted in accordance with the Declaration of Helsinki, and approved by the Institutional Review Board of the University of Utah (IRB_00123921).

Informed Consent Statement: Informed consent was obtained from all subjects involved in the study.

Data Availability Statement: Data presented in this library is freely available for public use. Library databases are available at AddBiomechanics, GitHub, and SimTK. The AddBiomechanics URL is: https://addbiomechanics.org/ (accessed on 4 March 2025). The GitHub URL is: https://github.com/nluttmer1/MeLLO-Data-Library (accessed on 4 March 2025). The SimTK URL is: https://simtk.org/projects/mello-library/ (accessed on 4 March 2025) [32].

Acknowledgments: The authors would like to thank Sasha McKee and Derrick Greer for their efforts to create the cart and wheelbarrow objects. We would also like to thank Brock Smith and Jaden Hunter for their help in processing VICON data.

Conflicts of Interest: The authors declare no conflicts of interest.

References

1. Feix, T.; Bullock, I.M.; Dollar, A.M. Analysis of human grasping behavior: Object characteristics and grasp type. *IEEE Trans. Haptics* **2014**, *7*, 311–323. [CrossRef] [PubMed]
2. Mandery, C.; Terlemez, Ö.; Do, M.; Vahrenkamp, N.; Asfour, T. The KIT whole-body human motion database. In Proceedings of the 2015 International Conference on Advanced Robotics (ICAR), Istanbul, Turkey, 27–31 July 2015; pp. 329–336.
3. Mandery, C.; Terlemez, Ö.; Do, M.; Vahrenkamp, N.; Asfour, T. Unifying representations and large-scale whole-body motion databases for studying human motion. *IEEE Trans. Robot.* **2016**, *32*, 796–809. [CrossRef]
4. Meixner, A.; Krebs, F.; Jaquier, N.; Asfour, T. An Evaluation of Action Segmentation Algorithms on Bimanual Manipulation Datasets. In Proceedings of the 2023 IEEE/RSJ International Conference on Intelligent Robots and Systems (IROS), Detroit, MI, USA, 1–5 October 2023; pp. 4912–4919.
5. Kang, S.; Ishihara, K.; Sugimoto, N.; Morimoto, J. Curriculum-based humanoid robot identification using large-scale human motion database. *Front. Robot. AI* **2023**, *10*, 1282299. [CrossRef]
6. Krebs, F.; Asfour, T. A bimanual manipulation taxonomy. *IEEE Robot. Autom. Lett.* **2022**, *7*, 11031–11038. [CrossRef]
7. Emami, M.; Bayat, A.; Tafazolli, R.; Quddus, A. A survey on haptics: Communication, sensing and feedback. *IEEE Commun. Surv. Tutor.* **2024**. [CrossRef]
8. Varalakshmi, B.; Thriveni, J.; Venugopal, K.; Patnaik, L. Haptics: State of the art survey. *Int. J. Comput. Sci. Issues* **2012**, *9*, 234.
9. El Saddik, A. The potential of haptics technologies. *IEEE Instrum. Meas. Mag.* **2007**, *10*, 10–17. [CrossRef]
10. Truong, T.E.; Luttmer, N.G.; Eshete, E.R.; Zaki, A.B.M.; Greer, D.D.; Hirschi, T.J.; Stewart, B.R.; Gregory, C.A.; Minor, M.A. Evaluating the Effect of Multi-Sensory Stimulation on Startle Response Using the Virtual Reality Locomotion Interface MS.TPAWT. *Virtual Worlds* **2022**, *1*, 62–81. [CrossRef]
11. Russo, M.; Lee, J.; Hogan, N.; Sternad, D. Mechanical effects of canes on standing posture: Beyond perceptual information. *J. neuroeng. Rehabil.* **2022**, *19*, 1–13. [CrossRef]
12. McClain, E.W. Simulation and Control of a Human Assistive Quadrupedal Robot. PhD Thesis, The University of Utah, Salt Lake City, UT, USA, 2022.
13. Zhu, W.; Ma, X.; Ro, D.; Ci, H.; Zhang, J.; Shi, J.; Gao, F.; Tian, Q.; Wang, Y. Human motion generation: A survey. *IEEE Trans. Pattern Anal. Mach. Intell.* **2023**, *46*, 2430–2449. [CrossRef]
14. Bassani, G.; Filippeschi, A.; Avizzano, C.A. A Dataset of Human Motion and Muscular Activities in Manual Material Handling Tasks for Biomechanical and Ergonomic Analyses. *IEEE Sens. J.* **2021**, *21*, 24731–24739. [CrossRef]
15. Geissinger, J.H.; Asbeck, A.T. Motion inference using sparse inertial sensors, self-supervised learning, and a new dataset of unscripted human motion. *Sensors* **2020**, *20*, 6330. [CrossRef] [PubMed]
16. Kang, P.; Zhu, K.; Jiang, S.; He, B.; Shull, P. HBOD: A Novel Dataset with Synchronized Hand, Body, and Object Manipulation Data for Human-Robot Interaction. In Proceedings of the 2023 IEEE 19th International Conference on Body Sensor Networks (BSN), Boston, MA, USA, 9–11 October 2023; pp. 1–4.
17. Maurice, P.; Malaisé, A.; Amiot, C.; Paris, N.; Richard, G.-J.; Rochel, O.; Ivaldi, S. Human movement and ergonomics: An industry-oriented dataset for collaborative robotics. *Int. J. Robot. Res.* **2019**, *38*, 1529–1537. [CrossRef]
18. Bhatnagar, B.L.; Xie, X.; Petrov, I.A.; Sminchisescu, C.; Theobalt, C.; Pons-Moll, G. Behave: Dataset and method for tracking human object interactions. In Proceedings of the IEEE/CVF Conference on Computer Vision and Pattern Recognition, 19–20 June 2022; pp. 15935–15946.
19. Wang, Y.; Truong, T.E.; Chesebrough, S.W.; Willemsen, P.; Foreman, K.B.; Merryweather, A.S.; Hollerbach, J.M.; Minor, M.A. Augmenting virtual reality terrain display with smart shoe physical rendering: A pilot study. *IEEE Trans. Haptics* **2020**, *14*, 174–187. [CrossRef]
20. Sabetian, P. Modular Cable-Driven Robot Development and Its Applications in Locomotion and Rehabilitation. Ph.D. Thesis, The University of Utah, Salt Lake City, UT, USA, 2019.

21. Duffell, L.D.; Hope, N.; McGregor, A.H. Comparison of kinematic and kinetic parameters calculated using a cluster-based model and Vicon's plug-in gait. *Proc. Inst. Mech. Eng. Part H J. Eng. Med.* **2014**, *228*, 206–210. [CrossRef]
22. Goldfarb, N.; Lewis, A.; Tacescu, A.; Fischer, G.S. Open source Vicon Toolkit for motion capture and Gait Analysis. *Comput. Methods Programs Biomed.* **2021**, *212*, 106414. [CrossRef]
23. Hollerbach, J.M. Introduction to Robotics: Chapter 7: Velocity and Acceleration. University of Utah. Available online: https://my.eng.utah.edu/~cs5310/files/chapter7.pdf (accessed on 29 January 2025).
24. Werling, K.; Bianco, N.A.; Raitor, M.; Stingel, J.; Hicks, J.L.; Collins, S.H.; Delp, S.L.; Liu, C.K. AddBiomechanics: Automating model scaling, inverse kinematics, and inverse dynamics from human motion data through sequential optimization. *PLoS ONE* **2023**, *18*, e0295152. [CrossRef]
25. Rajagopal, A.; Dembia, C.L.; DeMers, M.S.; Delp, D.D.; Hicks, J.L.; Delp, S.L. Full-body musculoskeletal model for muscle-driven simulation of human gait. *IEEE Trans. Biomed. Eng.* **2016**, *63*, 2068–2079. [CrossRef]
26. Foreman, K.B.; Wilson, C.; Dibble, L.E.; Merryweather, A.S. Training persons with Parkinson disease using an advanced CAVE virtual reality system. *FASEB J.* **2019**, *33*, 335.4. [CrossRef]
27. Arippa, F.; Leban, B.; Monticone, M.; Cossu, G.; Casula, C.; Pau, M. A study on lower limb asymmetries in Parkinson's disease during gait assessed through kinematic-derived parameters. *Bioengineering* **2022**, *9*, 120. [CrossRef]
28. Chesebrough, S.W. Robot-Assisted Gait Rehabilitation Using Virtual Reality with Torso Force Feedback. Ph.D. Thesis, The University of Utah, Salt Lake City, UT, USA, 2018.
29. Hollerbach, J.M.; Mills, R.; Tristano, D.; Christensen, R.R.; Thompson, W.B.; Xu, Y. Torso force feedback realistically simulates slope on treadmill-style locomotion interfaces. *Int. J. Robot. Res.* **2001**, *20*, 939–952. [CrossRef]
30. Stoica, P.; Moses, R.L. *Spectral Analysis of Signals*; Pearson Prentice Hall: Upper Saddle River, NJ, USA, 2005; Volume 452.
31. Luttmer, N.G.; Truong, T.E.; Boynton, A.M.; Carrier, D.; Minor, M.A. Treadmill based three tether parallel robot for evaluating auditory warnings while running. In Proceedings of the 2020 IEEE International Conference on Robotics and Automation (ICRA), Paris, France, 31 May–31 August 2020; pp. 9135–9142.
32. Luttmer, N.G.; Baum, N.I.; Flores-Gonzalez, J.; Hollerbach, J.M.; Minor, M.A. MeLLO Data Library (2025-present). GitHub. Available online: https://simtk.org/projects/mello-library/ (accessed on 4 March 2025).

Disclaimer/Publisher's Note: The statements, opinions and data contained in all publications are solely those of the individual author(s) and contributor(s) and not of MDPI and/or the editor(s). MDPI and/or the editor(s) disclaim responsibility for any injury to people or property resulting from any ideas, methods, instructions or products referred to in the content.

bioengineering

MDPI

Article

Exploring the Association of Hallux Limitus with Baropodometric Gait Pattern Changes

Natalia Tovaruela-Carrión [1], Ricardo Becerro-de-Bengoa-Vallejo [2], Marta Elena Losa-Iglesias [3], Daniel López-López [4,*], Juan Gómez-Salgado [5,6] and Javier Bayod-López [7]

1 Faculty of Nursing, Physiotherapy and Podiatry, University of Seville, 41009 Seville, Spain; ntovaruela@us.es
2 Faculty of Nursing, Physiotherapy and Podiatry, Complutense University of Madrid, 28040 Madrid, Spain; ribebeva@ucm.es
3 Faculty of Health Sciences, Universidad Rey Juan Carlos, 28922 Alcorcón, Spain; marta.losa@urjc.es
4 Research, Health and Podiatry Group, Department of Health Sciences, Faculty of Nursing and Podiatry, Industrial Campus of Ferrol, Universidade da Coruña, 15403 Ferrol, Spain
5 Department of Sociology, Social Work and Public Health, Faculty of Labour Sciences, Universidad de Huelva, 21004 Huelva, Spain; salgado@uhu.es
6 Safety and Health Postgraduate Program, Universidad Espíritu Santo, Guayaquil 092301, Ecuador
7 Applied Mechanics and Bioengineering Group (AMB), Aragon Institute of Engineering Research (I3A), Centro de Investigación Biomecánica en Red CIBER-BBN, Universidad de Zaragoza, 50009 Zaragoza, Spain; jbayod@unizar.es
* Correspondence: daniellopez@udc.es

Abstract: Background: Hallux limitus (HL) is a condition marked by the restricted dorsiflexion of the first metatarsophalangeal joint, causing pain and functional limitations, especially during the propulsive phase of walking. This restriction affects the gait, particularly in the final phase, and impairs foot stability and support. HL is more common in adults and leads to biomechanical and functional adaptations. The purpose of this study was to investigate the differences in the center of pressure between subjects with hallux limitus and those with healthy feet. **Methods:** A total of 80 participants (40 with bilateral HL and 40 healthy controls) aged 18 to 64 were selected from a biomechanics center at the Universidade da Coruña, Spain. The gait analysis focused on three key phases: initial contact, forefoot contact, and the loading response. Data were collected using a portable baropodometric platform and analyzed using IBM SPSS Statistics 29.0.2.0; statistical significance was set at $p < 0.05$, with a 95% confidence interval. **Results:** The gait analysis indicated that the case group exhibited statistically significant differences, showing lower values in the left foot load response during the foot contact time (77.83 ± 40.17) compared to the control group (100.87 ± 29.27) (p = 0. 010) and in the foot contact percentage (p = 0. 013) during the stance phase (10.02 ± 5.68) compared to the control group (13.05 ± 3.60). **Conclusions:** Bilateral HL causes subtle gait changes, with individuals showing greater contact time values in the total stance phase versus the control group. Early detection may improve quality of life and prevent complications.

Keywords: hallux limitus; gait analysis; gait patterns; stance phase gait

1. Introduction

The first metatarsophalangeal joint (IMTFJ) is extremely important in gait patterns—specifically in the terminal stance and pre-swing phases. In these phases, 40% to 60% of the body mass is sustained by the hallux, thus doubling the load that it supports with respect to the lesser toes [1]. The IMTFJ must offer the appropriate dorsiflexion (DF) required to produce the propulsion moment [2,3], and this range of dorsiflexion at the

IMTFJ typically averages 58° in normal subjects [2,4]. The concept of hallux limitus (HL) refers to a limitation in the dorsiflexion of the IMTFJ, which usually occurs in 1 out of 40 subjects over the age of 50, making it the main cause of foot arthritis, with an increasing incidence among the elderly population [5]. Senga et al., in their study, determined that the prevalence among people over 50 years of age was 26.7% [6], and, according to Bejarano-Pineda et al., it is as high as 73% in the population with end-stage ankle arthritis [7], with women being twice as likely to suffer from it [8]. The presence of HL is characterized by the appearance of hyperkeratosis in the area of the interphalangeal joint of the hallux, as well as under the head of the second metatarsal [9]. The early stages of HL occur with periods of painful synovitis and slight limitations in IMTFJ dorsiflexion, as osteophytes begin to develop due to arthritic degeneration, resulting in a significant dorsal bony protrusion that may cause friction with footwear and modify the gait [5,10]. When the disease is in a more advanced phase, neuropathic pain, paresthesia, and a positive Tinel sign as a result of the osteophytic compression of the dorsomedial cutaneous nerve are common. The advancement to hallux rigidus is linked to the drastic to total loss of joint functionality, chronic pain, and diminished quality of life [2,11,12]. Although previous studies report that a restriction in the DF movement of the IMTFJ linked to a pronated or highly pronated foot occurs due to biomechanical factors [13,14], there is currently still no agreement on the pathophysiology, cause, or treatment of HL [10,11,15], even though the etiology is considered multifactorial [16,17]

In spite of its clinical importance, the etiology and treatment of HL remain largely unclear [18]. The pathophysiology of HL is not well comprehended, with idiopathy being the most frequently noted etiology [19]. Lengthened metatarsals, hypermobility of the first ray, metatarsus primus elevatus, interphalangeal hallux valgus, being a woman, and having a family history have all been recognized as risk factors [4]. One of the possible etiological factors of HL that has been described is hindfoot eversion, which is associated with a higher degree of DF of the first ray [20].

A decreased range of IMTFJ motion when weight bearing and normal IMTFJ motion when not weight bearing is referred to as functional HL; this results in changes in gait patterns due to the limitation of closed-kinetic-chain joint movement, which restricts function during the terminal phase of gait by the obstruction of the third rocker (propulsive phase) [11,12,21]. The third rocker or forefoot rocker initiates when the heel begins to rise from the surface and ends when the entire foot is lifted from the toe area to begin the swing phase of the foot. At this point, it is important to have good movement in the metatarsophalangeal joints so that no type of support overload occurs in this area [22,23]. The obstruction of the third rocker causes a modification in the sagittal plane of the axis of the first radius; in accordance with the sagittal plane facilitation theory put forward by Dananberg [24], a dynamic limitation in the first MPJ during gait causes a lack of stability, forcing the body to compensate for these biomechanical changes. This leads to the center of mass shifting along the extrinsic and intrinsic structures of the foot to enhance the gait and conclude the propulsion phase [9,22]. Moreover, secondary compensations produced with the aim of improving joint movement to be able to carry out the last phase of walking can cause greater or lesser plantar pressure [12,23,25].

Individuals with HL frequently adopt compensatory gait patterns in order to reduce the discomfort and adjust to restricted mobility [26]. To counteract this limitation, they often shift their weight to the lateral side of the foot, resulting in the overloading of the lateral metatarsal heads, and sometimes push off using the lesser metatarsal heads [27,28], causing increased pressure on the lesser toes and hallux [29], while also showing decreased loading on the IMTFJ [30] and restricted hallux dorsiflexion during the stance and swing phases of gait. Previous pedobarographic studies have shown the increased loading of the lateral plantar areas and lesser metatarsal heads in patients with HL, most likely to avoid pain [31], suggesting compensatory movements in the foot and ankle to facilitate movement and avoid pain during push-off [32]. In addition to its role in locomotion, HL may influence the maintenance of balance. Postural control is a complex mechanism performed by the central nervous system and in which information transmitted by the musculoskeletal system is very important. The feet act as a link between the ground and the body; therefore, any alteration in them can influence the transmission of the forces required to maintain balance [33].

The center of pressure (COP) is described as the point that emerges from the aggregation of the ground reaction forces exerted on the plantar surface of the foot. The COP movement is recognized as an indicator of neuromuscular control while standing and walking and is thus suitable for the assessment of balance control, foot functionality, and the effectiveness of treatment [34]. Through the use of a force platform or pressure platform, this point can be calculated, and the path described by its movement during the test can be followed [31,35]. Despite this, there are aspects that are not clear in people with and without HL, such as the walking pattern and the area of the foot in contact with the surface (percentage), the duration in the foot contact area (milliseconds), and the frames within the foot area (images per second). Consequently, the aim of our research was to investigate the COP variations in subjects with and without HL. We proposed the hypothesis that participants with HL would exhibit an increase in the foot contact duration compared to normal foot contact without HL, as well as a medial shift in the COP during the stancephase.

2. Materials and Methods

2.1. Design and Sample

This research was carried out as a case–control study following the Strengthening the Reporting of Observational Studies in Epidemiology (STROBE) guidelines [36]. The participants were recruited through a consecutive non-random sample design in a biomechanical center at the Universidade da Coruña (Spain). The study was approved by the Universidade da Coruña Ethics Committee (consent no. 2024-0033), complying with the guidelines of the Declaration of Helsinki and Organic Law 3/2018 on the protection of personal data and guarantee of digital rights [37].

The sample was composed of 80 subjects (11 men and 69 women) aged 21–39 years (mean: 25.22 ± 4.45 SD). The case group was represented by 40 subjects that had bilateral HL and the control group by 40 subjects with healthy common feet.

For the HL group, the following inclusion criteria were taken into account: subjects aged between 18 and 64 years old, without diseases, not having had any surgery or trauma in the lower limbs, presenting bilateral HL, having signed the informed consent form, and participating in the project in all its phases. For the control group, the inclusion criteria were as follows: being between 18 and 64 years old, having no past surgical or traumatic history in the lower limbs, having feet that were bilaterally neutral, having completed the informed consent form, and agreeing to take part in all stages of the project. The exclusion criteria for both groups were as follows: subjects under 18 years of age and over 64 years of age, those with foot discomfort, patients on medication that could affect the final results of the study, pregnancy or breastfeeding, subjects with musculoskeletal disorders or neurological diseases, and individuals who either did not sign the consent form or were unable to comprehend the study guidelines.

2.2. Procedure

This research was performed by a skilled podiatrist specializing in biomechanical evaluation. The podiatrist interviewed the participants and provided information about all study details, such as the procedure and duration of the evaluation, as well as informing them that they could withdraw from participation at any time. This detailed explanation contributed to the high acceptance rate. The podiatrist then examined them to ensure that they met the inclusion criteria. The individuals were then weighed and their heights measured to determine their body mass index (BMI). Next, the podiatrist assessed the mobility of the hallux joint [38], and a standard clinical goniometer was employed to confirm the measurements [39]. The evaluation was conducted with the participant in a resting position, where the podiatrist needed to apply a force beneath the I metatarsal head (IMTH).

A force similar to the one applied to perform the DF of the hallux was utilized under the IMTH. A negative test (HL-) was deemed to occur if numerous movements were required to attain effective propulsion, and a positive test (HL+) was identified when the force necessary to execute the DF exceeded the one applied under the IMTH. A portable baropodometric platform (Figure 1) (Neo-Plate, Herbitas, Valencia, Spain) [40] was used in this study, according to the established protocol of Becerro de Bengoa Vallejo et al. [41].

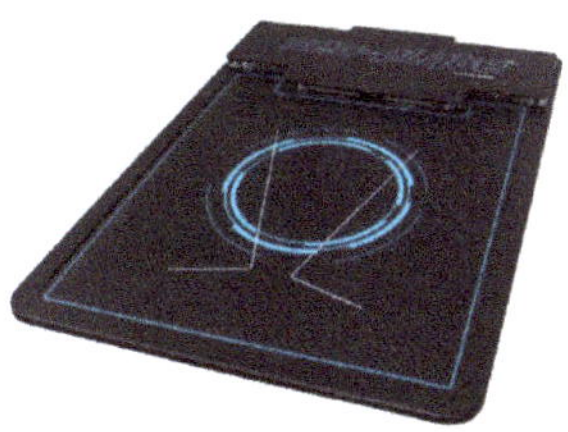

Figure 1. Neo-Plate platform used in this study.

All collected data were managed following confidentiality protocols and stored in a secure database. The data were coded to protect the participants' identities, and only the research team had access to the unidentifiable information.

2.3. Dynamic Baropodometric Analysis

A portable pressure platform with resistive sensors was employed with the following characteristics: measurements 40 × 40 cm, thickness of 8 mm, total weight of 4 kg, and 4096 resistive sensors. Measurement was carried out to the nearest 0.01 kPa for each sensor. Autocalibration was conducted before each onset. The Neo-Plate Version 1.12.28.0 for Windows software (Herbitas, Foiós, Valencia, Spain) was used to interpret the data, in accordance with the protocol of Becerro de Bengoa Vallejo et al., including a dynamic analysis focusing on the stance pattern of the gait (initial contact phase (ICP); forefoot contact phase (FFCP); flatfoot phase (FFP)), surface contact in foot area (percentage), time in foot contact area (milliseconds), and frames in foot area (images per second) [41]. The dynamics were generated for each foot variable by integrating the surface contact in the foot area (percentage), time in foot contact area (milliseconds), and frames in foot area (images per second).

2.4. Statistical Analysis

The G* Power 3.1.9.3 software (Heinrich-Heine-Universität Düsseldorf, Germany) was used to determine the sample size. The input parameters were tail(s) one, an effect size of 0.5, an α error of 0.05, power established by (1-β) of 0.7, and a distribution ratio for two groups established by N2/N = 1.

Statistical analyses were performed with IBM SPSS Statistics 29.0.2.0 for windows (Armonk, NY, USA). The Kolmogorov–Smirnov test was used to check the normality outcomes for all variables in static plantar measurement ($p < 0.05$). Independent t-tests were performed for the variables with a normal distribution. The Mann–Whitney "U" test was used for non-parametric phenomena to contrast groups with and without HL. The independent variables are presented as means, ranges from minimum to maximum, and standard deviation values.

3. Results

3.1. Sociodemographic Data

The sample consisted of 80 subjects, namely 40 with bilateral HL and 40 healthy controls, of whom 11 were men and 69 were women. The participants ranged in age from 21 to 39 years. A significant proportion of the subjects were overweight, with a BMI of 26.30 ± 5.26 kg/m^2, showing statistically significant differences ($p < 0.001$). The characteristics of all participants are detailed in Table 1.

Table 1. Main characteristics of total sample with and without bilateral hallux limitus.

Characteristics	Total Sample (n = 80) Mean ± SD (Range)	Case Group (n = 40) Mean ± SD (Range)	Control Group (n = 40) Mean ± SD (Range)	*p*-Value
Age (years)	25.22 ± 4.45 (21–39)	25.45 ± 4.34 (21–36)	25.00 ± 4.60 (21–39)	0.214 †
Weight (kg)	71.58 ± 13.69 (53–98)	76.75 ± 14.80 (56–98)	66.40 ± 10.30 (53–89)	**<0.002 †**
Height (cm)	165.15 ± 0.08 (150–185)	163.15 ± 0.08 (152–185)	166.15 ± 0.08 (150–185)	0.231 †
BMI (kg/m^2)	26.30 ± 5.26 (19.00–39.26)	28.58 ± 6.00 (21.08–39.26)	24.02 ± 3.06 (19.00–32.44)	**<0.001 †**
Sex, male/female (%)	11/69 (13.8/86.3)	7/33 (17.5/82.5)	4/36 (10/90)	0.518 ‡
Foot size	39.00 ± 2.26 (36–46)	38.83 ± 1.98 (36–44)	39.18 ± 2.53 (36–46)	0.600 †

Abbreviations: kg, kilogram; cm, centimeter; %, percentage; SD, standard deviation; N, number. † Mann–Whitney U test was used. ‡ Fisher exact test was used. In all analyses, $p < 0.05$ (with a 95% confidence interval) was considered statistically significant (bold).

3.2. Main Outcome Measure Data

As can be seen in the results presented in Table 2, during the gait analysis, the left foot minimum frame FFP was decreased in the subjects with bilateral HL (7.95 ± 4.06) compared to the control group in the left foot (10.30 ± 2.96), with a value of $p = 0.006$. Variations between the groups were noticeable in the time ($p = 0.010$), percentage ($p = 0.013$), and maximum frame in the left foot ICP, with 8.15 ± 4.25 in the case group and 10.50 ± 3.20 in the control group. However, statistically significant differences between the groups were not detected in the gait analysis of the lower left and right limbs.

Table 2. Main outcome measurements of gait analysis of total sample with and without bilateral hallux limitus.

Characteristic	Total Sample (n = 80) Mean ± SD (Range)	Case Group (n = 40) Mean ± SD (Range)	Control Group (n = 40) Mean ± SD (Range)	*p*-Value
Left foot FFCP (ms)	241.23 ± 57.22 (148–414)	243.78 ± 45.28 (178–335)	238.67 ± 67.59 (148–414)	0.349 †

Table 2. *Cont.*

Characteristic	Total Sample (n = 80) Mean ± SD (Range)	Case Group (n = 40) Mean ± SD (Range)	Control Group (n = 40) Mean ± SD (Range)	*p*-Value
Left foot FFCP (%)	33.21 ± 7.34 (20–54)	33.65 ± 6.77 (21–54)	32.78 ± 7.39 (20–48)	0.415 †
Left foot min frame FFCP	51.78 ± 8.71 (32–73)	51.95 ± 9.33 (32–73)	51.60 ± 8.15 (34–70)	0.555 †
Left foot max frame FFCP	76.24 ± 7.46 (58–91)	76.65 ± 7.38 (68–91)	75.82 ± 7.61 (58–89)	0.958 †
Left foot FFP (ms)	419.66 ± 90.39 (275–632)	433.03 ± 104.03 (275–632)	406.30 ± 73.23 (275–593)	0.196 †
Left foot FFP (%)	55.25 ± 8.75 (38–70)	56.33 ± 9.36 (41–70)	54.17 ± 8.06 (38–69)	0.359 †
Left foot min frame FFP	9.13 ± 3.72 (1–17)	7.95 ± 4.06 (1–13)	10.30 ± 2.96 (3–17)	**0.006 †**
Left foot max frame FFP	51.75 ± 8.72 (32–73)	51.90 ± 9.36 (32–73)	51.60 ± 8.15 (34–70)	0.514 †
Left foot ICP (ms)	89.35 ± 36.80 (9–167)	77.83 ± 40.17 (9–128)	100.87 ± 29.27 (29–167)	**0.010 †**
Left foot ICP (%)	11.54 ± 4.96 (1–21)	10.02 ± 5.68 (1–18)	13.05 ± 3.60 (4–21)	**0.013 †**
Left foot min frame ICP	0 ± 0.00 (0–0)	0 ± 0.00 (0–0)	0 ± 0.00 (0–0)	1.000 †
Left foot max frame ICP	9.33 ± 3.92 (1–17)	8.15 ± 4.25 (1–16)	10.50 ± 3.20 (3–17)	**0.009 †**
Right foot FFCP (ms)	261.50 ± 139.24 (148–748)	278.65 ± 173.85 (148–748)	244.35 ± 91.91 (158–455)	0.900 †
Right foot FFCP (%)	35.81 ± 17.56 (20–99)	37.63 ± 22.32 (21–99)	34.00 ± 10.93 (20–58)	0.896 †
Right foot min frame FFCP	49.76 ± 14.96 (1–71)	48.95 ± 18.40 (1–71)	50.58 ± 10.66 (30–68)	0.664 †
Right foot max frame FFCP	76.31 ± 8.41 (54–91)	77.23 ± 7.30 (68–89)	75.40 ± 9.40 (54–91)	0.527 †
Right foot FFP (ms)	404.57 ± 129.36 (0–602)	391.38 ± 157.12 (0–602)	417.77 ± 94.09 (254–561)	0.881 †
Right foot FFP (%)	53.40 ± 15.50 (0–70)	50.88 ± 19.01 (0–68)	55.93 ± 10.57 (34–70)	0.434 †
Right foot min frame FFP	8.63 ± 3.48 (1–18)	9.15 ± 3.32 (1–18)	8.10 ± 3.61 (1–14)	0.090 †
Right foot max frame FFP	49.76 ± 14.96 (1–71)	48.95 ± 18.40 (1–71)	50.58 ± 10.66 (30–68)	0.664 †
Right foot ICP (ms)	84.41 ± 34.42 (9.00–176)	89.58 ± 32.76 (9.00–176)	79.25 ± 35.67 (9.00–138)	0.078 †
Right foot ICP (%)	10.79 ± 4.59 (1–22)	11.50 ± 4.57 (1–22)	10.08 ± 4.54 (1–17)	0.282 †
Right foot min frame ICP	0 ± 0.00 (0–0)	0 ± 0.00 (0–0)	0 ± 0.00 (0–0)	1.000 †
Right foot max frame ICP	8.63 ± 3.48 (1–18)	9.15 ± 3.32 (1–18)	8.10 ± 3.61 (1–14)	0.090 †

Abbreviations: ICP, initial contact phase; FFCP, forefoot contact phase; FFP, flatfoot phase. ms, meters per second; kpa, kilopascal; %, percentage; SD, standard deviation; N, number. † Mann–Whitney U test was used. In all analyses, $p < 0.05$ (with a 95% confidence interval) was considered statistically significant (bold).

4. Discussion

The main objective of this case–control study was to investigate the COP differences in subjects with and without HL. To the best of our knowledge, this was an innovative study. It is important to emphasize that this was a preliminary exploration aimed at assessing the association between bilateral HL and gait alterations in comparison to healthy individuals. In this study, the protocol used by Becerro de Bengoa in previous research was followed [38,41]. Conducting the discussion was very difficult due to the novelty of this topic, and it was difficult to compare our results with those of other previous studies.

The findings indicated statistically significant variations in the ICP in the left foot in both groups. The results obtained in this research are in agreement with that of Canseco [42], which indicates that the restriction in the range of motion is the most noticeable at pre-swing and toe-off, when the dorsiflexion of the hallux is essential for the propulsion of the limb into the swing phase. These outcomes align with earlier research that suggests that the limited range of motion linked to IMTFJ osteoarthritis disrupts the natural propulsive function of the foot [39,43].

In this study, the group with bilateral HL reduced the contact area in terms of time and percentage. These results can be related to the study by Castro et al., consisting of an analysis of gait parameters in individuals with HL using Optogait [44], which highlighted the existence of alterations in the spatiotemporal aspects of gait compared to the control group. Differences were detected in the step length, the stride length for both the right and left feet, and the loading time. Canseco et al. also found gait alterations in subjects with HL compared to the control group, observing a prolonged support phase and a reduction in walking speed and stride length [42,45,46]. Therefore, according to these results, the presence of HL alters the dynamics of walking and affects its normal development.

In our study, significant differences were observed in the minimum frame in the forefoot contact phase for the left foot. Research has shown that the presence of HL causes greater plantar pressure to be generated under the hallux and therefore an increase in pressure on the rest of the forefoot [12,29,31]. Zammit et al., in their study, indicated that people with IMTFJ osteoarthritis displayed significantly greater maximum forces and peak pressures under the hallux and lesser toes [30].

Morasiewicz et al. conducted a study similar to ours but in subjects with a degenerative ankle injury (osteoarthritis), where they evaluated the change in balance and load distribution in the lower limbs in patients before and after ankle arthrodesis. They observed that the deformity, pain, and reduced range of motion affected the distribution of loads in the lower limbs [47]. In their study, the results showed that, after treatment with arthrodesis, they achieved almost a symmetrical distribution of loads, but with worse results than in the healthy group, and they concluded that this may have been due to the fact that the treatment only acted on the ankle, while, in these subjects, the movement of the toes, knee, and hip is restricted, altering the biomechanics of the neighboring joints. Therefore, long-term alterations of the foot and ankle, such as HL in this case, can lead to the central nervous system adapting to this condition, triggering compensatory mechanisms that can even affect other joints, altering the entire biomechanics of the lower limb and increasing the risk of secondary musculoskeletal problems due to changes in load distribution and joint function. This can limit the conditions for successful treatment if the pathology is detected at an advanced stage, preventing the musculoskeletal system from normalizing both statically and dynamically, thus highlighting the importance of our study and of detecting HL in time in order to prevent future complications.

A portable baropodometric platform was used in this research. Wearable technology, which helps to detect alterations in gait balance that may be related to foot pathologies, has been used in various studies on gait analysis with the aim of assessing body movement in individuals with and without biomechanical alterations. Other authors [44,46], using other different technological systems, have also found similar results, demonstrating that subjects with HL present gait disturbances. Therefore, the findings of these studies corroborate our outcomes, i.e., HL modifies the dynamic characteristics of walking.

Our study has some limitations; for example, the baropodometric platform could only record and identify vertical forces at a frequency of 60 Hz, and it would be interesting to use other frequencies and different forces in the capture and recording of force movement on the foot alone. In our study, only some parameters showed statistically significant differences between the groups, and most of them did not differ between the groups, so the biomechanical alteration observed was minor. Therefore, for future studies, it would also be interesting to assess other joints that may be altered as a consequence of HL. Biomechanical musculoskeletal lower-limb gait model data are of significant interest, since gait disturbances and loss of balance can cause falls, which are important to avoid. Therefore, for future studies, it would be interesting to evaluate other aspects with the aim of improving the gait in these subjects, through the premature compensation of the foot as a preventive measure. This is especially important in elderly subjects in order to avoid the risk of falls and improve the gait, thus enhancing their autonomy and quality of life. In our study, statistical power of 0.70 was used due to the limitations inherent in the available sample size and the characteristics of the studied population. Therefore, we will consider increasing the sample size in future studies to improve this aspect.

However, this study supplies information on a foot disorder for podiatrists and researchers regarding stance phase gait parameters in subjects with HL deformities. Deeper insight into the relationship between HL and modified gait biomechanics could provide the clinician with a more thorough evaluation of the condition as it pertains not only to hallux movement but also to its contribution to lower-extremity functionality. Continued research on this subject is important to facilitate early diagnosis and effective treatment for patients in order to improve their foot health and their general quality of life.

5. Conclusions

The existence of bilateral HL causes slight changes in gait analysis when compared to healthy individuals. Participants with bilateral HL, in contrast to the control group, demonstrated a reduced minimum frame FFP on the left foot. Differences in the time, percentage, and maximum frame in the left foot ICP were noted between the two groups, which may be associated with foot deformity. We believe that the early identification of these changes could enhance patients' quality of life and avert future complications. Therefore, it is necessary to continue with this line of research by analyzing new variables that may be related to the presence of HL.

Author Contributions: Conceptualization, N.T.-C., R.B.-d.-B.-V., M.E.L.-I., J.G.-S., D.L.-L. and J.B.-L.; Data curation, D.L.-L. and J.B.-L.; Formal analysis, N.T.-C., R.B.-d.-B.-V., M.E.L.-I., J.G.-S., D.L.-L. and J.B.-L.; Investigation, N.T.-C., R.B.-d.-B.-V., M.E.L.-I., J.G.-S., D.L.-L. and J.B.-L.; Methodology, N.T.-C., R.B.-d.-B.-V., M.E.L.-I., J.G.-S., D.L.-L. and J.B.-L.; Supervision, N.T.-C., R.B.-d.-B.-V., M.E.L.-I., J.G.-S., D.L.-L. and J.B.-L.; Writing—original draft, N.T.-C., R.B.-d.-B.-V., M.E.L.-I., J.G.-S., D.L.-L. and J.B.-L.; Writing—review and editing, N.T.-C., R.B.-d.-B.-V., M.E.L.-I., J.G.-S., D.L.-L. and J.B.-L. All authors have read and agreed to the published version of the manuscript.

Funding: This research was funded by the Spanish Ministry of Science and Innovation through the project PID2023-149353OB-I00.

Institutional Review Board Statement: The study was conducted in accordance with the Declaration of Helsinki, and approved by the Institutional Review Board at the University of A Coruña, under record number 2024-033.

Informed Consent Statement: Written informed consent was obtained from all participants involved in the study.

Data Availability Statement: The dataset supporting the conclusions of this article is available upon request to daniellopez@udc.es in the Research, Health and Podiatry Group, Department of Health Sciences, Faculty of Nursing and Podiatry, Industrial Campus of Ferrol, Universidade da Coruña, 15403, Ferrol, Spain.

Conflicts of Interest: All authors declare there are no conflicts of interest regarding the publication of this article and agree with this journal's copyright.

References

1. Coughlin, M.J.; Jones, C.P. Hallux valgus: Demographics, etiology, and radiographic assessment. *Foot Ankle Int.* **2007**, *28*, 759–777. [CrossRef] [PubMed]
2. Cuevas-Martínez, C.; Becerro-de-Bengoa-Vallejo, R.; Losa-Iglesias, M.E.; Casado-Hernández, I.; Turné-Cárceles, O.; Pérez-Palma, L.; Martiniano, J.; Gómez-Salgado, J.; López-López, D. Analysis of Static Plantar Pressures in School-Age Children with and without Functional Hallux Limitus: A Case-Control Study. *Bioengineering* **2023**, *10*, 628. [CrossRef] [PubMed]
3. Payne, C.; Chuter, V.; Miller, K. Sensitivity and Specificity of the Functional Hallux Limitus Test to Predict Foot Function. *J. Am. Podiatr. Med. Assoc.* **2002**, *92*, 269–271. [CrossRef]
4. Viehöfer, A.F.; Vich, M.; Wirth, S.H.; Espinosa, N.; Camenzind, R.S. The Role of Plantar Fascia Tightness in Hallux Limitus: A Biomechanical Analysis. *J. Foot Ankle Surg.* **2019**, *58*, 465–469. [CrossRef]
5. Kunnasegaran, R.; Thevendran, G. Hallux Rigidus: Nonoperative Treatment and Orthotics. *Foot Ankle Clin.* **2015**, *20*, 401–412. [CrossRef]
6. Senga, Y.; Nishimura, A.; Ito, N.; Kitaura, Y.; Sudo, A. Prevalence of and risk factors for hallux rigidus: A cross-sectional study in Japan. *BMC Musculoskelet. Disord.* **2021**, *22*, 786. [CrossRef]
7. Bejarano-Pineda, L.; Cody, E.A.; Nunley, J.A., II. Prevalence of Hallux Rigidus in Patients with End-Stage Ankle Arthritis. *J. Foot Ankle Surg.* **2021**, *60*, 21–24. [CrossRef]
8. Lam, A.; Chan, J.J.; Surace, M.F.; Vulcano, E. Hallux rigidus: How do I approach it? *World J. Orthop.* **2017**, *8*, 364–371. [CrossRef]
9. Sánchez-Gómez, R.; Becerro-de-Bengoa-Vallejo, R.; Losa-Iglesias, M.E.; Calvo-Lobo, C.; Navarro-Flores, E.; Palomo-López, P.; Romero-Morales, C.; López-López, D. Reliability Study of Diagnostic Tests for Functional Hallux Limitus. *Foot Ankle Int.* **2020**, *41*, 457–462. [CrossRef]
10. Shurnas, P.S. Hallux Rigidus: Etiology, Biomechanics, and Nonoperative Treatment. *Foot Ankle Clin.* **2009**, *14*, 1–8. [CrossRef]
11. Fung, J.; Sherman, A.; Stachura, S.; Eckles, R.; Doucette, J.; Chusid, E. Nonoperative Management of Hallux Limitus Using a Novel Forefoot Orthosis. *J. Foot Ankle Surg.* **2020**, *59*, 1192–1196. [CrossRef] [PubMed]
12. Cuevas-Martínez, C.; Becerro-de-Bengoa-Vallejo, R.; Losa-Iglesias, M.E.; Casado-Hernández, I.; Navarro-Flores, E.; Pérez-Palma, L.; Martiniano, J.; Gómez-Salgado, J.; López-López, D. Hallux Limitus Influence on Plantar Pressure Variations during the Gait Cycle: A Case-Control Study. *Bioengineering* **2023**, *10*, 772. [CrossRef] [PubMed]
13. Merker, J.; Hartmann, M.; Kreuzpointner, F.; Schwirtz, A.; Haas, J.P. Pathophysiology of juvenile idiopathic arthritis induced pes planovalgus in static and walking condition-A functional view using 3d gait analysis. *Pediatr. Rheumatol.* **2015**, *13*, 21. [CrossRef]
14. Okamura, K.; Egawa, K.; Ikeda, T.; Fukuda, K.; Kanai, S. Relationship between foot muscle morphology and severity of pronated foot deformity and foot kinematics during gait: A preliminary study. *Gait Posture* **2021**, *86*, 273–277. [CrossRef]
15. Vanore, J.V.; Christensen, J.C.; Kravitz, S.R.; Schuberth, J.M.; Thomas, J.L.; Weil, L.S.; Zlotoff, H.J.; Couture, S.D. Diagnosis and treatment of first metatarsophalangeal joint disorders. Section 2: Hallux rigidus. *J. Foot Ankle Surg.* **2003**, *42*, 124–136. [CrossRef]
16. Evans, R.D.L.; Averett, R.; Sanders, S. The Association of Hallux Limitus with the Accessory Navicular. *J. Am. Podiatr. Med. Assoc.* **2002**, *92*, 359–365. [CrossRef]
17. Tzioupis, C.; Oliveto, A.; Grabherr, S.; Vallotton, J.; Riederer, B.M. Identification of the retrotalar pulley of the Flexor Hallucis Longus tendon. *J. Anat.* **2019**, *235*, 757–764. [CrossRef]
18. Manfredi-Márquez, M.J.; Tavara-Vidalón, S.P.; Tavaruela-Carrión, N.; Gómez Benítez, M.Á.; Fernandez-Seguín, L.M.; Ramos-Ortega, J. Study of Windlass Mechanism in the Lower Limb Using Inertial Sensors. *Int. J. Environ. Res. Public Health* **2023**, *20*, 3220. [CrossRef]
19. Grady, J.F.; Axe, T.M.; Zager, E.J.; Sheldon, L.A. A Retrospective Analysis of 772 Patients with Hallux Limitus. *J. Am. Podiatr. Med. Assoc.* **2002**, *92*, 102–108. [CrossRef]
20. Zammit, G.V.; Menz, H.B.; Munteanu, S.E. Structural factors associated with hallux limitus/rigidus: A systematic review of case control studies. *J. Orthop. Sports Phys. Ther.* **2009**, *39*, 733–742. [CrossRef]
21. Clough, J.G. Functional hallux limitus and lesser-metatarsal overload. *J. Am. Podiatr. Med. Assoc.* **2005**, *95*, 593–601. [CrossRef] [PubMed]

22. Meyr, A.J.; Berkelbach, C.; Dreikorn, C.; Arena, T. Descriptive Quantitative Analysis of First Metatarsal Sagittal Plane Motion. *J. Foot Ankle Surg.* **2020**, *59*, 1244–1247. [CrossRef] [PubMed]
23. Padrón, L.; Bayod, J.; Becerro-de-Bengoa-Vallejo, R.; Losa-Iglesias, M.; López-López, D.; Casado-Hernández, I. Influence of the center of pressure on baropodometric gait pattern variations in the adult population with flatfoot: A case-control study. *Front. Bioeng. Biotechnol.* **2023**, *11*, 1147616. [CrossRef] [PubMed]
24. Dananberg, H.J. Functional hallux limitus and its relationship to gait efficiency. *J. Am. Podiatr. Med. Assoc.* **1986**, *76*, 648–652. [CrossRef]
25. Teyhen, D.S.; Stoltenberg, B.E.; Collinsworth, K.M.; Giesel, C.L.; Williams, D.G.; Kardouni, C.H.; Molloy, J.M.; Goffar, S.L.; Christie, D.S.; McPoil, T. Dynamic plantar pressure parameters associated with static arch height index during gait. *Clin. Biomech.* **2009**, *24*, 391–396. [CrossRef]
26. Miana, A.; Paola, M.; Duarte, M.; Nery, C.; Freitas, M. Gait and Balance Biomechanical Characteristics of Patients with Grades III and IV Hallux Rigidus. *J. Foot Ankle Surg.* **2022**, *61*, 452–455. [CrossRef]
27. Mulier, T.; Steenwerckx, A.; Thienpont, E.; Sioen, W.; Hoore, K.D.; Peeraer, L.; Dereymaeker, G. Results after cheilectomy in athletes with hallux rigidus. *Foot Ankle Int.* **1999**, *20*, 232–237. [CrossRef]
28. DeFrino, P.F.; Brodsky, J.W.; Pollo, F.E.; Crenshaw, S.J.; Beischer, A.D. First metatarsophalangeal arthrodesis: A clinical, pedobarographic and gait analysis study. *Foot Ankle Int.* **2002**, *23*, 496–502. [CrossRef]
29. Bryant, A.; Tinley, P.; Singer, K. A comparison of radiographic measurements in normal, hallux valgus, and hallux limitus feet. *J. Foot Ankle Surg.* **2000**, *39*, 39–43. [CrossRef]
30. Zammit, G.V.; Menz, H.B.; Munteanu, S.E.; Landorf, K.B. Plantar pressure distribution in older people with osteoarthritis of the first metatarsophalangeal joint (Hallux limitus/rigidus). *J. Orthop. Res.* **2008**, *26*, 1665–1669. [CrossRef]
31. Van Gheluwe, B.; Dananberg, H.J.; Hagman, F.; Vanstaen, K. Effects of hallux limitus on plantar foot pressure and foot kinematics during walking. *J. Am. Podiatr. Med. Assoc.* **2006**, *96*, 428–436. [CrossRef] [PubMed]
32. Stevens, J.; de Bot, R.T.A.L.; Hermus, J.P.S.; Schotanus, M.G.M.; Meijer, K.; Witlox, A.M. Gait analysis of foot compensation in symptomatic Hallux Rigidus patients. *Foot Ankle Surg. Off. J. Eur. Soc. Foot Ankle Surg.* **2022**, *28*, 1272–1278. [CrossRef] [PubMed]
33. Duarte, M.; Sternad, D. Complexity of human postural control in young and older adults during prolonged standing. *Exp. Brain Res.* **2008**, *191*, 265–276. [CrossRef] [PubMed]
34. Lugade, V.; Kaufman, K. Center of pressure trajectory during gait: A comparison of four foot positions. *Gait Posture* **2014**, *40*, 719–722. [CrossRef]
35. Bryant, A.R.; Tinley, P.; Cole, J.H. Plantar pressure and joint motion after the Youngswick procedure for hallux limitus. *J. Am. Podiatr. Med. Assoc.* **2004**, *94*, 22–30. [CrossRef]
36. Vandenbroucke, J.P.; von Elm, E.; Altman, D.G.; Gøtzsche, P.C.; Mulrow, C.D.; Pocock, S.J.; Poole, C.; Schlesselman, J.J.; Egger, M.; STROBE Initiative. Strengthening the Reporting of Observational Studies in Epidemiology (STROBE): Explanation and elaboration. *Int. J. Surg.* **2014**, *12*, 1500–1524. [CrossRef]
37. Parsa-Parsi, R.W.; Ellis, R.; Wiesing, U. Fifty years at the forefront of ethical guidance: The world medical association declaration of Helsinki. *South. Med. J.* **2014**, *107*, 405–406. [CrossRef]
38. Becerro-de-Bengoa-Vallejo, R.; Losa-Iglesias, M.E.; Rodriguez-Sanz, D. Static and Dynamic Plantar Pressures in Children with and without Sever Disease: A Case-Control Study. *Phys. Ther.* **2014**, *94*, 818–826. [CrossRef]
39. Menz, H.B.; Auhl, M.; Tan, J.M.; Buldt, A.K.; Munteanu, S.E. Centre of pressure characteristics during walking in individuals with and without first metatarsophalangeal joint osteoarthritis. *Gait Posture* **2018**, *63*, 91–96. [CrossRef]
40. Painceira-Villar, R.; García-Paz, V.; de Bengoa-Vallejo, R.B.; Losa-Iglesias, M.E.; López-López, D.; Martiniano, J.; Pereiro-Buceta, H.; Martínez-Jiménez, E.M.; Calvo-Lobo, C. Impact of Asthma on Plantar Pressures in a Sample of Adult Patients: A Case-Control Study. *J. Pers. Med.* **2021**, *11*, 1157. [CrossRef]
41. de Bengoa Vallejo, R.B.; Iglesias, M.E.L.; Zeni, J.; Thomas, S. Reliability and repeatability of the portable EPS-platform digital pressure-plate system. *J. Am. Podiatr. Med. Assoc.* **2013**, *103*, 197–203. [CrossRef]
42. Canseco, K.; Long, J.; Marks, R.; Khazzam, M.; Harris, G. Quantitative characterization of gait kinematics in patients with hallux rigidus using the Milwaukee foot model. *J. Orthop. Res.* **2008**, *26*, 419–427. [CrossRef]
43. Allan, J.J.; McClelland, J.A.; Munteanu, S.E.; Buldt, A.K.; Landorf, K.B.; Roddy, E.; Auhl, M.; Menz, H.B. First metatarsophalangeal joint range of motion is associated with lower limb kinematics in individuals with first metatarsophalangeal joint osteoarthritis. *J. Foot Ankle Res.* **2020**, *13*, 33. [CrossRef] [PubMed]
44. Castro-Méndez, A.; Canca-Sánchez, F.J.; Pabón-Carrasco, M.; Jiménez-Cebrián, A.M.; Córdoba-Fernández, A. Evaluation of Gait Parameters on Subjects with Hallux Limitus Using an Optogait Sensor System: A Case–Control Study. *Medicina* **2023**, *59*, 1519. [CrossRef] [PubMed]
45. Menz, H.B.; Auhl, M.; Tan, J.M.; Levinger, P.; Roddy, E.; Munteanu, S.E. Biomechanical Effects of Prefabricated Foot Orthoses and Rocker-Sole Footwear in Individuals with First Metatarsophalangeal Joint Osteoarthritis. *Arthritis Care Res.* **2016**, *68*, 603–611. [CrossRef]

46. Tarante, J.; Taranto, M.J.; Bryant, A.R.; Singer, K.P. Analysis of Dynamic Angle of Gait and Radiographic Features in Subjects with Hallux Abducto Valgus and Hallux Limitus. *J. Am. Podiatr. Med. Assoc.* **2007**, *97*, 175–188. [CrossRef]
47. Morasiewicz, P.; Konieczny, G.; Dejnek, M.; Urbański, W.; Dragan, S.Ł.; Kulej, M.; Dragan, S.F.; Pawik, Ł. Assessment of the distribution of load on the lower limbs and balance before and after ankle arthrodesis with the Ilizarov method. *Sci. Rep.* **2018**, *8*, 15693. [CrossRef]

Disclaimer/Publisher's Note: The statements, opinions and data contained in all publications are solely those of the individual author(s) and contributor(s) and not of MDPI and/or the editor(s). MDPI and/or the editor(s) disclaim responsibility for any injury to people or property resulting from any ideas, methods, instructions or products referred to in the content.

bioengineering

MDPI

Article

Gender Differences in Joint Biomechanics During Obstacle Crossing with Different Heights

Chenyan Wang [1,2], Yuan Guo [2], Weijin Du [2], Zhiqiang Li [3,4,5] and Weiyi Chen [2,*]

1 College of Mechanical Engineering, Taiyuan University of Technology, Taiyuan 030024, China; wangccccyyy@163.com
2 College of Artificial Intelligence, Taiyuan University of Technology, Taiyuan 030024, China; dwj18335100390@163.com (W.D.)
3 Shanxi Key Laboratory of Material Strength & Structural Impact, Taiyuan University of Technology, Taiyuan 030024, China; lizhiqiang@tyut.edu.cn
4 Shanxi Research Center of Basic Discipline of Mechanics, Taiyuan University of Technology, Taiyuan 030024, China
5 National Demonstration Center for Experimental Mechanics Education, Taiyuan University of Technology, Taiyuan 030024, China
* Correspondence: chenweiyi211@163.com

Abstract: Identifying gender-related gait changes offers valuable insights into the role of gender in motor control. It is anticipated that more difficult gait tasks (obstacle crossing) may reveal gender-specific effects on gait parameters. The present study aimed to explore the gait adaptations of male and female participants when stepping over obstacles of 0 cm, 13 cm, 19 cm, and 26 cm in height. A total of 12 male and 12 female participants were recruited. The Vicon motion capture system and AMTI force plates were utilized to obtain the gait parameters. Moreover, spatiotemporal parameters were investigated. Two-way repeated ANOVA (gender × obstacle height) and three-way repeated ANOVA (gender × obstacle height × leg) were performed to compare gait parameters, respectively. Correlations between maximum joint angle and obstacle height were also evaluated. Significant interactions were observed for leading leg swing time, maximum hip extension angle, maximum knee flexion angle, and maximum ankle plantarflexion angle (gender × obstacle height). There were some differences in gait parameters between males and females in the unobstructed gait, and these changes became more evident as obstacle height increased. This study also identified significant differences in gait parameters between leading and trailing legs when stepping over the obstacle.

Keywords: gait; gender; obstacles; kinematics; kinetics

1. Introduction

It is generally believed that there are inherent differences between the walking patterns of males and females [1]. The gender of a walking person can be recognized by observing the movement of their joints [2]. Certain diseases occur that are gender-specific, and this may be related to differences in walking mechanics [3]. However, some studies have indicated that there are no substantial differences in gait variables between males and females [4]. Although previous studies have reported gender-specific gait results, the present study provides a further comprehensive exploration of parameters, including spatiotemporal, joint kinematics, and kinetic parameters.

Tripping is a common cause of falls in adults [5], often occurring in the presence of fixed and visible obstacles. During everyday life, stepping over obstacles of different

 https://doi.org/10.3390/bioengineering12020189

heights (requiring the adjustment of gait parameters) occurs frequently, including walking over crossbars on the road or outdoor sports. Compared to unobstructed gait, crossing obstacles require more muscular, cognitive, and sensory demands; therefore, they may be associated with a higher risk of falls [6]. It is also necessary to integrate sensory information such as optical flow and proprioception when crossing obstacles in order to adequately plan and adjust these movements [7]. While approaching the obstacle, participants collected visual information (e.g., height and position of the obstacle) to adjust their foot position and successfully cross the obstacle [8]. If foot position was not adjusted in time, the presence of obstacles could be detrimental to stability. Stepping over the obstacle increased gait challenge, which increased systematically with an increase in obstacle height, and it was more challenging to fully describe the effect of task difficulty on gait characteristics. Adaptation to obstacle height when crossing an obstacle may reveal gait changes that are not apparent in unobstructed gait. In young adults, obstacle height produces a graded response, with higher obstacle height corresponding to longer stance, swing, and double limb support times [9]. Many studies have investigated the effects of obstacles on spatiotemporal parameters of a given population. In contrast, relatively little work has examined the interaction between gender and obstacle height. The strategies that males and females choose to adopt when crossing obstacle are still worthy of further exploration.

The purpose of this study was to assess the effect of gender and obstacle height on gait parameters. The parameters of interest were those that may differ between males and females due to structural differences. The first hypothesis was that females would exhibit different gait parameters (e.g., shorter stride length and slower speeds) compared to males in all gait conditions. The second hypothesis was that the spatiotemporal, kinematic, and kinetic parameters would alter for both genders at different obstacle heights. Moreover, it was also hypothesized that the difference between males and females would change as the height of the obstacle increased.

2. Materials and Methods

2.1. Participants

A total of 24 adults, 12 males (age 25.17 $\pm$ 2.44 years; mass 70.30 $\pm$ 7.59 kg; height 1.74 $\pm$ 0.05 m; BMI 23.09 $\pm$ 2.27 kg/m^2) and 12 females (age 26.50 $\pm$ 1.73 years; mass 53.71 $\pm$ 4.79 kg; height 1.60 $\pm$ 0.06 m; BMI 20.88 $\pm$ 1.75 kg/m^2), volunteered for this study. All participants were healthy and self-reported no history of joint injury, joint instability, or musculoskeletal disorders within the past six months. The protocol was approved by the University Research Ethics Committee, and informed consent was obtained from all participants prior to testing (Approval No. TYUT202105003).

2.2. Testing Protocol

Kinematic data were collected at 100 Hz using a 6-camera Vicon motion capture system (Vicon, Oxford, UK). The Vicon Plug-in Gait markers (16 light-reflecting markers of 14 mm diameter) were placed on the pelvis, shank, thigh, and foot to determine the kinematics of the extremity segments during gait. Participants wore tight shorts to ensure that all reflective markers were securely attached to the bony landmarks. Kinetic data were collected at 1000 Hz from two embedded force plates (AMTI, Watertown, MA, USA).

Prior to formal data collection, participants were instructed to walk for several minutes to familiarize themselves with the experiments. Participants were then instructed to complete an obstacle crossing at four different heights as follows: unobstructed, 13 cm (low), 19 cm (medium), and 26 cm (high). Additionally, participants completed all gait trials barefoot at a self-selected comfortable walking speed. In the obstacle-crossing condition, the obstacle was placed in the middle of two embedded force plates, and participants stepped over the obstacle without contacting it (Figure 1). The obstacle consisted of two adjustable upright standards and a plastic crossbar (2.5 cm in diameter, 1.0 m in length).

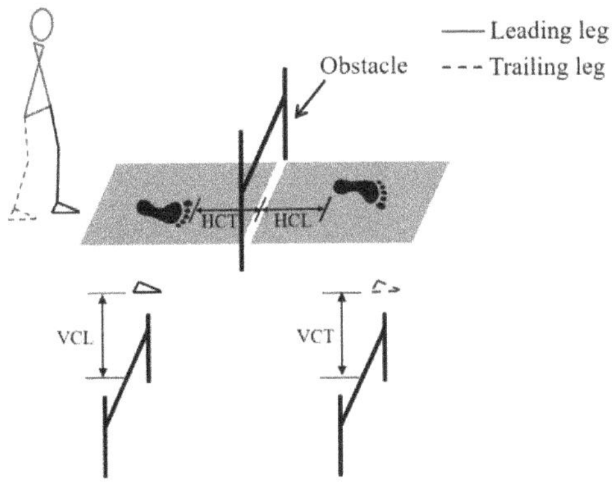

Figure 1. Schematic details of the obstacle. VCL: vertical distance between the obstacle and the left heel marker; VCT: vertical distance between the obstacle and the right heel marker; HCL: horizontal distance between the obstacle and the left heel marker; HCT: horizontal distance between the obstacle and the right toe marker.

In this experiment, the gait cycle was considered as two consecutive heel strikes of the right foot; thus, the left foot was the first foot to cross over the obstacle and was defined as the leading foot. Furthermore, the right foot's first contact and toe-off times were determined by evaluating the data from the first force plate, and the second contact time was ascertained by the coordinate change in the heel marker. Five trials were conducted for each gait condition, and three trials were randomly selected for further study.

2.3. Data Analysis

The complete gait cycle was time-normalized to 100 and an average of the three trials for each obstacle condition was obtained. Similarly, the swing phase of the leading leg and the stance phase of the gait cycle were time-normalized to 100, respectively.

The spatiotemporal gait characteristics including stride length, stride time, stance time, swing time, and speed were analyzed for all four gait conditions. In addition, the vertical heel-clearance of the leading foot (VCL) and trailing foot (VCT) was determined as the vertical distance between the obstacle and the left or right heel marker, respectively, when the heel was directly above the obstacle [10,11]. The horizontal clearance of the leading foot (HCL) was considered as the horizontal distance between the obstacle and the left heel marker at the moment of heel strike. Meanwhile, the horizontal clearance of the trailing foot (HCT) was regarded as the horizontal distance between the obstacle and the right toe marker at the moment of toe-off [12].

The ground reaction force (GRF) data were filtered using a zero-lag, fourth-order, low-pass Butterworth filter with a 20 Hz cut-off frequency [13]. The GRF data were normalized to bodyweight (% BW) to allow for the comparison between subjects and genders [14]. The GRF data were analyzed using eight values. Three values were identified for the medial-lateral component, the initially occurring positive peak (Fx_{PP}), and two consecutive negative peaks (Fx_{N1}, Fx_{N2}) of the stance phase. From the anterior–posterior curve, two peaks were determined, the initial braking force (Fy_{BF}) and propulsion force at the end of stance (Fy_{PF}). In addition, the vertical direction curve was characterized by two peaks, including the first peak at heel strike (Fz_{FP}) and the second peak toward the end of stance (Fz_{SP}) [15]. The downfall between the two peaks was also described (Fz_{DF}) [16].

2.4. Statistical Analysis

All statistical analyses were performed using SPSS 25.0 (SPSS Inc., Chicago, IL, USA), and the significance level was set at $p < 0.05$. A two-way repeated ANOVA was adopted to explore the influence of two main factors, gender (2 levels: male, female) and gait condition (4 levels: unobstructed, low, medium, high obstacle), as well as their interactive effect on spatiotemporal parameters. Similarly, for the assessment of the maximum joint angles of the trailing leg during the complete gait cycle and the values of GRF, a two-way repeated ANOVA was also used to investigate effects of gender and gait condition. To further examine the effects of gender group, gait condition, and leg (2 levels: leading leg, trailing leg) on the maximum hip/knee/ankle flexion angle during the swing phase, a three-way repeated ANOVA was performed. The Bonferroni post hoc test was used when statistical analyses showed significant interactions and main effects. Additionally, Spearman's rank order was applied to evaluate the relationship between the maximum joint angle of the trailing foot and obstacle height.

3. Results

3.1. Spatiotemporal Parameters

The effects of gender and obstacle height and the gender × obstacle interaction on the spatiotemporal parameters are presented in Table 1. Regarding the gender factor, the female group showed shorter stride length and lower speed than the male group. For the main effects of obstacle height, stride length, VCL, VCT, and HCL for stepping over the obstacle (low, medium, or high) were significantly higher than those of unobstructed gait. Moreover, there was a gender × obstacle interaction for the swing time of the trailing leg. The results indicated that when participants crossed obstacles (low, medium, or high), the swing time of the trailing leg was significantly increased in females compared to males ($p < 0.05$), while no effect of gender difference was shown in the unobstructed gait ($p > 0.05$).

Table 1. Mean and standard deviations of spatiotemporal parameters. The last three columns show the p-values for the main effects of the gender and obstacle height and the gender × obstacle interaction, respectively.

		Unobstructed	Low	Medium	High	Gender	Obstacle	Gender × Obstacle
Stride length (mm)	M	1269.3 (46.2)	1300.0 (53.5)	1295.4 (53.0)	1309.0 (68.4)	0.004	<0.001	0.300
	F	1195.2 (35.4)	1263.1 (51.5)	1236.0 (55.8)	1254.8 (43.3)			
Stride time (s)	M	1.15 (0.07)	1.30 (0.11)	1.35 (0.11)	1.48 (0.10)	0.104	<0.001	0.059
	F	1.15 (0.12)	1.39 (0.18)	1.46 (0.18)	1.66 (0.25)			
STT (s)	M	0.71 (0.04)	0.80 (0.06)	0.82 (0.07)	0.89 (0.07)	0.230	<0.001	0.309
	F	0.72 (0.07)	0.85 (0.11)	0.88 (0.11)	0.95 (0.19)			
SWL (s)	M	0.47 (0.03)	0.56 (0.05)	0.59 (0.05)	0.64 (0.04)	0.037	<0.001	0.018
	F	0.47 (0.04)	0.62 (0.08)	0.64 (0.08)	0.73 (0.10)			
Speed (mm/s)	M	1112.5 (74.0)	1004.6 (88.4)	965.0 (96.9)	888.4 (83.7)	0.016	<0.001	0.191
	F	1052.0 (108. 5)	922.9 (113.4)	856.7 (90.1)	770.1 (114.7)			
VCL (mm)	M	62.3 (12.1)	105.1 (47. 7)	112.1 (36.7)	129.3 (33.3)	0.988	<0.001	0.927
	F	56.4 (13.0)	104.6 (39.4)	114.7 (45.8)	132.3 (50.2)			
VCT (mm)	M	241.8 (23.5)	307.3 (47.2)	330.9 (46.6)	346.5 (59.2)	0.191	<0.001	0.770
	F	226.8 (14.1)	301.4 (38.3)	308.7 (38.9)	323.3 (41.5)			
HCL (mm)	M	166.4 (53.3)	188. 6 (46.9)	187.7 (32.7)	189.0 (36.8)	0.077	0.019	0.742
	F	176.2 (44.4)	220.4 (42.8)	216.7 (30.9)	217.5 (28.0)			
HCT (mm)	M	219.7 (40.5)	226.9 (32.7)	225.3 (32.1)	226.2 (34.1)	0.333	0.268	0.843
	F	202.8 (43.8)	216.3 (40.7)	208.8 (42.9)	218.8 (24.4)			

STT: Stance time of trialing leg; SWL: Swing time of leading leg; VCL: vertical heel-clearance of the leading foot; VCT: vertical heel-clearance of the trailing foot; HCL: horizontal clearance of the leading foot; HCT: horizontal clearance of the trailing foot; M: male; F: female.

3.2. Joint Angles

The lower extremity joint angles of the trailing leg for male and female participants during the complete gait cycle for unobstructed and medium obstacle gait are shown in Figure 2. The results showed similar trends in joint angles for male and female participants. Throughout most of the gait cycle, the medium obstacle gait demonstrated greater hip flexion, knee flexion, and ankle dorsiflexion angles during the second half of the gait cycle compared to the unobstructed gait.

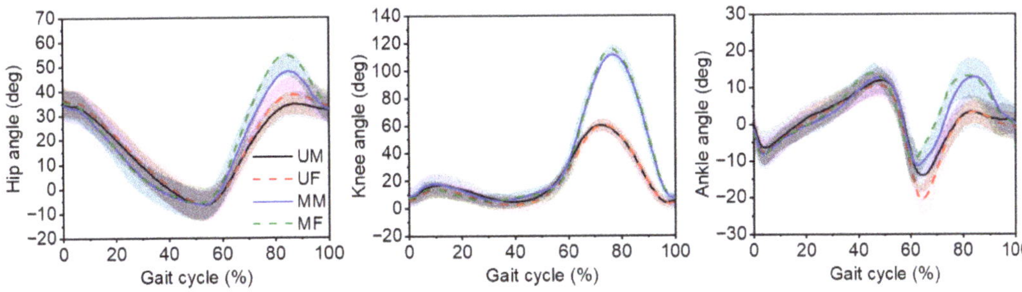

Figure 2. Trailing leg joint angles during the complete gait cycle for the unobstructed and medium obstacle gait. The shaded band shows standard deviation. UM: unobstructed gait for male participants; UF: unobstructed gait for female participants; MM: medium obstacle gait for male participants; MF: medium obstacle gait for female participants. Note: To increase the readability of the images, the joint angles when stepping over low and high obstacles are not shown in the figure.

The statistical analyses of the peak joint angle were listed in Table 2. For the main effects of obstacle height, the maximum hip flexion angle increased with the increase in the height of the obstacle. Regarding the gender × obstacle interactions (Figure 3), female participants had a higher knee flexion angle than male participants in the low obstacle gait condition, while no differences between genders were observed in the other obstacle conditions. Furthermore, a significant interaction was also observed for the maximum ankle plantarflexion angle.

Table 2. Mean and standard deviations of the peak joint angle of the trailing leg during the complete gait cycle. The last three columns show the p-values for the main effects of the gender and obstacle height and the gender × obstacle interaction, respectively.

		Unobstructed	Low	Medium	High	Gender	Obstacle	Gender × Obstacle
Max hip flexion	M	36.0 (5.8)	45.1 (7.2)	48.3 (7.8)	52.3 (8. 7)	0.063	<0.001	0.161
	F	39.1 (7.5)	52.8 (8.5)	55.7 (9.4)	59.0 (10.6)			
Max hip extension	M	6.9 (5.9)	8.2 (5.5)	7.1 (6.2)	6.5 (6.4)	0.701	<0.001	0.021
	F	6.5 (7.0)	7.0 (7.0)	6.3 (7.4)	4.7 (7.2)			
Max knee flexion	M	60.6 (4.7)	98.8 (8.0)	111.9 (7.4)	125.3 (7.0)	0.046	<0.001	0.019
	F	61.2 (4.8)	107.6 (4.0)	116.6 (4.7)	125.6 (7.0)			
Max ankle dorsiflexion	M	12.1 (3.8)	13.8 (4.1)	15.8 (3.7)	17.0 (4.7)	0.435	<0.001	0.141
	F	10.7 (3.7)	16.2 (4.6)	17.5 (4.7)	19.3 (5.5)			
Max ankle plantarflexion	M	15.4 (4.6)	12.6 (5.4)	13.2 (4.2)	12.3 (5.0)	0.084	< 0.001	0.006
	F	22.0 (4.9)	18.6 (8.5)	13.3 (5.5)	13.8 (4.7)			

M: male; F: female.

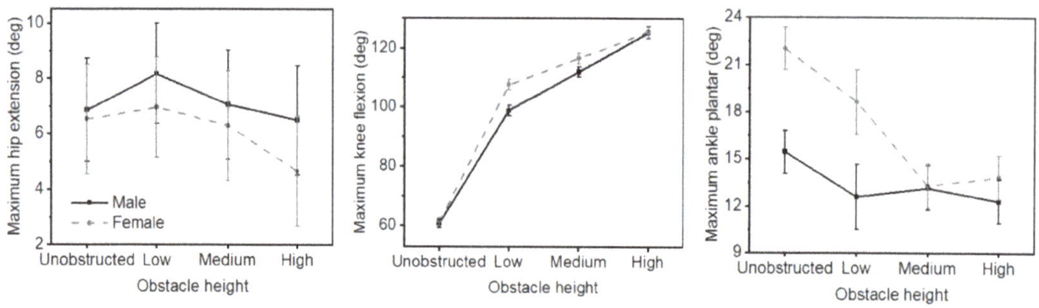

Figure 3. Gender × obstacle interaction for joint angle. Male participants (black solid line), female participants (gray dashed line). Error bars represent the standard error.

The lower extremity joint angles of the leading leg for male and female participants during the swing phase for unobstructed and medium obstacle gait are shown in Figure 4. The results indicated similar trends exist in joint angles for male and female participants. The results further showed that medium obstacle gait had greater hip and knee flexion angles during the swing phase compared to the unobstructed gait. However, when stepping over the obstacle, the ankle angle patterns of male and female participants changed during the terminal swing phase, that is, the ankle joint varied from dorsiflexion to plantarflexion.

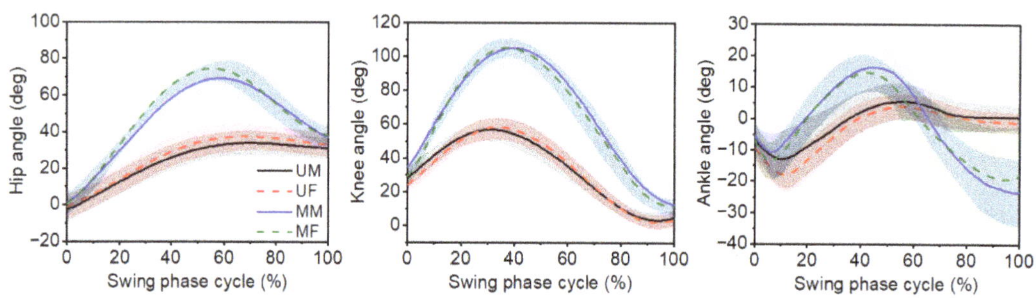

Figure 4. Leading leg joint angles during the swing phase for the unobstructed and medium obstacle gait. The shaded band shows standard deviation. UM: unobstructed gait for male participants; UF: unobstructed gait for female participants; MM: medium obstacle gait for male participants; MF: medium obstacle gait for female participants. Note: To increase the readability of the images, the joint angles when stepping over low and high obstacles are not shown in the figure.

The three-way repeated ANOVA revealed significant main effects for obstacle height on the maximum hip/knee flexion angles and ankle dorsiflexion angles (Figure 5). The leg had a significant main effect on the maximum hip/knee flexion angle. The angle of leading leg was significantly lower than that of the trailing leg in terms of maximum knee flexion angle; however, there was no significant difference between the leading and trailing leg in ankle flexion angle. Additionally, the results indicated that the hip flexion angle of the leading leg was greater than that of the trailing leg during the obstacle gait (low, medium, or high). No differences in hip flexion angle between the leading and trailing leg were observed for either male and female participants in the unobstructed gait.

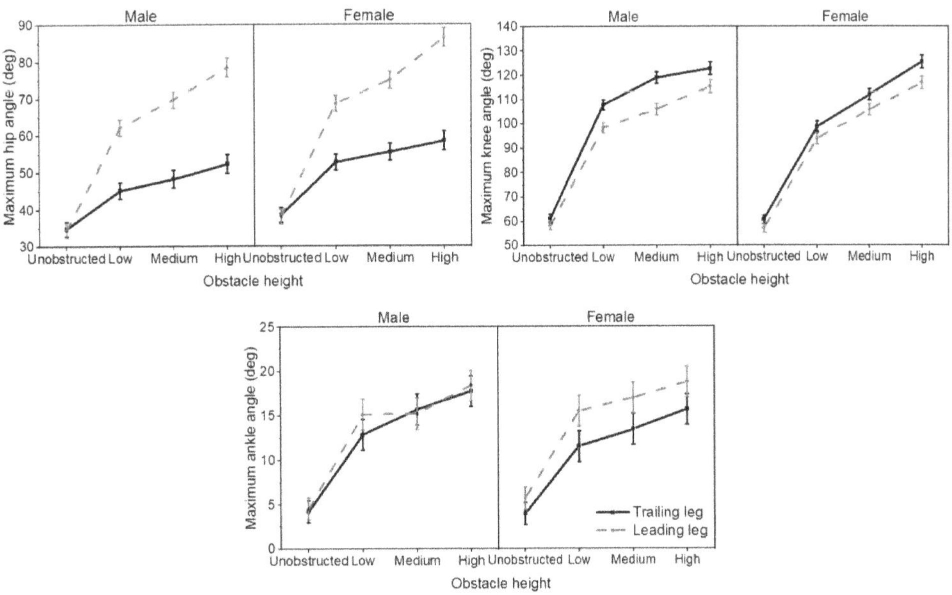

Figure 5. Gender × obstacle × leg interaction for joint angle. Trailing leg (black solid line), leading leg (gray dashed line). Error bars represent the standard error.

3.3. Relationship Between Joint Angle and Obstacle Height

The relationship between joint angle and obstacle height is shown in Table 3. The maximum hip flexion angle correlated with the obstacle height (r = 0.629/p < 0.001 for male and r = 0.632/p < 0.001 for female). The maximum knee flexion angle was significantly associated with obstacle height (r = 0.921/p < 0.001 for male and r = 0.932/p < 0.001 for female). Additionally, the maximum ankle dorsiflexion angle correlated with obstacle height (r = 0.436/p < 0.001 for male and r = 0.530/p < 0.001 for female).

Table 3. Correlation between the joint angle and obstacle height.

	Male		**Female**	
	r	p	r	p
Max hip flexion angle	0.629	<0.001	0.632	<0.001
Max knee flexion angle	0.921	<0.001	0.932	<0.001
Max ankle dorsiflexion angle	0.436	<0.001	0.530	<0.001

3.4. Ground Reaction Force

The GRF data along the medio-lateral (Fx), anterior–posterior (Fy), and vertical (Fz) directions during the stance phase are presented in Figure 6. The results indicated that the GRF curves of male and female participants had similar trends in the medio-lateral, anterior–posterior, and vertical directions. During the 28–66% of stance phase, the Fx in the medium obstacle gait was lower than that in the unobstructed gait. The braking force was greater during the first half of the stance phase when stepping over medium obstacle compared to the unobstructed gait. In addition, the medium obstacle gait had a higher propulsion force at the terminal stance phase than the unobstructed gait. During 1–28% and 75–100% of stance phase, the Fz in the medium obstacle gait was greater than that in the unobstructed gait.

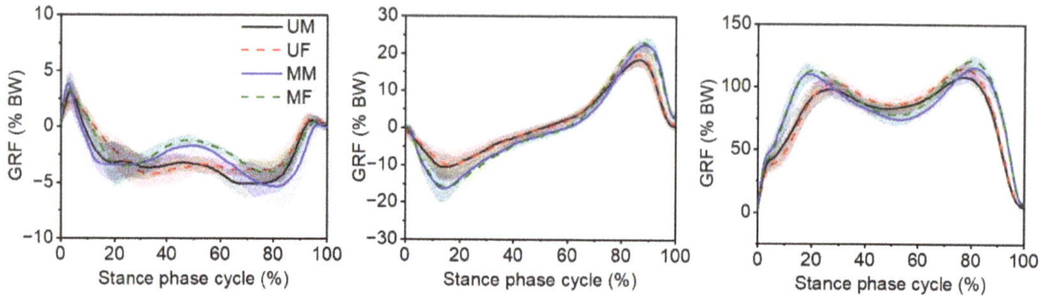

Figure 6. Ground reaction force (GRF) during the stance phase cycle under the unobstructed and medium obstacle gait. The shaded band shows standard deviation. UM: unobstructed gait for male participants; UF: unobstructed gait for female participants; MM: medium obstacle gait for male participants; MF: medium obstacle gait for female participants. Note: To increase the readability and simplicity of the images, the GRF when stepping over low and high obstacles is not shown in the figure.

The peak GRF variables for male and female participants in different gait conditions are shown in Table 4. Regarding the gender factor, male participants exhibited greater Fx_{N2} and lower Fz_{SP} than female participants. Moreover, the main effect of obstacle height was significant for the Fx_{PP}, Fx_{N1}, Fy_{BF}, Fy_{PF}, Fz_{FP}, Fz_{SP}, and Fz_{DF}. The interaction effects between gender and obstacle height on peak GRF variables were not statistically significant ($p > 0.05$).

Table 4. Mean and standard deviations of GRF values during the stance phase cycle. The last three columns show the *p*-values for the main effects of the gender and obstacle height and the gender × obstacle interaction, respectively.

GRF (% BW)		Unobstructed	Low	Medium	High	Gender	Obstacle	Gender × Obstacle
Fx_{PP}	M	3.26 (1.81)	3.39 (1.67)	4.01 (1.88)	4.08 (1.82)	0.600	0.005	0.501
	F	2.81 (1.21)	3.49 (1.20)	3.53 (1.18)	3.73 (0.93)			
Fx_{N1}	M	4.31 (0.95)	4.50 (1.19)	4.39 (1.26)	4.00 (1.21)	0.634	0.057	0.212
	F	4.50 (1.30)	3.94 (1.33)	4.04 (1.60)	3.79 (1.50)			
Fx_{N2}	M	5.42 (1.13)	5.62 (1.37)	5.63 (1.73)	5.40 (1.34)	0.032	0.990	0.326
	F	4.50 (0.95)	4.31 (1.44)	4.30 (0.99)	4.63 (1.11)			
Fy_{BF}	M	11.40 (2.92)	14.41 (2.79)	16.83 (3.16)	17.16 (3.04)	0.958	<0.001	0.094
	F	10.41 (4.05)	15.34 (4.31)	16.20 (4.30)	17.55 (4.49)			
Fy_{PF}	M	18.59 (1.89)	22.90 (1.92)	22.70 (2.09)	22.19 (1.47)	0.257	<0.001	0.302
	F	19.80 (3.41)	24.86 (3.76)	23.21 (2.53)	22.84 (2.90)			
Fz_{FP}	M	100.04 (7.78)	108.82 (8.44)	112.19 (8.37)	112.71 (7.67)	0.316	<0.001	0.577
	F	103.61 (8.26)	112.55 (7.33)	114.14 (7.76)	116.13 (9.26)			
Fz_{SP}	M	108.79 (4.74)	115.66 (7.59)	115.97 (9.57)	116.48 (7.63)	0.043	<0.001	0.259
	F	115.43 (4.85)	123.05 (8.66)	121.94 (8.53)	120.96 (8.90)			
Fz_{DF}	M	82.05 (5.39)	75.73 (4.68)	73.43 (6.06)	73.21 (5.74)	0.224	<0.001	0.632
	F	85.37 (6.63)	77.96 (6.66)	76.94 (8.14)	76.34 (8.51)			

Fx_{PP}: initially occurring positive peak on the medial-lateral curve; Fx_{N1}: first negative peak on the medial-lateral curve; Fx_{N2}: second negative peak on the medial-lateral curve; Fy_{BF}: initial braking force on the anterior–posterior curve; Fy_{PF}: propulsion force on the anterior–posterior curve; Fz_{FP}: first peak on the vertical curve; Fz_{SP}: second peak on the vertical curve; Fz_{DF}: downfall between the two peaks on the vertical curve; M: male; F: female.

4. Discussion

The purpose of this study was to investigate the effects of gender on the kinematics and kinetics of the lower extremity joints when stepping over unobstructed, low, medium, and high obstacles. There were more similarities than differences in gait spatiotemporal parameters, kinematics, and kinetics variables between males and females.

The stride length varied by gender, with females walking shorter strides, and similar results have been reported in overground walking studies on different genders [17,18]. The smaller stride length for females than males may be due to differences in height. There was no significant difference in stride time between male and female participants. Moreover, since gait speed is the quotient of stride length and stride time, it is not surprising that male participants exhibited significantly higher speeds than female participants [19]. The level of difficulty (i.e., obstacle heights) may affect the alertness of participants when performing the task, i.e., more caution is taken when stepping over taller obstacles [20]. During the obstacle crossing, participants adapted their gait to their physical condition by slowing down in order to perform the task cautiously. The reduced speed may be reflected in the reduced extrapolated center of mass, indicating that a conservative strategy was adopted when stepping over the obstacle, as confirmed by the absence of tripping in all gait conditions. Moreover, it has been suggested that there is a relationship between gait speed and the fear of falling [21], so the higher the obstacle, the slower the speed to avoid falling.

This result also indicated that more time was required (i.e., increased stride time) to cross the obstacle, and that an increase in the swing time of the leading leg was accompanied by an increase in the stance time of the trailing leg when stepping over the obstacle. The single leg stance phase, during which weight is redistributed, can be considered the most challenging step when the body is hovering over the obstacle [22]. It should be noted that this extended time of crossing the obstacle (i.e., single leg stance) may lead to a greater risk of falling in an unstable situation [23]. The interaction of gender and obstacle height based on the spatiotemporal parameters was also investigated. There was a significant difference in the leading leg swing time between male and female participants in the obstacle-crossing gait, but no such difference in the unobstructed gait. The results suggested that the overground gait condition was insufficient to reveal gender-related changes. However, differences were observed, not only for the high obstacle but also for the low and medium obstacle, suggesting that females may be more cautious when faced with difficult tasks. Mengarelli et al. revealed that female participants exhibit greater contraction activity and adopt a more complex muscular strategy during gait [24]. Muscle co-activation contributes to increasing limb stability during the double-to-single support transition [25]. It can be inferred that female participants require more muscle co-activation when facing more challenging obstacles. Therefore, it could be useful to develop separate movement patterns for males and females.

VCL and VCT are important parameters for detecting the success of crossing the obstacle. The progressive increase in VCL and VCT as a function of obstacle height in all male and female participants reflects their ability to recognize and adjust behaviors according to the level of task challenge. However, this strategy may be less efficient from an energetics perspective [26] and may place higher balance and stability demands on the leg [10]. Hence, the increased VCL and VCT could be an unstable behavior that may be dangerous when stepping over the obstacle, especially at higher obstacles. Controlling the trajectory of the trailing leg over an obstacle is a separate control process from that of the leading leg, and in the absence of visual use, the trailing leg is more likely to contact the obstacle and thus trip and fall [27]. In this study, the vertical heel-clearance of the trailing leg was higher than that of the leading leg, which may indicate that the trailing leg is more prone to tripping when crossing the obstacle.

Crossing the obstacle is mainly accomplished by flexing the three joints of the leading and trailing leg, even though the proximal joints, hip, and knee flex more than the ankle joint. Cho et al. reported that females showed a significantly greater hip flexion angle during walking [28]. Although not significant, the present study found similar results in that female participants had greater hip flexion angles in all gait conditions. This may be due to the structural differences that females exhibit at the hip and knee, which predispose them to having different movement patterns as well [29]. In addition, another focus of this study was to explore the interaction of gender and obstacle height on gait biomechanics. Male and female participants had similar knee flexion angles during walking, but only when stepping over low obstacles did the knee flexion angle change significantly in females compared to males. For the ankle plantarflexion angle, there was a significant difference between male and female participants during the unobstructed gait. However, as obstacle height increased, this difference gradually disappeared. This may be attributed to the fact that physiological and neuromuscular differences between males and females appear to influence the effects of different obstacle heights on lower extremity joint kinematics. Therefore, the choice of the potential small muscle training or rehabilitation means should be different in males and females.

In this study, there was a clear difference in ankle angles between the leading and trailing leg when stepping over the obstacle. Particularly in the terminal swing phase of the leading leg, the ankle joint changed from dorsiflexion to plantarflexion. The fact that there were differences in the ankle joint angle of the leading leg but not the trailing leg suggested a difference in crossing obstacle compared to the unobstructed gait. In general, these results imply that participants used different strategies to control their leading and trailing legs when stepping over the obstacle. Thus, the interaction of gender × obstacle × leg on joint angle during the swing phase was further investigated. The results showed that legs had a main effect on maximum hip/knee flexion angle. Additionally, legs and obstacle heights had an interaction effect on maximum hip flexion angle. This study indicated that the leading and trailing leg have some independence when stepping over obstacles. Furthermore, the different performance of the leading and trailing leg in crossing obstacle can be attributed to the fundamental phenomenon, which is that the leading leg relies on vision, while the trailing leg relies on memory [30,31].

The strong positive correlation between maximum knee flexion angle and obstacle height was observed in both male and female participants, so the higher the obstacle, the greater the knee flexion angle, which means more muscle forces are required. A moderate positive correlation was found between hip flexion/ankle dorsiflexion and obstacle height. The increased joint angles may be attributed to the result of adjusting joint kinematics when stepping over obstacle. It is presumed that prolonged obstacle crossing may accelerate muscle fatigue.

In this study, similar results were observed between males and females for the second peak of vertical GRF during the unobstructed gait, and in addition, females exhibited a greater second peak vertical GRF in obstacle crossing. The results of the present study also indicated that there was a significant difference between males and females in the second negative peak of medial-lateral GRF. Furthermore, as obstacle height increased, the GRF variables were significantly different from those of the unobstructed gait, except for the medial-lateral GRF variables (the first and second negative peaks). This study showed that during the first half and terminal portion of the stance phase, the braking/propulsion amplitudes in obstacle-crossing gait were greater than those in the unobstructed gait. It can be assumed that a greater effort is required to push the body's center of mass forward when stepping over the obstacle [32]. The first peak of the vertical GRF is primarily related to body mass and acceleration, while the second peak is associated with the altered neuromuscular control of the lower extremity [33]. Thus, the increase in the first and second vertical GRF peaks during the obstacle-crossing gait may be due to changes in body acceleration and neuromuscular control after seeing the obstacle.

There are some limitations to this study that must be acknowledged. This study did not address other kinetic variables (i.e., joint moments) and muscle activities during obstacle crossing. Combining kinematic variables, kinetic variables, and muscle activities may provide further insights into the effects on the lower extremity when stepping over obstacle. Moreover, the sample size for this study was relatively small, and more participants should be recruited for further study.

5. Conclusions

The current study extends the knowledge based on previous findings by not only reporting the differences between males and females in stepping over obstacle, but also by elucidating the interaction between gender and obstacle height. There were significant differences for certain gait parameters (e.g., stride length and speed) between males and females. The results also showed that the variability of some gait parameters between genders varied with obstacle height. The present study provides a window into further understanding the physiological changes that occur in both genders in response to different task difficulties that may not be apparent in the unobstructed gait.

Author Contributions: Conceptualization, C.W.; methodology, C.W., Y.G., and W.D.; formal analysis, W.D.; investigation, W.C.; data curation, W.D.; writing—original draft preparation, C.W.; writing—review and editing, Y.G., Z.L., and W.C.; supervision, Z.L.; funding acquisition, W.C. All authors have read and agreed to the published version of the manuscript.

Funding: This research was funded by a research grant from the National Natural Science Foundation of China (Grant number: 11632013).

Institutional Review Board Statement: The study was conducted in accordance with the Declaration of Helsinki, and it was approved by the University Research Ethics Committee of Taiyuan University of Technology (TYUT202105003).

Informed Consent Statement: Informed consent was obtained from all subjects involved in the study. Written informed consent has been obtained from the participants to publish this paper.

Data Availability Statement: The original contributions presented in this study are included in the article. Further inquiries can be directed to the corresponding author.

Conflicts of Interest: The authors declare no conflicts of interest.

Abbreviations

The following abbreviations are used in this manuscript:

STT	Stance time of trialing leg
SWL	Swing time of leading leg
VCL	Vertical heel-clearance of the leading foot
VCT	Vertical heel-clearance of the trailing foot
HCL	Horizontal clearance of the leading foot
HCT	Horizontal clearance of the trailing foot
UM	Unobstructed gait for male participants
UF	Unobstructed gait for female participants
MM	Medium obstacle gait for male participants
MF	Medium obstacle gait for female participants
Fx_{PP}	The initially occurring positive peak on the medial-lateral curve
Fx_{N1}	The first negative peak on the medial-lateral curve
Fx_{N2}	The second negative peak on the medial-lateral curve
Fy_{BF}	The initial braking force on the anterior–posterior curve
Fy_{PF}	The propulsion force on the anterior–posterior curve
Fz_{FP}	The first peak on the vertical curve
Fz_{SP}	The second peak on the vertical curve
Fz_{DF}	The downfall between the two peaks on the vertical curve

References

1. Smith, L.K.; Lelas, J.L.; Kerrigan, C. Gender differences in pelvic motions and center of mass displacement during walking: Stereotypes quantified. *J. Womens Health Gend. Based Med.* **2002**, *11*, 453–458. [CrossRef] [PubMed]
2. Cutting, J.E.; Proffitt, D.R.; Kozlowski, L.T. A biomechanical invariant for gait perception. *J. Exp. Psychol. Hum. Percept. Perform.* **1978**, *4*, 357–372. [CrossRef] [PubMed]
3. Boyer, K.A.; Beaupre, G.S.; Andriacchi, T.P. Gender differences exist in the hip joint moments of healthy older walkers. *J. Biomech.* **2008**, *41*, 3360–3365. [CrossRef] [PubMed]
4. Bhambhani, Y.; Maikala, R. Gender differences during treadmill walking with graded loads: Biomechanical and physiological comparisons. *Eur. J. Appl. Physiol.* **2000**, *81*, 75–83. [CrossRef] [PubMed]
5. Timsina, L.R.; Wiletts, J.L.; Brennan, M.J.; Marucci-Wellman, H.; Lombardi, D.A.; Courtney, T.K.; Verma, S.K. Circumstances of fall-related injuries by and gender among community-dwelling adults in the United States. *PLoS ONE* **2017**, *12*, e0176561. [CrossRef] [PubMed]
6. Chardon, M.; Barbieri, F.A.; Penedo, T.; Santos, P.C.R.; Vuillerme, N. The effects of experimentally-induced fatigue on gait parameters during obstacle crossing: A systematic review. *Neurosci. Biobehav. Rev.* **2022**, *142*, 104854. [CrossRef] [PubMed]
7. Billington, J.; Wilkie, R.M.; Wann, J.P. Obstacle avoidance and smooth trajectory control: Neural areas highlighted during improved locomotor performance. *Front. Behav. Neurosci.* **2013**, *18*, 9. [CrossRef] [PubMed]
8. Patla, A.E.; Greig, M. Any way you look at it, successful obstacle negotiation needs visually guided on-line foot placement regulation during the approach phase. *Neurosci. Lett.* **2006**, *397*, 110–114. [CrossRef] [PubMed]
9. Yamaji, S.; Demura, S.; Sugiura, H. Influence of degraded visual acuity from light-scattering goggles on obstacle gait. *Health* **2011**, *3*, 99–105. [CrossRef]
10. Angelini, M.J.; Kesler, R.M.; Petrucci, M.N.; Rosengren, K.S.; Horn, G.P.; Hsiao-Wecksler, E.T. Effects of simulated firefighting and asymmetric load carriage on firefighter obstacle crossing performance. *Appl. Ergon.* **2018**, *70*, 59–67. [CrossRef] [PubMed]
11. Muir, B.C.; Haddad, J.M.; van Emmerik, R.E.A.; Rietdyk, S. Changes in the control of obstacle crossing in middle age become evident as gait task difficulty increases. *Gait Posture* **2019**, *70*, 254–259. [CrossRef] [PubMed]
12. Park, K.; Rosengren, K.S.; Horn, G.P.; Smith, D.L.; Hsiao-Wecksler, E.T. Assessing gait changes in firefighters due to fatigue and protective clothing. *Saf. Sci.* **2011**, *49*, 719–726. [CrossRef]
13. Jafarnezhadgero, A.A.; Majlesi, M.; Azadian, E. Gait ground reaction force characteristics in deaf and hearing children. *Gait Posture* **2017**, *53*, 236–240. [CrossRef] [PubMed]
14. Moisio, K.C.; Sumner, D.R.; Shott, S.; Hurwitz, D.E. Normalization of joint moments during gait: A comparison of two techniques. *J. Biomech.* **2003**, *36*, 599–603. [CrossRef] [PubMed]
15. Andriacchi, T.P.; Ogle, J.A.; Galante, J.O. Walking speed as a basis for normal and abnormal gait measurements. *J. Biomech.* **1977**, *10*, 261–268. [CrossRef] [PubMed]
16. Liikavainio, T.; Isolehto, J.; Helminen, H.J.; Perttunen, J.; Lepola, V.; Kiviranta, I.; Arokoski, J.P.A.; Komi, P.V. Loading and gait symmetry during level and stair walking in asymptomatic subjects with knee osteoarthritis: Importance of quadriceps femoris in reducing impact force during heel strike. *Knee* **2007**, *14*, 231–238. [CrossRef] [PubMed]
17. Kerrigan, D.C.; Todd, M.K.; Della Croce, U. Gender differences in joint biomechanics during walking. *Am. J. Phys. Med. Rehabil.* **1998**, *77*, 2–7. [CrossRef] [PubMed]
18. Mckean, K.A.; Landry, S.C.; Hubley-Kozey, C.L.; Dunbar, M.J.; Stanish, W.D.; Deluzio, K.J. Gender differences exist in osteoarthritic gait. *Clin. Biomech.* **2007**, *22*, 400–409. [CrossRef] [PubMed]
19. Ko, S.U.; Tolea, M.I.; Hausdorff, J.M.; Ferrucci, L. Sex-specific differences in gait patterns of healthy older adults: Results from the Baltimore longitudinal study of aging. *J. Biomech.* **2011**, *44*, 1974–1979. [CrossRef] [PubMed]
20. Chou, L.S.; Kaufman, K.R.; Hahn, M.E.; Brey, R.H. Medio-lateral motion of the center of mass during obstacle crossing distinguishes elderly individuals with imbalance. *Gait Posture* **2003**, *18*, 125–133. [CrossRef] [PubMed]
21. Roche, N.; Chorin, F.; Gerus, P.; Deshayes, M.; Guerin, O.; Zory, R. Effects of age, gender, frailty and falls on spatiotemporal gait parameters: A retrospective cohort study. *Eur. J. Phys. Rehabil. Med.* **2021**, *57*, 923–930. [CrossRef] [PubMed]
22. Alcock, L.; Galna, B.; Hausdorff, J.M.; Lord, S.; Rochester, L. Gait adaptations in response to obstacle type in faller with Parkinson's disease. *Gait Posture* **2018**, *61*, 368–374. [CrossRef] [PubMed]
23. Ramachandran, A.K.; Rosengren, K.S.; Yang, Y.; Hsiao-Wecksler, E.T. Effect of Tai Chi on gait and obstacle crossing behaviors in middle-aged adults. *Gait Posture* **2007**, *26*, 248–255. [CrossRef] [PubMed]
24. Mengarelli, A.; Maranesi, E.; Barone, V.; Burattini, L.; Fioretti, S.; Nardo, F.D. Evaluation of gender-related differences in co-contraction activity of shank muscles during gait. *Annu. Int. Conf. IEEE. Eng. Med. Biol. Soc.* **2015**, *2015*, 6066–6069. [CrossRef] [PubMed]
25. Schmitz, A.; Silder, A.; Heiderscheit, B.; Mahoney, J.; Thelen, D.G. Differences in lower-extremity muscular activation during walking between healthy older and young adults. *J. Electromyogr. Kinesiol.* **2009**, *19*, 1082–1091. [CrossRef] [PubMed]

26. Jansen, S.E.M.; Toet, A.; Werkhoven, P.J. Human locomotion through a multiple obstacle environment: Strategy changes as a result of visual field limitation. *Exp. Brain. Res.* **2011**, *212*, 449–456. [CrossRef] [PubMed]
27. Chen, H.L.; Lu, T.W. Comparisons of the joint moments between leading and trailing limb in young adults when stepping over obstacles. *Gait Posture* **2006**, *23*, 69–77. [CrossRef] [PubMed]
28. Cho, S.H.; Park, J.M.; Kwon, O.Y. Gender differences in three dimensional gait analysis data from 98 healthy Korean adults. *Clin. Biomech.* **2004**, *19*, 145–152. [CrossRef] [PubMed]
29. Ferber, R.; Davis, I.M.; Williams, D.S. Gender differences in lower extremity mechanics during running. *Clin. Biomech.* **2003**, *18*, 350–357. [CrossRef] [PubMed]
30. Heijnen, M.J.H.; Romine, N.L.; Stumpf, D.M.; Rietdyk, S. Memory-guided obstacle crossing: More failures were observed for the trail limb versus lead limb. *Exp. Brain. Res.* **2014**, *232*, 2131–2142. [CrossRef] [PubMed]
31. Lajoie, K.; Bloomfield, L.W.; Nelson, F.J.; Suh, J.J.; Marigold, D.S. The contribution of vision, proprioception, and efference copy in storing a neural representation for guiding trail leg trajectory over an obstacle. *J. Neurophysiol.* **2012**, *107*, 2283–2293. [CrossRef] [PubMed]
32. Damavandi, M.; Dixon, P.C.; Pearsall, D.J. Ground reaction force adaptations during cross-slop walking and running. *Hum. Mov. Sci.* **2012**, *31*, 182–189. [CrossRef] [PubMed]
33. Behmaram, S.; Jalalvand, A.; Jahani, M.R. Effects of backpack-induced on gait ground reaction force characteristics in primary school children with flat-foot deformity. *J. Biomech.* **2021**, *129*, 110817. [CrossRef] [PubMed]

Disclaimer/Publisher's Note: The statements, opinions and data contained in all publications are solely those of the individual author(s) and contributor(s) and not of MDPI and/or the editor(s). MDPI and/or the editor(s) disclaim responsibility for any injury to people or property resulting from any ideas, methods, instructions or products referred to in the content.

bioengineering

MDPI

Article

Biomechanical Analysis of Cycle-Tempo Effects on Motor Control Among Jump Rope Elites

Qi Zhou [1,†], Yufeng Liu [1,*,†], Jianguo Kang [1], Xiuping Wang [1], Kai Zhang [1] and Gongbing Shan [2,*]

1 Department of Physical Education, Xinzhou Teachers' University, Xinzhou 034000, China; zhouqi@xztu.edu.cn (Q.Z.); tyxkjg@xztu.edu.cn (J.K.); wangxp@xztu.edu.cn (X.W.); xzsyzk@xztu.edu.cn (K.Z.)

2 Biomechanics Lab., Faculty of Arts & Science, University of Lethbridge, Lethbridge, AB T1K 3M4, Canada

* Correspondence: liuyf@xztu.edu.cn (Y.L.); g.shan@uleth.ca (G.S.)

† The authors contributed equally to this work.

Abstract: Jump rope is a widely applied basic training technique in various sports, yet it is understudied biomechanically. This study investigates the impact of cycle-tempo-induced motor control changes in elite jump rope athletes, addressing the biomechanical gap of cyclic skill control. The hypothesis posited two accelerations per jump cycle—one in front of and one behind the body—and anticipated that increased cycle frequency would alter the distribution of acceleration time within a cycle. Using 3D motion capture technology, 12 young elite jump rope athletes were analyzed at 100, 140, and 180 revolutions per minute (rpm). The kinematic parameters obtained confirmed the presence of two distinct accelerations per cycle. As tempo increased, the percentage of rear acceleration time increased from 9.58% at 100 rpm to 17.42% at 180 rpm, while front acceleration time decreased from 39.03% at 100 rpm to 31.40% at 180 rpm, along with peak velocities increasing from 12.94 m/s at 100 rpm to 22.74 m/s at 180 rpm significantly ($p < 0.01$). Rope trajectory analysis indicated a consistent movement pattern across tempos, primarily in the sagittal plane. Variations in skill control revealed shorter contact phases, decreasing from 61.53% at 100 rpm to 48.25% at 180 rpm, as well as a reduced vertical range of motion for the center of gravity (from 0.15 body height at 100 rpm to 0.06 body height at 180 rpm) and feet (from 0.05 body height at 100 rpm to 0.03 body height at 180 rpm) ($p < 0.05$). Significant reductions were also observed in the flexion/extension range of motion for the hip (from 22.31° at 100 rpm to 3.47° at 180 rpm), knee (from 49.31° at 100 rpm to 9.35° at 180 rpm), and ankle (from 52.99° at 100 rpm to 21.41° at 180 rpm) ($p < 0.01$). These findings enhance the understanding of motor control adaptations to different tempos and have practical implications for developing coaching programs aimed at optimizing performance, stability, and efficiency in jump rope training.

Keywords: biomechanical modeling; 3D motion analysis; rope trajectory; acceleration characteristics; contact time

1. Introduction

Jumping rope has long been widely applied as a versatile and practical method for enhancing athletic conditioning, balance, and coordination across various sports disciplines [1–3]. Its simplicity belies its effectiveness, making it a staple in training regimes worldwide [1–3]. Athletes, from amateur enthusiasts to elite professionals, incorporate jumping rope into their workouts to improve agility, endurance, and overall performance [4–7]. However, despite its extensive use, a significant gap exists in our understanding of how variations in jumping speed influence motor control patterns among athletes. A search conducted in November 2023 using the keywords "rope jump + speed-dependent motor control" in the Web of Science database returned no relevant results, highlighting a gap in research on this topic in relation to training practices.

The speed of rope jumping, normally quantified by revolutions per minute (rpm) [8,9], plays a pivotal role in performance. Athletes aiming to increase rpm encounter heightened physical demands [9–11], necessitating precise motor control to sustain rhythm, balance, and coordination. It is widely hypothesized that as jumping speed rises, distinct changes in motor control patterns occur, impacting both technique and efficiency.

The scarcity of published articles investigating speed-dependent motor control pattern changes in jumping rope underscores the significant research gap. While numerous studies have explored the benefits of jumping rope on athletic attributes such as jump strength, running speed, endurance, and agility [12–14], none have specifically addressed how increasing speed influences motor control strategies. This dearth of scientific evidence presents an unprecedented opportunity for pioneering research in the field.

Speed, as a temporal factor, is crucial for optimizing motor control in complex sports skills [15–18]. Therefore, understanding the nuances of motor control adaptations to varying jumping speeds is essential for optimizing training methods and enhancing athlete performance. By elucidating the relationship between speed and motor control, researchers can inform evidence-based coaching strategies tailored to the specific demands of jumping rope activities. Furthermore, insights gained from this research have the potential to extend beyond the realm of jumping rope to inform training practices in other sports and physical activities where speed and coordination are integral components.

To ensure reliable motor control pattern analysis, the quality of subjects is paramount [19–21]. Professional jumping rope athletes, distinguished by years of rigorous training and competition experience, offer an ideal cohort for examining speed-dependent motor control pattern changes. Their refined motor skills and consistent performance levels provide a stable baseline against which potential alterations in control patterns can be discerned. By studying this population, reliable results can be obtained, elucidating nuanced adaptations in motor control strategies at varying jumping speeds.

Rope jumping entails a cyclic movement. However, due to the absence of biomechanical quantification of this cyclic skill control, the acceleration characteristics within a cycle remain unclear. Drawing from practitioners' experiences, we hypothesize the presence of two accelerations in each jump cycle—one occurring in front of the body and the other behind the body. It is anticipated that the total time for rope movement within a complete cycle will decrease with increasing cycle frequency, along with both accelerations. Nonetheless, practitioners may find it intriguing to ascertain the relative change in control within a cycle, particularly the percentage change of acceleration times in a cycle. Building upon practitioners' experiences, we propose the second hypothesis for the current study: as cycle frequency increases, the percentage of acceleration time in front of the body will decrease, while the percentage behind the body will increase. Consequently, the primary aim of this investigation is to examine the alterations in speed-dependent motor control patterns among elite jumping rope athletes. Our objective is to elucidate the relationship between jumping speed variations and motor control alterations, thereby addressing the existing gap in coaching practice. The findings from this study carry practical implications for the development of targeted training programs designed to optimize athletic conditioning, balance, and coordination.

In short, this study aims to contribute novel insights into athletic training by examining the impact of rope tempo on motor control patterns among elite jumping rope athletes.

By bridging the gap between theory and practice, we aspire to inform evidence-based coaching strategies that optimize athletic performance and enhance the overall effectiveness of training programs.

2. Materials and Methods

2.1. Subjects

As elaborated in the introduction, a central goal of this study is to collect biomechanically appropriate kinematic data while minimizing any influence of the testing process. Consequently, individuals with stable skill control were required. Elite athletes, characterized by their well-trained motor-control stability resulting from extensive training, were deemed ideal candidates. It is important to note that recruiting elite participants for this type of study is particularly challenging due to their limited availability and other practical constraints. As a result, sample sizes in similar studies are typically small, ranging from 2 to 9 individuals [21]. In this pilot study, we made our best efforts to recruit as many elite participants as possible, resulting in a sample size of 12 male Chinese participants. Table 1 presents an overview of their physical attributes and relevant experiences. All participants had not experienced any sports injuries within the past year and were in good physical and mental condition during testing. The test protocol was thoroughly scrutinized and approved by the host university's ethics committee. Prior to the commencement of the study, participants were briefed on the testing procedures, signed consent forms, and voluntarily participated in the data collection process.

Table 1. Participants' anthropometrical and training information.

Age (Years)	Height (cm)	Weight (kg)	Training (Years)	Training (Hours/Week)	Level [1]
20.11 ± 2.4	170.24 ± 2.1	68.2 ± 3.4	4.5 ± 0.5	15.2 ± 2.1	1

[1] Chinese National Certificate System for Athlete Performance Level. In this system, the performance levels are classified as follows: 1 denotes professional athletes, 2 signifies pre-professional athletes, and 3 refers to individuals who achieve a placement within the top six positions in competitions conducted at the county level or higher [22].

2.2. Test Protocol

From a technical and performance standpoint, it is observed that the majority of proficient individuals with developed jumping rope skills maintain rope frequencies ranging between 100 rpm and 180 rpm [23,24]. Consequently, this study opts to commence at 100 rpm as a baseline, considering that jumpers at this frequency already demonstrate continuous, relatively stable, and refined rope-swinging techniques [23]. The tempo within the range of 92–100 rpm is regarded as optimal for rope jumping from an injury prevention standpoint, as it minimizes joint stress, particularly on the knees [11]. Beyond 100 rpm, as the jumping cycle accelerates, there is an increase in physical demands [11]. Notably, a frequency of 140 rpm serves as a critical threshold that jumpers and coaches should heed [1]. When assessing the physical demands of rope jumping, factors such as physiological readiness, coordination efficiency, and rope cycle need to be taken into account. Specifically, when the frequency surpasses 140 rpm, there are significant disparities in heart rate and oxygen consumption compared to frequencies below 140 rpm [1]; Quirk and Sinning [9] similarly observed notable increases in these parameters between 140 rpm and 160 rpm, with no significant distinctions between 120 rpm and 140 rpm. Additionally, these differences are absent across frequencies of 66, 84, 102, 120, and 132 [10]. Experienced jumpers typically adhere to a frequency of 138 rpm, with 140 rpm marking the lower threshold of the aerobic training frequency range for rope jumping [25]. In the majority of regions in China, approximately 180 rpm is regarded as the benchmark for middle school physical education rope jumping assessments. Achieving a speed of 180 rpm or higher is indicative of exceptional physical prowess, particularly concerning balance, reaction time, and coordination among young adolescents in China [26]. Moreover, a speed of 180 rpm meets the criteria for activating anaerobic energy systems through rope training [25]. Therefore, this study incorporates three representative frequencies, namely 100 rpm, 140 rpm, and 180 rpm.

The participants were guided through the three test tempos by a metronome, ensuring compliance with the required rhythms for each test condition. Before the commencement of the testing session, participants engaged in a ten-minute self-warm-up routine. Subsequently, participants executed three sets of rope jumping at frequencies of 100 rpm, 140 rpm, and 180 rpm, each lasting for 8 s. A 3 min rest interval was provided between frequency adjustments to allow participants to exert consistent physical effort (i.e., without experiencing fatigue) in completing all experimental tasks.

2.3. Three-Dimensional Motion Capture and Biomechanical Modeling

To capture the movement involved in jumping rope, a 3D motion-capture system with 13 high-speed cameras was utilized, incorporating 45 reflective soft markers (diameter = 9 mm), comprising 39 markers positioned on the body and 6 on the rope. Additionally, 2 camcorders (DV1 and DV2) were synchronized with the 3D motion-capture system to supply video references (Figure 1).

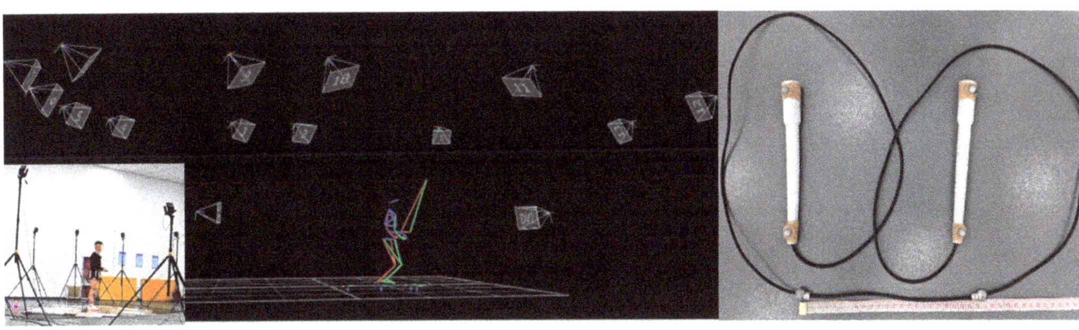

(a) (b) (c)

Figure 1. The setup of 3D motion capture: (**a**) camera setup, (**b**) an exemplary illustration of a captured instant of the 3D jumping rope with camera positions, and (**c**) the marker configuration on the rope.

The motion capture process employed a 13-high-speed-camera (200 frames/s) motion capture system (VICON MX40, Oxford Metrics Ltd., Oxford, UK). Extensive calibration procedures were conducted to minimize calibration residuals, following the guidelines provided by the manufacturer, resulting in an accuracy of <1 mm. Additionally, two CASIO video camcorders (100 Hz) synchronized with the VICON system were used to record all test trials, facilitating rapid visual assessments of trial quality.

The rope selected was constructed from PVC material designed for speed ropes, as it maximizes rope aerodynamics and can readily achieve speeds of 5 revolutions per second (i.e., 300 rpm) [25,27]. To standardize variables, the same jump rope was utilized for all participants, with a length extending from the feet to the upper chest. This length ensures optimal comfort for advanced jumpers without compromising body posture and technique during jumps, with rotational speeds of up to 240 rpm [25,27]. Two reflective soft markers were positioned in the middle of the jump rope, spaced 25 cm apart (Figure 1c), to prevent interference with the feet during jumps. Placing two reflective markers in the middle of the rope serves two purposes: firstly, to mitigate the impact of rope midpoint rebound on data integrity, and secondly, to ensure comprehensive and accurate data collection of rope revolutions. Additionally, four markers, two on each handle, were utilized to delineate the rope during jumping.

The strategic placement of 39 body markers facilitated the construction of a 15-segment biomechanical model [28,29], encompassing segments such as the head, upper and lower trunk, upper and lower arms, hands, thighs, shanks, and feet. The 15-segment model has been validated for assessing numerous complex sports skills in prior research [30–33]. The precise positioning of the 39 markers was conducted at specific anatomical landmarks on the subjects, including regions such as the temporal and posterior head regions, sternal end of the clavicle, xiphoid process of the sternum, C7 and T10 vertebrae, scapulae, iliac regions, acromion processes, epicondyles, and styloid processes of the radii and ulnae, among others. The use of 13 cameras and small markers provided subjects with substantial freedom of movement during motion capture, allowing them to closely replicate their trained "motor control style" to obtain their control patterns at different tempos.

2.4. Data Processing, Parameter Selection, and Statistical Analysis

To ensure stable control, we selected 5 revolutions near the midpoint of each 8 s data collection. The beginning of a revolution was defined as the midpoint of the rope at its lowest point in the vertical direction. This process resulted in a total of 180 revolutions of 3D data (3 tempos $\times$ 12 subjects $\times$ 5 revolutions = 180) for analysis. The raw motion capture data were processed using a five-point smoothing filter within the VICON software (Nexus 2.8.1, VICON Motion Systems, Oxford Metrics Ltd., Oxford, UK). This processing resulted in a dataset containing the 3D coordinates of 39 markers. These processed coordinates were then used to create a 15-segment biomechanical model [31,32] for analyzing the kinematics of rope jumping.

Biomechanical models provide a wide array of kinematic parameters, such as joint angles, velocities, accelerations, and more, derived from the 3D coordinates of captured markers on athletes to unveil control insights into complex sports skills [32–34]. However, it is imperative to select relevant data for the clear and concise communication of research findings. Focused reporting and discussion are essential principles in research writing [35,36], ensuring that the study's aims remain central. Therefore, researchers must carefully choose parameters aligned with their paper's focus to maintain coherence. Given the study's objective of quantifying the influence of rope revolution changes on control pattern variations, the primary outcomes focused on the velocity of the rope midpoint, rope handle, and big toe, as well as the timely coordination among these parameters, joint parameters, and center of gravity (COG) [16,37]. The secondary outcomes aimed to establish motor control patterns at different rope tempos, providing biomechanical insights for coaching practices.

The 3D coordinates of the rope midpoint were determined by averaging the coordinates of the two markers on the rope, each located 12.5 cm from the midpoint (Figure 1c). Speed and acceleration changes over time of the rope midpoint were calculated using frame-by-frame calculations of the average values in Microsoft Excel. Similarly, the averages of rope-handle markers and big toe markers were used to quantify the 3D excursions of the rope-handle point (center of cycle movement) and feet (dynamic distance to the ground), respectively. Additionally, two more calculated parameters, ROM (range of motion, determined by max–min) and % of a cycle time, were applied for kinematic analysis. This included the above parameters and the timely excursion of joint angles and COG obtained from the 15-segmental model quantification. With this approach, the potential control pattern changes induced by the tested tempos were quantitatively analyzed. To provide user-friendly results (e.g., minimizing the influence of body height in motor learning) for practitioners, normalization (% of body height) was applied to length-related parameters.

Statistical analysis was conducted on the data collected. Descriptive statistics, such as mean and standard deviations (mean ± SD), were calculated to demonstrate parameter characteristics. The normality of the data was evaluated using the Shapiro–Wilk test. If normality was confirmed, a one-way ANOVA was performed to identify changes in control patterns caused by variations in rope revolution frequency. All statistical analyses were carried out using IBM SPSS Statistics 23 (IBM Japan, Tokyo, Japan), with a significance level set at $p = 0.05$.

3. Results

3.1. Rope Trajectory

The rope cycle movement is quantified by the rope-handle point (center of cycle movement) and the rope midpoint (rope trajectory). The analysis shows that the rope trajectory is primarily in the sagittal plane (Figure 2), and this movement pattern is not influenced by the three tempos, as there were no significant differences among the rope-handle point and rope midpoint during cycle movement ($p > 0.05$).

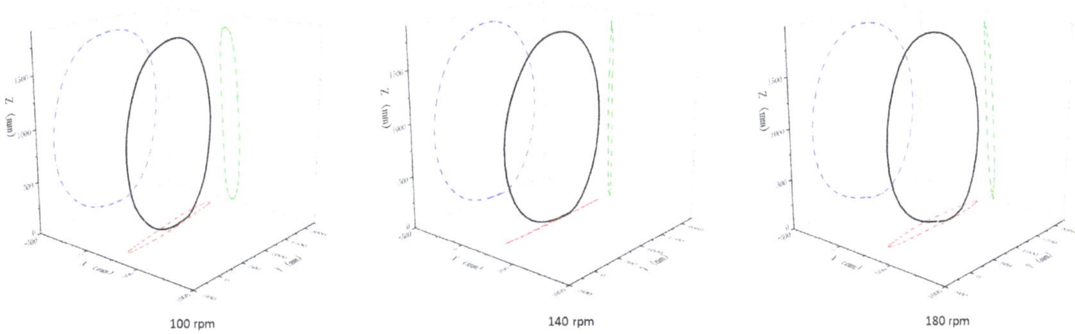

Figure 2. A 3D cycle trajectory (black) of the rope midpoint and its projections on 3 analysis planes (blue: sagittal plane, green: frontal plane, and red: transverse plane).

3.2. Rope Control Variation

As hypothesized, each rope cycle includes two accelerations, evidenced by two peaks in the velocity change-over-time curve for each cycle (Figure 3, left). The first peak occurs behind the body, termed rear-body acceleration (rear acceleration), and the second peak occurs in front of the body, termed front-body acceleration (front acceleration).

As rope tempo increases, the cycle time decreases significantly from 0.6 ± 0.01 s at 100 rpm to 0.43 ± 0.01 s at 140 rpm, reaching 0.33 ± 0.01 s at 180 rpm ($p < 0.01$). Correspondingly, the two peak velocities increase significantly from 13.39 ± 1.11 m/s at 100 rpm to 16.32 ± 1.13 m/s at 140 rpm, reaching 20.62 ± 0.73 m/s at 180 rpm ($p < 0.01$) for rear max velocity, and from 12.94 ± 1.20 m/s at 100 rpm to 16.88 ± 1.56 m/s at 140 rpm, reaching 22.74 ± 1.68 m/s at 180 rpm ($p < 0.01$) for front max velocity (Tables 2 and 3).

Regarding the relative time (% of a cycle) of the peak velocities, the results clearly show that the two peaks are close to the lowest point of the rope midpoint (Figure 3, left, and Table 2). However, significant differences ($p < 0.01$) are found only between 100 and 140 rpm, as well as between 100 and 180 rpm, not between 140 and 180 rpm ($p > 0.05$).

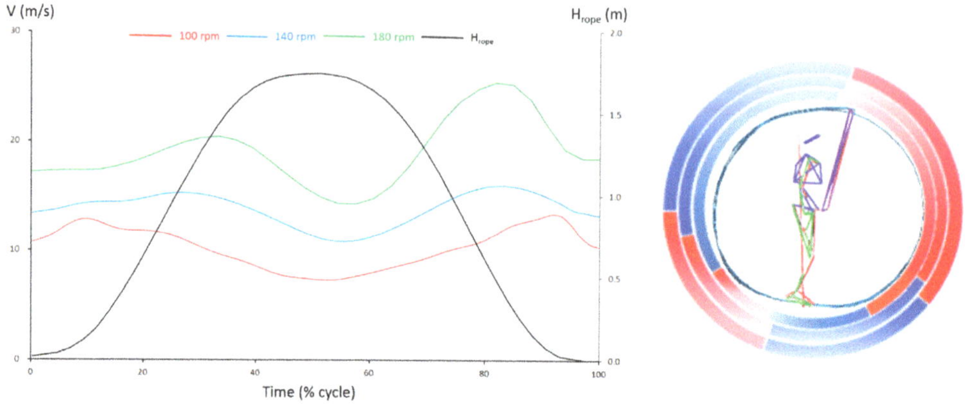

Figure 3. Variations in rope control within a cycle influenced by the three cycle tempos. The (**left panel**) illustrates the dynamic changes in rope-midpoint velocity during a cycle (H_{rope}: height of rope midpoint). Both the changes in absolute values and the time shifting of peak values are associated with variations in cycle tempo. The (**right panel**) depicts the spatial zones corresponding to the acceleration (red) and deceleration (blue) phases within a cycle. These relative phases are also influenced by the three cycle tempos (from inside to outside: 100 rpm, 140 rpm, and 180 rpm).

Table 2. Average and standard deviation (average ± SD) of the selected time–velocity variables associated with the influences of rope tempos on rope control.

Parameter	100 rpm	140 rpm	180 rpm
Cycle time (s)	0.60 ± 0.01	0.43 ± 0.01	0.33 ± 0.01
Rear V_{max} (m/s)	13.39 ± 1.11	16.32 ± 1.13	20.62 ± 0.73
Time at rear V_{max} (% of a cycle)	13.02 ± 4.20	21.76 ± 6.99	25.60 ± 5.60
Front V_{max} (m/s)	12.94 ± 1.20	16.88 ± 1.56	22.74 ± 1.68
Time at front V_{max} (% of a cycle)	89.17 ± 2.58	83.59 ± 4.77	85.06 ± 4.45

V_{max}: max velocity.

Table 3. Significance identified by *p*-value obtained from ANOVA with the probability of finding effects obtained from power analysis (*p*-value, probability) associated with the selected time–velocity parameters.

Parameter	100–140 rpm	140–180 rpm	100–180 rpm
Cycle time (s)	0.00, 1.00 **	0.00, 1.00 **	0.00, 1.00 **
Rear V_{max} (m/s)	0.00, 1.00 **	0.00, 1.00 **	0.00, 1.00 **
Time at rear V_{max} (% of a cycle)	0.00, 0.99 **		0.00, 1.00 **
Front V_{max} (m/s)	0.00, 1.00 **	0.00, 1.00 **	0.00, 1.00 **
Time at front V_{max} (% of a cycle)	0.01, 0.86 **		0.01, 0.82 **

V_{max}: max velocity, **: highly significant ($p \leq 0.01$).

The acceleration–time characteristics within a cycle reveal the reasons for the velocity variations influenced by rope tempos (Tables 4 and 5). In terms of magnitude, there are no significant differences among the rear accelerations ($p > 0.05$). However, the front acceleration increases significantly from 25.17 ± 13.73 m/s^2 at 100 rpm to 43.76 ± 15.70 m/s^2 at 140 rpm, reaching 86.66 ± 29.85 m/s^2 at 180 rpm ($p < 0.01$). Regarding timing, while there is no significant difference in the relative total acceleration time among the three tempos ($p > 0.05$), the rear acceleration time (9.58% ± 2.94%) at 100 rpm is significantly shorter than at 140 rpm (16.47% ± 5.38%) and 180 rpm (17.42% ± 4.68) ($p < 0.01$). Conversely, the front acceleration time (39.03% ± 8.63%) at 100 rpm is significantly longer than at 140 rpm (31.40% ± 5.57%) and 180 rpm (31.57% ± 5.70) ($p < 0.01$). There are no significant differences between 140 rpm and 180 rpm ($p > 0.05$). Figure 3 (left) illustrates these acceleration characteristics across the three tempos.

Table 4. Average and standard deviation (average ± SD) of the selected time–acceleration variables associated with the influences of rope tempos on rope control.

Parameter	100 rpm	140 rpm	180 rpm
Total acceleration time (% of a cycle)	48.61 ± 10.04	47.87 ± 6.97	48.99 ± 5.31
Average rear acceleration (m/s^2)	40.13 ± 17.18	43.87 ± 22.54	51.75 ± 20.25
Rear acceleration time (% of a cycle)	9.58 ± 2.94	16.47 ± 5.38	17.42 ± 4.68
Average front acceleration (m/s^2)	25.17 ± 13.73	43.76 ± 15.70	86.66 ± 29.85
Front acceleration time (% of a cycle)	39.03 ± 8.63	31.40 ± 5.57	31.57 ± 5.70

Table 5. Significance identified by p-value obtained from ANOVA test with the probability of finding effects obtained from power analysis (p-value, probability) associated with the selected time–acceleration parameters.

Parameter	100–140 rpm	140–180 rpm	100–180 rpm
Total acceleration time (% of a cycle)			
Average rear acceleration (m/s^2)			
Rear acceleration time (% of a cycle)	0.00, 0.81 **		0.00, 0.86 **
Average front acceleration (m/s^2)	0.00, 0.99 **	0.00, 1.00 **	0.00, 1.00 **
Front acceleration time (% of a cycle)	0.00, 0.80 **		0.00, 0.81 **

**: highly significant ($p \leq 0.01$).

3.3. Skill Control Variation

Figure 4 illustrates a typical example of skill control variation. As the rope tempo increases, the contact phase shortens, and the ROM (range of motion) of the COG (center of gravity) and feet in the vertical direction decrease. The movement patterns of the rope midpoint and rope-handle point remain unaffected by the different tempos.

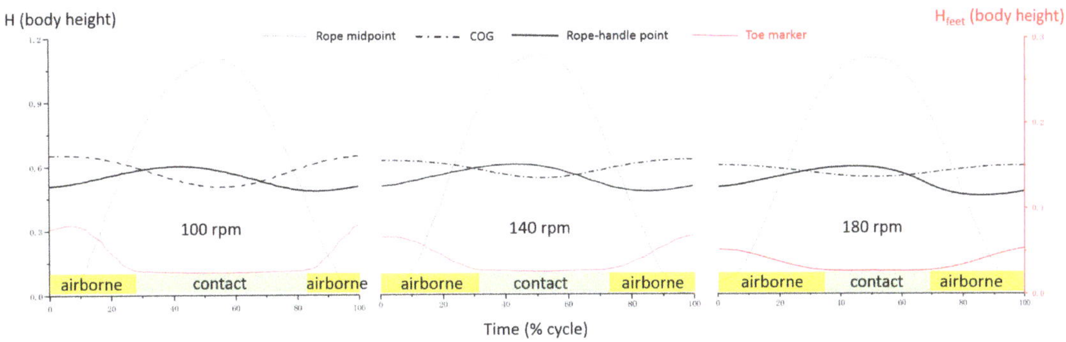

Figure 4. A typical position change over time for selected key markers. H (body height): height, H_{feet} (body height): feet height.

Statistical analysis reveals cycle-tempo-induced motor control changes, as shown in Figure 5. As the tempo increases, the contact time at 100 rpm (61.53% ± 9.03%) is significantly longer ($p < 0.01$) than at 140 rpm (50.97% ± 5.65%) and 180 rpm (48.25% ± 5.08%). There are no significant differences between 140 rpm and 180 rpm ($p > 0.05$) (Figure 5, left).

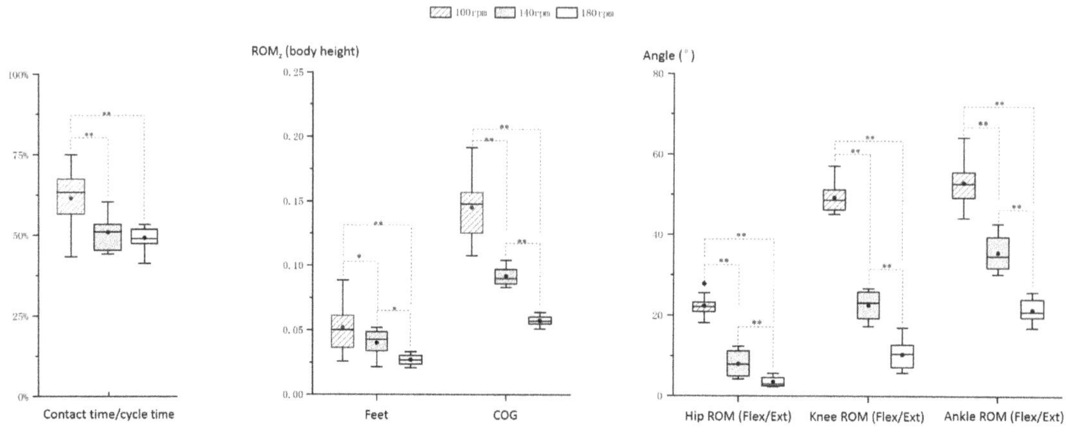

Figure 5. Selected skill control parameters significantly influenced by rope tempos. *: $p < 0.05$, **: $p < 0.01$, Flex/Ext: flexion/extension.

Regarding the ROM of feet and COG height (% of body height), both continuously decrease as tempo increases. The feet ROM decreases significantly from 0.05 ± 0.02 (body height) at 100 rpm to 0.04 ± 0.01 at 140 rpm, reaching 0.03 ± 0.00 at 180 rpm ($p < 0.05$). Similarly, the COG ROM decreases significantly from 0.15 ± 0.03 (% of body height) at 100 rpm to 0.09 ± 0.01 at 140 rpm, reaching 0.06 ± 0.00 at 180 rpm ($p < 0.01$) (Figure 5, middle).

The significant joint ROM changes are only found in lower limb joint flexion/extension. As tempo increased, the hip ROM decreased significantly from 22.31° ± 2.56° at 100 rpm to 8.00° ± 3.18° at 140 rpm, reaching 3.47° ± 1.22° at 180 rpm ($p < 0.05$). Similarly, the knee ROM decreased significantly from 49.31° ± 13.81° at 100 rpm to 22.55° ± 3.49° at 140 rpm, reaching 9.35° ± 3.37° at 180 rpm ($p < 0.01$) and the ankle ROM decreased significantly from 52.99° ± 5.60° at 100 rpm to 35.63° ± 4.16° at 140 rpm, reaching 21.41° ± 2.90° at 180 rpm ($p < 0.01$).

4. Discussion

The present study aimed to explore the impact of cycle-tempo-induced motor control changes in elite jump rope athletes. By examining the biomechanical aspects of rope jumping at various tempos, this research sought to fill a gap in the understanding of cyclic skill control in this athletic activity. The findings provide valuable insights into the relationship between jumping speed and motor control, offering practical implications for training and coaching practices.

4.1. Key Findings and Hypotheses Evaluation

The study's first hypothesis posited that each jump cycle includes two accelerations, one occurring in front of the body and the other behind it. The results have confirmed this hypothesis, revealing distinct velocity peaks in the velocity change-over-time curve for each cycle. These findings align with practitioners' observations, supporting the notion that the rope's movement entails significant accelerations at specific points within the cycle [25,38]. However, a novel aspect of this preliminary biomechanical study is that the two peak velocities are close to the lowest point of the rope midpoint, indicating that rear and front accelerations occur near the rope–foot intersection. This result highlights the unique timing characteristics of rope control, which should be emphasized in the skill learning and training process to increase learning/training efficiency [37]. This insight enhances the understanding of the skill control demands of jump rope, highlighting the importance of wrist control and its role in hand–foot coordination for optimizing performance.

The second hypothesis suggested that with increasing cycle frequency, the percentage of acceleration time in front of the body would decrease while the percentage behind the body would increase. The results have partially supported this hypothesis. While the relative total acceleration time did not vary significantly across tempos, the distribution of acceleration time between front and rear periods showed a two-stage change. Specifically, rear acceleration time increased significantly between 100 rpm and 140 rpm ($p = 0.00$) and remained relatively unchanged between 140 rpm and 180 rpm ($p > 0.05$). Similarly, front acceleration time decreased significantly between 100 rpm and 140 rpm ($p = 0.00$) and remained relatively unchanged between 140 rpm and 180 rpm ($p > 0.05$). This two-stage increase might suggest the existence of a critical tempo, beyond which the rear–front acceleration time ratio stabilizes at approximately 1:2. These findings imply that targeted timing control training could enhance training efficiency [39,40]. Further studies with larger samples are needed to validate these results.

4.2. Rope Trajectory and Training-Induced Control Adaptation

The analysis of rope trajectory indicated that the rope's movement predominantly occurs in the sagittal plane, with no significant differences among the three tempos. This consistency in movement pattern underscores the stability of the well-trained athletes' technique across varying speeds. The stability of the rope trajectory despite tempo changes suggests that elite athletes possess a high level of rope control that allows them to maintain consistent patterns under different tempo conditions. The results may indicate that rope jumping training helps trainees improve timely coordination between upper and lower limbs, especially between hands and feet. These preliminary biomechanical results provide direct evidence to support empirical findings from previous studies that suggest rope jumping improves dynamic coordination under various age and physical conditions [38,41–44].

Furthermore, the biomechanical analysis revealed that as rope tempos increased, the cycle time decreased significantly ($p = 0.00$), accompanied by a significant increase in peak velocities ($p = 0.00$) for both rear and front acceleration phases. This inverse relationship between cycle time and peak velocities indicates that higher tempos demand more rapid and forceful movements, exemplifying the basic physics principle: power = force $\times$ velocity in sport applications [45]. Specifically, the greater increase in front maximum velocity at higher tempos highlights the importance of increasing power control in this phase, which is crucial for successfully maintaining the rope's changing rhythm. To improve learning and training efficiency, this aspect should also be emphasized in coaching practice.

A further novel finding of the current study is the extremely low foot height at the rope–foot intersection point, particularly at 180 rpm. On average, this height is only 3% of the athlete's body height, translating to approximately 5 cm for an athlete who is 1.7 m tall. This observation explains why high tempos often lead to failure in practice, as both the time available for coordination and the allowable height decrease significantly ($p = 0.00$).

Lastly, combining the above results, increasing cycle-rope-tempo training improves timely acceleration control, limb coordination, and power generation and control. All of these characteristics are essential for enhancing athlete agility [46], especially in team sports [47]. From this perspective, this study provides biomechanical evidence explaining why rope jumping training can enhance athletic agility across various sports, as observed in previous studies [6,48–51]. The findings underscore the value of rope jumping as a training modality for developing the agility crucial for performance in a wide range of athletic disciplines.

4.3. Cycle-Tempo-Induced Body Control Pattern Changes

The skill control variation analysis demonstrated that increased rope tempos led to a shorter contact phase and reduced range of motion (ROM) for both the center of gravity (COG) and feet in the vertical direction. These changes suggest that athletes adapt to higher tempos by minimizing vertical displacement, which likely contributes to more efficient energy use and quicker cycle times. The unchanged movement patterns of the rope midpoint and rope-handle point across different tempos further emphasize the athletes' ability to maintain a consistent rope path while adapting to cycle-tempo variations. This newly unveiled control insight suggests a separation of upper and lower body control: the upper body maintains the consistency of the rope path regardless of rope-tempo variations, while the legs adapt to rope-tempo changes by reducing vertical movement of the feet and COG. This separation indicates the complexity and optimization of motor control developed through varied rope-tempo training, which enhances athletes' coordination abilities.

Currently, the literature lacks a consensus on the precise definition of joint-locking control. Based on the normal flexion/extension ROM of the hip, knee, and ankle in adult males [52], a cutoff value for joint locking/unlocking can be established at 10°—i.e., if the ROM is less than 10°, the joint is considered locked; otherwise, it is actively controlled. Using this cutoff value for joint locking identification, the ROM results of leg joints revealed new insights into lower limb control patterns: a hip–knee–ankle control strategy at 100 rpm, a knee–ankle control strategy at 140 rpm, and an ankle control strategy at 180 rpm. As rope tempo increases, the body becomes progressively stiffer, with the control pattern transitioning from multi-joint control to ankle-dominant control. This adaptation likely aids in maintaining stability and efficiency by limiting excessive joint motion under high-speed conditions. The results suggest that high-tempo training is beneficial for enhancing ankle power, potentially explaining why rope jumping is frequently utilized in sprinter and agility training across various sports [53–55].

4.4. Limitations, Practical Implications and Future Research

The current study, akin to numerous scholarly pursuits, presents constraints that necessitate contemplation. Notably, it embodies characteristics typical of a study with a limited sample size, which is susceptible to substantial biases. Small sample sizes are often inevitable in research involving skilled or elite athletes due to the limited availability of such subjects. However, one advantage is the high stability of control patterns developed through targeted training [32]. Typically, studies with small sample sizes in elite sports encompass 2 to 9 qualified subjects [56–60]. Our investigation adheres to this framework, albeit attempts were made to increase the sample size to 12 individuals.

An essential consideration in studies with a limited sample size revolves around whether the research objective emphasizes generalizable inferences or insights closely linked to practical scenarios. Our study is explicitly framed as a case-oriented inquiry, concentrating on furnishing intricate insights rather than deriving broad, generalizable conclusions. The case study methodology facilitates the examination of intricate units comprising numerous variables pertinent to the phenomenon under examination [61]. Grounded in authentic contexts, case studies furnish thorough and nuanced insights that can guide future research initiatives [61].

A further limitation pertains to the study's exclusive focus on elite males, raising questions regarding the extensibility of the findings to a broader populace. To fortify the reliability and relevance of these findings, forthcoming research should prioritize participant diversity, validating and potentially broadening the insights gleaned from this particular cohort.

The findings of this study have several practical implications for developing training programs aimed at enhancing athletic performance in jump rope. Understanding the specific motor control adjustments required at different tempos can inform evidence-based coaching strategies. Coaches can design targeted training drills that focus on improving acceleration control and optimizing joint ROM to enhance performance at varying speeds.

Future research should build on these findings by investigating the underlying neuromuscular mechanisms that facilitate these motor control adaptations. Additionally, exploring the impact of fatigue on motor control patterns and performance at different tempos could provide further insights into training and competition preparation. Longitudinal studies examining the effects of specific training interventions on motor control and performance in elite jump rope athletes would also be valuable.

5. Conclusions

This study offers a comprehensive biomechanical analysis of cycle-tempo-induced motor control changes in elite jump rope athletes. The findings confirm the presence of distinct acceleration phases within each jump cycle and reveal significant adjustments in motor control strategies as tempos increase. These insights enhance the understanding of the biomechanical demands of rope jumping and provide practical guidance for optimizing training and coaching practices. By bridging the gap between theory and practice, this research contributes to the development of evidence-based strategies that can enhance athletic performance and training effectiveness in jump rope.

Author Contributions: Conceptualization, Q.Z., Y.L., J.K. and G.S.; methodology, Q.Z., Y.L., X.W. and G.S.; validation, Q.Z., Y.L., J.K., X.W. and G.S.; formal analysis, Q.Z., Y.L., X.W. and G.S.; investigation, Q.Z., Y.L., J.K., X.W., K.Z. and G.S.; resources, Y.L.; data curation, Q.Z., Y.L., J.K., X.W. and K.Z.; writing—original draft preparation, Q.Z., Y.L. and G.S.; writing—review and editing, Q.Z., Y.L., J.K., X.W., K.Z. and G.S.; visualization, Q.Z., Y.L. and G.S.; supervision, Y.L. and G.S.; project administration, Y.L. and G.S.; funding acquisition, Q.Z. and Y.L. All authors have read and agreed to the published version of the manuscript.

Funding: This research project was supported by three grants from Shanxi Province, China: (1) Shanxi Higher Education Teaching Reform and Innovation Grant (Grant No.: J20231131), (2) 2023 Annual Grant of Xinzhou Science and Technology (Grant No.: 20230310), and (3) "Population Health Study: The Role of Rope Jumping in the Fitness Culture of Modern Chinese Society" at the Xinzhou Teachers' University (Grant No.: JG202401).

Institutional Review Board Statement: This study was carried out in accordance with the policy of the Ethical Committee of Xinzhou Teachers' University (protocol number: ECAXTU2022-12; approval period: 1 January to 31 December 2023).

Informed Consent Statement: Informed consent was obtained from all subjects involved in the study.

Data Availability Statement: The data presented in this study are available on request and after appropriate IRB approvals.

Acknowledgments: We would like to thank all the subjects of the study who donated their time and expertise.

Conflicts of Interest: The authors declare no conflicts of interest.

References

1. Solis, K.; Foster, C.; Thompson, N.; Cefalu, C. Aerobic requirements for and heart rate responses to variations in rope jumping techniques. *Physician Sportsmed.* **1988**, *16*, 121–128. [CrossRef] [PubMed]
2. Jahromi, M.S.; Gholami, M. The effect of jump-rope training on the physical fitness of 9 to 10 years old female students. *Adv. Appl. Sci. Res.* **2015**, *6*, 135–140.

3. Shkola, O.; Andriushchenko, T.; Zhamardiy, V.; Dubovoi, O.; Andreiev, P. Rope skipping as a means of increasing students' physical activity. *J. Educ. Teach. Trainers* **2022**, *13*, 301–309.
4. Orhan, S. Effect of weighted rope jumping training performed by repetition method on the heart rate, anaerobic power, agility and reaction time of basketball players. *Adv. Environ. Biol.* **2013**, *7*, 945–951.
5. Trecroci, A.; Cavaggioni, L.; Caccia, R.; Alberti, G. Jump rope training: Balance and motor coordination in preadolescent soccer players. *J. Sports Sci. Med.* **2015**, *14*, 792. [PubMed]
6. Pratama, N.E.; Mintarto, E.; Kusnanik, N.W. The influence of ladder drills and jump rope exercise towards speed, agility, and power of limb muscle. *J. Sports Phys. Educ.* **2018**, *5*, 22–29.
7. Dimarucot, H.C.; Soriano, G.P. Effectiveness of the multistage jumping rope program in enhancing the physical fitness levels among university students. *Int. J. Hum. Mov. Sports Sci.* **2020**, *8*, 235–239. [CrossRef]
8. Getchell, B.; Cleary, P. The caloric costs of rope skipping and running. *Physician Sportsmed.* **1980**, *8*, 55–60. [CrossRef]
9. Quirk, J.E.; Sinning, W.E. Anaerobic and aerobic responses of males and females to rope skipping. *Med. Sci. Sports Exerc.* **1982**, *14*, 26–29. [CrossRef] [PubMed]
10. Jette, M.; Mongeon, J.; Routhier, R. The energy cost of rope skipping. *J. Sports Med. Phys. Fit.* **1979**, *19*, 33–37.
11. Yamaguchi, H.; Yamamoto, K.; Edamatsu, C.; Hayata, G.; Miyakawa, T.; Onodera, S. Effect of Different Frequencies of Skipping Rope on Elastic Components of Muscle and Tendon in Human Triceps Surae. *Jpn. J. Phys. Fit. Sports Med.* **2002**, *51*, 185–192.
12. Singh, U.; Ramachandran, A.; Ramirez-Campillo, R.; Perez-Castilla, A.; Afonso, J.; Clemonte, F.; Oliver, J. Jump rope training effects on health-and sport-related physical fitness in young participants: A systematic review with meta-analysis. *J. Sports Sci.* **2022**, *40*, 1801–1814. [CrossRef] [PubMed]
13. Cengizel, Ç.; Öz, E.; Cengizel, E. Short-term plyometric and jump rope training effect on body profile and athletic performance in adolescent basketball players. *Int. J. Sport Stud. Health* **2022**, *5*, 132585.
14. Barrio, E.D.; Alvarez, C.; Thapa, R.K.; Ramachandran, A.K.; Singh, U.; Ramirez-Campillo, R. Jump rope training for health and fitness in school-age participants: Secondary analyses from a systematic review. *Int. J. Kinesiol. Sports Sci.* **2023**, *11*, 27–41. [CrossRef]
15. Shan, G.; Zhang, X. Soccer Scoring Techniques—A Biomechanical Re-Conception of Time and Space for Innovations in Soccer Research and Coaching. *Bioengineering* **2022**, *9*, 333. [CrossRef]
16. Zatsiorsky, V. *Biomechanics in Sport: Performance Enhancement and Injury Prevention*; John Wiley & Sons: Hoboken, NJ, USA, 2008.
17. Zhang, X.; Shan, G.; Liu, F.; Yu, Y. Jumping side volley in soccer—A biomechanical preliminary study on the flying kick and its coaching know-how for practitioners. *Appl. Sci.* **2020**, *10*, 4785. [CrossRef]
18. Shan, G.; Liu, Y.; Gorges, T.; Zhang, X.; Witte, K. Pilot Study on the Biomechanical Quantification of Effective Offensive Range and Ball Speed Enhancement of the Diving Header in Soccer: Insights for Skill Advancement and Application Strategy. *Appl. Sci.* **2024**, *14*, 946. [CrossRef]
19. Zhang, X.; Shan, G.; Liu, F.; Yong, S.; Meng, M. Diversity of Scoring, Ingenuity of Striking, Art of Flying-Conceptual and Systematical Identification of Soccer Scoring Techniques. *Phys. Act. Rev.* **2021**, *9*, 86–99. [CrossRef]
20. Bartlett, R.; Wheat, J.; Robins, M. Is movement variability important for sports biomechanists? *Sports Biomech.* **2007**, *6*, 224–243. [CrossRef]
21. Shan, G. The Practicality and Effectiveness of Soccer Scoring Techniques Revealed by Top Elite Soccer Scorers. *Phys. Act. Rev.* **2023**, *11*, 99–111. [CrossRef]
22. General Administration of Sport of China. National Standards for Athlete Technical Proficiency. 2010. Available online: https://www.gov.cn/gzdt/att/att/site1/20100226/001aa04b79580cf1b96001.pdf (accessed on 16 June 2022).
23. Li, W.B.; Chiu, W.H.; Feng, C.Z. The Effects of Sports Vision Control for Coordination—Biomechanical Analysis Based on the Action of Rope Skipping. *J. Jilin Inst. Phys. Educ.* **2016**, *32*, 41–48.
24. Liang, S.; Jing, L.; Sun, T.; Zong, X.; Wu, F. Upper Limb Kinematic Analysis of Rope Skipping. *Fujian Sports Sci. Technol.* **2023**, *42*, 93–96.
25. Lee, B. *Jump Rope Training*, 2nd ed.; Human Kinetics, Inc.: Champaign, IL, USA, 2003.
26. Ministry of Education of China. National Student Physical Health Standards. 2014. Available online: http://www.moe.gov.cn/s/8/A17/twys_left/moe_938/moe_792/s3273/201407/t20140708_171692.html (accessed on 16 July 2023).
27. Lee, B. Jump Rope Basics. *CrossFit J. Artic.* **2007**, *62*, 1–7.
28. Shan, G.; Bohn, C. Anthropometrical data and coefficients of regression related to gender and race. *Appl. Ergon.* **2003**, *34*, 327–337. [CrossRef] [PubMed]
29. Winter, D.A. *Biomechanics and Motor Control of Human Movement*; John Wiley & Sons: Hoboken, NJ, USA, 2009.
30. Shan, G.; Westerhoff, P. Full body kinematic characteristics of the maximal instep Soccer kick by male soccer players and parameters related to kick quality. *Sports Biomech.* **2005**, *4*, 59–72. [CrossRef]
31. Shan, G.; Visentin, P.; Zhang, X.; Hao, W.; Yu, D. Bicycle kick in soccer: Is the virtuosity systematically entrainable? *Sci. Bull.* **2015**, *60*, 819–821. [CrossRef]

32. Liu, Y.; Kong, J.; Wang, X.; Shan, G. Biomechanical analysis of Yang's spear turning-stab technique in Chinese martial arts. *Phys. Act. Rev.* **2020**, *8*, 16–22. [CrossRef]
33. Zhang, Z.; Li, S.; Wan, B.; Visentin, P.; Jiang, Q.; Dyck, M.; Li, H.; Shan, G. The influence of X-factor (trunk rotation) and experience on the quality of the badminton forehand smash. *J. Hum. Kinet.* **2016**, *53*, 9–22. [CrossRef] [PubMed]
34. Shan, G. Soccer Scoring Techniques: How Much Do We Know Them Biomechanically?—A State-of-the-Art Review. *Appl. Sci.* **2022**, *12*, 10886. [CrossRef]
35. Thomas, J.R.; Nelson, J.; Silverman, S. *Research Methods in Physical Activity*, 7th ed.; Human Kinetics, Inc: Champaign, IL, USA, 2022.
36. Kowalski, K.C.; McHugh, T.; Sabiston, C.; Ferguson, L. *Research Methods in Kinesiology*; Oxford University Press: Oxford, UK, 2018.
37. Magill, R.A. *Motor Learning Concepts and Applications*, 6th ed.; McGraw-Hill: Boston, MA, USA, 2001.
38. Curtis, D.M. *Rope Jumping and the Endurance, Leg Power, Agility, and Coordination of Children*; University of Illinois at Urbana-Champaign: Champaign, IL, USA, 1963.
39. Grondin, S.; Meilleur-Wells, G.; Lachance, R. When to start explicit counting in a time-intervals discrimination task: A critical point in the timing process of humans. *J. Exp. Psychol. Hum. Percept. Perform.* **1999**, *25*, 993. [CrossRef]
40. Mayer-Kress, G.; Liu, Y.T.; Newell, K.M. Time scales, difficulty/skill duality, and the dynamics of motor learning. *Adv. Exp. Med. Biol.* **2009**, *629*, 457–476.
41. Jeong, K.C.; Shin, J.G. Effects of Jump Rope Program on Motor Coordination of Children with Autistic Spectrum Disorder. *Res. J. Pharm. Technol.* **2017**, *10*, 2391–2394. [CrossRef]
42. Yang, X.; Lee, J.; Gu, X.; Zhang, X.X.; Zhang, T. Physical fitness promotion among adolescents: Effects of a jump rope-based physical activity afterschool program. *Children* **2020**, *7*, 95. [CrossRef] [PubMed]
43. Epure, M.; Bădău, D. Study on Improving Coordination Skills in Women's Basketball Game. *Discobolul-Phys. Educ. Sport Kinetotherapy J.* **2021**, *60*, 93–106.
44. Mischenko, N.; Kolokoltsev, M.; Romanova, E.; Vorozheikin, A.; Bolotin, A.; Vyazovichenko, Y.; Timchenko, N. «Help» methodology for improving coordination training effectiveness in acrobatics sports. *J. Phys. Educ. Sport* **2021**, *21*, 3504–3510.
45. Burkett, B. *Sport Mechanics for Coaches*; Human Kinetics: Champaign, IL, USA, 2010.
46. Sheppard, J.M.; Young, W.B. Agility literature review: Classifications, training and testing. *J. Sports Sci.* **2006**, *24*, 919–932. [CrossRef]
47. Paul, D.J.; Gabbett, T.J.; Nassis, G.P. Agility in team sports: Testing, training and factors affecting performance. *Sports Med.* **2016**, *46*, 421–442. [CrossRef]
48. Miller, J.M.; Hilbert, S.C.; Brown, L.E. Speed, quickness, and agility training for senior tennis players. *Strength Cond. J.* **2001**, *23*, 62. [CrossRef]
49. Turgut, E.; Colakoglu, F.; Guzel, N.; Karacan, S.; Baltaci, G. Effects of weighted versus standard jump rope training on physical fitness in adolescent female volleyball players: A randomized controlled trial. *Fiz. Rehabil.* **2016**, *27*, 108–115. [CrossRef]
50. İpekoğlu, G.; Erdogan, C.; Er, F.; Colakoglu, F.; Baltaci, G. Effect of 12 week neuromuscular weighted rope jump training on lower extremity reaction time. *Turk. J. Sport Exerc.* **2018**, *20*, 111–115. [CrossRef]
51. Malar, S.; Maniazhagu, D. Effect of circuit training combined with speed agility quickness drills and jump rope drills on agility. *Asian J. Appl. Sci. Technol. (AJAST)* **2022**, *6*, 111–121. [CrossRef]
52. Roaas, A.; Andersson, G.B. Normal range of motion of the hip, knee and ankle joints in male subjects, 30–40 years of age. *Acta Orthop. Scand.* **1982**, *53*, 205–208. [CrossRef]
53. Boccolini, G.; Costa, N.; Alberti, G. The effect of rope jump training on sprint, agility, jump and balance tests in young basketball players. In *Book of Abstracts of the 17th Annual Congress of the European College of Sport Science, 4–7th July, ECSS Bruges 2012–Belgium*; ECCS: Bruges, Belgium, 2012.
54. Makaruk, H. Acute effects of rope jumping warm-up on power and jumping ability in track and field athletes. *Pol. J. Sport Tour.* **2013**, *20*, 200–204. [CrossRef]
55. Miyaguchi, K.; Demura, S.; Omoya, M. Relationship between jump rope double unders and sprint performance in elementary schoolchildren. *J. Strength Cond. Res.* **2015**, *29*, 3229–3233. [CrossRef]
56. Cavanagh, P.R.; Andrew, G.; Kram, R.; Rodgers, M.; Sanderson, D.; Hennig, E. An approach to biomechanical profiling of elite distance runners. *J. Appl. Biomech.* **1985**, *1*, 36–62. [CrossRef]
57. Barris, S.; Farrow, D.; Davids, K. Increasing functional variability in the preparatory phase of the takeoff improves elite springboard diving performance. *Res. Q. Exerc. Sport* **2014**, *85*, 97–106. [CrossRef]
58. Ho, S.R.; Smith, R.; O'Meara, D. Biomechanical analysis of dragon boat paddling: A comparison of elite and sub-elite paddlers. *J. Sports Sci.* **2009**, *27*, 37–47. [CrossRef]
59. Gløersen, Ø.; Myklebust, H.; Hallén, J.; Federolf, P. Technique analysis in elite athletes using principal component analysis. *J. Sports Sci.* **2018**, *36*, 229–237. [CrossRef] [PubMed]

60. Hébert-Losier, K.; Supej, M.; Holmberg, H.C. Biomechanical factors influencing the performance of elite alpine ski racers. *Sports Med.* **2014**, *44*, 519–533. [CrossRef] [PubMed]
61. Hamel, J.; Dufour, S.; Fortin, D. *Case Study Methods*; Sage Publications: New York, NY, USA, 1993.

Disclaimer/Publisher's Note: The statements, opinions and data contained in all publications are solely those of the individual author(s) and contributor(s) and not of MDPI and/or the editor(s). MDPI and/or the editor(s) disclaim responsibility for any injury to people or property resulting from any ideas, methods, instructions or products referred to in the content.

bioengineering

MDPI

Article

Older Fallers' Comprehensive Neuromuscular and Kinematic Alterations in Reactive Balance Control: Indicators of Balance Decline or Compensation? A Pilot Study

Ringo Tang-Long Zhu [1,2], Timmi Tim Mei Hung [1], Freddy Man Hin Lam [3], Jun-Zhe Li [1], Yu-Yan Luo [1], Jingting Sun [4], Shujun Wang [1,2] and Christina Zong-Hao Ma [1,2,*]

[1] Department of Biomedical Engineering, The Hong Kong Polytechnic University, Hong Kong SAR 999077, China; ringo-tanglong.zhu@connect.polyu.hk (R.T.-L.Z.); timmei-timmi.hung@connect.polyu.hk (T.T.M.H.); junzhe.li@connect.polyu.hk (J.-Z.L.); yuyan-laura.luo@connect.polyu.hk (Y.-Y.L.); shu-jun.wang@polyu.edu.hk (S.W.)

[2] Research Institute for Smart Ageing, The Hong Kong Polytechnic University, Hong Kong SAR 999077, China

[3] Department of Rehabilitation Sciences, The Hong Kong Polytechnic University, Hong Kong SAR 999077, China; freddy-mh.lam@polyu.edu.hk

[4] Future Architecture and Urban Research Institute, Tongji Architectural Design (Group) Co., Ltd., Shanghai 200092, China; 3002_sunny@tongji.edu.cn

* Correspondence: czh.ma@polyu.edu.hk; Tel.: +852-2766-7671; Fax: +852-2334-2429

Abstract: Background: Falls and fall consequences in older adults are global health issues. Previous studies have compared postural sways or stepping strategies between older adults with and without fall histories to identify factors associated with falls. However, more in-depth neuromuscular/kinematic mechanisms have remained unclear. This study aimed to comprehensively investigate muscle activities and joint kinematics during reactive balance control in older adults with different fall histories. **Methods**: This pilot observational study recruited six community-dwelling older fallers (≥1 fall in past one year) and six older non-fallers, who received unpredictable translational balance perturbations in randomized directions and intensities during standing. The whole-body center-of-mass (COM) displacements, eight dominant-leg joint motions and muscle electrical activities were collected, and analyzed using the temporal and amplitude parameters. **Results**: Compared to non-fallers, fallers had significantly: (a) smaller activation rate of the ankle dorsiflexor, delayed activation of the hip flexor/extensor, larger activation rate of the knee flexor, and smaller agonist-antagonist co-contraction in lower-limb muscles; (b) larger knee/hip flexion angles, longer ankle dorsiflexion duration, and delayed timing of recovery in joint motions; and (c) earlier downward COM displacements and larger anteroposterior overshooting COM displacements following unpredictable perturbations ($p < 0.05$). **Conclusions**: Compared to non-fallers, fallers used more suspensory strategies for reactive standing balance, which compensated for inadequate ankle/hip strategies but resulted in prolonged recovery. A further longitudinal study with a larger sample is still needed to examine the diagnostic accuracies and training values of these identified neuromuscular/kinematic factors in differentiating fall risks and preventing future falls of older people, respectively.

Keywords: community-dwelling; older adults; falls; reactive balance; perturbation; electromyographic (EMG); co-contraction index (CCI); kinematics; postural sways

1. Introduction

Falls and fall consequences in older adults burden society heavily and are global health issues [1]. Annually, around one in three older adults falls, one in ten older adults has fall-related injuries, and 684,000 fall-related deaths happen worldwide [1,2]. However, even the multi-factorial fall-prevention management has shown relatively limited success in fall reduction, especially in older adults with fall histories, i.e., fallers [3]. Given that balance and gait disorders are the second leading causes of falls except accidents [1], some in-depth physiological alterations of balance control in older fallers that have remained unidentified may be modifiable to prevent older adults' future falls more effectively.

Several balance control strategies with the involvement of lower limbs have been proposed, based on the analyses of kinematics (i.e., postural sways, joint motions) and neuromuscular activities (i.e., electromyographic [EMG] signals). The feet-in-place strategy is commonly employed to keep the whole-body center of mass (COM) within the base of support (BOS) when external perturbations are not large; this comprises a single or a combination of the ankle strategy, hip strategy, and suspensory strategy (bending knees to lower the COM for stability) [4]. The stepping strategy is used to establish a new BOS when the feet-in-place strategy is not enough to overcome the increasing perturbation intensity [4,5]. Compared to young adults, older adults tended to rely more on the proximal lower-limb joint motions and muscles than the distal ones, and may use the stepping strategy for reactive/compensatory/automatic balance control following unpredictable perturbations [6]. Apart from the age-related changes in the responses of multiple muscles/joints, prior studies have also shown the interaction effects of age with the perturbation direction and perturbation intensity on balance control strategies [6–8]. Nevertheless, the identified age-related kinematic and neuromuscular alterations underlying reactive balance control may not be directly indicative of fall risks, due to the potential existence of the confounding factor of age. Specific investigations and comparisons of the older adults with and without fall histories (i.e., fallers vs. non-fallers, and excluding the confounding factor of age) are therefore warranted to identify further balance control alterations in older individuals who are prone to falls, and to identify the fall-related factors.

Previous studies have intensively analyzed the stepping strategies and whole-body postural sways to compare the reactive balance control between fallers vs. non-fallers [9–15], while there has been less focus on the differences in specific joint motions or muscle activities [16–18]. Firstly, lower-limb muscle activities during reactive balance control have primarily been examined within a restricted number of lower-limb muscles, i.e., the ankle dorsiflexor/plantarflexor [16–18], knee flexor/extensor [16,18], and hip abductor [18]. The differences in hip adductor and hip flexor/extensor activation between fallers and non-fallers remain unknown. Secondly, prior investigations of lower-limb muscle activities have examined only one single EMG parameter in each study [16–18]. Fallers were reported to exhibit longer EMG onset latency of the ankle dorsiflexor following anterior translational perturbations during standing [17], longer EMG onset latencies of the hip abductor and knee flexor in the weight-bearing leg following lateral shoulder-impact perturbations during standing [18], and no significantly different agonist-antagonist co-contraction index (CCI) of the ankle dorsiflexor-plantarflexor or knee flexor-extensor following optical flow perturbations during walking as compared to non-fallers [16]. The existing analysis of timing and amplitude characteristics of EMG signals may have been insufficient, since only the delayed muscular reaction was identified to differentiate fallers from non-fallers [17,18]. Thirdly, regarding joint kinematics, interestingly, no prior studies seemed to have compared them in fallers vs. non-fallers during reactive balance control, to the best of authors' knowledge. Although fallers exhibited a decreased range of motion in lower-limb joints than non-fallers [19], it has been unclear whether the lower-limb joint motions during reactive balance control differ between fallers and non-fallers or not. More comprehensive analyses of lower-limb muscle activities and joint kinematics are needed to facilitate the understanding of older fallers' balance control strategies.

Reactive balance control strategies are influenced by both the perturbation direction and perturbation intensity [5,20], while there is still insufficient evidence on how fallers and non-fallers respond differently to diverse directions or intensities of balance perturbations. Regarding the perturbation intensity, a previous study reported that fallers and non-fallers' differences in stepping strategy were more pronounced following a higher intensity of mediolateral perturbation [10], whereas another study did not observe an interaction effect of fall history and perturbation intensity on the reactive stepping strategy following unpredictable anterior perturbations [21]. Regarding the perturbation direction, prior studies also reported inconsistent differences in postural sway between fallers and non-fallers when responding to the unpredictable anteroposterior [13,21] or mediolateral [9,13,18,22] perturbations. The underlying reasons for these inconsistent findings have not been thoroughly understood/explained. Analyzing neuromuscular responses and joint kinematics during reactive balance control can potentially help better explain how the fall-prone older adults respond to varied levels of threats of suddenly losing balance. This may also provide useful insights for clinical assessments or even interventional enhancement of reactive balance.

The main aim of this study was therefore to explore the older fallers' neuromuscular and kinematic alterations of lower limbs during reactive balance control as compared to non-fallers. Specifically, this study had the research question of how EMG/angle signals varied among the eight different dominant-leg muscles/joint motions, different fall histories, directions, and intensities of unpredictable translational perturbations. In addition, the study investigated how the COM displacements varied among the six different postural sway directions (i.e., forward/backward, medial/lateral, and upward/downward), different fall histories, perturbation directions, and perturbation intensities. The temporal parameters including onset latency, time to peak, and burst duration, together with the amplitude parameters including rate of rise, peak amplitude, and/or agonist-antagonist CCI were analyzed for these signals. We hypothesized that the analyzed parameters during reactive balance control would be affected by the interaction of fall history, muscle/joint motion/postural sway direction, perturbation direction, and perturbation intensity. Furthermore, for the effects of fall history, based on the previously available findings related to aging [4,6,7,16,19,23] and fall histories [16–18], we extrapolated that fallers would have delayed timing and larger amplitudes of proximal muscles' activation/joint motions as compared to non-fallers following a high intensity of unpredictable anterior or lateral balance perturbation.

2. Materials and Methods

2.1. Study Design and Participants

This study was a pilot observational cross-sectional study. Participants were recruited through convenience sampling. Inclusion criteria were: (1) aged 65 years old or over, (2) living in the community independently and able to walk for 400 m without any assistance, and (3) fallers (with at least one fall within the past one year) or non-fallers (with no fall within the past one year), matched for age and sex. Exclusion criteria were: (1) being hospitalized or living in a nursing home for more than six months in the past year; (2) experiencing fall(s) due to traffic or occupational accidents; (3) being diagnosed with cognitive impairment or severe systemic disease (e.g., neuromuscular, renal, hepatic, orthopedic, vestibular, or cardiopulmonary disorders) that impacts or limits physical activities; and (4) participated in any structured exercise training or strengthening exercises within the past one year. A total of twelve older participants were finally eligible for this study. Before being tested, each participant read and signed an informed consent form to participate in this study (Ethics approval agency: Institutional Review Board, The Hong Kong Polytechnic University; Ethical reference number: HSEARS20201230002). Each participant underwent the experiment once, involving subjective assessments and perturbation trials.

2.2. Subjective Assessments

Collection of demographic data (e.g., age, sex, height, body mass), medical history, and fall history was first conducted, followed by assessments using questionnaires/scales. A fall was defined as an event that resulted in coming to rest inadvertently on the ground or floor or other lower level and not resulting from an intrinsic or overwhelming hazard [24]. The short Falls Efficacy Scale-International (FES-I) and the Chinese version of the Physical Activity Scale for the Elderly (PASE-C) were used for the measurement of a participant's fear of falling and physical activity level, respectively [25,26]. The Mini-Balance Evaluation System Test (Mini-BEST) was used to assess a participant's functional balance performance, including anticipatory postural control, reactive postural control, sensory orientation, and dynamic gait [27]. The Mini-BEST was selected due to its established reliability and validity [28] together with its comprehensive evaluation of various balance dimensions, particularly for the sub-item of reactive balance, making it more relevant to the topic of this study than other clinical assessments (e.g., Timed Up and Go test, Berg Balance Scale). Then the participant's dominant leg was determined through the use of three tests: the balance recovery test, the ball-kick test, and the step-up test [5,29]. The leg that was used more frequently for stepping after being nudged forward, kicking a ball, and stepping onto a stair across a total of nine trials (three trials for each test) was identified as the dominant leg [5,29]. All subjective assessments were conducted by the same examiner.

2.3. Perturbation Trials

2.3.1. Experimental Set-Up

A moving-platform perturbation system was used to induce the unpredictable translational perturbations (Figure 1), with technical details reported in a previous study [5]. Briefly, the platform can move horizontally at a random starting time, with random moving direction and random moving distance/velocity/acceleration (related to different intensities) to constitute an unpredictable balance perturbation to the participant standing on it. The whole-body kinematics were collected using an 8-camera motion capture system (Nexus 2.11, Vicon Motion Systems Ltd., Yarnton, UK) that sampled at 250 Hz. An eight-channel Trigno Wireless Biofeedback System (Delsys Inc., Natick, MA, USA) that sampled at 2000 Hz was used to record muscular electrical activities. The data collection was synchronized for the three systems [5].

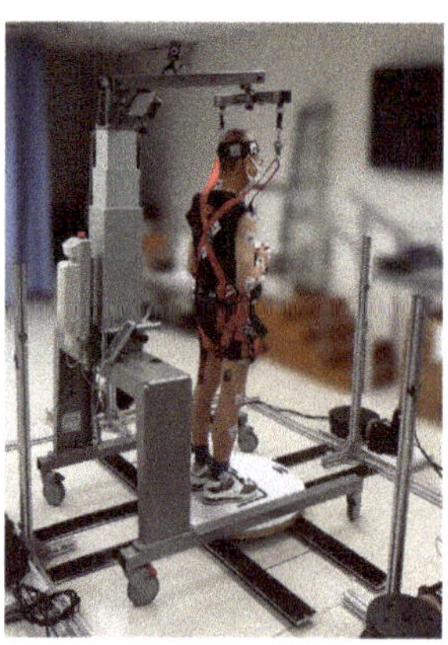

Figure 1. The moving-platform perturbation system being used by a participant.

2.3.2. Protocol of Perturbation Trials

The procedure for the perturbation trials was firstly explained to the participant. Participants were asked in advance to wear their daily footwear, except for impractical shoes, such as sandals, high heels, ballet shoes and slippers. Each participant was given an identical set of tight shirt and shorts, to optimize the Vicon motion capture and the placement of retroreflective markers and EMG sensors. Before the perturbation trials, EMG sensors and retroreflective markers were placed on the participant. The eight wireless surface EMG sensors were placed on the eight dominant-leg muscles, according to the recommendation of the Surface ElectroMyoGraphy for the Non-Invasive Assessment of Muscles (SENIAM) project (Table A1 in Appendix A) [30]. The major muscles relevant to eight ankle, knee and hip joint motions were selected, including the tibialis anterior (TA), gastrocnemius medialis (GM), rectus femoris (RF), long head of bicep femoris (BF), sartorius (SA), gluteus maximus (GMax), gluteus medius (GMed), and adductor magnus (AM). A standard skin preparation procedure, including shaving, cleaning, and slightly abrading with alcohol wipes, was performed before attaching the EMG electrodes. The sensors were applied to the skin with double-sided tape (Trigno Sensor Adhesive Interface, Delsys, Boston, MA, USA), with medical tape to enhance fixation. Then a set of 39 retroreflective markers were attached to the bony landmarks of the head, torso, left and right upper limbs, pelvis, and left and right lower limbs [31]. All placements were conducted by the same examiner.

The participant was then instructed to stand with two feet wearing shoes and shoulder-width apart on the middle of the platform, holding a light rod at waist level and close to the trunk to keep the arms from blocking the reflective markers. The participant was told to stand naturally and look forward at the beginning, try best to maintain balance if feeling the perturbation, and then return to the original foot position marked by the dark-colored tapes as quickly as possible if the foot moved. A safety harness system (PG-360, Physio Gait Dynamic Unweighting System, Healthcare International Ltd., Langley, WA, USA) was equipped on each participant as a safety measure during the perturbation.

Each participant then experienced four trials (each consisted of 12 random perturbations) covering a total of 48 unpredictable balance perturbations (4 directions × 4 intensities × 3 repetitions), with 5 min of rest after each trial. The platform moved horizontally in a pre-determined direction and intensity first, then remained stationary for 12 s, and was finally pulled back to its original position. The triggering time, directions (anterior, posterior, medial, and lateral), and intensities (highest, high, low, and lowest) were randomized and blinded to the participant. The anterior, posterior, medial, and lateral perturbations induced the participant's backward, forward, lateral, and medial loss of balance, respectively. Based on the human's limits of stability in different directions and our pilot study results in young adults [5], the highest intensity for the anterior, posterior, medial, and lateral directions corresponded to the platform's moving distances of 2.67%, 4.00%, 5.33% and 5.33% of each participant's height, respectively. Based on the trajectory of the reflective marker placed on the platform, the displacement, velocity, and acceleration of platform movement for each intensity are presented in Table A2 of Appendix A. Videos were recorded in real time during all perturbation trials to enable further manual observation and analysis of balance control strategies. Regardless of whether feet-in-place strategies or stepping strategies were used, the dominant-leg muscle activities and joint motions were focused on and analyzed for all participants.

2.4. Data Processing

Kinematic data, including the whole body's COM, the dominant-leg hip, knee, and ankle joint motions were first processed using the Plug-in Gait full body model. Then the kinematic data and the raw EMG data of dominant-leg muscles were further processed as described below in a custom MATLAB program MATLAB 2019b, The MathWorks, Inc., Natick, MA, USA). The kinematic data were subtracted by the mean signal value of the 1000-ms baseline interval before the start of each perturbation for normalization. To obtain the COM displacement relative to the base of support (BOS), the COM displacement was further subtracted by the displacement of the moving platform [5]. The raw EMG signals were zeroed to the mean value of the entire perturbation trial [32,33], full-wave rectified, and low-pass filtered at 4 Hz with a bi-directional 4th order Butterworth filer to obtain the envelope [32], then further divided by the mean signal value of the 1000-ms baseline interval before the start of the perturbation trial for normalization [5,20].

Temporal parameters, including the onset latency, time to peak, and burst duration, together with amplitude parameters, including the peak amplitude, rate of rise, and/or agonist-antagonist CCI were analyzed through a custom MATLAB algorithm (Figure 2). Within 2 s after the start of each perturbation, the onset was detected as the first point in time when the corresponding signal value exceeded five times the standard deviation (SD) over the mean baseline value (mean + 5 SD), and the peak was identified as the point with the maximum signal value after the onset [5,20,34]. The reason for detecting onset and peak within 2 s after a perturbation was because participants were observed to recover balance within this duration following perturbations in the pilot study, and the kinematic or EMG reactions within this duration were considered meaningful to resist the sudden balance loss. Within 9 s after the start of each perturbation, the offset was identified as the first point in time after the onset, when the corresponding signal value dropped below five times the standard deviation over the mean baseline value (mean + 5 SD) [35]. The baseline for onset or offset detection was the 1000-ms interval of a signal before the start of each perturbation. The onset latency indicated the time delay from the start of perturbation to the signal onset, the time to peak indicated that from the start of perturbation to the signal peak, and the burst duration indicated that from the signal onset to offset. The rate of rise was determined as the gradient of the signal rise within a 50-ms period following the onset [5,20]. The agonist-antagonist CCI within the duration from two muscles' later EMG onset to two muscles' earlier EMG offset was calculated based on the formula in Figure 2 [16,36,37]. When the onset of a signal was absent within 2 s after a perturbation, the onset latency, time to peak, and burst duration were filled with 2000 ms, 2000 ms, and 0 ms, respectively; while the peak amplitude, rate of rise, and agonis-antagonist CCI were all filled with 0. For each parameter, the mean value of the three perturbations with the same direction and intensity was used in further statistical analyses.

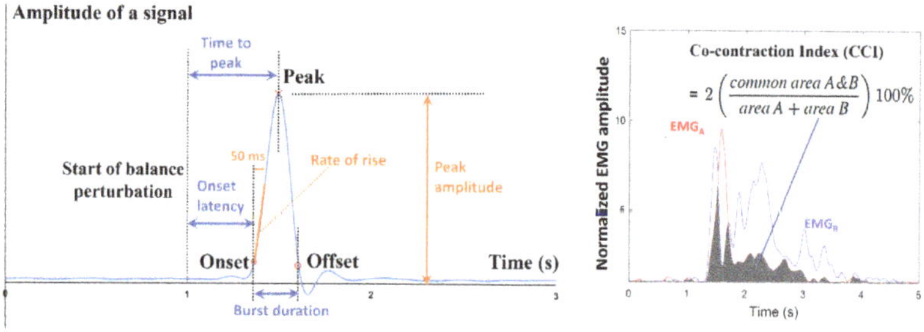

Figure 2. Illustrations of the analyzed temporal and amplitude parameters. **EMG**: electromyographic.

2.5. Statistical Analyses

The statistical analyses were performed using SPSS (version 25.0), with the significance level set as 0.05. To examine differences in baseline subjective assessment data between fallers and non-fallers, independent sample t tests or Mann-Whitney U tests were used based on the data normality for continuous variables, and Chi-square tests were used for categorical variables. For each parameter (i.e., onset latency, time to peak, peak amplitude, burst duration, peak amplitude, rate of rise, and/or agonist-antagonist CCI), a four-way analysis of variance (ANOVA) and post hoc pairwise comparisons with Bonferroni corrections were conducted to examine the effects of two fall statuses, four perturbation directions, four perturbation intensities, and six postural sway directions/eight dominant-leg joint motions/eight dominant-leg muscles/four dominant-leg muscle pairs. With samples of equal size, the ANOVAs were considered robust, even when the assumptions of normality and homogeneity were not fully met [38]. Given the objectives, this study focused on the interaction effects of fall history with other factor(s), the main effects of fall history when there were no significant interactions, and the simple effects of fall history when there were significant interactions. Results regarding the simple effects of the factor(s) that had interactions with fall history are presented in Tables A3–A5 of Appendix A.

3. Results

3.1. Subjective Assessment Results

No adverse incidents happened during any of the experiments. In the faller group, two participants experienced recurrent falls and four had a single fall in the past year before the perturbation trials. There was no significant difference in the number of medications, age, body mass, height, foot length, BMI, short FES-I score or the PASE-C score between the participating older fallers and older non-fallers (Table 1). Nevertheless, the Mini-BEST score of fallers was significantly lower than that of non-fallers ($p < 0.05$).

Table 1. Subjective assessment results (categorical variable: ratio; continuous variable: mean ± SD) of twelve participants.

	Faller ($n = 6$, 3 Males and 3 Females)	Non-Faller ($n = 6$, 3 Males and 3 Females)	Significance (p Value)
Number of falls	1.3 ± 0.5	0	/
Number of medications	1.0 ± 1.1	0.3 ± 0.5	0.279
Age (year)	71.5 ± 4.6	69.2 ± 2.9	0.316
Body mass (kg)	55.6 ± 8.4	61.4 ± 13.0	0.381
Height (cm)	157.9 ± 8.7	162.0 ± 7.9	0.406
BMI (kg/m^2)	22.2 ± 2.0	23.3 ± 4.4	0.587
Leg length (cm)	77.3 ± 6.3	80.8 ± 4.6	0.297
Dominant leg (right/left)	5/1	6/0	0.296
Short FES-I (score)	12.2 ± 2.4	11.5 ± 6.0	0.332
PASE-C (score)	139.5 ± 73.2	148.1 ± 34.6	0.802
Mini-BEST (score)	23.3 ± 1.5	26.0 ± 0.9	**0.004**

BMI: body mass index. **FES-I**: Falls Efficacy Scale-International. **PASE-C**: Physical Activity Scale of Elderly-Chinese. **Mini-BEST**: Mini-Balance Evaluation System Test.

3.2. Balance Control Strategies

Fallers were more likely to have stepping responses than non-fallers. The unpredictable translational perturbations mainly induced feet-in-place strategies (567/576, 98.4%), and three participants (3/12, 25.0%) showed stepping responses following nine perturbations (9/576, 1.6%). Specifically, following three highest-intensity medial perturbations, one non-faller exhibited responses of the non-dominant leg, including stepping toward the perturbation direction, performing leg abduction, and elevating the leg (3/576, 0.5%). One faller took a backward step using the non-dominant leg together with several small steps, following a highest-intensity anterior perturbation (1/576, 0.2%). The other faller stepped backward using the non-dominant leg, following the highest-intensity (2/576, 0.3%) and high-intensity (1/576, 0.2%) anterior perturbations. Additionally, this individual stepped toward the perturbation direction using both legs in response to a low-intensity posterior perturbation (1/576, 0.2%), and with the non-dominant leg in response to a highest-intensity medial perturbation (1/576, 0.2%).

3.3. COM Displacements

The mean changes in COM displacements over time ($n = 12$, Figure 3) together with the onset latency, time to peak, peak amplitude, and burst duration of COM displacement (mean ± SD; Figure 4) are displayed for each postural sway direction, each perturbation intensity, and each perturbation direction in participating older fallers and older non-fallers.

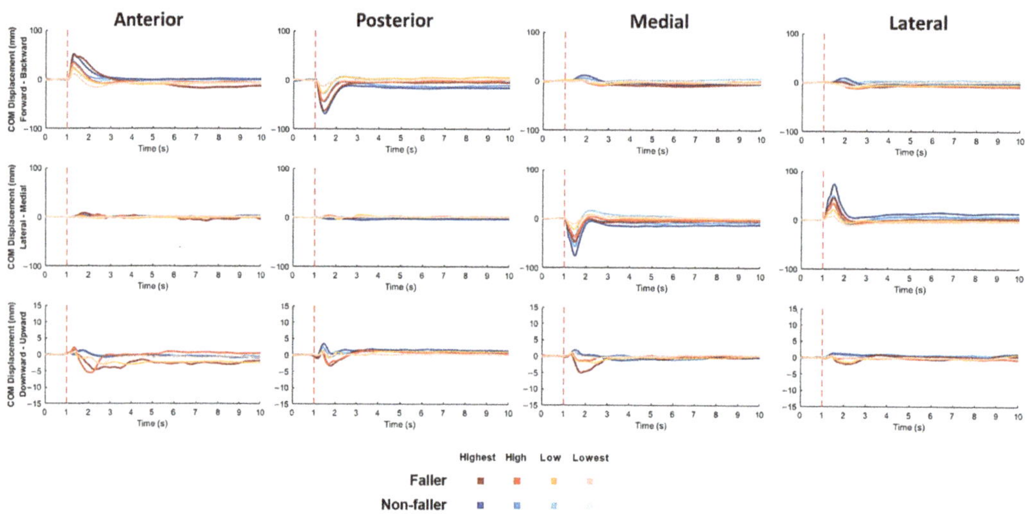

Figure 3. Mean forward/backward, medial/lateral, and upward/downward COM displacements in fallers ($n = 6$) and non-fallers ($n = 6$) following perturbations with different directions and intensities. The red dotted line denotes the start of balance perturbation. **COM**: center of mass.

Regarding the onset latency of COM displacement, there was a significant interaction between "fall history" and "postural sway direction" factors ($p < 0.05$). Significant simple effects of fall history showed that fallers had a longer onset latency in the backward direction, but had shorter onset latencies in the forward and downward directions compared to non-fallers ($p < 0.05$, Figure 4).

Regarding the time to peak COM displacement, a significant interaction was also found between "fall history" and "postural sway direction" factors ($p < 0.05$). Significant simple effects of fall history showed that fallers had a longer time to peak COM displacement in the backward direction, but had a shorter time to peak in the downward direction compared to non-fallers ($p < 0.05$; Figure 4).

Regarding the peak COM displacement, a significant interaction of fall history with other factors was observed (fall history × direction × postural sway direction, $p < 0.05$). Significant simple effects of fall history showed that fallers had larger peak COM displacements in the forward and downward directions following anterior perturbations, in the backward direction following posterior perturbations, and in the forward direction following both medial and lateral perturbations ($p < 0.05$; Figure 4).

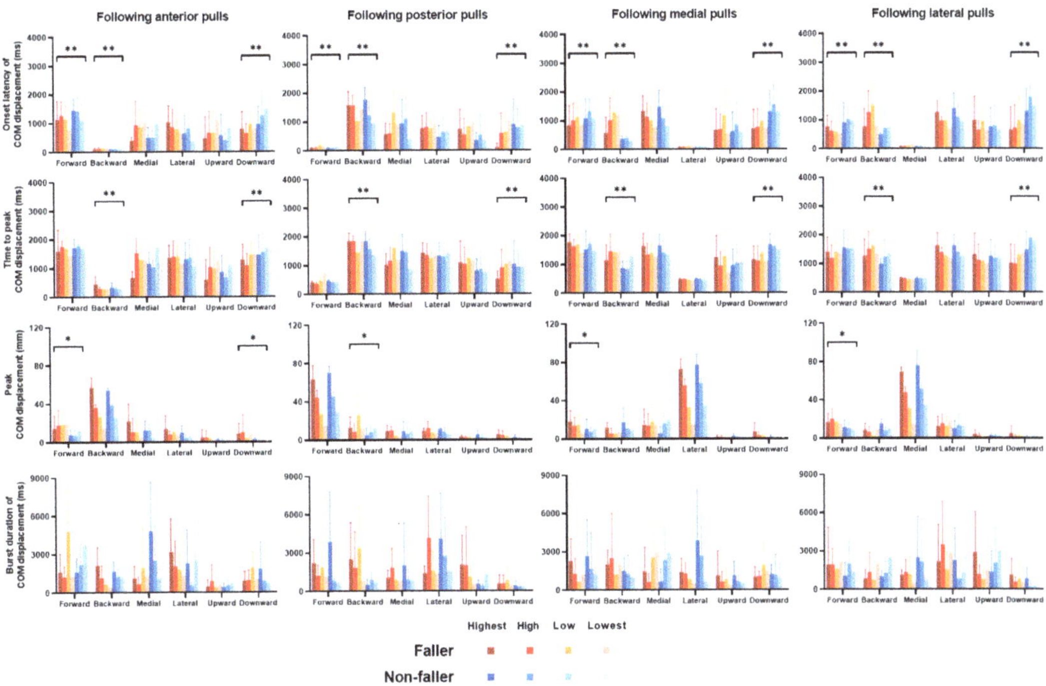

Figure 4. Onset latencies, time to peak, peak amplitudes, and burst durations of COM displacements in six postural sway directions (n = 6, mean ± SD). Significant effects of fall history are indicated by the ┌┐ ($p < 0.05$). ** denotes the significant effect of fall history at a certain postural sway direction ("fall history × postural sway direction" interaction). * denotes the significant effect of fall history at a certain postural sway direction and following a certain direction of perturbation ("fall history × postural sway direction × direction" interaction). **COM**: center of mass. **SD**: standard deviation.

Regarding the burst duration of COM displacement, there was no significant interaction of fall history with any other factor. No significant main effect of fall history was observed on this parameter either (Figure 4).

3.4. Dominant-Leg Joint Motions

The mean changes of dominant-leg joint motions over time (Figure 5) together with the angle onset latency, time to peak angle, peak angle, and angle burst duration (mean ± SD; Figure 6) are displayed for each joint motion, each perturbation intensity, and each perturbation direction in fallers and non-fallers.

Regarding the angle onset latency, a significant interaction of fall history with other factors was observed (fall history × direction × joint motion, $p < 0.05$). Significant simple effects of fall history showed that compared to non-fallers, fallers had longer onset latencies of hip adduction, hip extension, and knee extension following anterior perturbations, and a longer onset latency of ankle plantarflexion following medial perturbations ($p < 0.05$; Figure 6).

Regarding the time to peak angle, a significant interaction of fall history with other factors was also observed (fall history × direction × joint motion, $p < 0.05$). Significant simple effects of fall history showed that fallers had longer time to peak hip adduction, hip flexion, hip extension, and knee extension following anterior perturbations, longer time to peak ankle plantarflexion following medial perturbations, but shorter time to peak ankle plantarflexion following lateral perturbations as compared to non-fallers ($p < 0.05$; Figure 6).

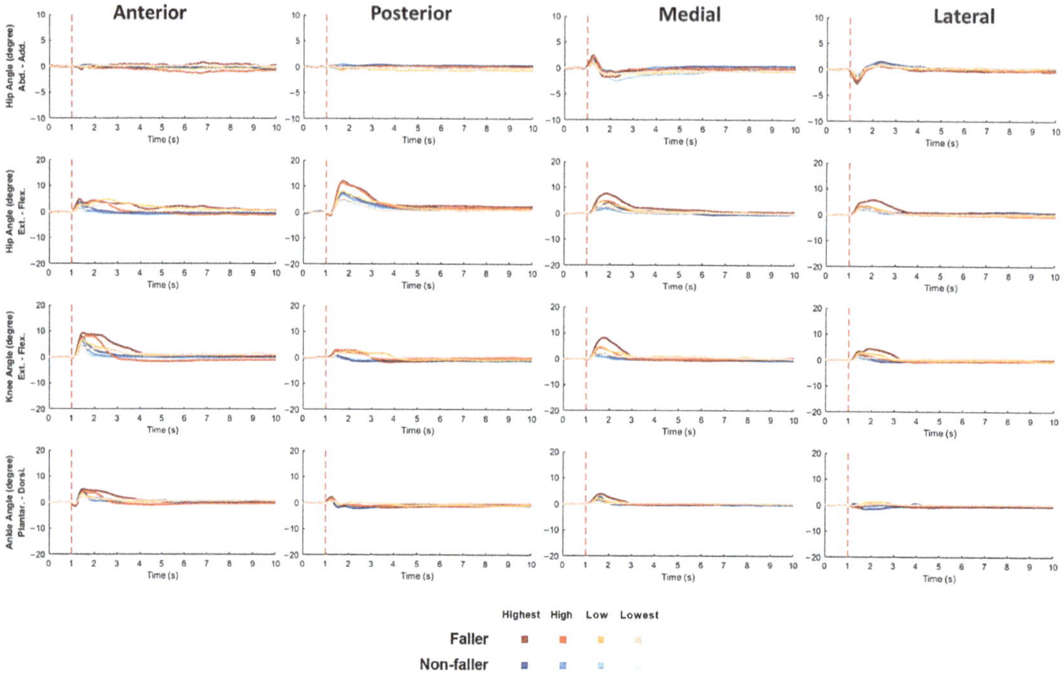

Figure 5. Mean change for each of the eight dominant-leg joint motions in fallers (n = 6) and non-fallers (n = 6) following perturbations with different directions and intensities. The red dotted line denotes the start of balance perturbation. **Add**: adduction. **Abd**: abduction. **Flex**: flexion. **Ext**: extension. **Dorsi**: dorsiflexion. **Plantar**: plantarflexion.

Regarding the peak angle, there was a significant interaction between "fall history" and "joint motion" factors ($p < 0.05$). Significant simple effects of fall history showed that fallers had larger peak hip flexion and knee flexion than non-fallers following unpredictable perturbations ($p < 0.05$; Figure 6).

Regarding the angle burst duration, a significant interaction was also observed between "fall history" and "joint motion" factors ($p < 0.05$). The significant simple effect of fall history showed that fallers had a longer burst duration of ankle dorsiflexion than non-fallers following unpredictable perturbations ($p < 0.05$; Figure 6).

3.5. EMG Signals of Dominant-Leg Muscles

The mean changes of EMG signals over time (Figure 7) together with the EMG onset latency, rate of EMG rise, time to peak EMG amplitude, EMG burst duration, and agonist-antagonist CCI (mean ± SD; Figure 8) are presented for each dominant-leg muscle (pair), each perturbation intensity, and each perturbation direction in fallers and non-fallers.

Regarding the EMG onset latency, there was a significant interaction between "fall history" and "muscle" factors ($p < 0.05$). Significant simple effects of fall history showed that the fallers' EMG onset latencies were longer for the hip flexor and hip extensor compared to non-fallers following unpredictable perturbations ($p < 0.05$; Figure 8).

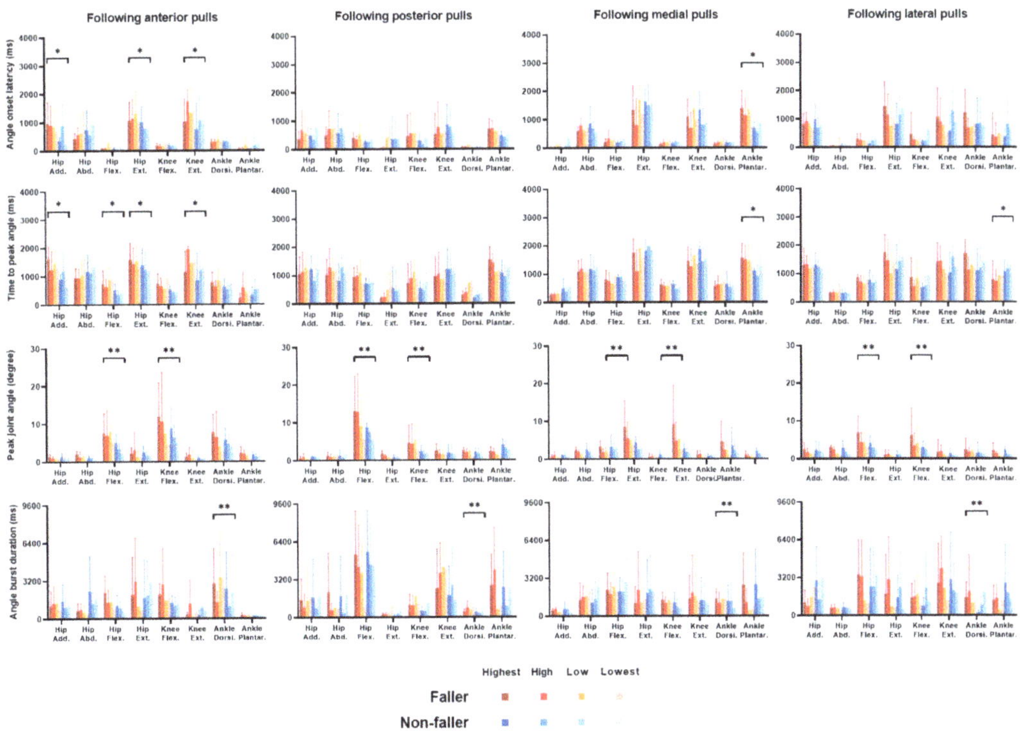

Figure 6. Onset latencies, time to peak, peak amplitudes, and burst durations of hip, knee, and ankle joint motions ($n = 6$, mean $\pm$ SD). Significant effects of fall history are indicated by the ⌐¬ ($p < 0.05$). * denotes the significant effect of fall history at a certain joint motion and following a certain direction of perturbation ("fall history × joint motion × direction" interaction). ** denotes the significant effect of fall history at a certain joint motion ("fall history × joint motion" interaction). **Add**: adduction. **Abd**: abduction. **Flex**: flexion. **Ext**: extension. **Dorsi**: dorsiflexion. **Plantar**: plantarflexion. **SD**: standard deviation.

Regarding the rate of EMG rise, there was also a significant interaction between "fall history" and "muscle" factors ($p < 0.05$). Significant simple effects of fall history showed that the fallers' rate of EMG rise was smaller for the ankle dorsiflexor, but was larger for the knee flexor as compared to non-fallers following unpredictable perturbations ($p < 0.05$; Figure 8).

Regarding the time to peak EMG amplitude, there was no significant interaction of fall history with any other factor. The significant main effect of fall history showed that fallers had longer time to peak EMG amplitudes of lower-limb muscles as compared to non-fallers following unpredictable perturbations ($p < 0.05$; Figure 8).

Regarding the EMG burst duration, a significant interaction between "fall history" and "muscle" factors was observed ($p < 0.05$). Significant simple effects of fall history showed that fallers had longer EMG burst durations of the hip abductor and ankle dorsiflexor, but had a shorter one of the hip flexor than non-fallers following unpredictable perturbations ($p < 0.05$; Figure 8). In addition, there was a significant interaction between "fall history" and "direction" factors ($p < 0.05$). Significant simple effects of fall history showed that fallers had longer EMG burst durations following the anterior and posterior perturbations, but had a shorter one following the medial perturbations compared to non-fallers ($p < 0.05$; Figure 8).

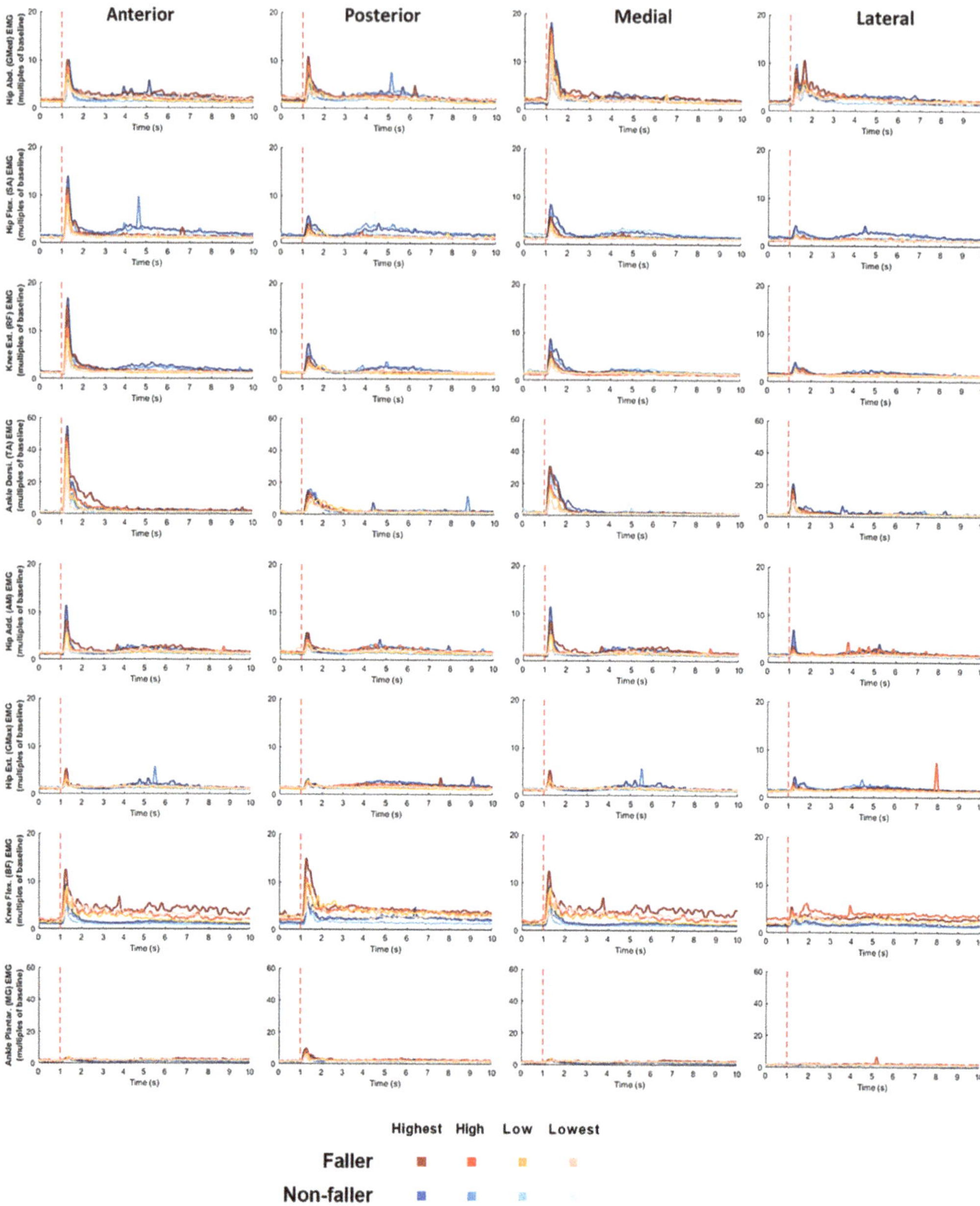

Figure 7. Mean EMG signal change for each of the eight dominant-leg muscles in fallers (n = 6) and non-fallers (n = 6) following perturbations with different directions and intensities. The red dotted line denotes the start of balance perturbation. **EMG**: electromyographic. **GMed**: gluteus medius. **SA**: sartorius. **RF**: rectus femoris. **TA**: tibialis anterior. **AM**: adductor magnus. **GMax**: gluteus maximus. **BF**: biceps femoris. **GM**: gastrocnemius medialis. **Add**: adductor. **Abd**: abductor. **Flex**: flexor. **Ext**: extensor. **Dorsi**: dorsiflexor. **Plantar**: plantarflexor.

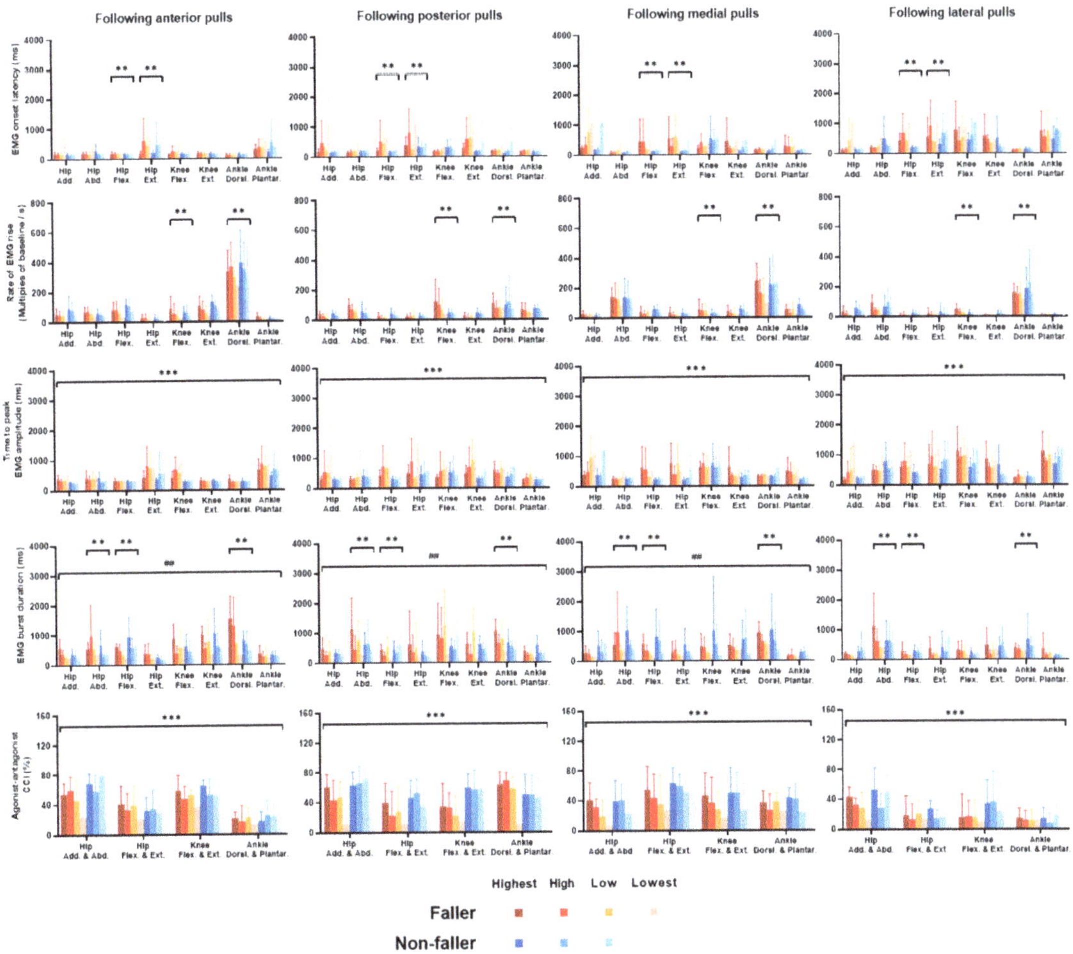

Figure 8. Onset latencies, rate of rise, time to peak, burst durations, and agonist-antagonist CCIs of EMG signals for eight dominant-leg muscles (n = 6, mean ± SD). Significant effects of fall history are indicated by the ⎴ ($p < 0.05$). *** denotes the significant main effect of fall history (no interaction of "fall history" and any other factor). ** denotes the significant effect of fall history at a certain muscle ("fall history × muscle" interaction). ## denotes the significant effect of fall history following a certain direction of perturbation ("fall history × direction" interaction). **EMG**: electromyographic. **CCI**: co-contraction index. **SD**: standard deviation. **Add**: adductor. **Abd**: abductor. **Flex**: flexor. **Ext**: extensor. **Dorsi**: dorsiflexor. **Plantar**: plantarflexor.

Regarding the time to peak EMG amplitude, no significant interaction was observed between fall history and any other factor. The significant main effect of fall history showed that fallers had smaller agonist-antagonist CCIs in the investigated muscle pairs than non-fallers following unpredictable perturbations ($p < 0.05$; Figure 8).

4. Discussion

This study comprehensively examined the effects of fall history on reactive standing balance in community-dwelling older adults, by focusing on dominant-leg muscle activities and joint motions. Partially in line with our hypotheses, the effects of "fall history" on the investigated outcomes during reactive balance control interacted with the "muscle/joint motion/postural sway direction" and "perturbation direction" but not with the "perturbation intensity". Specifically, compared to older non-fallers, older fallers demonstrated slowed activation of ankle/hip muscles while tending to use a suspensory strategy for reactive balance control, as supported by a series of neuromuscular alterations and joint kinematics. These new insights reflect possible reasons for fallers' decreased balance capability and indicate their utilization of prolonged and enlarged (and even overreacted) compensatory strategies for preserving postural stability [19]. Developing some future assessment tools based on the identified parameters may be helpful to screen and identify the fallers from non-fallers in the community-dwelling adults. Furthermore, interventions targeting these identified fall-related alterations may lead to more effective solutions for improving reactive balance control and preventing recurrent falls in older fallers. Details are discussed below.

4.1. Fallers Tended to Use Suspensory Strategies Following Unpredictable Perturbations: Neuromuscular and Kinematic Mechanisms

The primary finding of this study was that fallers have tended to use the suspensory strategy to maintain standing balance following unpredictable translational perturbations as compared to non-fallers. This strategy enabled fallers to promptly compensate for their insufficient initiation of ankle and hip strategies, but it led to their prolonged and overacted balance recovery. This finding provides insights into the specific decline in reactive balance control and compensation strategies among the older adults with fall histories and poor overall balance performance (i.e., low Mini-BEST scores).

Fallers exhibited decreased activation in the ankle dorsiflexor and hip flexor/extensor as compared to non-fallers. This could be attributed to the potential degradation in any components along the sensorimotor pathway, including sensory input (feedback from external perturbation), central organization, and motor output [6]. Ankle dorsiflexor's activation immediately following the start of perturbation has been in the first line to resist the sudden loss of balance [5]. With ageing, humans may shift from a distal-to-proximal strategy to a proximal-to-distal strategy to maintain balance, compensating for the difficulties of generating sufficient ankle torque [39]. This study further proved that this phenomenon was more pronounced in older fallers than older non-fallers. On the other hand, fallers showed delayed EMG onset timing of the hip flexor/extensor and reduced EMG burst duration of the hip flexor as compared to non-fallers. These alterations could partly restrict the initiation of the hip strategy, which is the second line of defense against sudden loss of balance. The delayed activation of hip muscles may be explained by previous morphological observations, where fallers were found to have reduced density of skeletal muscle fibers and increased intramuscular adipose issues in the gluteus muscles as compared to non-fallers [40]. A prior study also reported delayed neuromuscular activation in reactive standing balance, with fallers exhibiting later EMG onset timing of the hip abductor and knee flexor in the loading leg than non-fallers following unpredictable lateral perturbations exerted on the shoulder [18]. The discrepancy in the affected muscles could be attributed to the different perturbation methods.

A series of kinematic and neuromuscular alterations in fallers when facing unpredictable translational balance perturbations have indicated their prominent use of suspensory strategies as compared to non-fallers. In the absence of sufficient ankle and hip muscle activation, fallers utilized the suspensory strategy, i.e., the third strategy to resist sudden loss of balance, by lowering the COM to increase the limit of stability and absorb the external perturbation [41–43]. This is evident from their earlier onset and peak timing of downward COM displacement compared to non-fallers. The increased activation rate of the knee flexor, generally decreased agonist-antagonist co-contraction of the lower-limb muscles, and larger knee/hip flexion in fallers may have facilitated this strategy. Interestingly, our findings differ from a prior study that reported no differences in postural sway timing or amplitude between fallers and non-fallers following lateral shoulder-impact perturbations [18], suggesting that different body segment perturbations may elicit distinct reactive balance control strategies. Additionally, while previous research linked greater co-contraction to more joint stability and poorer balance control [44,45], this study observed that older fallers were able to reduce agonist-antagonist co-contractions of lower-limb muscles and achieve larger knee/hip flexion for a suspensory strategy. On top of them, this study has observed that fallers showed longer activation durations of the ankle dorsiflexor and hip abductor, together with a longer ankle dorsiflexion duration than non-fallers, which may be necessary for maintaining a knee bending posture during the suspensory strategy.

Fallers' balance control strategies in the current study, however, have required a prolonged recovery time and caused overreactions. This is evidenced by their neuromuscular and kinematic alterations, as described below. Firstly, fallers' delayed time to peak activation may suggest reduced motor unit recruitment and firing rate in response to external perturbations [23]. Secondly, fallers showed longer time to peak hip flexion angle following anterior perturbations, longer burst durations of ankle dorsiflexion following all perturbations, and delayed timing of recovery joint motions following anterior/medial perturbations than non-fallers. Thirdly, fallers showed larger overshooting postural sways when recovering to initial positions following unpredictable anteroposterior perturbations. This is indicated by their larger forward peak COM displacements following sudden backward balance loss (induced by anterior perturbations) and larger backward ones following sudden forward balance loss (induced by posterior perturbations) as compared to non-fallers. These findings indicate that sudden perturbations could pose greater challenges to older fallers. Fallers' more prominent overshoots of backward postural sways, as compared to non-fallers, have also been previously reported following anterior waist-pull perturbations [46]. Additionally, a prior study found that fallers had more variable and delayed recovery steps than non-fallers in perturbed walking [11], which could be corroborated by this study's observation of fallers' larger overshooting postural sways and delayed timing of overshooting lower-limb joint motions. The slowed but exaggerated postural adjustments seem to reveal the ineffective strategies used by the older adults with fall histories for reactive balance control, aligning with their poorer overall balance performance, as shown by the lower Mini-BEST scores.

This study also observed large within-group variations in some of the analyzed parameters during reactive balance control. For example, although the faller group was identified to exhibit longer EMG onset latencies in hip muscles than the non-faller group, the within-group variations were large, as indicated by the standard deviations. This reflects the fact that even individuals with the same fall status may respond differently during reactive balance control. On the one hand, a previous study reported that fallers had a higher variation in walking stability than non-fallers after unpredictable perturbations [11]. Given its potential in differentiating fall status, the variability of reactive balance performance should not be neglected. On the other hand, analysis of individual variations in reactive balance control within the faller group (e.g., coefficient of variation) could be also crucial for understanding personalized balance intervention requirements, which merits further investigation.

4.2. *Fallers Had Altered Responses to Different Perturbation Directions*

The secondary finding of this study was that fall history showed interaction effects with perturbation direction, but not with perturbation intensity, on the older adults' neuromuscular and kinematic responses during reactive balance control.

Fallers have shown distinct responses to anteroposterior and mediolateral perturbations as compared to non-fallers. Regarding kinematics, a previous study reported fallers' larger COM path displacement as compared to non-fallers following the mediolateral translational perturbations [9]. This study has further revealed that fallers' larger postural sways were specifically in the forward direction following the mediolateral perturbations. These responses could be partly attributed to fallers' delayed timing of recovery joint motions compared to non-fallers following the medial perturbation. Regarding the neuromuscular responses, fallers have exhibited longer EMG burst durations in dominant-leg muscles following anteroposterior perturbations as compared to non-fallers. This could also explain fallers' overshooting postural sways. Additionally, this could explain why fallers had more non-dominant leg stepping following anteroposterior perturbations than non-fallers, as more body weight was loaded on the dominant leg. Conversely, fallers have exhibited shorter EMG burst durations of dominant-leg muscles than non-fallers following medial perturbations, resulting in fallers' fewer non-dominant leg steps following medial perturbations compared to non-fallers.

Notably, this study has found no differences in the responses of fallers compared to non-fallers to varied intensities of unpredictable perturbations. Previous studies reported inconsistent results regarding the interaction effect of fall history and perturbation intensity on the stepping characteristics following waist-pull perturbations [10,21]. The finding of this study has further built on the evidence of unpredictable translational perturbations and suggested that fallers' neuromuscular/kinematic responses to the different intensities of perturbations, which primarily induced feet-in-place strategies, were similar to those of non-fallers.

4.3. Strengths and Limitations

To the best of authors' knowledge, this study offers a preliminary but more in-depth exploration of the differences in eight major lower-limb muscles' activation or lower-limb joint kinematics during reactive balance control between older fallers and older non-fallers. With the comprehensive analyses of temporal and amplitude characteristics of these investigated signals, this study has built knowledge upon the prior investigations that focused on a limited number of muscles and EMG parameters, and has addressed the gap of limited research on joint kinematics in fallers vs. non-fallers. The mechanisms of fall-prone older adults' decline of reactive balance control and compensatory strategies could be better understood with the findings of this study.

This study has several limitations that shall be acknowledged, and the findings shall be interpreted with caution. (1) Given the small sample sizes of recruited older fallers and older non-fallers, it should be noted that the findings of this pilot study using four-way ANOVAs can provide only preliminary insights. Results of alternative analyses for the "fall history" factor, using independent sample t-tests for normally distributed data and Mann-Whitney U tests for non-normally distributed data, are presented in Supplementary Table S1. In addition, this study did not specifically analyze the recurrent fallers' neuromuscular/kinematic strategies in reactive balance control, which demands further studies with larger sample sizes. (2) This study did not ensure that the faller and non-faller groups had matched ranges of motion in the investigated joints or muscle strength, which may confound the identified between-group differences in reactive balance performance. Additionally, this study only focused on reactive balance control in fall-prone people. It is important to note that the causes of loss of balance or falls are not confined to this and are multi-factorial (e.g., environmental factors). (3) Although diagnosis of cognitive impairment was an exclusion criterion for this study and the testers ensured participants understood task instructions, a clinical scale such as the Montreal Cognitive Assessment (MoCA) should be used to better quantify the older participants' cognitive function in future research. (4) The cut-off frequency used for EMG low-pass filtering in this study may not be optimal for all of the investigated eight leg muscles. Further attempts are warranted to determine the cut-off frequency for processing each respective muscle's EMG signal based on the frequency spectrum analysis. Additionally, this study did not conduct maximal voluntary contraction tests but used the baseline EMG signal value in unperturbed standing for EMG amplitude normalization. It is therefore important to note that the rate of EMG rise and agonist-antagonist CCI in this study reflected the extent to which the perturbation task utilized the activation required for normal standing rather than the maximal activation. (5) This study did not explore gender-specific variations in balance control by having equal representation of male and female participants in a group. Future studies could consider specifically examining the gender-specific difference in older people with a larger sample size to address this issue.

4.4. Implications for Clinical Practice and Future Resesarch

This study has preliminary implications for assessing and training reactive balance control in future applications. On the one hand, the identified fall-related kinematic and neuromuscular factors may inform clinical practice. Reactive balance training may need to be prescribed more for the community-dwelling older adults with fall histories in the future, considering their generally delayed peak activation of lower-limb muscles. A recent review has reported that perturbation-based balance training and stepping training can improve the slowed reaction time in response to sudden loss of balance [47]. This is a promising future avenue, as fallers' degradation in neuromuscular timing can be modified. Our findings further imply that more focus/efforts may need to be put into the ankle and hip muscle power (or reaction speed) training in older fallers to improve their reactive balance control performance. Although the proximal hip and knee muscles were previously reported to be more affected by aging following unpredictable perturbations [48], the findings of this study may suggest that the training of ankle muscles should not be ignored, especially in older fallers.

On the other hand, with the advancement of wearable sensors and real-time monitoring systems, future studies could also consider employing these tools to improve balance assessment and training in fall-prone individuals. Real-time monitoring and analysis of the reaction speed (e.g., EMG onset latency, rate of EMG rise) of an older client's ankle dorsiflexor or hip flexor/extensor for reactive balance control may potentially enhance the fall-risk assessment on top of the current reactive balance test. The EMG-based biofeedback may potentially enhance power training for ankle or hip muscles, while the quantitative results on muscle reaction speed may help therapists offer more personalized feedback and guidance during reactive balance training.

Nonetheless, we acknowledge that these implications need validation in future longitudinal studies with larger sample sizes, where the diagnostic accuracy of slower activation in ankle and hip muscles in differentiating older adults' fall risks, as identified in this pilot study, should be examined.

5. Conclusions

This pilot study found that older fallers' kinematic and neuromuscular alterations in resisting unpredictable translational perturbations could be indicators of both the decline and the compensation of reactive balance control. Compared to non-fallers, fallers had a decreased activation rate in the ankle dorsiflexor and delayed activation in the hip flexor/extensor, thereby resorting to the suspensory strategy for quickly responding to external perturbations. The increased activation rate of knee flexor, decreased agonist-antagonist co-contraction of lower-limb muscles, enlarged knee and hip flexion, and earlier downward postural sways in fallers could be the basis of their prioritizing of suspensory strategies as compared to non-fallers. However, fallers' balance control strategies required prolonged recovery in lower-limb joint motions and caused overreactions in postural sways. A further longitudinal study with a larger sample is merited to verify these fall-related factors, which could enhance the identification of fall-prone people and provide insights for more targeted fall-prevention strategies.

Supplementary Materials: The following supporting information can be downloaded at: https://www.mdpi.com/article/10.3390/bioengineering12010066/s1, Table S1: Temporal and amplitude parameters of EMG, joint motion, and COM displacement signals in older fallers and older non-fallers.

Author Contributions: R.T.-L.Z.: Conceptualization, Methodology, Software, Validation, Formal analysis, Investigation, Data Curation, Writing—Original Draft, Visualization; T.T.M.H.: Formal analysis, Investigation, Writing—Original Draft; F.M.H.L.: Writing—Review and Editing; J.-Z.L.: Investigation; Y.-Y.L.: Investigation; J.S.: Writing—Review and Editing; S.W.: Writing—Review and Editing; C.Z.-H.M.: Conceptualization, Methodology, Resources, Writing—Review and Editing, Supervision, Project administration, Funding acquisition. All authors have read and agreed to the published version of the manuscript.

Funding: This work was supported by the Research Institute for Smart Ageing, The Hong Kong Polytechnic University [P0038945]; The Hong Kong Polytechnic University [P0034491]; and Associated Money, The Hong Kong Polytechnic University [G4Y56R006 to R.T.L.Z].

Institutional Review Board Statement: The study was conducted in accordance with the Declaration of Helsinki, and approved by the Ethics approval agency: Institutional Review Board, The Hong Kong Polytechnic University (Ethical reference number: HSEARS20201230002; Date of approval: 1 December 2020).

Informed Consent Statement: Informed consent was obtained from all subjects involved in the study.

Data Availability Statement: Data are contained within the article and Appendix A.

Conflicts of Interest: J.S. is employed by the Future Architecture and Urban Research Institute, Tongji Architectural Design (Group) Co., Ltd. The other authors declare no conflicts of interest.

List of Abbreviations

Abbreviation	Full Name
AM	Adductor Magnus
ANOVA	Analysis of Variance
BF	Long Head of Bicep Femoris
CCI	Co-Contraction Index
COM	Center of Mass
EMG	Electromyographic
FES-I	Falls Efficacy Scale-International
MG	Medial Gastrocnemius
GMax	Gluteus Maximus
GMed	Gluteus Medius
Mini-BEST	Mini-Balance Evaluation System Test
PASE-C	Chinese Version of The Physical Activity Scale for the Elderly
RF	Rectus Femoris
SA	Sartorius
SD	Standard Deviation
SENIAM	Surface Electromyography for the Non-Invasive Assessment of Muscles
TA	Tibialis Anterior

Appendix A

Table A1. Eight investigated dominant leg muscles and placement locations for EMG sensors.

Muscle	Location of EMG and MMG Sensor Placement
Hip adductor: Adductor magnus (AM)	Halfway between the pubic tubercle and the medial femoral epicondyle
Hip abductor: Gluteus medius (GMed)	Halfway between the iliac crest to the greater trochanter
Hip flexor: Sartorius (SA)	At 8 cm distal from the ASIS towards the medial epicondyle of the femur
Hip extensor: Gluteus maximus (GMax)	Halfway between the sacral vertebrae and the greater trochanter
Knee flexor: Long head of bicep femoris (BF)	Halfway between the ischial tuberosity and the lateral epicondyle of tibia
Knee extensor: Rectus femoris (RF)	Halfway between the anterior superior iliac spine (ASIS) and the superior border of the patella
Ankle dorsiflexor: Tibialis anterior (TA)	At 1/3 on the line between the tip of fibula and the tip of medial malleolus
Ankle plantarflexor: Gastrocnemius medialis (GM)	On the most prominent bulge of the muscle

Table A2. Platform movement profiles of different perturbations ($n = 12$).

Perturbation Direction	Perturbation Intensity	Mean of Maximum Displacements (mm)	Mean of Maximum Velocities (m/s)	Mean of Maximum Accelerations (m/s^2)
Anterior	Highest	59	0.40	4.3
	High	43	0.31	3.4
	Low	29	0.21	2.3
	Lowest	13	0.10	1.1
Posterior	Highest	79	0.33	3.7
	High	56	0.26	2.8
	Low	37	0.18	1.9
	Lowest	18	0.09	1.0
Medial	Highest	110	0.37	4.7
	High	82	0.29	3.7
	Low	54	0.20	2.5
	Lowest	28	0.11	1.4
Lateral	Highest	113	0.35	4.3
	High	86	0.26	3.2
	Low	55	0.19	2.3
	Lowest	25	0.09	1.1

Table A3. Significant results for the analyzed COM displacement parameters.

Parameter	Onset Latency of COM Displacement	Time to Peak COM Displacement	Peak COM Displacement
Significant interaction effect of "fall history" and other factor(s) in four-way ANOVAs	fall history × postural sway direction	fall history × postural sway direction	fall history × direction × postural sway direction
All significant results of post hoc pairwise comparisons within the postural sway direction & perturbation direction factor	**fallers**: lateral < backward	**fallers**: upward < forward	**fallers**: **A**: upward & downward & lateral & medial & forward < backward; upward & downward & lateral < forward; upward < medial **P**: upward & downward & medial & lateral < backward < forward; upward < lateral **M**: upward & downward & backward < forward & medial < lateral **L**: upward & downward & backward < lateral & forward < medial
	non-fallers: backward & lateral & upward < forward < downward; medial < downward	**non-fallers**: backward & upward & lateral & medial < downward; backward & upward < forward	**non-fallers**: **A**: downward & upward & lateral & medial & forward < backward; downward & upward < medial & forward **P**: downward & upward & medial & lateral & backward < forward; downward & upward < backward; downward < lateral **M**: downward & upward < forward & backward & medial < lateral **L**: downward & upward < backward & forward & lateral < medial

A: anterior perturbations. **P**: posterior perturbations. **M**: medial perturbations. **L**: lateral perturbations. **COM**: center-of-mass.

Table A4. Significant results for the analyzed angle parameters.

Parameter	Angle Onset Latency	Time to Peak Angle	Peak Angle	Angle Burst Duration
Significant interaction effect of "fall history" and other factor(s) in four-way ANOVAs	fall history × direction × joint motion	fall history × direction × joint motion	fall history × joint motion	fall history × joint motion
All significant results of post hoc pairwise comparisons within the joint motion & perturbation direction factor	**fallers**: **A**: ankle plantarflexion & hip flexion & knee flexion & ankle dorsiflexion & hip abduction & hip adduction < knee extension; ankle plantarflexion & hip flexion & knee flexion & ankle dorsiflexion < hip adduction & hip extension; ankle plantarflexion & hip flexion & knee flexion < hip abduction **P**: ankle dorsiflexion < knee extension & hip adduction & hip abduction & ankle plantarflexion **M**: hip adduction & ankle dorsiflexion & knee flexion & hip flexion & hip abduction < hip extension & ankle plantarflexion; hip adduction & ankle dorsiflexion & knee flexion & hip flexion < knee extension; hip adduction & ankle dorsiflexion < hip abduction **L**: hip abduction & hip flexion & knee flexion < knee extension & hip adduction & ankle dorsiflexion & hip extension; ankle plantarflexion < hip extension	**fallers**: **A**: ankle plantarflexion & knee flexion < hip abduction & hip adduction & hip extension & knee extension; ankle dorsiflexion & hip flexion < hip adduction & hip extension & knee extension **P**: hip extension & ankle dorsiflexion < knee extension & hip abduction & hip adduction & ankle plantarflexion **M**: hip adduction < hip flexion & hip abduction & knee extension & ankle plantarflexion & hip extension; knee flexion & ankle dorsiflexion < hip abduction & knee extension & ankle plantarflexion & hip extension; hip flexion < knee extension & ankle plantarflexion & hip extension; hip abduction < hip extension **L**: hip abduction & knee flexion & hip flexion < knee extension & hip adduction & ankle dorsiflexion & hip extension; ankle plantarflexion < hip adduction & ankle dorsiflexion & hip extension	**fallers**: hip extension & knee extension & hip adduction & ankle plantarflexion & hip abduction < ankle dorsiflexion < knee flexion < hip flexion	**fallers**: hip abduction & hip adduction & ankle plantarflexion & hip extension < hip flexion; hip abduction & hip adduction & ankle plantarflexion < knee extension

Table A4. *Cont.*

Parameter	Angle Onset Latency	Time to Peak Angle	Peak Angle	Angle Burst Duration
All significant results of post hoc pairwise comparisons within the joint motion & perturbation direction factor	**non-fallers**: **A**: hip flexion & ankle plantarflexion & knee flexion & ankle dorsiflexion & hip adduction < knee extension; hip flexion & ankle plantarflexion & knee flexion & ankle dorsiflexion < hip abduction; hip flexion & ankle plantarflexion & knee flexion < hip extension **P**: ankle dorsiflexion < hip adduction & hip extension & hip abduction & knee extension **M**: ankle dorsiflexion & knee flexion & hip flexion & hip adduction & hip abduction & ankle plantarflexion & knee extension < hip extension; ankle dorsiflexion < hip abduction **L**: hip abduction < ankle plantarflexion & hip adduction & ankle dorsiflexion & knee extension & hip extension; hip flexion < hip adduction & ankle dorsiflexion & knee extension & hip extension; knee flexion & ankle plantarflexion < hip extension	**non-fallers**: **A**: ankle plantarflexion & knee flexion & hip flexion < hip adduction & knee extension & hip extension & hip abduction; ankle dorsiflexion < knee extension & hip extension & hip abduction **P**: ankle dorsiflexion < knee flexion & hip extension & hip flexion & hip abduction & ankle plantarflexion & hip adduction & knee extension; knee flexion & hip extension < ankle plantarflexion & hip adduction & knee extension; hip flexion < knee extension **M**: knee flexion & hip adduction & ankle dorsiflexion < ankle plantarflexion & hip abduction & knee extension & hip extension; hip flexion & ankle plantarflexion < knee extension & hip extension; hip abduction < hip extension **L**: hip abduction < knee flexion & ankle plantarflexion & hip adduction & ankle dorsiflexion & knee extension & hip extension; hip flexion & knee flexion < hip adduction & ankle dorsiflexion & knee extension & hip extension	**non-fallers**: hip extension & knee extension & hip adduction & hip abduction & ankle plantarflexion & ankle dorsiflexion < hip flexion; hip extension & knee extension & hip adduction & hip abduction < knee flexion; hip extension & knee extension < ankle dorsiflexion	**non-fallers**: ankle dorsiflexion & knee flexion & hip abduction & hip extension & ankle plantarflexion & hip adduction & knee extension < hip flexion

A: anterior perturbations. **P**: posterior perturbations. **M**: medial perturbations. **L**: lateral perturbations.

Table A5. Significant results for the analyzed electromyographic (EMG) signal parameters.

Parameter	EMG Onset Latency	Rate of EMG Rise	EMG Burst Duration
Significant interaction effect of "fall history" and other factor(s) in four-way ANOVAs	fall history × muscle	fall history × muscle	fall history × muscle; fall history × direction
All significant results of post hoc pairwise comparisons within the muscle & perturbation direction factor	**fallers**: ankle dorsiflexor < knee flexor & ankle plantarflexor & knee extensor & hip flexor & hip adductor & hip extensor; hip abductor < hip adductor & hip extensor; knee flexor < hip extensor	**fallers**: hip extensor & hip adductor & hip flexor & ankle plantarflexor & knee extensor & knee flexor & hip abductor < ankle dorsiflexor; hip extensor & hip adductor & hip flexor & ankle plantarflexor & knee extensor < hip abductor; hip extensor < knee flexor	**fallers**: Within **muscle** factor: ankle plantarflexor & hip adductor & hip extensor & hip flexor < hip abductor & ankle dorsiflexor; ankle plantarflexor & hip adductor & hip extensor < knee flexor; ankle plantarflexor & hip adductor < knee extensor Within **perturbation direction** factor: lateral & medial < posterior & anterior
	non-fallers: ankle dorsiflexor < hip extensor & knee flexor; hip flexor & hip abductor < knee flexor	**non-fallers**: hip extensor & knee flexor & hip adductor & ankle plantarflexor & hip flexor & knee extensor & hip abductor < ankle dorsiflexor; hip extensor & knee flexor & hip adductor & ankle plantarflexor < hip abductor	**non-fallers**: Within **muscle** factor: ankle plantarflexor & hip extensor & hip adductor < ankle dorsiflexor; ankle plantarflexor < knee extensor & hip abductor. Within **perturbation direction** factor: lateral < medial

References

1. World Health Organization. Falls. Available online: https://www.who.int/news-room/fact-sheets/detail/falls# (accessed on 30 April 2023).
2. Moreland, B.; Kakara, R.; Henry, A. Trends in nonfatal falls and fall-related injuries among adults aged ≥ 65 years—United States, 2012–2018. *Morb. Mortal. Weekly Rep.* **2020**, *69*, 875. [CrossRef] [PubMed]
3. de Vries, O.J.; Peeters, G.M.E.E.G.; Elders, P.J.M.; Muller, M.; Knol, D.L.; Danner, S.A.; Bouter, L.M.; Lips, P. Multifactorial Intervention to Reduce Falls in Older People at High Risk of Recurrent Falls: A Randomized Controlled Trial. *Arch. Intern. Med.* **2010**, *170*, 1110–1117. [CrossRef] [PubMed]
4. Kasahara, S.; Saito, H. Mechanisms of postural control in older adults based on surface electromyography data. *Hum. Mov. Sci.* **2021**, *78*, 102803. [CrossRef]
5. Tong, C.Y.; Zhu, R.T.; Ling, Y.T.; Scheeren, E.M.; Lam, F.M.; Fu, H.; Ma, C.Z. Muscular and Kinematic Responses to Unexpected Translational Balance Perturbation: A Pilot Study in Healthy Young Adults. *Bioengineering* **2023**, *10*, 831. [CrossRef]
6. Manchester, D.; Woollacott, M.; Zederbauer-Hylton, N.; Marin, O. Visual, vestibular and somatosensory contributions to balance control in the older adult. *J. Gerontol.* **1989**, *44*, M118–M127. [CrossRef]
7. Allum, J.H.; Carpenter, M.G.; Honegger, F.; Adkin, A.L.; Bloem, B.R. Age-dependent variations in the directional sensitivity of balance corrections and compensatory arm movements in man. *J. Physiol.* **2002**, *542*, 643–663. [CrossRef]
8. Ma, C.Z.-H.; Lee, W.C.-C. A wearable vibrotactile biofeedback system improves balance control of healthy young adults following perturbations from quiet stance. *Hum. Mov. Sci.* **2017**, *55*, 54–60. [CrossRef] [PubMed]

9. Batcir, S.; Shani, G.; Shapiro, A.; Alexander, N.; Melzer, I. The kinematics and strategies of recovery steps during lateral losses of balance in standing at different perturbation magnitudes in older adults with varying history of falls. *BMC Geriatr.* **2020**, *20*, 249. [CrossRef] [PubMed]
10. Bair, W.-N.; Prettyman, M.G.; Beamer, B.A.; Rogers, M.W. Kinematic and behavioral analyses of protective stepping strategies and risk for falls among community living older adults. *Clin. Biomech.* **2016**, *36*, 74–82. [CrossRef] [PubMed]
11. Gerards, M.H.; Meijer, K.; Karamanidis, K.; Grevendonk, L.; Hoeks, J.; Lenssen, A.F.; McCrum, C. Adaptability to balance perturbations during walking as a potential marker of falls history in older adults. *Front. Sports Act. Living* **2021**, *3*, 132. [CrossRef]
12. Sturnieks, D.L.; Menant, J.; Delbaere, K.; Vanrenterghem, J.; Rogers, M.W.; Fitzpatrick, R.C.; Lord, S.R. Force-Controlled Balance Perturbations Associated with Falls in Older People: A Prospective Cohort Study. *PLoS ONE* **2013**, *8*, e70981. [CrossRef]
13. Maki, B.E.; Holliday, P.J.; Topper, A.K. A Prospective Study of Postural Balance and Risk of Falling in An Ambulatory and Independent Elderly Population. *J. Gerontol.* **1994**, *49*, M72–M84. [CrossRef] [PubMed]
14. Tantisuwat, A.; Vachalathiti, R.; Hiengkaew, V.; Assantachai, P. Stepping Responses during Forward and Backward Fall Recovery between Thai Elderly Fallers and Non-fallers. *J. Phys. Ther. Sci.* **2011**, *23*, 373–379. [CrossRef]
15. Mille, M.-L.; Johnson-Hilliard, M.; Martinez, K.M.; Zhang, Y.; Edwards, B.J.; Rogers, M.W. One step, two steps, three steps more... directional vulnerability to falls in community-dwelling older people. *J. Gerontol. Ser. A Biomed. Sci. Med. Sci.* **2013**, *68*, 1540–1548. [CrossRef]
16. Thompson, J.D.; Plummer, P.; Franz, J.R. Age and falls history effects on antagonist leg muscle coactivation during walking with balance perturbations. *Clin. Biomech.* **2018**, *59*, 94–100. [CrossRef] [PubMed]
17. Studenski, S.; Chandler, J. Postural Responses and Effector Factors in Persons with Unexplained Falls: Results and Methodologic Issues. *J. Am. Geriatr. Soc.* **1991**, *39*, 229–234. [CrossRef] [PubMed]
18. Claudino, R.; Dos Santos, M.J.; Mazo, G.Z. Delayed Compensatory Postural Adjustments After Lateral Perturbations Contribute to the Reduced Ability of Older Adults to Control Body Balance. *Motor Control* **2017**, *21*, 425–442. [CrossRef]
19. Lin, S.-I.; Woollacott, M.H. Postural muscle responses following changing balance threats in young, stable older, and unstable older adults. *J. Mot. Behav.* **2002**, *34*, 37–44. [CrossRef]
20. Zhu, R.T.; Lyu, P.Z.; Li, S.; Tong, C.Y.; Ling, Y.T.; Ma, C.Z. How Does Lower Limb Respond to Unexpected Balance Perturbations? New Insights from Synchronized Human Kinetics, Kinematics, Muscle Electromyography (EMG) and Mechanomyography (MMG) Data. *Biosensors* **2022**, *12*, 430. [CrossRef]
21. Rogers, M.W.; Hedman, L.D.; Johnson, M.E.; Cain, T.D.; Hanke, T.A. Lateral Stability During Forward-Induced Stepping for Dynamic Balance Recovery in Young and Older Adults. *J. Gerontol. Ser. A* **2001**, *56*, M589–M594. [CrossRef]
22. Fujimoto, M.; Bair, W.N.; Rogers, M.W. Center of pressure control for balance maintenance during lateral waist-pull perturbations in older adults. *J. Biomech.* **2015**, *48*, 963–968. [CrossRef] [PubMed]
23. de Freitas, P.B.; Knight, C.A.; Barela, J.A. Postural reactions following forward platform perturbation in young, middle-age, and old adults. *J. Electromyogr. Kinesiol.* **2010**, *20*, 693–700. [CrossRef] [PubMed]
24. Tinetti, M.E.; Speechley, M.; Ginter, S.F. Risk factors for falls among elderly persons living in the community. *N. Engl. J. Med.* **1988**, *319*, 1701–1707. [CrossRef] [PubMed]
25. Yardley, L.; Beyer, N.; Hauer, K.; Kempen, G.; Piot-Ziegler, C.; Todd, C. Development and initial validation of the Falls Efficacy Scale-International (FES-I). *Age Ageing* **2005**, *34*, 614–619. [CrossRef] [PubMed]
26. Ku, P.-W.; Sun, W.; Chen, L.-J. Reliability and Validity of the Chinese Version of the Physical Activity Scale for the Elderly. *Sport Exerc. Res.* **2013**, *15*, 309–319. [CrossRef]
27. King, L.; Horak, F. On the Mini-BESTest: Scoring and the Reporting of Total Scores. *Phys. Ther.* **2013**, *93*, 571–575. [CrossRef] [PubMed]
28. Godi, M.; Franchignoni, F.; Caligari, M.; Giordano, A.; Turcato, A.M.; Nardone, A. Comparison of reliability, validity, and responsiveness of the mini-BESTest and Berg Balance Scale in patients with balance disorders. *Phys. Ther.* **2013**, *93*, 158–167. [CrossRef]
29. Hoffman, M.; Schrader, J.; Applegate, T.; Koceja, D. Unilateral postural control of the functionally dominant and nondominant extremities of healthy subjects. *J. Athl. Train.* **1998**, *33*, 319–322. [PubMed]
30. Hermens, H.J.; Freriks, B.; Disselhorst-Klug, C.; Rau, G. Development of recommendations for SEMG sensors and sensor placement procedures. *J. Electromyogr. Kinesiol.* **2000**, *10*, 361–374. [CrossRef]
31. Vicon Motion Systems Limited. Plug-In Gait Reference Guide. Available online: https://docs.vicon.com/display/Nexus212/Plug-in+Gait+Reference+Guide (accessed on 20 April 2022).
32. Kim, D.; Hwang, J.-M. The center of pressure and ankle muscle co-contraction in response to anterior-posterior perturbations. *PLoS ONE* **2018**, *13*, e0207667. [CrossRef]
33. Konrad, P. The Abc of Emg. In *A Practical Introduction to Kinesiological Electromyography*; Noraxon Inc.: Scottsdale, AZ, USA, 2005; Volume 1, pp. 30–35.

34. Ling, Y.T.; Ma, C.Z.; Shea, Q.T.; Zheng, Y.-P. Sonomechanomyography (SMMG): Mapping of Skeletal Muscle Motion Onset during Contraction Using Ultrafast Ultrasound Imaging and Multiple Motion Sensors. *Sensors* **2020**, *20*, 5513. [CrossRef] [PubMed]
35. Hesam-Shariati, N.; Trinh, T.; Thompson-Butel, A.G.; Shiner, C.T.; McNulty, P.A. A longitudinal electromyography study of complex movements in Poststroke therapy. 1: Heterogeneous changes despite consistent improvements in clinical assessments. *Front. Neurol.* **2017**, *8*, 340. [CrossRef] [PubMed]
36. Di Nardo, F.; Morano, M.; Strazza, A.; Fioretti, S. Muscle Co-Contraction Detection in the Time-Frequency Domain. *Sensors* **2022**, *22*, 4886. [CrossRef]
37. Falconer, K. Quantitative assessment of cocontraction at the ankle joint in walking. *Electromyogr. Clin. Neurophysiol.* **1985**, *25*, 135–148.
38. Portney, L.G. *Foundations of Clinical Research: Applications to Evidence-Based Practice*; FA Davis: Philadelphia, PA, USA, 2020.
39. Woollacott, M.H. 8 Age-Related Changes in Posture and Movement. *J. Gerontol.* **1993**, *48*, 56–60. [CrossRef]
40. Inacio, M.; Ryan, A.S.; Bair, W.-N.; Prettyman, M.; Beamer, B.A.; Rogers, M.W. Gluteal muscle composition differentiates fallers from non-fallers in community dwelling older adults. *BMC Geriatr.* **2014**, *14*, 37. [CrossRef] [PubMed]
41. Nijhuis, L.B.O.; Bloem, B.R.; Carpenter, M.G.; Allum, J.H.J. Incorporating voluntary knee flexion into nonanticipatory balance corrections. *J. Neurophysiol.* **2007**, *98*, 3047–3059. [CrossRef]
42. Cheng, K.B. Does knee motion contribute to feet-in-place balance recovery? *J. Biomech.* **2016**, *49*, 1873–1880. [CrossRef] [PubMed]
43. Kasahara, S.; Saito, H.; Anjiki, T.; Osanai, H. The effect of aging on vertical postural control during the forward and backward shift of the center of pressure. *Gait Posture* **2015**, *42*, 448–454. [CrossRef] [PubMed]
44. Schulz, B.W.; Jongprasithporn, M.; Hart-Hughes, S.J.; Bulat, T. Effects of step length, age, and fall history on hip and knee kinetics and knee co-contraction during the maximum step length test. *Clin. Biomech.* **2013**, *28*, 933–940. [CrossRef]
45. Falk, J.; Strandkvist, V.; Pauelsen, M.; Vikman, I.; Nyberg, L.; Röijezon, U. Increased co-contraction reaction during a surface perturbation is associated with unsuccessful postural control among older adults. *BMC Geriatr.* **2022**, *22*, 438. [CrossRef]
46. Ho, C.Y.; Bendrups, A.P. Ankle Reflex Stiffness During Unperceived Perturbation of Standing in Elderly Subjects. *J. Gerontol. Ser. A* **2002**, *57*, B344–B350. [CrossRef] [PubMed]
47. Bhagwat, A.P.; Deodhe, N.P. The Effect of Perturbation-Based Balance Training vs Step Training on Reaction Time in Older Persons: A Review. *Cureus* **2023**, *15*, e48104. [CrossRef]
48. Hall, C.D.; Jensen, J.L. Age-related differences in lower extremity power after support surface perturbations. *J. Am. Geriatr. Soc.* **2002**, *50*, 1782–1788. [CrossRef]

Disclaimer/Publisher's Note: The statements, opinions and data contained in all publications are solely those of the individual author(s) and contributor(s) and not of MDPI and/or the editor(s). MDPI and/or the editor(s) disclaim responsibility for any injury to people or property resulting from any ideas, methods, instructions or products referred to in the content.

bioengineering

MDPI

Article

Reliability and Accuracy of Standard Reference Procedures for Measurements of Trunk and Arm Postures in Ergonomics

Carl M. Lind [1,*], Ida-Märta Rhen [1,2,3] and Mikael Forsman [1,2,4]

1 Unit of Occupational Medicine, Institute of Environmental Medicine, Karolinska Institutet, 171 77 Stockholm, Sweden
2 Centre for Occupational and Environmental Medicine, Stockholm County Council, 113 65 Stockholm, Sweden
3 Department of Industrial and Materials Science, Chalmers University of Technology, 412 96 Gothenburg, Sweden
4 School of Engineering Sciences in Chemistry, Biotechnology and Health, KTH Royal Institute of Technology, 141 57 Stockholm, Sweden
* Correspondence: carl.lind@ki.se

Abstract: Adequate reference procedures for obtaining the reference zero-angle position are important for precise and accurate posture measurements, but few studies have systematically investigated these. A limited number of previous studies suggest differences in accuracy between procedures, with some causing an underestimation of the true arm elevation angle when sensors are taped to the skin. The reliability of commonly used reference procedures for the measurement of the trunk posture is also not well explored, and alternative procedures may improve precision. Based on this identified gap, this study evaluated the test–retest reliability of the N-position (I-pose), i.e., the standard procedure for recording trunk postures, and compared it with two new alternative procedures. Additionally, the accuracy of the N-position for measuring arm elevation angles was compared with one alternative procedure. A total of 40 participants (22 women and 18 men) aged 26–70 years performed the reference procedures in a laboratory setting. Postures were recorded using a smart workwear system equipped with two inertial measurement units (IMUs) embedded in pockets within the workwear. For the trunk posture, the N-position showed a slight lack of test–retest reliability, while one of the alternative procedures demonstrated better test–retest reliability. For the arm posture, the N-position, which does not include lateral trunk inclination, resulted in a substantial underestimation of the arm elevation angle of approximately 15°, which is a novel finding. In contrast, the posture involving trunk inclination closely matched the targeted reference, with a difference of less than 2°. This study underscores the importance of selecting appropriate reference procedures to ensure precise and accurate posture measurements.

Keywords: measurement error; measurement bias; work postures; calibration procedures; posture assessment; standard posture; plumb line test; normal standing position; inclinometry; wearables

1. Introduction

Musculoskeletal disorders (MSDs) of the lower back and neck are significant global health concerns, accounting for approximately 95 million disability-adjusted life years (DALYs) annually, while other musculoskeletal disorders collectively account for over 33 million DALYs worldwide [1]. Shoulder pain is prevalent globally with a seven-day prevalence of up to approximately 34% and a 12-month prevalence of up to around 55% [2].

The economic burden of work-related musculoskeletal disorders (WMSDs) and occupational accidents and diseases has been estimated at 3.3% of the gross domestic product in the European Union and 3.9% of the global gross domestic product [3]. WMSDs contribute to increased risks of short- and long-term work absenteeism, a reduced work capacity, and a premature exit from the labor market [4–6]. WMSDs are multifactorial, with both physical and psychosocial risk factors playing a role [7–9]. Important physical risk factors include strenuous postures and movements [7,10–16], strenuous and repetitive manual handling [7,10,12,16–22], and whole-body and hand–arm vibrations [7,10,23,24]. Accurate and precise measurements of these risk factors are important for establishing exposure–effect relationships and for risk assessment [25–29].

1.1. Sensor-Based Motion Capture Devices in Risk Prevention

Recent advancements in microelectronics have facilitated the increased use of sensor-based measurement instruments, such as triaxial accelerometers and inertial measurement units (IMUs), in research and occupational health practice. These tools enable more accurate assessments of work postures [27], complementing the traditional assessment that primarily relies on observation-based tools [25,26,30–32], enabling extended measurement durations from a few minutes to several hours or full workdays, providing more representative exposure measurements.

To increase the ease of use, motion devices can be integrated into workwear and connected to systems that enable the automated analysis and real-time monitoring of workers [27,33,34]. Examples of such sensor-based solutions include stretchable textile sensors attached on the outer surface of the workwear [35,36] and IMUs placed in embedded pockets in the workwear [37–40]. Stretchable textile sensors can be used to distinguish gross physical activity types [35,36], but generally exhibit lower accuracy compared to IMUs embedded in workwear. Embedding motion devices such as IMUs into workwear eliminates the need for skin attachment using tape or straps, which sometimes can be inconvenient and sensitive, as it may require partial undressing, access to private spaces, and anatomical knowledge for precise sensor placement.

1.2. Review of Reference Procedures for Accurate and Reliable Sensor-Based Measurements of Sagittal Trunk Inclination and Arm Elevation

In addition to accurate instrumentation, precise reference postures (i.e., procedures for obtaining the reference zero-angle position, typically a neutral body posture) are essential for obtaining accurate and reliable measurements and to make studies inter-comparable. While several studies have assessed, e.g., the reliability and inter-rater reliability of instruments and methods to assess the range of motion, such as for lumbar flexion [41–43], and the accuracy of inertia-based wearable motion capture systems against marker-based motion capture systems [44–47], less attention has been given to evaluating the reliability of reference positions for a neutral position for the trunk and upper arm. Ideally, a reference procedure (i.e., reference positions or postures and other arrangements such as instructions, assistance, and the use of assisting objects like chairs and external loads) should not only provide accurate and reliable measurements but also be practical for use in both laboratory and field studies.

To record the neutral posture for the trunk, arms, and head (or neck), Aarås and Stranden [48] proposed an upright, well-balanced position where the shoulders are relaxed and the upper arms hang naturally alongside the body without holding an external load. This reference procedure allows for simultaneous zero-posture recordings of the trunk, head, and arms.

The posture is often referred to as the natural, normal, or standard posture, the normal stance [49,50], or the N-position, N-posture, or I-pose [51] (hereafter to be referred to as the

N-position). Variations of the N-position have been widely used in ergonomics research to establish the reference zero-angle position for both the trunk (see Table 1) and the upper arm (see Table 2).

As shown in Table 1, the N-position appears to be the most used zero posture. Among the variations of the N-position, some studies specify that the feet should be close together or shoulder width apart; while some describe subjects looking forward, others specify using a visual mark or point at eye level. An alternative variation of the N-position, referred to as the Toe-position in this article, was used in studies by Fan et al. [52] and Forsman et al. [53], where subjects returned to the N-position from a toe stand.

Table 1. Reference posture used to record a neutral trunk posture, indicating 0° trunk inclination or flexion. All studies were conducted in real work environments, and the selection was based on those identified by Lind et al. [27].

Reference Posture	
Standing upright	**Reference posture not reported** [1]
[13,40,54–89]	[46,90–102]

Note: [1] not reported or information cannot be found.

The N-position appears to be the dominant posture for recording the reference zero-angle position for the trunk posture. It is also used to establish the reference zero-angle position for the upper arm, alongside other reference procedures, as summarized in Table 2. While the N-position does not involve lateral trunk inclination or typically require the use of an external dumbbell, most other reference procedures include these elements, typically using a 2 kg dumbbell. One of these procedures, referred to here as the "Stockholm procedure", involves lateral trunk inclination and an external weight and is performed either standing or seated [44,89,103–105].

Table 2. Reference posture used to record a neutral arm posture, indicating 0° arm elevation. All studies were conducted in real work environments, and the selection was based on those identified by Lind et al. [27].

Lateral Trunk Inclination				No Lateral Trunk Inclination					Posture Not Reported
Standing		Seated		Standing			Seated		
weight	no weight	weight	no weight	weight	no weight	not reported	weight	no weight	
[89]	[106]	[52–57,64,67, 74,83,88,91, 104,106–118]	-	[119]	[14,75,79,120]	[65,70,71,73,76–78,87,121,122]	[103,123–125]	-	[46,80,84,86,93,95, 97–99,101,102,126–132] [1]

Note: [1] a weight was used.

However, the peer-reviewed literature provides limited information on the reproducibility and accuracy of these reference postures and similar approaches for measuring neutral trunk- and arm postures. Additionally, alternative procedures may offer improved reliability. Aarås and Stranden [48] evaluated the reliability of the N-position reference posture for the head and arms in five participants, reporting an average deviation from the midpoint of less than 1° for the head posture, 1.2° for arm flexion (i.e., arm elevation in the sagittal plane, forward), and 0.9° for arm abduction (i.e., arm elevation in the frontal plane, sideways). In a more recent study [69], median group differences before and after measurements were 3.8° for trunk sagittal inclination and 1.8° for trunk lateral inclination (Nastaran, Raffler. 2020. e-mail message to author, August 25). In our research, we have observed that this posture can occasionally be challenging to consistently adopt without postural divergence. While sensor-based inclinometers provide highly accurate measurements, calibration-related errors of approximately 4° in the reference posture can be unacceptably large, potentially obscuring actual improvements following an intervention [133]. To our knowledge, no study in the ergonomics literature has systematically evaluated the reliability of this reference posture for trunk angles on a larger sample or the reliability of alternative procedures.

With regard to the arm posture, Dahlqvist et al. [106,134] observed considerable differences between reference positions involving lateral (sideways) trunk inclination when a seated posture with an external weight was compared to standing reference positions without an external weight. For example, Dahlqvist et al. [134] reported group root mean square differences of 8.5° and 14° for the left and right arms, respectively. Furthermore, Jackson et al. [105] evaluated the accuracy of upper arm inclinometry against visually projected lines between 30° and 150°, with incremental steps of 30°. The inclinometers (triaxial accelerometers) were taped to the arm and a seated reference position with lateral trunk inclination with an external weight was used as the reference position (0° arm elevation). They reported that the inclinometers systematically underestimated the arm elevation angle, for example, by 13.5° and 11.1° on average at 90° arm abduction and arm flexion, respectively. The divergences were potentially attributed (at least partly) to soft tissue artifacts [105,135,136], and the authors presented conversion equations to allow for correction for the bias. Notably, this bias was not observed by Hansson [137] who, in a letter to the editor, reported an average divergence of $\leq$1° for the right and left arms when the participants held their arms at what was judged to be 90°.

1.3. Summary of Identified Research Gap

The identified literature highlights a lack of research on the reliability of reference postures for arm and trunk measurements. Additionally, it remains unclear whether the bias in arm elevation measurements reported by Jackson et al. [105] persists when motion capture devices are placed in the pockets of workwear, allowing for slight movement, rather than being taped directly to the arm.

1.4. Research Objective

Given these research gaps, the aim of this study was to evaluate the reliability of three reference positions for sagittal (forward/backward) trunk inclination and the accuracy of two reference positions for arm inclinometry using motion capture devices embedded in workwear.

2. Materials and Methods

2.1. Subjects

The study population (Table 3) comprised 22 women and 18 men, recruited from a working population pool at three organizations located in the Stockholm Region, Sweden. To ensure a broad working-age sample, the inclusion criteria required participants to be 18 years or older, currently employed or enrolled as students, and free from physical conditions, such as pain, disorders, or impairments that could hinder the execution of the reference procedures. Thirty-seven participants reported right-hand dominance and three reported left-hand dominance. Twenty participants had a BMI $\geq$ 23.0, and eleven had a BMI $\geq$ 25.0. There were no statistically significant differences in age or stature between these groups and the rest of the population. The study was approved by the Regional Ethics Committee in Stockholm, Sweden (2017/1586-31/4 and 2019-01206), and all participants provided written informed consent prior to participation.

Table 3. Summary of participant characteristics (SD, standard deviation).

Demographic Variables	Women, Mean (SD)	Men, Mean (SD)
N	22	18
Age (years)	42.0 (13.4)	42.5 (10.7)
Body mass (kg)	61.3 (9.7)	76.8 (10.6)
Stature (cm)	164.0 (6.5)	178.7 (8.4)
BMI (kg/m^2)	22.7 (2.8)	24.0 (2.2)

2.2. Instrumentation

Postural data for the trunk and upper arms were recorded using the Smart Workwear System [37,38]. The system included a stretchy workwear shirt (Model 9418, LiteWork, Snickers Workwear, Hultafors Group Sverige AB, Bollebygd, Sweden; fabric: 58% polyamid and 42% polyester 37.5®; mass: 165 g/m^2) customized into a short-sleeved shirt with embedded pockets on the trunk and arms for IMUs (LPMS-B2, LP Research, Tokyo, Japan; dimensions: 39 × 39 × 8 mm; mass: 12 g). Participants were individually fitted with appropriately sized shirts (XS–L) to accommodate their body dimensions. To measure the trunk inclination, a single IMU was placed in the trunk pocket positioned on the upper back at the level of thoracic vertebrae 1–2 [45,52] (Figure 1). To measure the right upper arm elevation angle, a single IMU was placed in a pocket of the workwear enabling the upper edge of the IMU to be positioned approximately distal to the medial deltoideus muscle insertion [39,40,138] (Figure 1). The IMUs (Figure 1D) transmitted real-time data via Bluetooth to an Android 8.0 smartphone (Galaxy A5 2017, Samsung, Seoul, Republic of Korea), and the data were analyzed using the ErgoRiskLogger application, as described elsewhere [38]. Since the study focused on static postures, the IMU sampling rate was set to 25 Hz. The 3-axis accelerometer in the IMUs was set to a range, per axis, of ±4 G, and the 3-axis gyroscope was set to ±500°/s. A 16-bit resolution was used, followed by an extensive complementary Kalman filter (that is, a sensor fusion filter) to obtain the orientation of the sensor. As this study concerned static postures, it mainly used the accelerometer signals. According to the specification of the IMU, the static angle error was below 0.5°. More information on the Smart Workwear System is reported elsewhere [38].

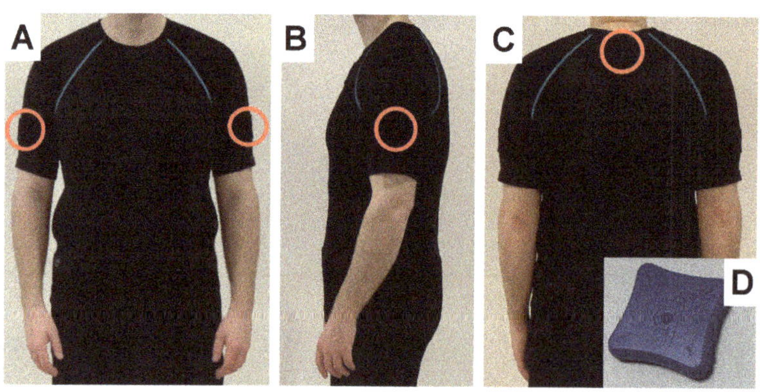

Figure 1. Positions of the inertial measurement units (IMUs) (here highlighted with red circles) from the anterior view (**A**), the lateral view (**B**), and the posterior view (**C**). The motion tracking device (i.e., the IMU) used (**D**).

2.3. Experimental Protocol

Four different reference positions were performed in a fixed order (Figures 2 and 3). Trunk postures were assessed using three of the four positions, and arm postures were assessed using two positions. As shown in Figure 2, the evaluation began with recordings of the N-position, followed by the Stockholm-position. Subsequently, static arm elevation angles were recorded at a set angle of 90°. The N-position was then repeated. Finally, the Balance-position was repeated twice, and the session concluded with two repetitions of the Toe-Position.

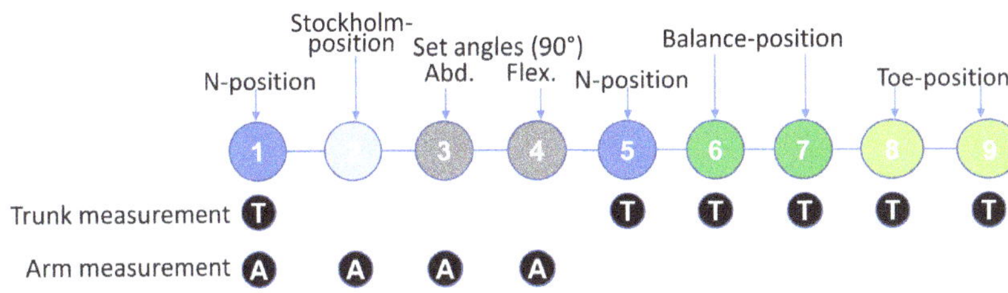

Figure 2. The order of the reference procedures and set angle trials.

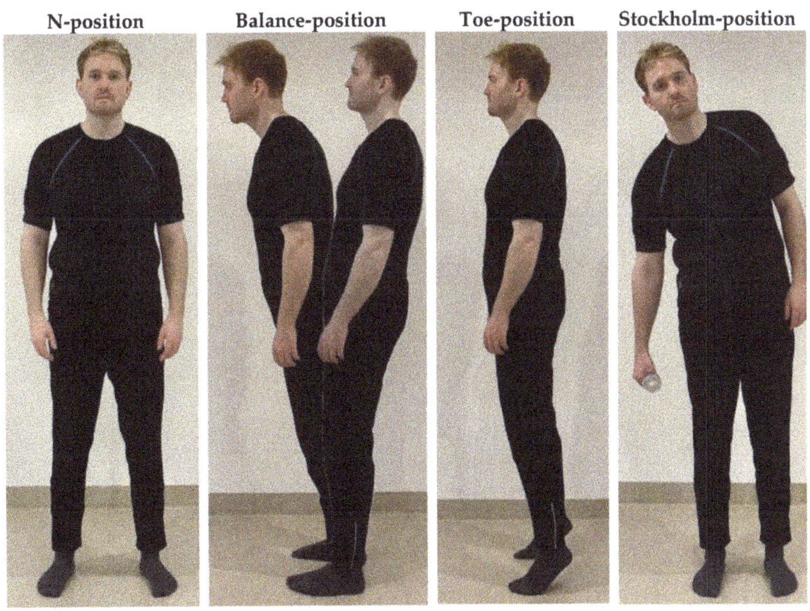

N-position	Balance-position	Toe-position	Stockholm-position
Standing upright, looking forward at approximately eye level, with relaxed arms hanging downward, relaxed fingers, and palms facing the body.	Standing upright, slightly incline the trunk forward and backward, then stabilize in a fully balanced position.	Standing upright, looking forward at eye level. Rise up onto the toes, then slowly return to a fully balanced position with the entire shoe sole resting flat on the floor.	Standing with a lateral trunk inclination, with a relaxed right arm hanging downward without touching the hip, holding a 2 kg dumbbell with the palm facing the body.

Figure 3. Description of the four reference procedures.

The set angle procedure involved holding the upper arm still for 5 s in a 90° arm elevation (abduction), followed by another 90° arm elevation (flexion), with assistance from an instructor. The set angles were performed with a straight arm, maintaining a straight elbow and wrist, with the palm facing downward. The instructor (one of two physiotherapists) aligned the participants' right arm by positioning the midline of the humerus parallel to the targeted abduction and inclination angles guided by the set angles printed on a large paper sheet (100 × 135 cm). This approach was modeled after the procedure described by Jackson et al. [105], but instead of visual projection, printed lines were used to eliminate the spatial distortion observed during preliminary pilot tests. Consistent with Jackson et al. [105], this assisted positioning was assumed to represent the "true" angle of the upper arm.

To record the postures of the trunk and arm in the version of the ErgoRiskLogger application we used, a global (original) reference recording was first made (the first N-position shown in Figure 2), and the other recordings were derived from this as a base. For arm postures, the global (original) value for the Stockholm-position was derived by subtracting the angular elevation difference (delta) between the global reference recording (i.e., 1st N-position) and the Stockholm-position. To illustrate this, if an elevation angle of 15° was recorded for the Stockholm-position, this value was equal to the difference compared to the global reference recording (i.e., 1st N-position). In the same way, the measured elevation at the set angle of 90° arm abduction and 90° arm flexion for the Stockholm-position was estimated as the individually measured angle in the global reference recording, with the addition of the individual delta.

2.4. Data Analysis

The data were checked for normality using the Shapiro–Wilk test ($\alpha = 0.05$) and by visually inspecting histograms. For non-normally distributed data, the Wilcoxon signed-rank test was applied, while the paired samples t-test was used for normally distributed data.

For the trunk posture, the average trunk sagittal inclination angle was compared pairwise among the reference procedures using the Wilcoxon signed-rank test, as one of the three pairs was non-normally distributed.

The test–retest reliability was evaluated through pairwise comparisons among the three reference procedures using the Wilcoxon signed-rank test, as all three pairs were non-normally distributed.

For the arm posture, the differences in the arm elevation between the N-position and the Stockholm-position were compared pairwise at the set angles of 90° abduction and 90° flexion using the paired samples *t*-test.

Statistical analyses were performed using MATLAB R2023b Update 4 (The MathWorks, Inc., Natick, MA, USA), while normality tests were conducted using R (The R Foundation, version 2024.09.0). The significance level was set at $\alpha = 0.01$.

3. Results

The results are based on 240 recordings of trunk postures and 160 recordings of arm postures, encompassing all 40 participants with no missing data.

3.1. Trunk Posture

The group mean differences in trunk inclination angles in the sagittal plane relative to the N-position are shown in Table 4. At the group level, the Balance-position resulted in a slightly more forward trunk inclination angle relative to the N-position (0.44°), while the Toe-position resulted in a slightly more backward trunk inclination angle (−0.33°); however, these differences were not statistically significant ($p > 0.01$).

Table 4. Group mean differences in trunk angles in the sagittal plane (forward/backward) relative to the N-position and the statistical differences (Wilcoxon signed-rank test) of the group differences.

Angular Differences			Statistical Differences		
N-position	**Balance-position**	**Toe-position**	**N-position vs. Balance-position**	**N-position vs. Toe-position**	**Balance-position vs. Toe-position**
Ref.	0.44°	−0.33°	$p = 0.095$	$p = 0.622$	$p = 0.067$

Notes: Angular differences with positive values indicate a forward sagittal trunk inclination relative to the reference, and negative values indicate a backward sagittal trunk inclination relative to the reference.

Trunk Posture—Reliability

The test–retest reliability of the reference postures for trunk angles in the sagittal plane is presented in Table 5, based on data from 40 subjects, each performing two repetitions of each position (no missing values). The group mean absolute difference for the N-position and the Balance-position was 1.60° and 1.56°, respectively, with individual maximum differences exceeding 5°. The Toe-position demonstrated the lowest group mean absolute difference at 0.72°, i.e., the highest test–retest reliability, significantly higher than the two other reference postures ($p < 0.005$).

Table 5. Average absolute test–retest differences in the sagittal trunk inclination (forward/backward) of the reference positions to record a neutral trunk angle, first versus second trial, expressed as the mean (standard deviation, SD), and the statistical differences (Wilcoxon signed-rank test) of the group mean differences. The results are based on 40 subjects, each performing two repetitions of each reference position.

Absolute Group Differences (SD) for 1st vs. 2nd Recording			Statistical Differences		
N-position	**Balance-position**	**Toe-position**	**N-position vs. Balance-position**	**N-position vs. Toe-position**	**Balance-position vs. Toe-position**
1.60° (1.37°)	1.56° (1.29°)	0.72° (0.54°)	$p = 0.717$	$p < 0.005$	$p < 0.001$

3.2. *Arm Posture*

Arm Posture—Accuracy

The corresponding values for the N-position and Stockholm-position at the 90° set angle for abduction and flexion are displayed in Figure 4 and Appendix A.

For arm abduction, using the N-position as a reference resulted in an average elevation angle of 74.1° (SD 4.7), which is 15.9° lower than the assumed true angle. In comparison, the Stockholm-position produced an average elevation angle of 88.3° (SD of 5.5), which was 1.7° lower than the assumed true angle.

For arm flexion, the N-position yielded an average elevation angle of 74.4° (SD of 3.9), which was 15.6° lower than the assumed true angle. In comparison, the Stockholm-position resulted in an average elevation angle of 88.6° (SD of 4.7), i.e., 1.4° lower than the assumed true angle. Hence, the Stockholm-position consistently yielded values that were substantially closer to the assumed true angle, and the angular differences between the N-position and the Stockholm-position at the 90° set angle were statistically significant (paired samples t-test) for both arm abduction and arm flexion ($p < 0.001$).

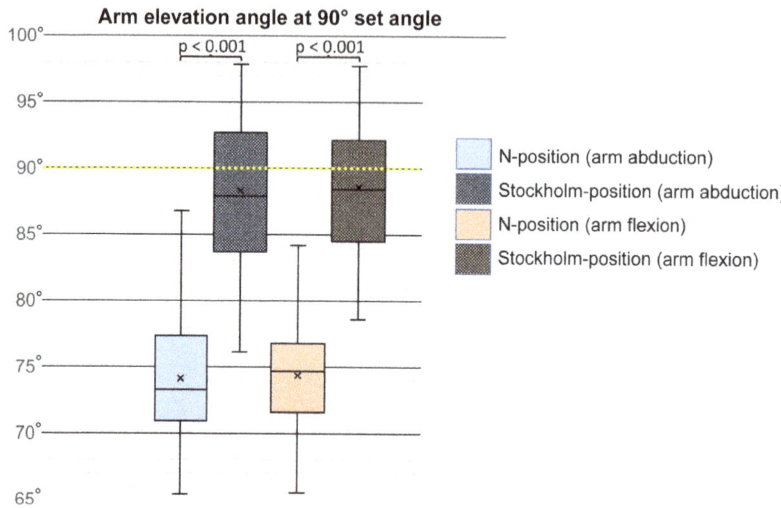

Figure 4. Box plots of arm elevation angles (abduction and flexion) at 90° set angles (yellow dotted line) for the two reference positions: N-position and Stockholm-position. The box represents the interquartile range (25th to 75th percentiles) and the median, while the mean is marked with an "x". Vertical lines extending from the box indicate adjacent values, which are the most extreme values within 1.5 times the interquartile range for each group.

4. Discussion

4.1. General Summary of the Findings

This study, which included 40 subjects, evaluated commonly used reference procedures for obtaining the reference zero-angle positions for measurements of trunk and arm postures. The findings support the conclusion that the choice of reference procedure is critical, as it can significantly affect the reliability and accuracy of technical measurements using sensor-based inclinometers.

For recordings of trunk postures, the results of this study suggest that the test–retest reliability can be improved by replacing the commonly used reference posture (referred to as the N-position) with an alternative reference procedure (referred to as the Toe-position) where the participants arrive at a balanced upright posture from a toe stance.

For recordings of arm postures, the results show that the commonly used N-position, performed in an upright posture without lateral inclination, can lead to substantial and systematic underestimation of arm elevation angles relative to the reference, with errors of approximately 15° for both abduction and flexion if the bias is not corrected. In contrast, the use of an alternative reference procedure (position), i.e., the upright Stockholm-position, which involves lateral trunk inclination and the use of an external weight, resulted in group mean values that closely matched the reference angles, with deviations of less than 2°. These findings highlight the importance of incorporating lateral trunk inclination, and possibly an external weight, to improve measurement accuracy.

4.2. General Interpretation of the Results and Comparisons with Related Literature

This study contributes to the identified research gap by providing new information on the reliability of a commonly used procedure for achieving accurate recordings of a neutral trunk posture, based on a relatively large and diverse sample of men and women spanning various age groups.

4.2.1. Trunk Sagittal Inclination

Regarding trunk postures, the group mean (absolute) test–retest differences in the trunk sagittal inclination in the current study were smaller for all three positions evaluated (i.e., all $\leq 1.60^{\circ}$) compared to the median group differences of 3.8° in the study by Raffler et al. [69]. Notably, Raffler et al. [69] measured the postures before and after the measurement of work activities, which lasted about 1–2 h. One potential reason for the difference could be related to changes in the position of the motion device, which can occur, especially during prolonged use, dynamic activities, or when motion devices are insufficiently secured. The group mean (absolute) test–retest differences in the trunk sagittal inclination in the current study, especially for the Toe-position (0.72°), were close to the test–retest values for the neck (head) of 0.85° reported by Aarås and Stranden [48].

4.2.2. Arm Elevation

Concerning arm postures, contrary to findings from earlier studies by Bernmark and Wiktorin [44], Jackson et al. [105], Lind and Forsman [139], and the related study by Lind et al. [140], this study did not confirm a considerable bias in arm posture recordings at a 90° arm elevation. Instead, and in agreement with what was reported by Hansson [137], who used a seated reference posture, the observed values in the current study closely approximated the assumed true angle, with only slightly lower values of <2°. This can be compared with the difference from the assumed true angle noted by Jackson et al. [105], which averaged 13.5° and 11.1° at a 90° arm abduction and arm flexion, respectively. Previous research has developed equations to harmonize data across different instruments and calculations [52,53,141] or to correct inaccuracies potentially caused by soft tissue artifacts and reference procedures [105]. The large underestimation of arm elevation angles (approximately 15°) is likely caused by the arm, although relaxed, being more abducted when leaning against the body.

4.3. Strengths and Limitations

It should be noted that this study is limited to the sagittal trunk inclination and arm elevation. Although these are the most common exposure metrics for postures of the trunk and upper arm in the ergonomics literature related to WMSD outcomes [27], future studies are needed to explore the reference position in relation to, e.g., trunk sagittal inclination.

Regarding reference procedures for obtaining the reference zero-angle position for the trunk, while the study's findings suggest that the reliability can be improved through alternative procedures, the accuracy of these reference positions was not directly evaluated. Furthermore, it is debated which posture truly represents the "natural" or "neutral" upright posture [49,50]. However, since high accuracy depends on precision, some conclusions can still be drawn regarding the potential advantages of adopting alternative procedures to enhance both the reliability and overall measurement accuracy. A potential limitation was that the reference procedures were not performed in a randomized order, which could introduce learning effects, particularly for reference positions performed later. However, all participants were already familiarized with the reference procedures from a prior trial [140], with the exception of the Balance-position and Toe-position. Therefore, it seems unlikely that the relatively higher test–retest reliability observed for the Toe-position was due to learning effects.

With respect to reference procedures for obtaining the reference zero-angle position for the arm, while the results provide important findings, the accuracy was evaluated only at a 90° arm elevation angle (flexion and abduction). Consequently, the bias may vary in magnitude at other angles. Furthermore, additional information is necessary to develop conversion equations for correcting bias, particularly for the N-position, which resulted in substantial bias. Although only the standing version of the Stockholm procedure was included in this study, preliminary findings from a related study suggest that the differences between the standing and seated variations are small [140].

Additionally, the global (original) reference recording for arm abduction and flexion for the Stockholm-position was derived by subtracting the angular elevation difference between the first N-position and the Stockholm-position (as described in Section 2.3). This approach was necessitated by limitations in the version of the Smart Workwear System used. Preferably, another global (original) reference recording should have been obtained when having the participants stand in the Stockholm-position. The present method introduces an approximation in determining the angle between the Stockholm-position and the 90° arm elevations. Nevertheless, this adjustment likely has a negligible effect on the abduction angle recorded at the 90° set angle, and a negligible-to-minimal effect on the flexion angle. Future studies are, however, recommended to further investigate this.

A strength of this study is the inclusion of a relatively large and diverse sample of subjects, encompassing both women and men across a wide age range (26–70 years). This improves the generalizability to other populations. The stature and body mass of the women in this study were slightly lower than those reported among a Swedish female working population [142] with a median stature of 167.3 cm and median body mass of 64 kg. This stature approximates that of US women aged 40–49 years (162.6 cm) but with a higher body mass (75.2 kg) [143]. The men's stature and body mass were approximately equal to the median stature of 177.9 cm and body mass of 75 kg among a Swedish male working population [142]. This stature approximates that of US men aged 40–49 years (176.5 cm), who have a higher body mass (90.5 kg) [143].

All measurements were recorded with static (isometric) postures, without involving any movement. The potential improvement in the measurement accuracy that can be attributed to having the sensors embedded in tight workwear (as opposed to taped) may differ during tasks involving high movement velocities, especially if the fit of the workwear is loose in some parts where the sensors are embedded, as pointed out by Hoareau et al. [144].

4.4. Practical Implications and Future Research

The bias attributed to reference procedures seems to have been underestimated, especially as measurements from technical measurement instruments such as IMUs and accelerometers are often regarded as having superior accuracy and precision when compared to self-reports and systematic observations [54,145–148].

The main implication of this study is that an upright neutral position is not recommended for recording the neutral position of the upper arm. Instead, the reference position should include lateral trunk inclination. As a result, findings from studies that assume that the N-position represents zero arm elevation (without additional corrective measures) may not be directly comparable to those that use other reference positions. Furthermore, it is questionable whether the N-position should be used at all for recording arm postures without corrections. Given the relatively common use of the N-position, as shown in Table 2, caution is warranted when interpreting the results of studies that did not account for the bias associated with the N-position as observed in the current study. This also underscores the need for conversion methods to convert data obtained from different reference procedures, particularly when one involves trunk inclination and the other does not.

While the current study demonstrated that a posture including trunk inclination and an external load can yield relatively accurate arm elevation angles (both abduction and flexion), the divergent results from the related study by Lind et al. [140], as well as findings from Jackson et al. [105], Bernmark and Wiktorin [44], and Lind and Forsman [139], underscore the need for further research to better understand the reasons behind these discrepancies. The results of the current study highlight the need for the conversion of postures obtained using different reference positions to ensure accuracy and comparability between studies.

To improve the test–retest reliability in recording a neutral trunk position, and consequently the accuracy of the N-position, future studies could explore the feasibility and efficiency of increasing the number of measurements, allowing for the calculation of an average value based on multiple recordings taken before and after the work activity, or alternatively, consider using the Toe-position.

5. Conclusions

The choice of reference procedures for obtaining reference zero-angle positions can significantly impact the reliability and accuracy of technical measurements using sensor-based inclinometers. For recordings of a zero-angle trunk position in the sagittal plane, the commonly used N-position (or N-posture, or I-pose) was observed to exhibit some imprecision. An alternative posture, where participants arrived at the N-position from a toe stand, improved the test–retest reliability.

For recordings of arm elevation, the N-position was compared with an alternative procedure (the Stockholm-position), which includes lateral trunk inclination. The N-position resulted in a substantial average bias of 15°, raising concerns about its use without adjustments to mitigate this error. In contrast, the Stockholm-position demonstrated higher accuracy, with deviations averaging less than 2°, making it the superior option of the two.

The findings of this study can guide the selection of appropriate reference procedures for both field and laboratory applications. Additionally, the findings highlight the importance of incorporating lateral trunk inclination when recording the reference zero-angle position of the arm.

Author Contributions: Conceptualization, C.M.L., I.-M.R. and M.F.; data curation, C.M.L.; methodology, C.M.L., I.-M.R. and M.F.; formal analysis, C.M.L. and M.F.; investigation, C.M.L. and I.-M.R.; writing—original draft preparation, C.M.L.; writing—review and editing, C.M.L., I.-M.R. and M.F.; project administration, C.M.L.; funding acquisition, C.M.L., I.-M.R. and M.F. All authors have read and agreed to the published version of the manuscript.

Funding: This research was funded by AFA Insurance (Afa Försäkring), grant numbers 180098 and 180254.

Institutional Review Board Statement: The study was conducted in accordance with the Declaration of Helsinki and approved by the Regional Ethics Committee in Stockholm, Sweden (2017/1586–31/4 and 2019-01206).

Informed Consent Statement: Informed consent was obtained from all participants involved in the study and from the person in the figures showing the system and reference procedures.

Data Availability Statement: The raw data supporting the conclusions of this article will be made available by the authors on request.

Acknowledgments: Johan Eriksson is gratefully acknowledged for his contribution to the data collection. We would also like to express our gratitude to the participants.

Conflicts of Interest: The authors declare no conflicts of interest. The funders had no role in the design of the study; in the collection, analyses, or interpretation of data; in the writing of the manuscript; or in the decision to publish the results.

Appendix A

Table A1. Mean (SD) arm elevation angles (abduction and flexion) at 90° set angles for two reference positions: N-position and Stockholm-position.

Arm Abduction		Arm Flexion	
N-position	**Stockholm-position**	**N-position**	**Stockholm-position**
74.1 (4.7)	88.3 (5.5)	74.4 (3.9)	88.6 (4.7)

References

1. Kassebaum, N.J.; Arora, M.; Barber, R.M.; Bhutta, Z.A.; Brown, J.; Carter, A.; Casey, D.C.; Charlson, F.J.; Coates, M.M.; Coggeshall, M.; et al. Global, regional, and national disability-adjusted life-years (DALYs) for 315 diseases and injuries and healthy life expectancy (HALE), 1990–2015: A systematic analysis for the Global Burden of Disease Study 2015. *Lancet* **2016**, *388*, 1603–1658. [CrossRef]
2. Lucas, J.; van Doorn, P.; Hegedus, E.; Lewis, J.; van der Windt, D. A systematic review of the global prevalence and incidence of shoulder pain. *BMC Musculoskelet. Disord.* **2022**, *23*, 1073. [CrossRef]
3. Tompa, E.; Mofidi, A.; van den Heuvel, S.; van Bree, T.; Michaelsen, F.; Jung, Y.; Porsch, L.; van Emmerik, M. *The Value of Occupational Safety and Health and the Societal Costs of Work-Related Injuries and Diseases*; Publications Office of the European Union: Luxembourg, 2019. [CrossRef]
4. Sundstrup, E.; Andersen, L.L. Joint association of physical and psychosocial working conditions with risk of long-term sickness absence: Prospective cohort study with register follow-up. *Scand. J. Public Health* **2021**, *49*, 132–140. [CrossRef] [PubMed]
5. Pedersen, J.; Bjorner, J.B.; Andersen, L.L. Physical work demands and expected labor market affiliation (ELMA): Prospective cohort with register-follow-up among 46 169 employees. *Scand. J. Public Health* **2022**, *48*, 641–650. [CrossRef] [PubMed]
6. Badarin, K.; Hemmingsson, T.; Hillert, L.; Kjellberg, K. The impact of musculoskeletal pain and strenuous work on self-reported physical work ability: A cohort study of Swedish men and women. *Int. Arch. Occup. Environ. Health* **2022**, *95*, 939–952. [CrossRef]
7. NRC. *Musculoskeletal Disorders and the Workplace: Low Back and Upper Extremities*; National Academies Press: Washington, DC, USA, 2001. [CrossRef]
8. Widanarko, B.; Legg, S.; Devereux, J.; Stevenson, M. The combined effect of physical, psychosocial/organisational and/or environmental risk factors on the presence of work-related musculoskeletal symptoms and its consequences. *Appl. Ergon.* **2014**, *45*, 1610–1621. [CrossRef] [PubMed]
9. Hauke, A.; Flintrop, J.; Brun, E.; Rugulies, R. The impact of work-related psychosocial stressors on the onset of musculoskeletal disorders in specific body regions: A review and metaanalysis of 54 longitudinal studies. *Work Stress* **2011**, *25*, 243–256. [CrossRef]
10. NIOSH. *Musculoskeletal Disorders and Workplace Factors*; National Institute for Occupational Safety and Health: Cincinnati, OH, USA, 1997.
11. Hoogendoorn, W.E.; Bongers, P.M.; de Vet, H.C.; Douwes, M.; Koes, B.W.; Miedema, M.C.; Ariëns, G.A.; Bouter, L.M. Flexion and rotation of the trunk and lifting at work are risk factors for low back pain: Results of a prospective cohort study. *Spine* **2000**, *25*, 3087–3092. [CrossRef] [PubMed]
12. da Costa, B.R.; Vieira, E.R. Risk factors for work-related musculoskeletal disorders: A systematic review of recent longitudinal studies. *Am. J. Ind. Med.* **2010**, *53*, 285–323. [CrossRef]
13. Gupta, N.; Bjerregaard, S.S.; Yang, L.; Forsman, M.; Rasmussen, C.L.; Rasmussen, C.D.N.; Clays, E.; Holtermann, A. Does occupational forward bending of the back increase long-term sickness absence risk? A 4-year prospective register-based study using device-measured compositional data analysis. *Scand. J. Work Environ. Health* **2022**, *48*, 651–661. [CrossRef] [PubMed]
14. Gupta, N.; Rasmussen, C.L.; Forsman, M.; Søgaard, K.; Holtermann, A. How does accelerometry-measured arm elevation at work influence prospective risk of long-term sickness absence? *Scand. J. Work Environ. Health* **2022**, *48*, 137–147. [CrossRef] [PubMed]
15. Versloot, A.H.C.; Jackson, J.A.; van Rijn, R.M.; Elbers, R.G.; Søgaard, K.; Macri, E.M.; Koes, B.; Burdorf, A.; Chiarotto, A.; Gerger, H. Physical and psychosocial work-related exposures and the occurrence of disorders of the shoulder: A systematic review update. *Appl. Ergon.* **2024**, *118*, 104277. [CrossRef] [PubMed]
16. Jahn, A.; Andersen, J.H.; Christiansen, D.H.; Seidler, A.; Dalbøge, A. Occupational mechanical exposures as risk factor for chronic low-back pain: A systematic review and meta-analysis. *Scand. J. Work Environ. Health* **2023**, *49*, 453–465. [CrossRef]
17. van Rijn, R.M.; Huisstede, B.M.; Koes, B.W.; Burdorf, A. Associations between work-related factors and the carpal tunnel syndrome--a systematic review. *Scand. J. Work Environ. Health* **2009**, *35*, 19–36. [CrossRef] [PubMed]
18. Garg, A.; Boda, S.; Hegmann, K.T.; Moore, J.S.; Kapellusch, J.M.; Bhoyar, P.; Thiese, M.S.; Merryweather, A.; Deckow-Schaefer, G.; Bloswick, D.; et al. The NIOSH lifting equation and low-back pain, part 1: Association with low-back pain in the BackWorks prospective cohort study. *Hum. Factors* **2014**, *56*, 6–28. [CrossRef] [PubMed]

19. Garg, A.; Kapellusch, J.M.; Hegmann, K.T.; Moore, J.S.; Boda, S.; Bhoyar, P.; Thiese, M.S.; Merryweather, A.; Deckow-Schaefer, G.; Bloswick, D.; et al. The NIOSH lifting equation and low-back pain, Part 2: Association with seeking care in the backworks prospective cohort study. *Hum. Factors* **2014**, *56*, 44–57. [CrossRef] [PubMed]
20. Hoozemans, M.J.; Knelange, E.B.; Frings-Dresen, M.H.; Veeger, H.E.; Kuijer, P.P. Are pushing and pulling work-related risk factors for upper extremity symptoms? A systematic review of observational studies. *Occup. Environ. Med.* **2014**, *71*, 788–795. [CrossRef] [PubMed]
21. Kozak, A.; Schedlbauer, G.; Wirth, T.; Euler, U.; Westermann, C.; Nienhaus, A. Association between work-related biomechanical risk factors and the occurrence of carpal tunnel syndrome: An overview of systematic reviews and a meta-analysis of current research. *BMC Musculoskelet. Disord.* **2015**, *16*, 231. [CrossRef] [PubMed]
22. Fox, R.R.; Lu, M.L.; Occhipinti, E.; Jaeger, M. Understanding outcome metrics of the revised NIOSH lifting equation. *Appl. Ergon.* **2019**, *81*, 102897. [CrossRef] [PubMed]
23. Nilsson, T.; Wahlström, J.; Burström, L. Hand-arm vibration and the risk of vascular and neurological diseases—A systematic review and meta-analysis. *PLoS ONE* **2017**, *12*, e0180795. [CrossRef] [PubMed]
24. Burström, L.; Nilsson, T.; Wahlström, J. Whole-body vibration and the risk of low back pain and sciatica: A systematic review and meta-analysis. *Int. Arch. Occup. Environ. Health* **2015**, *88*, 403–418. [CrossRef]
25. Rose, L.M.; Eklund, J.; Nord Nilsson, L.; Barman, L.; Lind, C.M. The RAMP package for MSD risk management in manual handling—A freely accessible tool, with website and training courses. *Appl. Ergon.* **2020**, *86*, 103101. [CrossRef]
26. Lind, C.M.; Forsman, M.; Rose, L.M. Development and evaluation of RAMP II—A practitioner's tool for assessing musculoskeletal disorder risk factors in industrial manual handling. *Ergonomics* **2020**, *63*, 477–504. [CrossRef]
27. Lind, C.M.; Abtahi, F.; Forsman, M. Wearable Motion Capture Devices for the Prevention of Work-Related Musculoskeletal Disorders in Ergonomics-An Overview of Current Applications, Challenges, and Future Opportunities. *Sensors* **2023**, *23*, 4259. [CrossRef] [PubMed]
28. Lind, C.M.; Rose, L.M. Shifting to proactive risk management: Risk communication using the RAMP tool. *Agron. Res.* **2016**, *14*, 513–524.
29. Cantley, L.F.; Taiwo, O.A.; Galusha, D.; Barbour, R.; Slade, M.D.; Tessier-Sherman, B.; Cullen, M.R. Effect of systematic ergonomic hazard identification and control implementation on musculoskeletal disorder and injury risk. *Scand. J. Work Environ. Health* **2014**, *40*, 57–65. [CrossRef] [PubMed]
30. Lind, C.M.; Forsman, M.; Rose, L.M. Development and evaluation of RAMP I—A practitioner's tool for screening of musculoskeletal disorder risk factors in manual handling. *Int. J. Occup. Saf. Ergon.* **2019**, *25*, 165–180. [CrossRef]
31. Eliasson, K.; Lind, C.M.; Nyman, T. Factors influencing ergonomists' use of observation-based risk-assessment tools. *Work* **2019**, *64*, 93–106. [CrossRef]
32. Lowe, B.D.; Dempsey, P.G.; Jones, E.M. Ergonomics assessment methods used by ergonomics professionals. *Appl. Ergon.* **2019**, *81*, 102882. [CrossRef]
33. Lind, C.M. A Rapid Review on the Effectiveness and Use of Wearable Biofeedback Motion Capture Systems in Ergonomics to Mitigate Adverse Postures and Movements of the Upper Body. *Sensors* **2024**, *24*, 3345. [CrossRef]
34. Lind, C.M. Effectiveness of Sensors-Based Augmented Feedback in Ergonomics to Reduce Adverse Biomechanical Exposure in Work-Related Manual Handling-A Rapid Review of the Evidence. *Sensors* **2024**, *24*, 6977. [CrossRef]
35. Esfahani, M.I.M.; Nussbaum, M.A.; Kong, Z.Y. Using a smart textile system for classifying occupational manual material handling tasks: Evidence from lab-based simulations. *Ergonomics* **2019**, *62*, 823–833. [CrossRef] [PubMed]
36. Mokhlespour Esfahani, M.I.; Nussbaum, M.A. Classifying Diverse Physical Activities Using "Smart Garments". *Sensors* **2019**, *19*, 3133. [CrossRef] [PubMed]
37. Lind, C.M.; Sandsjö, L.; Mahdavian, N.; Högberg, D.; Hanson, L.; Diaz Olivares, J.A.; Yang, L.; Forsman, M. Prevention of Work-Related Musculoskeletal Disorders Using Smart Workwear—The Smart Workwear Consortium. In *Human Systems Engineering and Design*; Ahram, T., Karwowski, W., Taiar, R., Eds.; Springer Nature: Cham, Switzerland, 2019; Volume 876, pp. 477–483. [CrossRef]
38. Lind, C.M.; Diaz-Olivares, J.A.; Lindecrantz, K.; Eklund, J. A Wearable Sensor System for Physical Ergonomics Interventions Using Haptic Feedback. *Sensors* **2020**, *20*, 6010. [CrossRef]
39. Lind, C.M.; Yang, L.; Abtahi, F.; Hanson, L.; Lindecrantz, K.; Lu, K.; Forsman, M.; Eklund, J. Reducing postural load in order picking through a smart workwear system using real-time vibrotactile feedback. *Appl. Ergon.* **2020**, *89*, 103188. [CrossRef] [PubMed]
40. Lind, C.M.; De Clercq, B.; Forsman, M.; Grootaers, A.; Verbrugghe, M.; Van Dyck, L.; Yang, L. Effectiveness and usability of real-time vibrotactile feedback training to reduce postural exposure in real manual sorting work. *Ergonomics* **2023**, *66*, 198–216. [CrossRef] [PubMed]
41. Saur, P.M.; Ensink, F.B.; Frese, K.; Seeger, D.; Hildebrandt, J. Lumbar range of motion: Reliability and validity of the inclinometer technique in the clinical measurement of trunk flexibility. *Spine* **1996**, *21*, 1332–1338. [CrossRef] [PubMed]

42. Tyson, S. A Systematic Review of Methods to Measure Posture. *Phys. Ther. Rev.* **2003**, *8*, 45–50. [CrossRef]
43. Fraeulin, L.; Holzgreve, F.; Brinkbäumer, M.; Dziuba, A.; Friebe, D.; Klemz, S.; Schmitt, M.; Theis, A.A.; Tenberg, S.; van Mark, A.; et al. Intra- and inter-rater reliability of joint range of motion tests using tape measure, digital inclinometer and inertial motion capturing. *PLoS ONE* **2020**, *15*, e0243646. [CrossRef] [PubMed]
44. Bernmark, E.; Wiktorin, C. A triaxial accelerometer for measuring arm movements. *Appl. Ergon.* **2002**, *33*, 541–547. [CrossRef] [PubMed]
45. Korshøj, M.; Skotte, J.H.; Christiansen, C.S.; Mortensen, P.; Kristiansen, J.; Hanisch, C.; Ingebrigtsen, J.; Holtermann, A. Validity of the Acti4 software using ActiGraph GT3X+accelerometer for recording of arm and upper body inclination in simulated work tasks. *Ergonomics* **2014**, *57*, 247–253. [CrossRef]
46. Schall, M.C., Jr.; Fethke, N.B.; Chen, H.; Oyama, S.; Douphrate, D.I. Accuracy and repeatability of an inertial measurement unit system for field-based occupational studies. *Ergonomics* **2016**, *59*, 591–602. [CrossRef]
47. Yang, L.; Grooten, W.J.A.; Forsman, M. An iPhone application for upper arm posture and movement measurements. *Appl. Ergon.* **2017**, *65*, 492–500. [CrossRef] [PubMed]
48. Aarås, A.; Stranden, E. Measurement of postural angles during work. *Ergonomics* **1988**, *31*, 935–944. [CrossRef]
49. Barra-López, M.E. The standard posture is a myth: A scoping review. *J. Rehabil. Med.* **2024**, *56*, jrm41899. [CrossRef] [PubMed]
50. Xue, R.; Liu, D.; Shen, Y. The differences in whole-body sagittal alignment between different postures in young, healthy adults. *BMC Musculoskelet. Disord.* **2020**, *21*, 696. [CrossRef]
51. Lee, W.; Lin, J.H.; Bao, S. Inter-rater reliability of an inertial measurement unit sensor-based posture-matching method: A pilot study. *Int. J. Ind. Ergon.* **2020**, *80*, 103025. [CrossRef]
52. Fan, X.; Lind, C.M.; Rhen, I.M.; Forsman, M. Effects of Sensor Types and Angular Velocity Computational Methods in Field Measurements of Occupational Upper Arm and Trunk Postures and Movements. *Sensors* **2021**, *21*, 5527. [CrossRef]
53. Forsman, M.; Fan, X.; Rhen, I.-M.; Lind, C.M. Mind the gap—Development of conversion models between accelerometer- and IMU-based measurements of arm and trunk postures and movements in warehouse work. *Appl. Ergon.* **2022**, *105*, 103841. [CrossRef]
54. Juul-Kristensen, B.; Hansson, G.A.; Fallentin, N.; Andersen, J.H.; Ekdahl, C. Assessment of work postures and movements using a video-based observation method and direct technical measurements. *Appl. Ergon.* **2001**, *32*, 517–524. [CrossRef] [PubMed]
55. Byström, J.U.; Hansson, G.A.; Rylander, L.; Ohlsson, K.; Källrot, G.; Skerfving, S. Physical workload on neck and upper limb using two CAD applications. *Appl. Ergon.* **2002**, *33*, 63–74. [CrossRef] [PubMed]
56. Christmansson, M.; Medbo, L.; Hansson, G.Å.; Ohlsson, K.; Unge Byström, J.; Möller, T.; Forsman, M. A case study of a principally new way of materials kitting—An evaluation of time consumption and physical workload. *Int. J. Ind. Ergon.* **2002**, *30*, 49–65. [CrossRef]
57. Arvidsson, I.; Arvidsson, M.; Axmon, A.; Hansson, G.Å.; Johansson, C.R.; Skerfving, S. Musculoskeletal disorders among female and male air traffic controllers performing identical and demanding computer work. *Ergonomics* **2006**, *49*, 1052–1067. [CrossRef] [PubMed]
58. Freitag, S.; Ellegast, R.; Dulon, M.; Nienhaus, A. Quantitative measurement of stressful trunk postures in nursing professions. *Ann. Occup. Hyg.* **2007**, *51*, 385–395. [CrossRef] [PubMed]
59. Hermanns, I.; Raffler, N.; Ellegast, R.P.; Fischer, S.; Göres, B. Simultaneous field measuring method of vibration and body posture for assessment of seated occupational driving tasks. *Int. J. Ind. Ergon.* **2008**, *38*, 255–263. [CrossRef]
60. Raffler, N.; Hermanns, I.; Sayn, D.; Göres, B.; Ellegast, R.; Rissler, J. Assessing combined exposures of whole-body vibration and awkward posture--further results from application of a simultaneous field measurement methodology. *Ind. Health* **2010**, *48*, 638–644. [CrossRef] [PubMed]
61. Ribeiro, D.C.; Sole, G.; Abbott, J.H.; Milosavljevic, S. Cumulative postural exposure measured by a novel device: A preliminary study. *Ergonomics* **2011**, *54*, 858–865. [CrossRef]
62. Fethke, N.B.; Gant, L.C.; Gerr, F. Comparison of biomechanical loading during use of conventional stud welding equipment and an alternate system. *Appl. Ergon.* **2011**, *42*, 725–734. [CrossRef]
63. Freitag, S.; Fincke-Junod, I.; Seddouki, R.; Dulon, M.; Hermanns, I.; Kersten, J.F.; Larsson, T.J.; Nienhaus, A. Frequent bending—An underestimated burden in nursing professions. *Ann. Occup. Hyg.* **2012**, *56*, 697–707. [CrossRef]
64. Jonker, D.; Rolander, B.; Balogh, I.; Sandsjö, L.; Ekberg, K.; Winkel, J. Rationalisation in public dental care—Impact on clinical work tasks and mechanical exposure for dentists—A prospective study. *Ergonomics* **2013**, *56*, 303–313. [CrossRef]
65. Ciccarelli, M.; Straker, L.; Mathiassen, S.E.; Pollock, C. Posture variation among office workers when using different information and communication technologies at work and away from work. *Ergonomics* **2014**, *57*, 1678–1686. [CrossRef] [PubMed]
66. Freitag, S.; Seddouki, R.; Dulon, M.; Kersten, J.F.; Larsson, T.J.; Nienhaus, A. The effect of working position on trunk posture and exertion for routine nursing tasks: An experimental study. *Ann. Occup. Hyg.* **2014**, *58*, 317–325. [CrossRef]
67. Wahlström, J.; Bergsten, E.; Trask, C.; Mathiassen, S.E.; Jackson, J.; Forsman, M. Full-Shift Trunk and Upper Arm Postures and Movements Among Aircraft Baggage Handlers. *Ann. Occup. Hyg.* **2016**, *60*, 977–990. [CrossRef]

68. Raffler, N.; Ellegast, R.; Kraus, T.; Ochsmann, E. Factors affecting the perception of whole-body vibration of occupational drivers: An analysis of posture and manual materials handling and musculoskeletal disorders. *Ergonomics* **2016**, *59*, 48–60. [CrossRef] [PubMed]
69. Raffler, N.; Rissler, J.; Ellegast, R.; Schikowsky, C.; Kraus, T.; Ochsmann, E. Combined exposures of whole-body vibration and awkward posture: A cross sectional investigation among occupational drivers by means of simultaneous field measurements. *Ergonomics* **2017**, *60*, 1564–1575. [CrossRef]
70. Yu, D.; Dural, C.; Morrow, M.M.; Yang, L.; Collins, J.W.; Hallbeck, S.; Kjellman, M.; Forsman, M. Intraoperative workload in robotic surgery assessed by wearable motion tracking sensors and questionnaires. *Surg. Endosc.* **2017**, *31*, 877–886. [CrossRef] [PubMed]
71. Vignais, N.; Bernard, F.; Touvenot, G.; Sagot, J.-C. Physical risk factors identification based on body sensor network combined to videotaping. *Appl. Ergon.* **2017**, *65*, 410–417. [CrossRef]
72. Arias, O.E.; Umukoro, P.E.; Stoffel, S.D.; Hopcia, K.; Sorensen, G.; Dennerlein, J.T. Associations between trunk flexion and physical activity of patient care workers for a single shift: A pilot study. *Work* **2017**, *56*, 247–255. [CrossRef] [PubMed]
73. Zare, M.; Biau, S.; Brunet, R.; Roquelaure, Y. Comparison of three methods for evaluation of work postures in a truck assembly plant. *Ergonomics* **2017**, *60*, 1551–1563. [CrossRef]
74. Heiden, M.; Zetterberg, C.; Mathiassen, S.E. Trunk and upper arm postures in paper mill work. *Appl. Ergon.* **2019**, *76*, 90–96. [CrossRef]
75. Jorgensen, M.B.; Gupta, N.; Korshoj, M.; Lagersted-Olsen, J.; Villumsen, M.; Mortensen, O.S.; Skotte, J.; Sogaard, K.; Madeleine, P.; Samani, A.; et al. The DPhacto cohort: An overview of technically measured physical activity at work and leisure in blue-collar sectors for practitioners and researchers. *Appl. Ergon.* **2019**, *77*, 29–39. [CrossRef] [PubMed]
76. Thamsuwan, O.; Galvin, K.; Tchong-French, M.; Kim, J.H.; Johnson, P.W. A feasibility study comparing objective and subjective field-based physical exposure measurements during apple harvesting with ladders and mobile platforms. *J. Agromedicine* **2019**, *24*, 268–278. [CrossRef] [PubMed]
77. Thamsuwan, O.; Galvin, K.; Tchong-French, M.; Aulck, L.; Boyle, L.N.; Ching, R.P.; McQuade, K.J.; Johnson, P.W. Comparisons of physical exposure between workers harvesting apples on mobile orchard platforms and ladders, part 1: Back and upper arm postures. *Appl. Ergon.* **2020**, *89*, 103193. [CrossRef]
78. Zare, M.; Bodin, J.; Sagot, J.C.; Roquelaure, Y. Quantification of Exposure to Risk Postures in Truck Assembly Operators: Neck, Back, Arms and Wrists. *Int. J. Environ. Res. Public Health* **2020**, *17*, 6062. [CrossRef] [PubMed]
79. Holtermann, A.; Fjeldstad Hendriksen, P.; Greby Schmidt, K.; Jagd Svendsen, M.; Nørregaard Rasmussen, C.D. Physical Work Demands of Childcare Workers in Denmark: Device-Based Measurements and Workplace Observations Among 199 Childcare Workers from 16 Day Nurseries. *Ann. Work Expo. Health* **2020**, *64*, 586–595. [CrossRef]
80. Robert-Lachaine, X.; Larue, C.; Denis, D.; Delisle, A.; Mecheri, H.; Corbeil, P.; Plamondon, A. Feasibility of quantifying the physical exposure of materials handlers in the workplace with magnetic and inertial measurement units. *Ergonomics* **2020**, *63*, 283–292. [CrossRef]
81. Khan, M.I.; Bath, B.; Kociolek, A.; Zeng, X.; Koehncke, N.; Trask, C. Trunk Posture Exposure Patterns among Prairie Ranch and Grain Farmers. *J. Agromedicine* **2020**, *25*, 210–220. [CrossRef] [PubMed]
82. Porta, M.; Pau, M.; Orrù, P.F.; Nussbaum, M.A. Trunk Flexion Monitoring among Warehouse Workers Using a Single Inertial Sensor and the Influence of Different Sampling Durations. *Int. J. Environ. Res. Public Health* **2020**, *17*, 7117. [CrossRef]
83. Wilhelmsson, S.; Andersson, M.; Arvidsson, I.; Dahlqvist, C.; Hemsworth, P.H.; Yngvesson, J.; Hultgren, J. Physical workload and psychosocial working conditions in Swedish pig transport drivers. *Int. J. Ind. Ergon.* **2021**, *83*, 103124. [CrossRef]
84. Schall, M.C., Jr.; Zhang, X.; Chen, H.; Gallagher, S.; Fethke, N.B. Comparing upper arm and trunk kinematics between manufacturing workers performing predominantly cyclic and non-cyclic work tasks. *Appl. Ergon.* **2021**, *93*, 103356. [CrossRef]
85. Brents, C.; Hischke, M.; Reiser, R.; Rosecrance, J. Trunk Posture during Manual Materials Handling of Beer Kegs. *Int. J. Environ. Res. Public Health* **2021**, *18*, 7380. [CrossRef] [PubMed]
86. Kim, J.H.; Vaughan, A.; Kincl, L. Characterization of Musculoskeletal Injury Risk in Dungeness Crab Fishing. *J. Agromedicine* **2022**, *28*, 309–323. [CrossRef]
87. Nunes, M.L.; Folgado, D.; Fujão, C.; Silva, L.; Rodrigues, J.; Matias, P.; Barandas, M.; Carreiro, A.V.; Madeira, S.; Gamboa, H. Posture Risk Assessment in an Automotive Assembly Line Using Inertial Sensors. *IEEE Access* **2022**, *10*, 83221–83235. [CrossRef]
88. Rolander, B.; Forsman, M.; Ghafouri, B.; Abtahi, F.; Wåhlin, C. Measurements and observations of movements at work for warehouse forklift truck operators. *Int. J. Occup. Saf. Ergon.* **2022**, *28*, 1840–1848. [CrossRef]
89. Fan, X.; Forsman, M.; Yang, L.; Lind, C.M.; Kjellman, M. Surgeons' physical workload in open surgery versus robot-assisted surgery and nonsurgical tasks. *Surg. Endosc.* **2022**, *36*, 8178–8194. [CrossRef] [PubMed]
90. Hess, J.A.; Hecker, S.; Weinstein, M.; Lunger, M. A participatory ergonomics intervention to reduce risk factors for low-back disorders in concrete laborers. *Appl. Ergon.* **2004**, *35*, 427–441. [CrossRef]

91. Kazmierczak, K.; Mathiassen, S.E.; Forsman, M.; Winkel, J. An integrated analysis of ergonomics and time consumption in Swedish "craft-type' car disassembly. *Appl. Ergon.* **2005**, *36*, 263–273. [CrossRef] [PubMed]
92. Nowak, J.; Erbe, C.; Hauck, I.; Groneberg, D.A.; Hermanns, I.; Ellegast, R.; Ditchen, D.; Ohlendorf, D. Motion analysis in the field of dentistry: A kinematic comparison of dentists and orthodontists. *BMJ Open* **2016**, *6*, e011559. [CrossRef]
93. Schall, M.C., Jr.; Fethke, N.B.; Chen, H. Working postures and physical activity among registered nurses. *Appl. Ergon.* **2016**, *54*, 243–250. [CrossRef] [PubMed]
94. Kozak, A.; Freitag, S.; Nienhaus, A. Evaluation of a Training Program to Reduce Stressful Trunk Postures in the Nursing Professions: A Pilot Study. *Ann. Work Expo. Health* **2017**, *61*, 22–32. [CrossRef]
95. Granzow, R.F.; Schall, M.C., Jr.; Smidt, M.F.; Chen, H.; Fethke, N.B.; Huangfu, R. Characterizing exposure to physical risk factors among reforestation hand planters in the Southeastern United States. *Appl. Ergon.* **2018**, *66*, 1–8. [CrossRef] [PubMed]
96. Hauck, I.; Erbe, C.; Nowak, J.; Hermanns, I.; Ditchen, D.; Ellegast, R.; Oremek, G.; Groneberg, D.A.; Ohlendorf, D. Kinematic posture analysis of orthodontists in their daily working practice. *J. Orofac. Orthop.* **2018**, *79*, 389–402. [CrossRef]
97. Merino, G.; da Silva, L.; Mattos, D.; Guimarães, B.; Merino, E. Ergonomic evaluation of the musculoskeletal risks in a banana harvesting activity through qualitative and quantitative measures, with emphasis on motion capture (Xsens) and EMG. *Int. J. Ind. Ergon.* **2019**, *69*, 80–89. [CrossRef]
98. Merkus, S.L.; Lunde, L.K.; Koch, M.; Waersted, M.; Knardahl, S.; Veiersted, K.B. Physical capacity, occupational physical demands, and relative physical strain of older employees in construction and healthcare. *Int. Arch. Occup. Environ. Health* **2019**, *92*, 295–307. [CrossRef]
99. Fethke, N.B.; Schall, M.C., Jr.; Chen, H.; Branch, C.A.; Merlino, L.A. Biomechanical factors during common agricultural activities: Results of on-farm exposure assessments using direct measurement methods. *J. Occup. Environ. Hyg.* **2020**, *17*, 85–96. [CrossRef] [PubMed]
100. Bijanzadeh, A.; Hermanns, I.; Ellegast, R.; Fraeulin, L.; Holzgreve, F.; Mache, S.; Groneberg, D.A.; Ohlendorf, D. A kinematic posture analysis of neurological assistants in their daily working practice-a pilot study. *J. Occup. Med. Toxicol.* **2020**, *15*, 36. [CrossRef] [PubMed]
101. Loske, D.; Klumpp, M.; Keil, M.; Neukirchen, T. Logistics Work, Ergonomics and Social Sustainability: Empirical Musculoskeletal System Strain Assessment in Retail Intralogistics. *Logistics* **2021**, *5*, 89. [CrossRef]
102. Zhao, J.; Obonyo, E.; Bilén, S.G. Wearable Inertial Measurement Unit Sensing System for Musculoskeletal Disorders Prevention in Construction. *Sensors* **2021**, *21*, 1324. [CrossRef]
103. Ettinger, L.; Kincl, L.; Johnson, P.; Carter, C.; Garfinkel, S.; Karduna, A. Workday Arm Elevation Exposure: A Comparison Between Two Professions. *IISE Trans. Occup. Ergon. Hum. Factors* **2013**, *1*, 119–127. [CrossRef]
104. Hanvold, T.N.; Wærsted, M.; Mengshoel, A.M.; Bjertness, E.; Veiersted, K.B. Work with prolonged arm elevation as a risk factor for shoulder pain: A longitudinal study among young adults. *Appl. Ergon.* **2015**, *47*, 43–51. [CrossRef] [PubMed]
105. Jackson, J.A.; Mathiassen, S.E.; Wahlström, J.; Liv, P.; Forsman, M. Is what you see what you get? Standard inclinometry of set upper arm elevation angles. *Appl. Ergon.* **2015**, *47*, 242–252. [CrossRef] [PubMed]
106. Dahlqvist, C.; Nordander, C.; Forsman, M.; Enquist, H. Self-recordings of upper arm elevation during cleaning—Comparison between analyses using a simplified reference posture and a standard reference posture. *BMC Musculoskelet. Disord.* **2018**, *19*, 402. [CrossRef] [PubMed]
107. Hansson, G.Å.; Balogh, I.; Unge Byström, J.; Ohlsson, K.; Nordander, C.; Asterland, P.; Sjölander, S.; Rylander, L.; Winkel, J.; Skerfving, S. Questionnaire versus direct technical measurements in assessing postures and movements of the head, upper back, arms and hands. *Scand. J. Work Environ. Health* **2001**, *27*, 30–40. [CrossRef] [PubMed]
108. Balogh, I.; Ohlsson, K.; Hansson, G.Å.; Engström, T.; Skerfving, S. Increasing the degree of automation in a production system: Consequences for the physical workload. *Int. J. Ind. Ergon.* **2006**, *36*, 353–365. [CrossRef]
109. Jonker, D.; Rolander, B.; Balogh, I. Relation between perceived and measured workload obtained by long-term inclinometry among dentists. *Appl. Ergon.* **2009**, *40*, 309–315. [CrossRef] [PubMed]
110. Jonker, D.; Rolander, B.; Balogh, I.; Sandsjö, L.; Ekberg, K.; Winkel, J. Mechanical exposure among general practice dentists in Sweden and possible implications of rationalisation. *Ergonomics* **2011**, *54*, 953–960. [CrossRef] [PubMed]
111. Heilskov-Hansen, T.; Svendsen, S.W.; Thomsen, J.F.; Mikkelsen, S.; Hansson, G.Å. Sex differences in task distribution and task exposures among Danish house painters: An observational study combining questionnaire data with biomechanical measurements. *PLoS ONE* **2014**, *9*, e110899. [CrossRef] [PubMed]
112. Simonsen, J.G.; Dahlqvist, C.; Enquist, H.; Nordander, C.; Axmon, A.; Arvidsson, I. Assessments of Physical Workload in Sonography Tasks Using Inclinometry, Goniometry, and Electromyography. *Saf. Health Work* **2018**, *9*, 326–333. [CrossRef]
113. Unge, J.; Ohlsson, K.; Nordander, C.; Hansson, G.Å.; Skerfving, S.; Balogh, I. Differences in physical workload, psychosocial factors and musculoskeletal disorders between two groups of female hospital cleaners with two diverse organizational models. *Int. Arch. Occup. Environ. Health* **2007**, *81*, 209–220. [CrossRef]

114. Nordander, C.; Ohlsson, K.; Balogh, I.; Hansson, G.Å.; Axmon, A.; Persson, R.; Skerfving, S. Gender differences in workers with identical repetitive industrial tasks: Exposure and musculoskeletal disorders. *Int. Arch. Occup. Environ. Health* **2008**, *81*, 939–947. [CrossRef] [PubMed]
115. Wahlström, J.; Mathiassen, S.E.; Liv, P.; Hedlund, P.; Ahlgren, C.; Forsman, M. Upper arm postures and movements in female hairdressers across four full working days. *Ann. Occup. Hyg.* **2010**, *54*, 584–594. [CrossRef] [PubMed]
116. Åkesson, I.; Balogh, I.; Hansson, G.Å. Physical workload in neck, shoulders and wrists/hands in dental hygienists during a work-day. *Appl. Ergon.* **2012**, *43*, 803–811. [CrossRef] [PubMed]
117. Balogh, I.; Ohlsson, K.; Nordander, C.; Bjork, J.; Hansson, G.A. The importance of work organization on workload and musculoskeletal health—Grocery store work as a model. *Appl. Ergon.* **2016**, *53 Pt A*, 143–151. [CrossRef]
118. Wærsted, M.; Enquist, H.; Veiersted, K.B. Hairdressers' shoulder load when blow-drying—Studying the effect of a new blow dryer design on arm inclination angle and muscle pain. *Int. J. Ind. Ergon.* **2019**, *74*, 102839. [CrossRef]
119. Nourollahi-Darabad, M.; Afshari, D.; Dianat, I.; Jodakinia, L. Long-duration assessment of upper arm posture and motion and their association with perceived symptoms among bakery workers. *Int. J. Ind. Ergon.* **2020**, *80*, 103029. [CrossRef]
120. Palm, P.; Gupta, N.; Forsman, M.; Skotte, J.; Nordquist, T.; Holtermann, A. Exposure to Upper Arm Elevation During Work Compared to Leisure Among 12 Different Occupations Measured with Triaxial Accelerometers. *Ann. Work Expo. Health* **2018**, *62*, 689–698. [CrossRef] [PubMed]
121. Bruno Garza, J.L.; Eijckelhof, B.H.W.; Johnson, P.W.; Raina, S.M.; Rynell, P.W.; Huysmans, M.A.; van Dieën, J.H.; van der Beek, A.J.; Blatter, B.M.; Dennerlein, J.T. Observed differences in upper extremity forces, muscle efforts, postures, velocities and accelerations across computer activities in a field study of office workers. *Ergonomics* **2012**, *55*, 670–681. [CrossRef] [PubMed]
122. Thamsuwan, O.; Galvin, K.; Tchong-French, M.; Aulck, L.; Boyle, L.N.; Ching, R.P.; McQuade, K.J.; Johnson, P.W. Comparisons of physical exposure between workers harvesting apples on mobile orchard platforms and ladders, part 2: Repetitive upper arm motions. *Appl. Ergon.* **2020**, *89*, 103192. [CrossRef]
123. Moriguchi, C.S.; Carnaz, L.; Alencar, J.F.; Miranda Júnior, L.C.; Granqvist, L.; Hansson, G.; Gil Coury, H.J. Postures and movements in the most common tasks of power line workers. *Ind. Health* **2011**, *49*, 482–491. [CrossRef] [PubMed]
124. Moriguchi, C.S.; Carnaz, L.; Miranda Júnior, L.C.; Marklin, R.W.; Gil Coury, H.J. Are posture data from simulated tasks representative of field conditions? Case study for overhead electric utility workers. *Ergonomics* **2012**, *55*, 1382–1394. [CrossRef]
125. Moriguchi, C.S.; Carnaz, L.; Veiersted, K.B.; Hanvold, T.N.; Hæg, L.B.; Hansson, G.; Cote Gil Coury, H.J. Occupational posture exposure among construction electricians. *Appl. Ergon.* **2013**, *44*, 86–92. [CrossRef]
126. Arvidsson, I.; Hansson, G.Å.; Mathiassen, S.E.; Skerfving, S. Changes in physical workload with implementation of mouse-based information technology in air traffic control. *Int. J. Ind. Ergon.* **2006**, *36*, 613–622. [CrossRef]
127. Buchholz, B.; Park, J.S.; Gold, J.; Punnett, L. Subjective ratings of upper extremity exposures: Inter-method agreement with direct measurement of exposures. *Ergonomics* **2008**, *51*, 1064–1077. [CrossRef] [PubMed]
128. Hess, J.A.; Kincl, L.; Amasay, T.; Wolfe, P. Ergonomic evaluation of masons laying concrete masonry units and autoclaved aerated concrete. *Appl. Ergon.* **2010**, *41*, 477–483. [CrossRef] [PubMed]
129. Arvidsson, I.; Balogh, I.; Hansson, G.; Ohlsson, K.; Åkesson, I.; Nordander, C. Rationalization in meat cutting—Consequences on physical workload. *Appl. Ergon.* **2012**, *43*, 1026–1032. [CrossRef]
130. Douphrate, D.I.; Fethke, N.B.; Nonnenmann, M.W.; Rosecrance, J.C.; Reynolds, S.J. Full shift arm inclinometry among dairy parlor workers: A feasibility study in a challenging work environment. *Appl. Ergon.* **2012**, *43*, 604–613. [CrossRef]
131. Kersten, J.T.; Fethke, N.B. Radio frequency identification to measure the duration of machine-paced assembly tasks: Agreement with self-reported task duration and application in variance components analyses of upper arm postures and movements recorded over multiple days. *Appl. Ergon.* **2019**, *75*, 74–82. [CrossRef] [PubMed]
132. Veiersted, K.B.; Gould, K.S.; Osteras, N.; Hansson, G.A. Effect of an intervention addressing working technique on the biomechanical load of the neck and shoulders among hairdressers. *Appl. Ergon.* **2008**, *39*, 183–190. [CrossRef]
133. Mathiassen, S.E.; Paquet, V. The ability of limited exposure sampling to detect effects of interventions that reduce the occurrence of pronounced trunk inclination. *Appl. Ergon.* **2010**, *41*, 295–304. [CrossRef]
134. Dahlqvist, C.; Hansson, G.Å.; Forsman, M. Validity of a small low-cost triaxial accelerometer with integrated logger for uncomplicated measurements of postures and movements of head, upper back and upper arms. *Appl. Ergon.* **2016**, *55*, 108–116. [CrossRef]
135. Jackson, J.A.; Mathiassen, S.E.; Wahlström, J.; Liv, P.; Forsman, M. Digging deeper into the assessment of upper arm elevation angles using standard inclinometry. *Appl. Ergon.* **2015**, *51*, 102–103. [CrossRef]
136. Peters, A.; Galna, B.; Sangeux, M.; Morris, M.; Baker, R. Quantification of soft tissue artifact in lower limb human motion analysis: A systematic review. *Gait Posture* **2010**, *31*, 1–8. [CrossRef] [PubMed]
137. Hansson, G. Letter to the editor. Re: Is what you see what you get? Standard inclinometry of set upper arm elevation angles. *Appl. Ergon.* **2015**, *48*, 109–110. [CrossRef] [PubMed]

138. Hansson, G.A.; Arvidsson, I.; Ohlsson, K.; Nordander, C.; Mathiassen, S.E.; Skerfving, S.; Balogh, I. Precision of measurements of physical workload during standardised manual handling. Part II: Inclinometry of head, upper back, neck and upper arms. *J. Electromyogr. Kinesiol.* **2006**, *16*, 125–136. [CrossRef]
139. Lind, C.M.; Forsman, M. Accuracy of a posture measurement system for practitioners. In Proceedings of the 47th Nordic Ergonomics and Human Factors Society Conference, Lillehammer, Norway, 1–4 November 2015.
140. Lind, C.M.; Fan, X.; Rhen, I.M.; Forsman, M. *Does Posture Matter—Accuracy of Standard Calibration Procedures for Arm Inclinometry [Manuscript in Preparation]*; Institute of Environmental Medicine, Karolinska Institutet: Stockholm, Sweden, 2024.
141. Forsman, M.; Fan, X.; Rhén, I.M.; Lind, C.M. Concerning a Work Movement Velocity Action Level Proposed in "Action Levels for the Prevention of Work-Related Musculoskeletal Disorders in the Neck and Upper Extremities: A Proposal" by Inger Arvidsson et al. (2021). *Ann. Work Expo. Health* **2022**, *66*, 130–131. [CrossRef] [PubMed]
142. Hanson, L.; Sperling, L.; Gard, G.; Ipsen, S.; Olivares Vergara, C. Swedish anthropometrics for product and workplace design. *Appl. Ergon.* **2009**, *40*, 797–806. [CrossRef] [PubMed]
143. Fryar, C.D.; Carroll, M.D.; Gu, Q.; Afful, J.; Ogden, C.L. Anthropometric Reference Data for Children and Adults: United States, 2015–2018. In *Vital & Health Statistics. Series 3, Analytical and Epidemiological Studies*; Centers for Disease Control and Prevention National Center for Health Statistics: Hyattsville, MD, USA, 2021; pp. 1–44.
144. Hoareau, D.; Fan, X.; Abtahi, F.; Yang, L. Evaluation of In-Cloth versus On-Skin Sensors for Measuring Trunk and Upper Arm Postures and Movements. *Sensors* **2023**, *23*, 3969. [CrossRef] [PubMed]
145. Stock, S.R.; Fernandes, R.; Delisle, A.; Vézina, N. Reproducibility and validity of workers' self-reports of physical work demands. *Scand. J. Work Environ. Health* **2005**, *31*, 409–437. [CrossRef]
146. Koch, M.; Lunde, L.K.; Gjulem, T.; Knardahl, S.; Veiersted, K.B. Validity of Questionnaire and Representativeness of Objective Methods for Measurements of Mechanical Exposures in Construction and Health Care Work. *PLoS ONE* **2016**, *11*, e0162881. [CrossRef]
147. Barriera-Viruet, H.; Sobeih, T.M.; Daraiseh, N.; Salem, S. Questionnaires vs observational and direct measurements: A systematic review. *Theor. Issues Ergon. Sci.* **2006**, *7*, 261–284. [CrossRef]
148. Nyman, T.; Rhén, I.M.; Johansson, P.J.; Eliasson, K.; Kjellberg, K.; Lindberg, P.; Fan, X.; Forsman, M. Reliability and Validity of Six Selected Observational Methods for Risk Assessment of Hand Intensive and Repetitive Work. *Int. J. Environ. Res. Public Health* **2023**, *20*, 5505. [CrossRef] [PubMed]

Disclaimer/Publisher's Note: The statements, opinions and data contained in all publications are solely those of the individual author(s) and contributor(s) and not of MDPI and/or the editor(s). MDPI and/or the editor(s) disclaim responsibility for any injury to people or property resulting from any ideas, methods, instructions or products referred to in the content.

bioengineering

MDPI

Article

Digitalized 3D Spinal Decompression and Correction Device Improved Initial Brace Corrections and Patients' Comfort Among Adolescents with Idiopathic Scoliosis: A Single-Centre, Single-Blinded Randomized Controlled Trial

Yi Jie [1,2,3,†], Mengyao Li [2,3,†], Anqin Dong [2,3], Yu-Yan Luo [1], Chang-Liang Luo [1], Jing Li [2], Pengyuan Zheng [2,3], Xinmin Zhang [4], Man Sang Wong [1,*], Christina Zong-Hao Ma [1,5,6,*] and Ming Zhang [1,5]

1 Department of Biomedical Engineering, The Hong Kong Polytechnic University, Hong Kong SAR, China; yi620.jie@connect.polyu.hk (Y.J.); yuyan-laura.luo@connect.polyu.hk (Y.-Y.L.); chang-liang.luo@connect.polyu.hk (C.-L.L.); ming.zhang@polyu.edu.hk (M.Z.)
2 Department of Rehabilitation Medical Engineering, The Fifth Affiliated Hospital of Zhengzhou University, Zhengzhou 450052, China; mengyao0930@outlook.com (M.L.); anqindong@163.com (A.D.); jingliljlj@163.com (J.L.); medp7123@126.com (P.Z.)
3 Research Institute of Rehabilitation Medicine, Henan Academy of Innovations in Medical Science, Zhengzhou 450000, China
4 Zhengzhou Feilong Medical Equipment Co., Ltd., Zhengzhou 450000, China; 17737316777@163.com
5 Research Institute for Sports Science and Technology, The Hong Kong Polytechnic University, Hong Kong SAR, China
6 Research Institute for Smart Ageing, The Hong Kong Polytechnic University, Hong Kong SAR, China
* Correspondence: m.s.wong@polyu.edu.hk (M.S.W.); czh.ma@polyu.edu.hk (C.Z.-H.M.); Tel.: +852-2766-7680 (M.S.W.); +852-2766-7671 (C.Z.-H.M.); Fax: +852-2334-2429 (M.S.W. & C.Z.-H.M.)
† These authors contributed equally to this work.

Abstract: This study aimed to evaluate the efficacy of a novel three-dimensional (3D) spinal decompression and correction device in improving the in-brace correction and patient comfort level for adolescents with idiopathic scoliosis (AIS), and to assess the impact of the number of vertebrae involved in the scoliotic curve on the correction's effectiveness. A single-centre, single-blinded randomized controlled trial (RCT) was conducted in 110 AIS patients aged 10–18 years who were randomly allocated into four groups receiving 0–3 days of device intervention. Each session lasted for 30 min and was conducted twice daily. Significant improvements were observed in both the in-brace correction ratio and patient comfort level, particularly in the 2- and 3-day intervention groups ($p < 0.001$). The number of involved vertebrae for a scoliotic curve was positively correlated with the in-brace correction ratio in the no intervention (or 0-day) and 1-day intervention groups, while this correlation varied in the 2- and 3-day intervention groups. These findings suggested that the prolonged use of the 3D device could improve the correction ratios and patient comfort, while the role of vertebrae involvement in predicting the initial correction may require further exploration to optimize personalized treatment strategies in future clinical practice.

Keywords: adolescent idiopathic scoliosis (AIS); in-brace correction; patient comfort; prognosis; vertebral number; 3D spinal decompression and correction; randomized controlled trial

1. Introduction

Scoliosis is a common skeletal deformity affecting adolescents worldwide [1], and is characterized by the lateral curvature and rotation of the spine [2]. This condition not only affects the appearance of the affected individuals [3], but may also have long-term effects on their respiratory function and cardiac health [4,5]. Treatment options for scoliosis primarily include surgical and non-surgical approaches, with the non-surgical treatment often involving the use of spinal orthoses or braces, particularly for scoliotic cases with mild-to-moderate severity [6,7].

Brace treatment has been an effective method to prevent the progression of scoliosis and, as a result, to avoid the need for surgical intervention. Extensive research supports the positive role of brace treatments in delaying or reversing the progression of scoliosis [6–9]. However, its success rate can be influenced by various factors, including the design of the brace, the duration of wearing time by the patient, and patient adherence [10–12]. Nevertheless, the patient's comfort when wearing the brace is a key factor affecting patient compliance [13]. Patient discomfort, including that caused by the excessive friction and pressure from brace and the psychological distress related to one's self-image, can significantly impact the effectiveness of the treatment [13]. Discomfort when wearing the brace not only reduces the duration of wearing time by the patient but also directly affects the correction outcomes, ultimately deteriorating the effectiveness of the treatment [14]. It is essential to develop an approach to address the discomfort issue and improve brace treatment outcomes.

The effectiveness of in-brace correction has been considered as an important basis for predicting the final corrective outcomes for scoliosis. Van den Bogaart et al. assessed the predictive factors of brace treatment in AIS in a review, and reported that an insufficient initial correction within the brace is strongly correlated with treatment failure [15]. This indicates that the effectiveness of the initial correction is a key indicator of the success or failure of brace treatment. Research by Xu et al. demonstrated that the initial correction rate (ICR) within the brace (or in-brace correction) can serve as a predictor for the effectiveness of brace treatment, and that a higher ICR is associated with a higher probability of successful treatment outcomes [16]. All these studies support the adoption of in-brace correction to evaluate and predict the effectiveness of a brace to correct scoliotic curvature during the initial fitting in patients with AIS. In addition to in-brace correction, there might also be some additional factors contributing to the effectiveness of brace treatment outcomes, including the number of vertebrae in a scoliotic curve, which has not been studied before and merits further exploration.

To further improve brace treatment effectiveness, this study conducted a single-centre double-blinded randomized controlled trial (RCT) and explored the effectiveness of a novel 3D spinal decompression correction device in treating patients with adolescent idiopathic scoliosis (AIS). It was hypothesized that this device could enhance the in-brace correction efficiency and improve patient comfort by employing longitudinal traction, lateral three-point corrective force, and axial rotational adjustments. This study also assessed the impact of the number of vertebrae involved in a scoliotic curvature on the in-brace correction ratio and explored whether the developed treatment protocol with the device could mitigate the influence of vertebral number discrepancies on correction outcomes. This approach is expected to provide more effective non-surgical treatment options than the existing ones for patients with AIS.

2. Materials and Methods

2.1. Study Design

This single-centre, double-blinded (for outcome assessors and statisticians) RCT was conducted from May 2023 to February 2024 in the Department of Rehabilitation Medical Engineering at The Fifth Affiliated Hospital of Zhengzhou University. The research protocol was approved by the Ethics Committee of The Fifth Affiliated Hospital of Zhengzhou University (Reference number: KY2022028; Date: 23 June 2022) and followed the tenets of the Declaration of Helsinki. Signed informed consent forms were obtained from all participants and their guardians before the study. This study was retrospectively registered on 15 May 2024 in the World Health Organization (WHO) International Clinical Trials Registry Platform (ICTRP)—Chinese Clinical Trial Registry (Reference number: ChiCTR2400084383).

2.2. Participants

All patients were recruited at the outpatient clinic of the Department of Rehabilitation Medical Engineering at The Fifth Affiliated Hospital of Zhengzhou University. Patients diagnosed with AIS who met the eligibility criteria were recruited. Clinical diagnoses were made by a spine specialist with over 10 years of clinical experience. The inclusion criteria were as follows: 10–18 years old, diagnosed with AIS, met the criteria for brace treatment (a Cobb angle between 20 and 45 degrees), and a Risser sign grade of 0–4. The exclusion criteria were as follows: with a history of cardiovascular disease, neuromuscular disorder, psychiatric disorder, or prior conservative intervention for scoliosis.

A total of 110 patients diagnosed with scoliosis met the eligibility criteria and participated in this study. Researchers obtained the written informed consent from patients and their guardians at the outpatient clinic before data collection.

2.3. Randomization and Blinding

Randomization was conducted in a 1:1:1:1 ratio. The randomization sequence was prepared in advance by an independent statistician. The opaque envelopes containing the allocated intervention group numbers were also prepared by the same independent statistician. The original randomization list was kept confidential by the independent statistician and was not disclosed to the researchers. The random envelopes were opened in the presence of at least two individuals when the patients were recruited at the outpatient clinic. Due to the nature of the study, the blinding of therapists and AIS participants was not feasible. However, the study maintained blinding for the outcome assessors and data analysts to ensure their impartiality during patient evaluation and data analysis.

2.4. Intervention

The research team has developed an innovative 3D spinal decompression and correction device for patients with AIS. This device comprised a control platform, a longitudinal traction cable/band, a lateral three-point correction assembly, and an axial rotational adjustment mechanism located on the treatment bed. The device operated by alternately applying the corrective longitudinal traction force, lateral three-point force, and rotational force. It can be adapted to correct various types of scoliosis with different Cobb angles in patients with AIS. Specifically, the two pairs of pneumatical pressure pads (correction and counteracting/stabilizing pads) of the lateral three-point correction assembly had inflatable air bladders. The embedded force transducers in the bladders could measure and display the instantaneous lateral passive force being applied. The available longitudinal traction force generated by the traction cable/band ranged from 0 to 666 N, and the lateral corrective force generated by the three-point corrective component ranged from 0 to 500 N. The distraction impulse was 58.1 N/s, and the time error between generating longitudinal traction and lateral passive force was within 0.6 s. The traction intensity, traction mode (static or intermittent), pulling angle, and traction duration could be selected in the user interface system (Figure 1).

During the intervention, patients received a 28-min digitalized 3D scoliosis correction intervention session consisting of 7 intervention cycles, as instructed by the same certified physical therapist. Each 4-min intervention cycle included, firstly, a 2-min stretching phase with gradually increasing longitudinal traction forces and decreasing lateral corrective forces (reaching the maximum and minimum values at the end of the trial, respectively), followed by a 2-min resting phase with gradually decreasing longitudinal traction forces and increasing lateral corrective forces (reaching the minimum and maximum values at the end of the trial). The provision of longitudinal traction was derived from the treatment protocol of mechanical spinal traction for patients with low back pain [17], initiating at an intensity that did not exceed 50% of the participant's body weight [18] and maintaining an angle that was parallel to the spine (pulling angle = 0 degree). The lateral corrective forces were manually applied to patients, with reference to each patient's coronal radiographies and the three-point pressure system [19], by adjusting the position of the pressure pads on the apical vertebra directly or on the corresponding ribs. Reactive forces were also applied to the upper and end vertebrae and pelvis using pressure pads to prevent body shifting, following the guidelines of the three-point pressure system. The provision of lateral corrective force adhered to the criteria that equalled to 330 N or the maximum lateral corrective force that each patient could tolerate, whichever was the smaller force value.

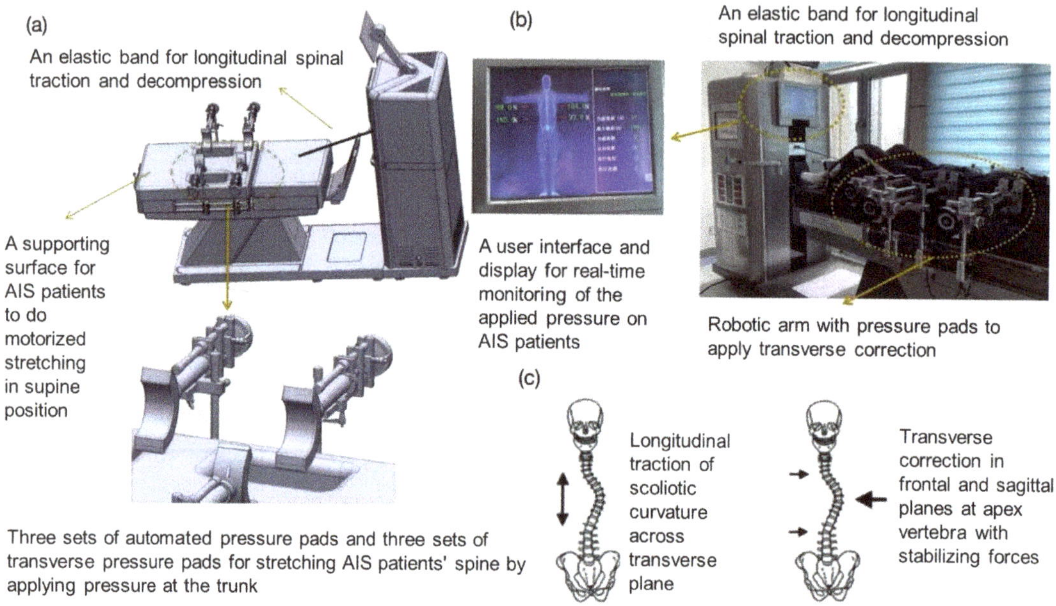

Figure 1. Diagram of the 3D spinal decompression and correction device: (**a**) schematic diagram of the novel 3D spinal decompression and correction device; (**b**) an example of applying automated spinal longitudinal traction, lateral correction, and axial rotation protocol in a patient with AIS; and (**c**) application of longitudinal traction and transverse correction on a scoliotic curve.

In this study, AIS participants were randomly assigned to one of four groups. The control group received no device treatment (Group 1, no intervention or 0-day group); the first experimental group underwent 1 day of treatment with the device (Group 2, 1-day group); the second experimental group received 2 consecutive days of treatment with the device (Group 3, 2-day group); and the third experimental group received 3 consecutive days of treatment with the device (Group 4, 3-day group). The dosage of the device treatment was twice per day, with each session lasting for approximately 30 min. All device treatments were completed the day before the fitting of the orthotic braces.

All orthotic braces were designed by a senior certified orthotist with 20 years of clinical experience using computer-aided design (CAD) software (Version18.0.4, Orthotics and Prosthetics CAD, Canfit™, Vorum, Vancouver, BC, Canada). The design criterion was to achieve a correction of the patient's in-brace Cobb angle to zero degrees, indicating a full correction, in the software simulation. The orthotic brace was finalized and adjusted by the same senior certified orthotist, who also provided guidance on its wearing to each of the AIS participants. After achieving the optimal fit, an in-brace X-ray was taken for each participant to measure the in-brace Cobb angle (Figure 2).

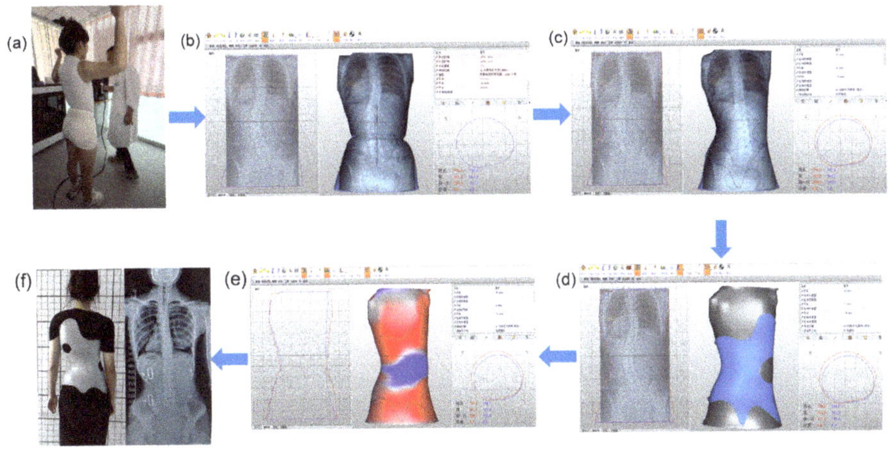

Figure 2. Manufacturing process of the scoliosis brace based on CAD/CAM for each AIS participant: (**a**) scanning of a patient with AIS; (**b**) importing the scanned model and the patient's X-ray into the software for brace design; (**c**) computer-aided simulation of the correction outcome; (**d**) illustration of the brace's appearance; (**e**) computer-aided simulation of the pressure applied by the brace on the patient's body surface; and (**f**) brace fitting and in-brace X-ray of the same patient with AIS. Explanation of lines and regions in (**b–e**): the red line represents the original spinal model contour, and the blue line represents the adjusted contour. In (**b**), before design adjustments, the red and blue lines overlap. In (**e**), the red regions indicate areas of pressure applied by the brace, with darker shades representing higher pressure levels, while blue regions represent areas where pressure has been relieved. White regions correspond to areas with no significant pressure adjustment.

2.5. Outcome Measures

2.5.1. Primary Outcomes

This study focused on two primary outcomes:

1. In-brace Correction Ratio: Immediately after the patients wore the spinal braces, an X-ray examination was conducted to measure the in-brace Cobb angle (Figure 3a). The in-brace correction ratio was calculated using the following equation:

$$\text{In-Brace Correction Ratio} = (\text{Pre-brace Cobb Angle} - \text{In-brace Cobb Angle})/(\text{Pre-brace Cobb Angle}) \quad (1)$$

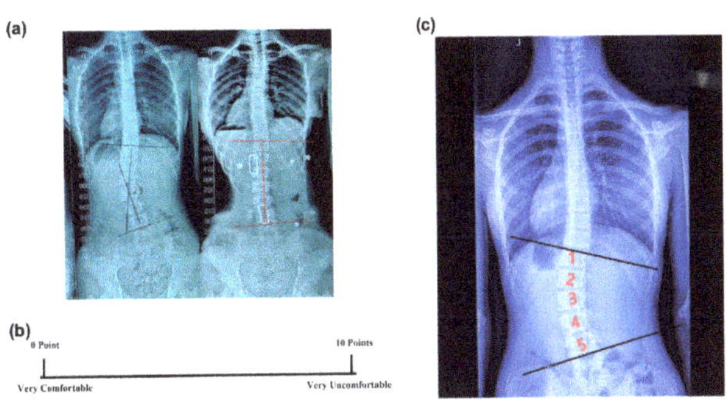

Figure 3. Primary and secondary outcome measures: (**a**) measurement of the pre-brace Cobb angle and in-brace Cobb angle; (**b**) comfort level assessed using a visual analogue scale (VAS); and (**c**) number of vertebrae within a scoliotic curvature.

This ratio could provide a quantitative measure of how effectively the brace corrected the scoliosis curvature (Figure 3a).

2. Visual Analogue Scale (VAS): After fitting the brace, the VAS was used to assess a subject's comfort level [20]. The scale ranged from 0 to 10, with 0 meaning very comfortable and 10 meaning very uncomfortable (Figure 3b). This rating was given independently by the patient to ensure an unbiased assessment of their comfort level while wearing the brace.

2.5.2. Secondary Outcomes

The number of vertebrae involved in a scoliotic curve based on the Cobb angle measurement was also analyzed. It was measured by counting the number of all the vertebrae from the upper end vertebra to the lower end vertebra of a scoliotic curve on the X-ray (Figure 3c). Whether the variations in the number of vertebrae affected the in-brace correction ratio, and whether the treatment with the device could mitigate this impact, were examined. Additionally, the correlation between the number of vertebrae and the correction ratio was analyzed.

2.6. Statistical Analysis

All statistical analyses of the collected data were performed using the IBM SPSS Statistics 26.0 software package (IBM Corp; Armonk, NY, USA). The normality of the variables was assessed using the Kolmogorov–Smirnov test. Analyses of variance (ANOVAs) were conducted to compare the differences in the in-brace correction ratios and comfort scores at baseline among the four groups. Post-hoc comparisons were performed using the least significant difference (LSD) method to identify the existence of specific between-group significant differences whenever a significant F-test result was obtained in the ANOVA.

Subjects were also divided into two groups based on the number of vertebrae involved in the scoliosis curvature: one group included individuals with a vertebral count below the median, and the other included those with a vertebral count above the median. The Mann–Whitney U test was then used to compare the in-brace correction ratios between these two groups. Pearson's correlation analysis was used to explore the relationship between the number of vertebrae and the in-brace correction ratio. A two-tailed p-value of less than 0.05 was considered statistically significant.

3. Results

3.1. Participant Characteristics

As shown in Figure 4, between 1 May 2023 and 27 February 2024, a total of 141 patients were assessed for eligibility, of whom 116 met the inclusion criteria and did not meet the exclusion criteria. Finally, a total of 110 eligible patients participated in the study, as 6 patients refused to participate and withdrew from the study (Figure 4).

The baseline characteristics of the participants are presented in Table 1. The mean age of the entire cohort was 14.40 (standard deviation [SD] = 1.94) years. There were 83 (72%) female patients and 32 (28%) male patients, with an average age of 14.27 (SD = 1.96) years and 14.74 (SD = 2.08) years, respectively. During the trial, the per-protocol analysis included 110 patients: 30 (27%) in the control, or 0-day, group; 28 (25%) in the 1-day intervention group; 24 (22%) in the 2 day intervention group; and 28 (25%) in the 3 day intervention group. The Kolmogorov–Smirnov test indicated that the study variables were normally distributed across the four groups at baseline ($p > 0.05$), allowing for the use of an ANOVA to assess the baseline characteristics of the patients. This analysis further confirmed that the characteristics were balanced across the four control and experimental groups.

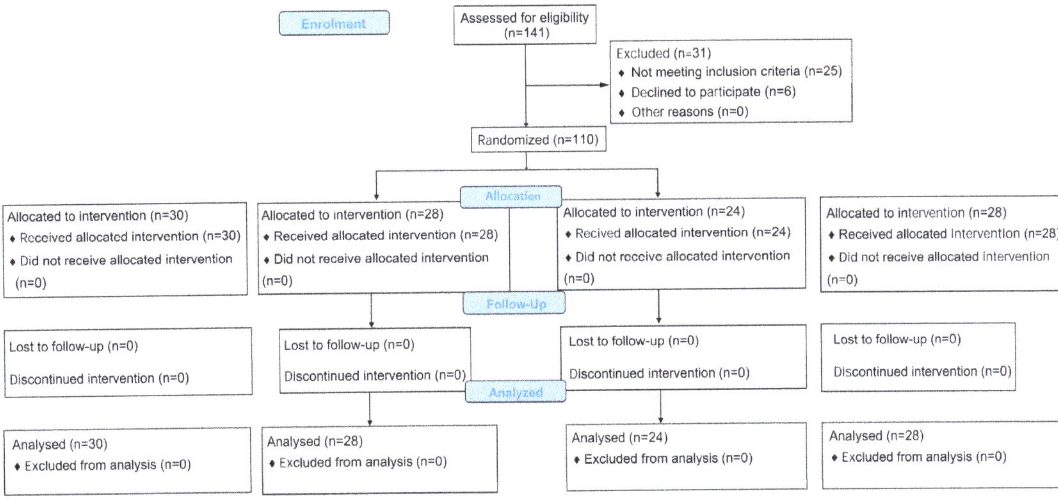

Figure 4. CONSORT 2010 flow diagram of this study.

Table 1. Baseline characteristics of the patients (n = 110).

Subject Demographics	0-Day Control (n = 30)	1-Day Intervention (n = 28)	2-Day Intervention (n = 24)	3-Day Intervention (n = 28)	p-Value (ANOVA)
Age (years), Mean (SD)	13.97 (2.03)	14.14 (1.60)	14.79 (2.65)	14.71 (1.60)	0.325
Gender, n (%)					
Female	20 (18.20%)	23 (20.90%)	17 (15.50%)	23 (20.90%)	
Male	10 (9.09%)	5 (4.55%)	7 (6.36%)	5 (4.55%)	
Curve type, n (%)					
STC	3 (2.73%)	2 (1.82%)	6 (5.45%)	5 (4.55%)	
SL/TLC	12 (10.91%)	9 (8.18%)	8 (7.27%)	5 (4.55%)	
DC	15 (13.64%)	17 (15.45%)	10 (9.09%)	18 (16.36%)	
Risser Sign, Mean (SD)	2.60 (1.16)	2.71 (1.08)	2.81 (1.17)	2.79 (0.96)	0.940
Cobb angle, Mean (SD)					
T Cobb angle	24.78 (7.22)	25.89 (7.08)	28.58 (9.16)	29.36 (6.89)	0.091
L/TL Cobb angle	25.52 (7.24)	27.27 (7.95)	28.39 (7.18)	30.74 (7.32)	0.104

(SD: standard deviation; T: thoracic curvature; L: lumbar curvature; TL: thoracolumbar curvature.)

3.2. In-Brace Correction Ratios

As shown in Figure 5, for the thoracic scoliosis curves, the mean in-brace correction ratio was significantly improved in the 2-day intervention (0.83 ± 0.76) and 3-day intervention (0.81 ± 0.11) groups as compared with the 0-day control group (0.68 ± 0.13) ($p < 0.01$). Additionally, the mean in-brace correction ratio was significantly different between the 1-day intervention (0.70 ± 0.12) and 3-day intervention (0.81 ± 0.11) groups ($p < 0.05$).

Similarly, for the lumbar and thoracolumbar curves, the in-brace correction ratio was significantly increased in the 2-day intervention (0.85 ± 0.11) and 3-day intervention (0.85 ± 0.13) groups compared with the 0-day control group (0.69 ± 0.19) ($p < 0.05$). No significant differences were observed in other pairwise comparisons (Figure 5).

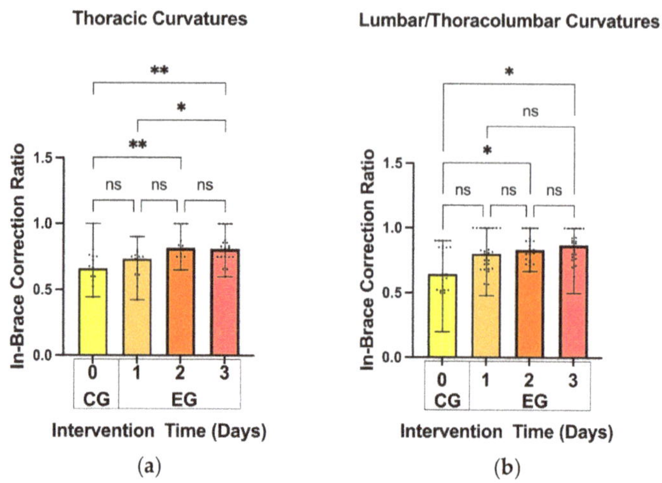

Figure 5. Comparison of the in-brace correction ratios among different control and experimental groups for the (**a**) thoracic and (**b**) lumbar/thoracolumbar curvatures. (Note: ns: no significance; *: $p < 0.05$; **: $p < 0.01$; CG: control group; EG: experimental group).

3.3. Patient Comfort Level While Wearing the Fitted Brace

The results of the ANOVAs and LSD post-hoc tests revealed significant differences regarding the patients' comfort levels while wearing the fitted brace. In particular, the mean comfort score was substantially increased in the 2-day intervention (6.96 ± 1.31, 36.2% increase) and 3-day intervention (7.43 ± 1.48, 45.4% increase) groups as compared with the 0-day control group (5.11 ± 1.10) ($p < 0.001$). Significant improvements in the mean comfort score were also observed in the 2-day intervention (6.96 ± 1.31, 21.0% increase; $p < 0.01$) and 3-day intervention (7.43 ± 1.48, 29.2% increase; $p < 0.001$) groups compared with the 1-day intervention group (5.75 ± 1.40) (Figure 6).

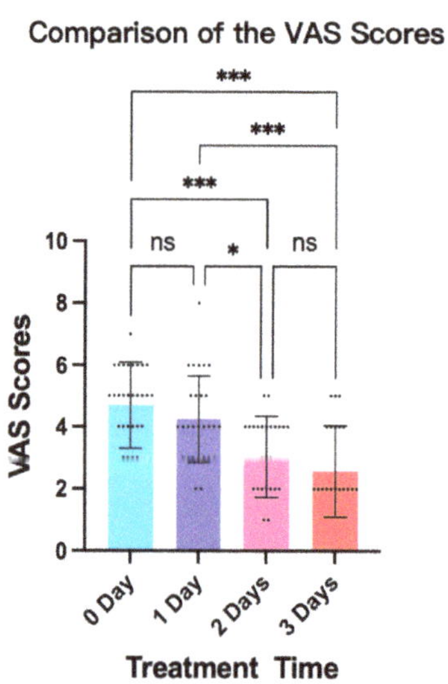

Figure 6. Comparison of the VAS scores of patients' comfort levels. (Note: ns: no significance; *: $p < 0.05$; ***: $p < 0.001$).

3.4. Impact of the Number of Vertebrae Involved in Scoliosis Curvature on the In-Brace Correction's Effectiveness

The participants with thoracic scoliosis had a median number of seven vertebrae within a scoliotic curvature, while those with lumbar/thoracolumbar curves had a median number of six. Based on these medians, subjects were further divided into different groups: thoracic curves (number of vertebrae <7 and ≥7) and lumbar/thoracolumbar curves (number of vertebrae <6 and ≥6). Due to the lack of significant differences between the control group and 1-day intervention group and between the 2-day and 3-day intervention groups, the analysis was further divided into two broader categories for comparison: 0–1 day of intervention vs. 2–3 days of intervention (Figure 7a).

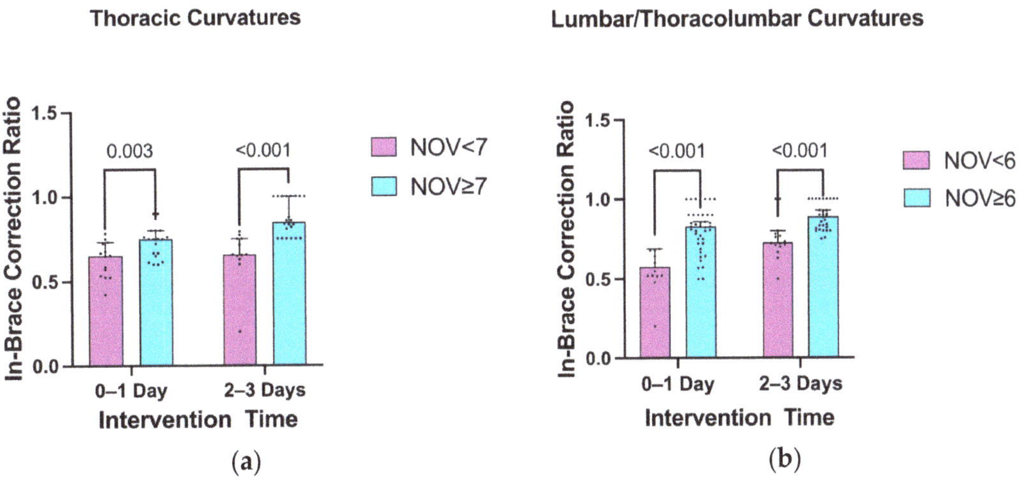

Figure 7. Comparison of the in-brace correction ratio in the (**a**) thoracic and (**b**) lumbar/thoracolumbar curvatures with various numbers of vertebrae (NOV).

For the 0–1-day intervention group, patients with thoracic curves involving ≥7 vertebrae had a significantly better in-brace correction ratio than those with <7 vertebrae ($p = 0.003$). Similarly, in the 2–3-day intervention group, patients with ≥7 vertebrae in their thoracic curves also showed a significantly better correction ratio than those with <7 vertebrae ($p < 0.001$). A similar pattern was observed in the lumbar/thoracolumbar curve groups. In both the 0–1-day and 2–3-day intervention groups, patients with ≥6 vertebrae in their lumbar/thoracolumbar curves exhibited significantly better in-brace correction ratios than those with <6 vertebrae ($p < 0.001$) (Figure 7b).

Correlation tests confirmed that, for patients receiving 0–1 day of the intervention, there was a low positive correlation between the number of vertebrae and the initial in-brace correction ratio for both the thoracic (r = 0.248, $p = 0.004$) and the lumbar/thoracolumbar (r = 0.075, $p = 0.049$) curves. For patients receiving 2–3 days of the intervention, there was a low positive correlation between the number of vertebrae and the initial in-brace correction effectiveness for the lumbar/thoracolumbar curves (r = 0.220, $p < 0.001$), whereas no correlation was observed for the thoracic curves (Figure 8).

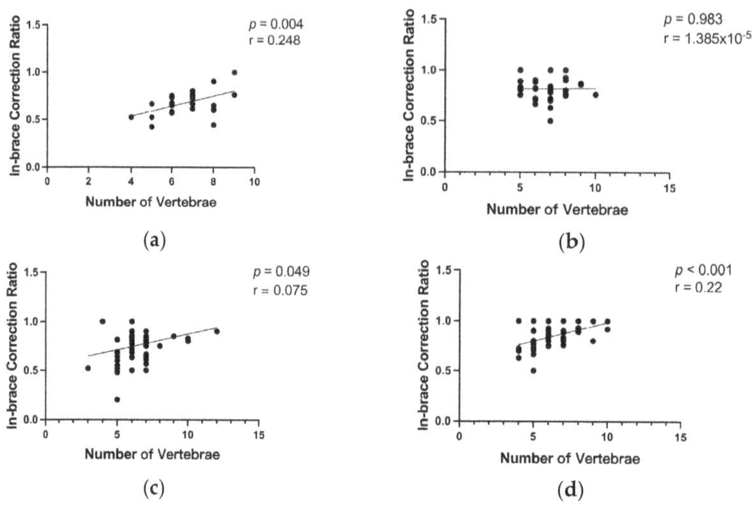

Figure 8. Correlation between the number of vertebrae and the in-brace correction ratio in (**a**) thoracic curves for the 0–1-day intervention group; (**b**) thoracic curves for the 2–3-day intervention group; (**c**) lumbar/thoracolumbar curves for the 0–1-day intervention group; and (**d**) lumbar/thoracolumbar curves for the 2–3-day intervention group.

4. Discussion

This study evaluated the therapeutic effects of an innovative 3D spinal decompression and correction device in patients with AIS and explored the impact of the number of vertebrae within the scoliotic curvature on the effectiveness of the in-brace correction by conducting a single-centre, double-blinded RCT on 110 patients with AIS. By preliminarily integrating the traditional brace therapy with more advanced assistive robotic technology, this study delved into a new domain in the conservative treatment of scoliosis, offering a more effective and user-friendly treatment option. Although the current results are preliminary, the current study still provides valuable insights for the future development and optimization of treatment strategies. More details can be found below.

The primary finding of this study is that applying the novel 3D spinal decompression and correction device in patients with AIS could significantly enhance in-brace correction ratios. Notable improvements in the in-brace correction ratios were observed for both the thoracic and the lumbar/thoracolumbar curves. In particular, the treatments lasting for more than 2 consecutive days demonstrated more significant effects than that of no treatment or only 1 day of treatment in participants. This could be explained by increased spinal flexibility [21], which was supported by our previous pilot study that showed that the proposed treatment could significantly increase the flexibility of the trunk in forward bending and lateral bending tests in patients with AIS [22]. A previous systematic review also supported that, among all factors, increased spinal flexibility has been a favourable predictive factor for improved initial in-brace corrections [23]. This review supported our hypothesis and the positive effect of the developed treatment protocol on treating scoliosis. To further verify this finding, future studies may consider utilizing some non-invasive evaluation techniques, such as ultrasound imaging [24–26] and photogrammetry [27], to evaluate and compare the difference in scoliotic curvature before and after the treatment. While the thoracic in-brace correction ratio continued to increase after receiving the treatment for more than two days (i.e., 1-day vs. 3-day treatment), there was no significant difference for the lumbar/thoracolumbar curves. This may be because traction and lateral forces have a more direct impact on the soft tissues of the lumbar spine, allowing for quick results with short-term treatments [28]. However, for the thoracic spine, traction appeared to take a longer time to be effective. Additionally, due to the ribs, the effect of lateral forces in releasing the soft tissues of the thoracic spine gradually improved as treatment progressed [29]. Future studies need to further investigate treatment dosage and changes in soft tissues during the treatment process to validate our hypothesis.

The secondary finding of this study is that AIS patients' comfort level during the initial brace fitting, as measured directly using a VAS, significantly improved after receiving treatment with the novel 3D spinal decompression and correction device. This improvement was especially evident in patients who received more than two days of treatment, which may also be related to the increased spinal flexibility following the treatment. The combination of traction with substantial lateral corrective forces allows for the stretching of the original tense paravertebral muscle contractures, thus reducing the discomfort of affected muscles during the initial brace fitting. Previous studies have reported that discomfort while wearing a brace affected the treatment outcome due to excessive friction and pressure [13] and reduced wearing time [14] in patients with AIS. The improved appearance and wearing comfort level of the brace can significantly improve patients' psychological acceptance and compliance [30]. A systematic review by Negrini et al. also indicated that brace treatment did not significantly improve the quality of life or mental health status of adolescents [7]. While the VAS is a commonly used tool to assess comfort levels, it is important to note that its results can be influenced by individual differences, such as pain tolerance, mood, and personal perceptions, which may limit its reliability and standardization [20]. Therefore, future studies may need to cross-validate the findings with additional assessment methods to provide a more comprehensive evaluation of treatment effectiveness. The positive findings of the current study supported the feasibility of reducing patients' discomfort levels during their initial brace fitting by utilizing this novel 3D spinal decompression and correction technology. Significantly improved comfort of patients during the initial brace fitting can help them adapt to the brace treatment more quickly. This improvement is expected to enhance patients' acceptance of brace treatment, increase compliance, elongate effective brace wearing times, and ultimately, enhance the overall effectiveness of conservative brace treatments for scoliosis. Further studies are still needed to explore and identify an optimal treatment protocol that balances not only treatment outcomes but also cost-effectiveness for patients. Long-term studies investigating the patient compliance in wearing the braces after receiving the developed novel 3D spinal decompression and correction treatment could also be conducted in the future.

It is also interesting to observe that a greater number of vertebrae involved within a scoliotic curvature has been associated with improved effectiveness of in-brace correction in patients with AIS. This is in line with a previous study that evaluated and reported a significant, negative correlation between the coronal deformity angle ratio (C-DAR) and in-brace correction ($r = -0.69$), indicating that in-brace correction is less effective in patients with a higher C-DAR [31]. The finding of the current study further supported that a reduced number of vertebrae may contribute to a smaller coronal deformity angle ratio, leading to reduced effectiveness of in-brace corrections. This may be due to the fact that fewer vertebrae within one scoliotic curvature may lead to a shorter lever arm and/or reduced space to provide the corrective force or pressure via the brace. This finding suggests that the patient's anatomical spinal characteristics, particularly the number of vertebrae within one specific scoliosis curvature, need to be carefully revised and considered when developing treatment plans.

There are several limitations that need to be acknowledged for this pilot study. Firstly, all the braces were designed using a CAD system and simulated within the computer system to ensure that the simulated effects could achieve full correction of the spine. However, there were discrepancies between the computer simulations and the actual initial fitting results. Such differences may be related to the varied muscular states of different patients' trunks, and it is anticipated that the developed device could potentially reduce these discrepancies to some extent. Secondly, the sample size was relatively small for a clinical trial, and only a single medical centre was involved in data collection. Further validation is still required through larger-scale and multi-centre studies. Additionally, this study lacks a long-term follow-up to monitor the prolonged compliance with brace wearing and long-term changes in the Cobb angle in participating patients with AIS. A muti-centre RCT with a large sample size, long-term follow-up, and high-quality study design will be conducted in the future to identify the optimal treatment for patients with AIS.

5. Conclusions

In summary, the results of this study supported the notion that using the novel 3D spinal decompression and correction device can significantly enhance and in-brace correction's effectiveness and a patient's comfort level when wearing the brace in patients with AIS. Additionally, the number of vertebrae was positively correlated with the effectiveness of the in-brace correction during the initial fitting of spinal orthosis for patients with AIS. The findings of this pilot study could provide important clinical guidance for future treatment of scoliosis and offer valuable insights for future studies and clinical practice in this field.

Author Contributions: Y.J. contributed to the study's conception, study design, data collection and analysis, data interpretation, and the draft of the manuscript. M.L. contributed to data collection and analysis, data interpretation, and the draft of the manuscript. A.D. and Y.-Y.L. contributed to data collection and analysis, data interpretation, and editing the manuscript. C.-L.L., J.L. and P.Z. contributed to data analysis, data interpretation, and editing the manuscript. X.Z. contributed to system development and editing the manuscript. M.S.W. and M.Z. contributed to data interpretation, project supervision, and editing the manuscript. C.Z.-H.M. contributed to study conception, study design, data analysis and interpretation, project supervision, and the draft of the manuscript. All authors have read and agreed to the published version of the manuscript.

Funding: The project was supported by the National Key R&D Program of China (grant number 2022YFC360170) and the Henan Provincial Key Discipline of Rehabilitation Engineering (grant number NA). The APC was funded by the National Key R&D Program of China and the Henan Provincial Key Discipline of Rehabilitation Engineering.

Institutional Review Board Statement: The study was conducted in accordance with the Declaration of Helsinki and approved by the Fifth Affiliated Hospital of Zhengzhou University (Reference number: KY2022028; Date: 23 June 2022). This study was registered on the World Health Organization International Clinical Trials Registry Platform (ICTRP) via the Chinese Clinical Trial Registry [ChiCTR, Reference No.: ChiCTR2400084383; Date: 15 May 2024; Website: https://www.chictr.org.cn/showproj.html?proj=224119 (accessed on 26 November 2024)].

Informed Consent Statement: Informed consent was obtained from all subjects involved in the study. Written informed consent was obtained from the patients to publish this paper.

Data Availability Statement: The data that support the findings of this study are available from the corresponding authors upon reasonable request.

Acknowledgments: The authors would like to thank all the AIS patients who volunteered to participate in this study.

Conflicts of Interest: X.Z. is serving as the CEO of the Zhengzhou Feilong Medical Equipment Co., Ltd., which developed and optimized the 3D spinal decompression and correction device used in this study. The other authors declare no conflicts of interest.

References

1. Gorman, K.F.; Julien, C.; Moreau, A. The genetic epidemiology of idiopathic scoliosis. *Eur. Spine J.* **2012**, *21*, 1905–1919. [CrossRef] [PubMed]
2. Weinstein, S.L.; Dolan, L.A.; Cheng, J.C.; Danielsson, A. Adolescent idiopathic scoliosis. *Lancet* **2008**, *371*, 1527–1537. [CrossRef] [PubMed]
3. Savvides, P.; Gerdhem, P.; Grauers, A.; Danielsson, A.; Diarbakerli, E. Self-Experienced Trunk Appearance in Individuals with and Without Idiopathic Scoliosis. *Spine* **2020**, *45*, 522–527. [CrossRef] [PubMed]
4. Koumbourlis, A.C. Scoliosis and the respiratory system. *Paediatr. Respir. Rev.* **2006**, *7*, 152–160. [CrossRef]
5. Lang, C.; Wang, R.; Chen, Z.; He, S.; Zou, Q.; Wu, J.; Zhu, X. Incidence and Risk Factors of Cardiac Abnormalities in Patients with Idiopathic Scoliosis. *World Neurosurg.* **2019**, *125*, e824–e828. [CrossRef]

6. Weinstein, S.L.; Dolan, L.A.; Wright, J.G.; Dobbs, M.B. Effects of Bracing in Adolescents with Idiopathic Scoliosis. *N. Engl. J. Med.* **2013**, *369*, 1512–1521. [CrossRef]
7. Negrini, S.; Minozzi, S.; Bettany-Saltikov, J.; Chockalingam, N.; Grivas, T.B.; Kotwicki, T.; Maruyama, T.; Romano, M.; Zaina, F. Braces for idiopathic scoliosis in adolescents. *Cochrane Database Syst. Rev.* **2015**, *2015*, CD006850. [CrossRef]
8. Grivas, T.B.; Wade, M.H.; Negrini, S.; O'Brien, J.P.; Maruyama, T.; Hawes, M.C.; Rigo, M.; Weiss, H.R.; Kotwicki, T.; Vasiliadis, E.S.; et al. SOSORT consensus paper: School screening for scoliosis. Where are we today? *Scoliosis* **2007**, *2*, 17. [CrossRef]
9. Herring, J.A.; Katz, D.E.; Browne, R.H.; Kelly, D.M.; Birch, J.G. Brace wear control of curve progression in adolescent idiopathic scoliosis. *J. Bone Jt. Surg. Am.* **2010**, *92*, 1343–1352. [CrossRef]
10. Rahimi, S.; Kiaghadi, A.; Fallahian, N. Effective factors on brace compliance in idiopathic scoliosis: A literature review. *Disabil. Rehabil. Assist. Technol.* **2020**, *15*, 917–923. [CrossRef]
11. El Hawary, R.; Zaaroor-Regev, D.; Floman, Y.; Lonner, B.S. Brace treatment in adolescent idiopathic scoliosis: Risk factors for failure—A literature review. *Spine J.* **2019**, *19*, 1917–1925. [CrossRef] [PubMed]
12. Thompson, R.M.; Hubbard, E.W.; Jo, C.-H.; Virostek, D.; Karol, L.A. Brace Success Is Related to Curve Type in Patients with Adolescent Idiopathic Scoliosis. *J. Bone Jt. Surg.* **2017**, *99*, 923–928. [CrossRef] [PubMed]
13. Liu, S.; Ho, L.Y.; Beygi, B.H.; Wong, M.S. Effectiveness of Orthotic Treatment on Clinical Outcomes of the Patients with Adolescent Idiopathic Scoliosis Under Different Wearing Compliance Levels: A Systematic Review. *JBJS Rev.* **2023**, *11*, e23. [CrossRef] [PubMed]
14. Karol, L.A.; Virostek, D.; Felton, K.; Wheeler, L. Effect of Compliance Counseling on Brace Use and Success in Patients with Adolescent Idiopathic Scoliosis. *J. Bone Jt. Surg.* **2016**, *98*, 9–14. [CrossRef] [PubMed]
15. Bogaart, M.v.D.; van Royen, B.J.; Haanstra, T.M.; de Kleuver, M.; Faraj, S.S.A. Predictive factors for brace treatment outcome in adolescent idiopathic scoliosis: A best-evidence synthesis. *Eur. Spine J.* **2019**, *28*, 511–525. [CrossRef]
16. Aulisa, A.G.; Galli, M.; Giordano, M.; Falciglia, F.; Careri, S.; Toniolo, R.M. Initial In-Brace Correction: Can the Evaluation of Cobb Angle Be the Only Parameter Predictive of the Outcome of Brace Treatment in Patients with Adolescent Idiopathic Scoliosis? *Children* **2022**, *9*, 338. [CrossRef]
17. El-Zayat, A.R.; Gomah, W.; Aldesouky, A.H. Spinal decompression therapy as an alternative modality for management of low back pain and radicular pain caused by lumbar disc herniation or protrusion. *Egypt. Rheumatol. Rehabil.* **2019**, *46*, 183–188. [CrossRef]
18. Pergolizzi, J.V., Jr.; Clair, D.F. 2 Prospective Evaluation of the Efficacy of Spinal Decompression via the DRX9000 for Chronic Low Back Pain. *J. Pain Pract.* **2008**, 2–8.
19. Karam, J.A.; Eid, R.; Kreichati, G.; Abiad, R.; Kharrat, K.; Ghanem, I.B. Optimizing the vertical position of the brace thoracic pad: Apical rib or apical vertebra? *Orthop. Traumatol. Surg. Res.* **2019**, *105*, 727–731. [CrossRef]
20. Pearson, E.J.M. Comfort and its measurement—A literature review. *Disabil. Rehabil. Assist. Technol.* **2009**, *4*, 301–31020094301. [CrossRef]
21. He, C.; To, M.K.-T.; Cheung, J.P.-Y.; Cheung, K.M.-C.; Chan, C.-K.; Jiang, W.-W.; Zhou, G.-Q.; Lai, K.K.-L.; Zheng, Y.-P.; Wong, M.-S. An effective assessment method of spinal flexibility to predict the initial in-orthosis correction on the patients with adolescent idiopathic scoliosis (AIS). *PLoS ONE* **2017**, *12*, e0190141. [CrossRef] [PubMed]
22. Jie, Y.; Ma, W.M.; Zhang, M. *The Usefulness of a Dual-period System with Distraction and Lateral Force Application for Spinal Correction and Flexibility in Adolescent Idiopathic Scoliosis*; The International Research Society of Spinal Deformities (IRSSD): Hong Kong, China, 2024; p. 94.
23. Peeters, C.M.; van Hasselt, A.J.; Wapstra, F.H.; Jutte, P.C.; Kempen, D.H.; Faber, C. Predictive Factors on Initial in-brace Correction in Idiopathic Scoliosis: A Systematic Review. *Spine* **2022**, *47*, E353–E361. [CrossRef] [PubMed]
24. Yang, D.; Lee, T.; Lai, K.; Wong, Y.; Wong, L.; Yang, J.; Lam, T.; Castelein, R.; Cheng, J.; Zheng, Y. A novel classification method for mild adolescent idiopathic scoliosis using 3D ultrasound imaging. *Med. Nov. Technol. Devices* **2021**, *11*, 100075. [CrossRef]
25. Yang, D.; Lee, T.T.-Y.; Lai, K.K.-L.; Lam, T.-P.; Chu, W.C.-W.; Castelein, R.M.; Cheng, J.C.-Y.; Zheng, Y.-P. Semi-automatic ultrasound curve angle measurement for adolescent idiopathic scoliosis. *Spine Deform.* **2022**, *10*, 351–359. [CrossRef]
26. Wang, L.; Xia, N.; Wang, C.; Zheng, Q.; Ma, C.Z.; Youssef, A.S.A.; Zhang, C.; Deng, Y.; Zhu, G.; Huang, X. Optimized scheme for paired transverse corrective forces in S-shaped scoliosis via ultrasound and application in Cheneau brace: A pilot study. *Prosthet. Orthot. Int.* **2022**, *46*, 42–49. [CrossRef]
27. Zheng, Q.; Xie, L.; Xu, J.; Xia, N.; Ma, C.Z. A feasibility study of applying two-dimensional photogrammetry for screening and monitoring of patients with adolescent idiopathic scoliosis in clinical practice. *Sci. Rep.* **2023**, *13*, 14273. [CrossRef]
28. Vanti, C.; Panizzolo, A.; Turone, L.; A Guccione, A.; Violante, F.S.; Pillastrini, P.; Bertozzi, L. Effectiveness of Mechanical Traction for Lumbar Radiculopathy: A Systematic Review and Meta-Analysis. *Phys. Ther.* **2021**, *101*, pzaa231. [CrossRef]
29. Karimi, M.; Rabczuk, T.; Luthfi, M.; Pourabbas, B.; Esrafilian, A. An evaluation of the efficiency of endpoint control on the correction of scoliotic curve with brace: A case study. *Acta Bioeng. Biomech.* **2019**, *21*, 3–10. [CrossRef]

30. Rahman, T.; Bowen, J.R.; Takemitsu, M.; Scott, C. The Association Between Brace Compliance and Outcome for Patients with Idiopathic Scoliosis. *J. Pediatr. Orthop.* **2005**, *25*, 420–422. [CrossRef]
31. Lang, C.; Huang, Z.; Zou, Q.; Sui, W.; Deng, Y.; Yang, J. Coronal deformity angular ratio may serve as a valuable parameter to predict in-brace correction in patients with adolescent idiopathic scoliosis. *Spine J.* **2019**, *19*, 1041–1047. [CrossRef]

Disclaimer/Publisher's Note: The statements, opinions and data contained in all publications are solely those of the individual author(s) and contributor(s) and not of MDPI and/or the editor(s). MDPI and/or the editor(s) disclaim responsibility for any injury to people or property resulting from any ideas, methods, instructions or products referred to in the content.

bioengineering

MDPI

Article

Around-Body Versus On-Body Motion Sensing: A Comparison of Efficacy Across a Range of Body Movements and Scales

Katelyn Rohrer [1,2], Luis De Anda [1], Camila Grubb [1,2], Zachary Hansen [1,2], Jordan Rodriguez [1,2], Greyson St Pierre [3], Sara Sheikhlary [1,4], Suleyman Omer [4], Binh Tran [5], Mehrail Lawendy [4], Farah Alqaraghuli [3], Chris Hedgecoke [4], Youssif Abdelkeder [4], Rebecca C. Slepian [1,6], Ethan Ross [6], Ryan Chung [6] and Marvin J. Slepian [1,3,4,6,*]

1 Arizona Center for Accelerated Biomedical Innovation, University of Arizona, Tucson, AZ 85724, USA; katelynrohrer@arizona.edu (K.R.); lad44@arizona.edu (L.D.A.); cdgrubb@arizona.edu (C.G.); zacharysehansen@arizona.edu (Z.H.); jerodriguez@arizona.edu (J.R.); sheikhlary@arizona.edu (S.S.); beccaslepian@arizona.edu (R.C.S.)
2 Department of Computer Science, College of Science, University of Arizona, Tucson, AZ 85721, USA
3 Department of Chemical Engineering, College of Engineering, University of Arizona, Tucson, AZ 85721, USA; gstpierre@arizona.edu (G.S.P.); farahalqaraghuli@arizona.edu (F.A.)
4 Department of Biomedical Engineering, College of Engineering, University of Arizona, Tucson, AZ 85721, USA; somer4@arizona.edu (S.O.); mlawendy@arizona.edu (M.L.); chedgecoke@arizona.edu (C.H.); youssifwafa@email.arizona.edu (Y.A.)
5 Department of Cellular and Molecular Medicine, College of Medicine, University of Arizona, Tucson, AZ 85721, USA; bttran@arizona.edu
6 Department of Medicine, Sarver Heart Center, University of Arizona, Tucson, AZ 85721, USA; ecross1@arizona.edu (E.R.); chungr@arizona.edu (R.C.)
* Correspondence: slepian@arizona.edu

Abstract: Motion is vital for life. Currently, the clinical assessment of motion abnormalities is largely qualitative. We previously developed methods to quantitatively assess motion using visual detection systems (around-body) and stretchable electronic sensors (on-body). Here we compare the efficacy of these methods across predefined motions, hypothesizing that the around-body system detects motion with similar accuracy as on-body sensors. Six human volunteers performed six defined motions covering three excursion lengths, small, medium, and large, which were analyzed via both around-body visual marker detection (MoCa version 1.0) and on-body stretchable electronic sensors (BioStamp version 1.0). Data from each system was compared as to the extent of trackability and comparative efficacy between systems. Both systems successfully detected motions, allowing quantitative analysis. Angular displacement between systems had the highest agreement efficiency for the bicep curl and body lean motion, with 73.24% and 65.35%, respectively. The finger pinch motion had an agreement efficiency of 36.71% and chest abduction/adduction had 45.55%. Shoulder abduction/adduction and shoulder flexion/extension motions had the lowest agreement efficiencies with 24.49% and 26.28%, respectively. MoCa was comparable to BioStamp in terms of angular displacement, though velocity and linear speed output could benefit from additional processing. Our findings demonstrate comparable efficacy for non-contact motion detection to that of on-body sensor detection, and offers insight as to the best system selection for specific clinical uses based on the use-case of the desired motion being analyzed.

Keywords: motion capture; motion analysis; on-body sensing; around-body sensing; wearable sensors; stretchable electronics; marker tracking; human locomotion

1. Introduction

Human motion is vital for life. In a wide variety of disease states, mobility is often compromised, either due to direct pathology involving neuromuscular and skeletal function, or indirectly via systemic functional, biochemical, or inflammatory alterations [1–6]. To aid in overall disease management, motion analysis has emerged as a potential diagnostic tool to guide both direct mobility rehabilitation as well as systemic therapies impacting mobility [7–9]. Great strides have been made in recent years in improving both the accessibility and usability of motion analysis systems, as well as in defining optimal specific use applications [10–12]. In recent years there has been a transition from strict hospital and facility-based motion labs to a wide range of portable and wearable technologies being employed [13,14]. Based on this technological evolution, motion analysis today may be broadly categorized as either "around-body", i.e., via non-contact observation/detection systems, or "on-body", via a range of wearable sensors detecting attached subject motion [14,15]. Our group has been involved in the development and testing of both of these types of systems, including on-body sensors utilizing stretchable electronics containing accelerometers and gyroscopes [16] as well as around-body systems utilizing visual marker detection and computational motion tracking [17]. It has become clear from this work, and the work of others, that each form of motion detection has functional nuanced differences, as to the ability to detect motion at a range of distances and involving differing geometric scales, with specific characteristics potentially favoring particular situational use [18–21].

The BioStamp (MC 10, Lexington, MA, USA) is an example of a portable, small-footprint on-body motion sensor, well suited for out-of-hospital home use, developed and studied in collaboration with our group [22]. The BioStamp is a wearable, conformal patch fabricated with pliant materials and containing stretchable electronics, capable of measuring motion with six degrees of freedom [22]. The BioStamp contains embedded accelerometers and gyroscopes, able to record acceleration and angular velocity [22]. In previous work we described details of this sensor system and demonstrated its ability to capture motion, as well as define a "motion envelope" for a given limb movement [22]. In other work we demonstrated the ability of the BioStamp to delineate signatures of specific motion tasks [23]. In general, the BioStamp provides detailed motion information, appearing to function best for the capture and quantitation of motion for the specific focal body region to which it is applied.

In contrast, the Mobile Motion Capture Analysis (MoCa) is an example of a low cost, video-based around-body motion tracking system able to detect and quantitate movement in a non-contact fashion [17,24]. MoCa uses brightly colored inexpensive markers (<=10 mm^2 in size) and a smart-phone video camera to track positional movement. In prior work, we described this system and defined its operating parameters and boundaries in terms of distance tracked, marker identification and discrimination, and the effect of illumination and speed on motion detection [17]. Overall, MoCa appears well suited for the capture and quantitation of large region motions.

While both of these systems offer great advantages for out-of-hospital motion detection, what remains unknown is their comparative efficacy over a range of motions. In an effort to guide operational choice and the translation of these systems for the best situational and clinical use it is vital to define how these systems compare as to the detection of movements of differing size body components, e.g., whole body vs. limbs vs. digits. Over what size region is each best suited for motion detection? How well is each suited to detect, capture, and quantitate angular displacement, angular velocity, and linear speed? Over what speed of motion? In this present study, we conducted a comparative study to define and clarify these differences. We hypothesized that around-body motion detection with the MoCa system will provide similar data to that of the wearable on-body BioStamp system, though with identifiable differences in specific use cases and conditions. As a first step, we examined the ability of each system to detect and track specific, defined identical movements. Next, we examined the ability of each system to quantitate motion across differing movement excursions or "sizes", herein defined in terms of dimensional areas, i.e., as small (<1 sq ft), medium (1–5 sq ft), and large (6–10 sq ft). We then compared the efficacy of each system across motion endpoint variables for each of these movement sizes, with efficacy defined in terms of angular displacement, angular velocity, and linear speed. We then examined the effect of the speed of movement on the comparative efficacy of each system. Finally, we discuss our findings in the context of translatable clinical utility as to which each type of system is best.

In summary, the contributions of this work are as follows: MoCa, a novel computer-vision "around-body" motion analysis system is compared to BioStamp, an established gyroscopic and accelerometer IMU. Meaningful angular and linear data are extracted out of both systems and compared against one another. Their statistical results are analyzed in the context of the medical domain, and next steps are outlined for the applicability of either system in a clinical application.

2. Materials and Methods

2.1. Materials

Six volunteers were enrolled in this study, 3 male, 3 female, ages 15–30, all providing informed consent, under study approval by UA IRB 2107032177.

Around-body testing via MoCa: General materials included neon pink or green construction paper, a ruler and tape measures, a metronome, and Apple iPhone 8, XR, or newer models. Pink, orange, and green markers were used as identification points. Markers were cut from construction paper as 2 mm squares for small movements and 10 mm squares for medium and large movements (Table 1). A low-stick adhesive was affixed to the back of each marker to allow direct skin adhesion, or adhesion on top of an affixed BioStamp. A smartphone camera with 1080 p resolution, recording at 60 frames per second, was used to track each movement, ensuring that the video produced was of high quality to accurately record the motion. The phone was supported by a variable-length tripod.

Table 1. Existing movement size categories (small, medium, and large), the reps per second for both slow and fast paces use, and the movement area required in square feet per size.

Movement Size	Slow Pace (×3)	Fast Pace (×3)	Movement Area Requirement	MoCa Stamp Size
Small	1 rep/1 s	3 reps/1 s	1 sq ft	2 × 2 mm
Medium	1 rep/6 s	1 rep/2 s	5 sq ft	10 × 10 mm
Large	1 rep/6 s	1 rep/2 s	10 sq ft	10 × 10 mm

On-body testing via BioStamps: The BioStampRC® (Model No. BRCS01) and kit (charging station for stamps, adhesive strips, recording tablet (Samsung Galaxy Tab. A), and conductive gel), were obtained from MC10, Inc. (Lexington, MA, USA). The BioStamp is a thin, pliable device containing stretchable electronics directly applied to the skin surface (3.4 cm × 6.6 cm × 0.45 cm; weight = 7 g). The BioStamp is controlled via an embedded microcontroller for recording bio-signals and the transmission of data via WiFi to the MC10 Investigator Portal or broadcasting wirelessly via Bluetooth to the MC10 Discovery app, pre-loaded on an Android™ tablet. Prior to the application of BioStamp to a subject, the sensor was configured to select the measurement modality (3 axis accelerometer, 3 axis gyroscope, ECG, EMG, or combination), sampling frequency (50–250 Hz), and measurement range (±2–16 G for accel.; ±250–4000°/s for gyro). Once configured, the BioStamp was applied to the subject and was selected to start or stop recording and sync data from the tablet. Data were then uploaded to the cloud where they could be accessed and downloaded from the MC10 Investigator Portal website. Participants were supported by a table and/or chair to perform recorded movements.

As to metrics, the BioStamp recorded in 3 dimensions and 62.5 Hz whereas MoCa recorded in 2 dimensions and the camera recording settings were set to 60 frames per second in HD (1080 × 1920 pixels) quality.

At most, five BioStamps were used to measure movements. The BioStamps were controlled by a tablet and cell phone combination from the BioStamps kit. The combination links to a docking stand that synchronized the in-use BioStamps, as well as uploaded data from the BioStamps to the associated website, MC10. The BioStamps were attached to the subject with surgical tape and medical wrap.

2.2. Experimental Methods

Subjects performed 6 standard movements in 30 s increments at slow and fast paces. Each movement was repeated three times at each speed for a total of six runs per standard movement per subject. These movements were simultaneously recorded with the MoCa and BioStamp systems. The six standard movements were categorized based on area requirements: (1) small movements (<1 sq ft)—finger pinch, (2) medium movements (1–5 sq ft)—bicep curl, chest abduction/adduction, shoulder abduction/adduction, and shoulder flexion/extension, and (3) large movements (>5 sq ft)—body lean (Table 2).

Table 2. Categorization of movements into movement sizes. The movement sizes (small, medium, and large) are differentiated by movement area (sq ft) required to perform the movement.

Movement Size	Movement Area Requirement	Movements
Small	1 sq ft	Finger Pinch
Medium	5 sq ft	Bicep Curl Chest Abduction/Adduction Shoulder Abduction/Adduction Shoulder Flexion/Extension
Large	1 rep/6 s	Body Lean

2.3. Generic Protocol

To compare the efficacy of MoCa to BioStamp, the protocol outlined in Figure 1 was employed; each trial recorded MoCa and BioStamp data simultaneously. Once repeated, the raw data from both systems were processed and compared.

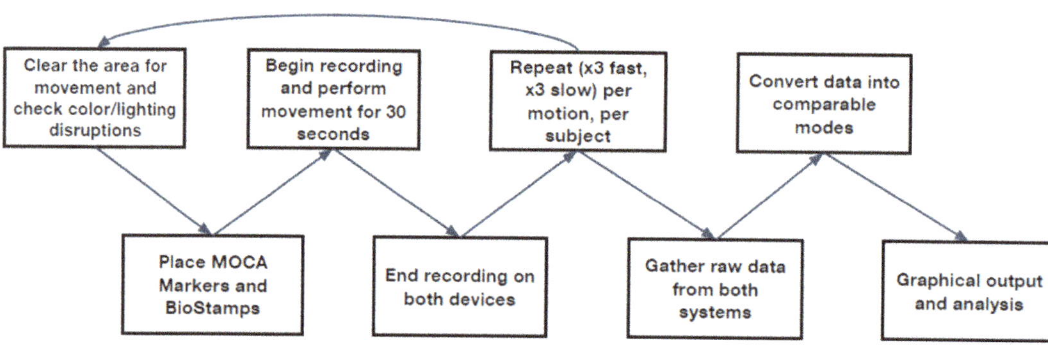

Figure 1. Outlined steps for recording the runs for both MoCa and BioStamp. The procedure covers the setting up of the area for recording the data transformation into graphs.

To set up the MoCa system, two cameras were placed at the same height as the pivot marker and parallel to the subject. The primary tracking camera was placed perpendicular to the primary axis of movement for the test motion, and the secondary camera was placed directly to the left or right of the subject to ensure that the third axis of motion remained stable. Next, the identification markers were set up by placing different color markers on pivot, endpoint, and intermediate locations as per the directions for each motion. These markers were required to be directly facing the primary camera and remained primarily visible to the camera in order to consistently record axis movement. Once both systems were set up, the subject performed the movement for 30 s at both fast and slow speeds (Table 1). The speed of movement was controlled by the time per repetition (Table 1). At the end of the movement, the subject returned to the starting position and waited for all motion capture devices to stop recording.

For the BioStamp system, sensors were placed based on the subject at defined reproducible locations. BioStamps were secured bilaterally with medical tape and subsequently wrapped in gauze to ensure no part of the stamp would move or detach from the subject's skin during the study.

2.3.1. Finger Pinch (FingerP) Movement Protocol

To setup MoCa, a pink 2 mm marker was placed on the lateral tip of the index finger, and another pink marker was placed on the fingernail of the thumb. A green 2 mm marker was placed on the hand between the thumb and index finger (Figure 2). The finger pinch movement required two BioStamps. The BioStamps used for this movement were placed on the index finger and thumb of the subject's dominant hand, with the tab side of the BioStamp pointing towards the tip of each finger (Figure 3). Both BioStamps were secured adjacent to the fingernail.

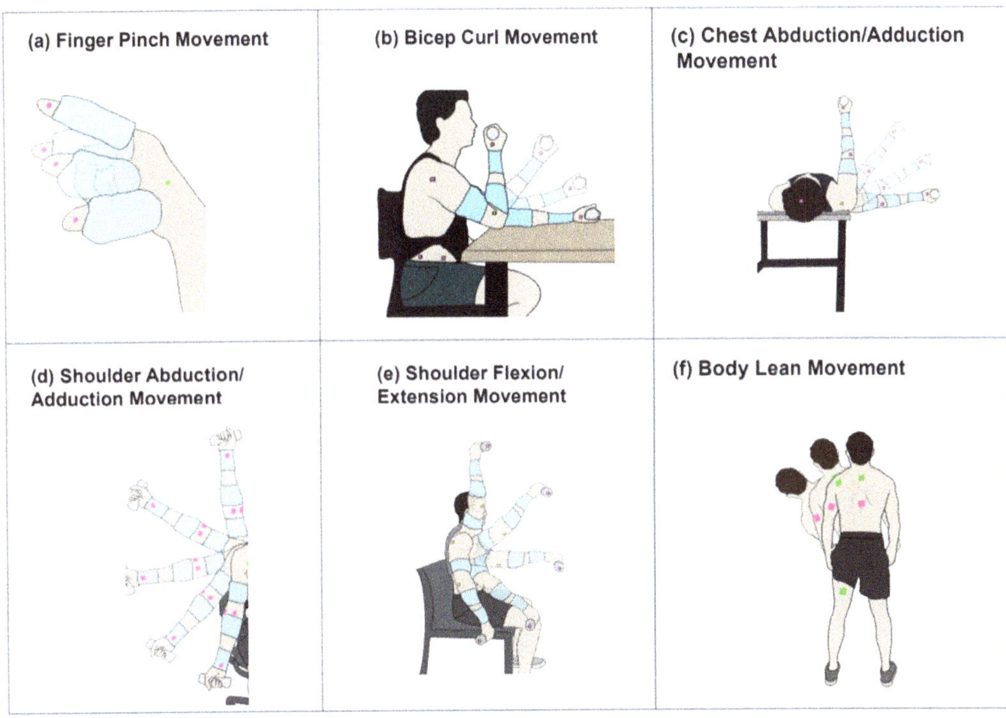

Figure 2. Locations of MoCa markers per six predefined motions: (**a**) finger pinch movement, (**b**) bicep curl movement, (**c**) chest abduction/adduction movement, (**d**) shoulder abduction/adduction movement, (**e**) shoulder flexion/extension movement, and (**f**) body lean movement. Sequential images outline the complete movement excursion per motion with variously colored MoCa markers indicating marker positions.

A table and chair were set up in the testing area, with the table directly in front of the chair. The subject was instructed to sit in a chair with a proper upright posture. The subject then rested their dominant arm on the edge of the table (Figure 2). The subject started with their fingers about 2–3 inches apart in an 'open' position, and when instructed to begin, performed the finger pinch for 30 s at a slow pace (1 rep/s) and a fast pace (3 reps/s) (Table 1).

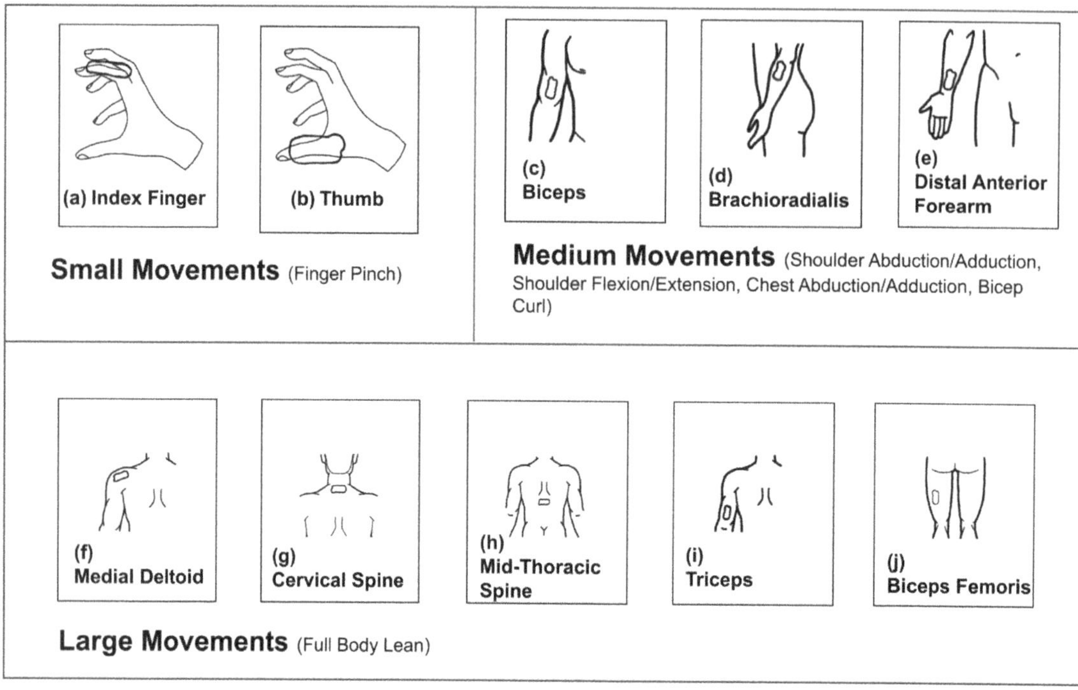

Figure 3. Location of BioStamp placement per motion categorized by excursion length (small, medium, and large). Small movements require two stamps: (**a**) index finger and (**b**) thumb. Medium movements require three stamps placed on (**c**) biceps, (**d**) brachioradialis, and (**e**) distal anterior forearm. Large movements require the most stamps with stamps placed on the (**f**) medial deltoid, (**g**) the cervical spine, (**h**) mid-thoracic spine, (**i**) triceps, and (**j**) biceps femoris.

2.3.2. Bicep Curl (BicepC) Movement Protocol

To setup MoCa, one 10 mm pink marker was placed on the side of the 2 lb. weight facing the camera, held in the dominant hand. The other 10 mm pink marker was placed on the deltoid muscle on the dominant side, just below the acromion. The 10 mm green marker was placed on the lateral epicondyle of the elbow on the dominant side (Figure 2). Three BioStamps were used for the bicep curl movement, placed on top of the bicep, brachioradialis, and distal anterior forearm (Figure 3).

A table and chair were set up in the testing area with the table directly in front of the chair where the subject sat. The subject sat with an upright posture, resting their dominant elbow on the edge of the table (Figure 2). The subjects started with the back of their dominant hand resting on the table. While keeping their elbow on the table, the subject performed a standard bicep curl with a 2 lb. weight in hand. They performed the bicep curl movement for 30 s at a slow pace (1 rep/6 s) and a fast pace (1 rep/2 s) (Table 1).

2.3.3. Chest Abduction/Adduction (ChestAA) Movement Protocol

MoCa required four 10 mm × 10 mm markers for the chest abduction/adduction movement: two pink, one green, and one orange. One of the pink markers was placed on the side of the dumbbell facing the camera during the movement. The other pink marker was placed on the top of the subject's head. The green marker was placed on the top of the subject's shoulder at the acromion on the dominant side and an orange marker was placed on the brachioradialis on the top part of the arm that was facing the camera (Figure 2). This movement required three BioStamps. They were placed on the top of the bicep, brachioradialis, and distal anterior forearm (Figure 3).

The movement (medium) was performed for 30 s at a slow pace (1 rep/6 s) and fast pace (1 rep/2 s) (Table 1). A table was set up where the subject lay on the table flat on their back. The dominant arm hung off the edge of the table straight out to the side parallel to the ground to allow a full range of movement. They extended the dominant arm out past the edge of the table. To perform this movement the subject started with their arm flat out to the side with the 2 lb. weight in their hand. When the 30 s movement period began, the subject rotated their arm by 90° to be directly in front of their body (Figure 2).

2.3.4. Shoulder Abduction/Adduction (ShoulderAA) Movement Protocol

MoCa required four 10 mm × 10 mm markers for the shoulder abduction/adduction movement: two pink, one green, and one orange. One of the pink markers was placed on the medial side of the wrist. The other pink marker was placed on the front of the subject's lateral aspect of the hip on the dominant side. The green marker was placed on the front of the subject's deltoid muscle on the dominant side, just below the acromion, and an orange marker was placed on the elbow joint on the inside forward-facing part of the arm that was facing the camera (Figure 2). This movement required three BioStamps. The BioStamp locations were on top of the bicep, brachioradialis, and distal interior (Figure 3).

The movement (medium) was performed for 30 s at a slow pace (1 rep/6 s) and fast pace (1 rep/2 s) (Table 1). A table and chair were set up where the subject sat with proper posture. The subject started the position as described above with the arm flat down to the side of their body, pronated, with the 2 lb. weight in their hand. When the 30 s movement period began, the subject raised their arm to their side, rotating in the shoulder by 180° such that their arm was directly up in the air (Figure 2).

2.3.5. Shoulder Flexion/Extension (ShoulderFE) Movement Protocol

MoCa required four 10 mm × 10 mm markers for the shoulder flexion/extension movement: two pink, one green, and one orange. The pink markers identify the endpoints of the movement, the green identifies the pivot locations, and the orange markers identify intermediate locations. One of the pink markers was placed on the side of the dumbbell facing the camera. The other pink marker was placed on the side of the lateral aspect of the hip on the dominant side. The green marker was placed on the side of the deltoid muscle on the dominant side, just below the acromion, and an orange marker was placed outside the elbow on the dominant side (Figure 2). This movement required three BioStamps. The BioStamp locations were on top of the bicep, brachioradialis, and distal anterior forearm (Figure 3).

The movement (medium) was performed for 30 s at a slow pace (1 rep/6 s) and a fast pace (1 rep/2 s) (Table 1). The subject sat in a chair with proper posture. The dominant arm hung to the side of their body with the top of the hand facing forward and the palm facing backward. When the 30 s movement period begins, the subject will raise their arm in front of themselves, rotating in the shoulder by 180° to where the arm is directly up in the air (Figure 2).

2.3.6. Body Lean (BodyL) Movement Protocol

MoCa required five 10 mm × 10 mm markers for the body lean movement: two pink, two green, and one orange. All of the markers were placed directly on top of the BioStamps for this movement (Figure 2f). The pink markers were positioned on the tricep and bicep femoris BioStamps and the medial deltoid BioStamp. The green markers, identifying two pivot locations, were placed on the cervical spine and mid-thoracic spine BioStamps. This movement required five BioStamps, the most of all movements. The BioStamp locations used for this movement are on top of the medial deltoid, cervical spine, mid-thoracic spine, triceps, and bicep femoris (Figure 3).

The movement (large) was performed for 30 s at a slow pace (1 rep/8 s) and a fast pace (1 rep/4 s) (Table 1). To begin the experiment, a 10 ft × 10 ft test area was cleared and the subject stood with proper posture in the middle. When the 30 s movement period began, the subject leaned their body to the dominant side, keeping the tips of the fingers touching the side of the leg (Figure 2). The tips of the fingers moved up and down the leg as the movement was performed.

2.4. MoCa Statistical Methods

MoCa data were collected via video recordings (.mp4 or .mov) which were gathered and renamed for convenience. The MoCa markers were tracked using a color detection program on each frame of the video which outputted coordinate data in pixels. Angles (degrees) were found between two or three markers. To obtain angles from three markers, the standard law of cosine was applied. To obtain angles from two markers, the initial position of the non-pivot marker was used as a "ghost point" to mimic a third stamp position. Next, the law of cosines was used to find the angle between the two tracked markers and the new "ghost point". Because the law of cosines only calculates the absolute angle, the resulting angle was manually inverted when the moving marker crossed its original position in x/y, as it represents a negative displacement from the initial angle. The derivative of the angular displacement outputted angular velocity (degrees per second). Linear speed was calculated by determining the displacement of the markers over time. First, each pixel recorded was converted into meters using manual measurements for each subject's trial. Multiple measurements were manually recorded via a tape measure. The distance in meters between each stamp was recorded for each trial. These measurements were then used to scale the pixels to meters. Displacement was computed as the Euclidian distance between consecutive positions in meters. This displacement was then divided by the time difference between frames to yield linear speed in meters per second (m/s). The full MoCa statistical steps are shown in Figure 4. In addition to the full motion data, the maximum angular displacement was calculated by averaging the top 5% of the highest angular displacements values.

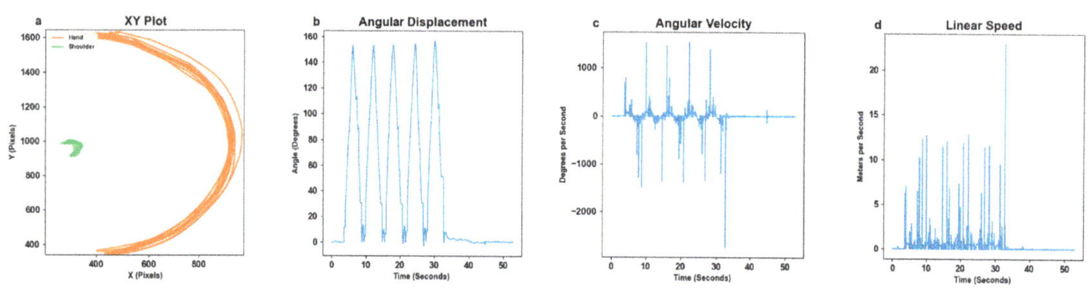

Figure 4. Complete data conversion process, from raw MoCa data to the final endpoint variables, subplots (**a–d**) representing data from the same trial. (**a**) Positional tracking of individual MoCa markers on the hand, elbow, and shoulder. (**b**) Angular displacement calculated by applying the cosine function to the angles formed by the markers. (**c**) Angular velocity derived from the original angles. (**d**) Linear speed calculated from positional data.

2.5. BioStamp Statistical Methods

Raw data collected from BioStamps were uploaded to the MC10 BioStamp website where files are stored. We downloaded and renamed them for convenience. Each BioStamp outputs three axes of angular velocity (°/s) and linear acceleration (g) [25]. We gathered angular velocity from the BioStamp marker that moved the most, as it captured the most relevant movement in reference to the motion at hand. To enhance the quality and accuracy of the gyroscope angular velocity measurements, a low-pass Butterworth filter was applied. The purpose of this filtering step is to make angular velocity comparable to MoCa by reducing high-frequency noise that can obscure the true signal of interest. Acceleration data inherently capture the constant force of gravity. In order to isolate gravitational acceleration from raw acceleration data, we applied a low-pass filter with a smoothing factor $\alpha = 0.9$.

The gravitation component at each time step was calculated by incorporating the previous gravity estimate with the current acceleration data. This resulting gravity vector accounts for changes in sensor orientation and is subtracted from the raw acceleration to obtain linear acceleration [26]. The 3-dimensional linear speed of the sensor (m/s) was calculated by integrating the acceleration in each axis (m/s^2) over time and then computing the Euclidian norm of the resulting vectors across each time interval [27]. For the X, Y, and Z axes on each BioStamp, angular velocity (°/s) was integrated to obtain angular displacement (°). The full data conversion process and each metric at each step are shown in Figure 5. In addition to the full motion data, the maximum angular displacement was calculated by averaging the top 5% of the highest angular displacements values.

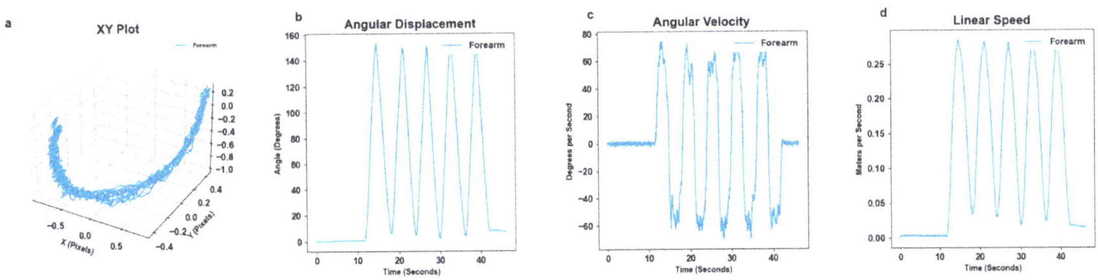

Figure 5. Full data conversion steps from obtaining raw BioStamp data into the final endpoint variables subplots (**a**–**d**) are from the same trial. (**a**) Marker tracking collected along the X, Y, and Z axes in pixels. (**b**) Angular displacement obtained through further integration. (**c**) Angular velocity integrated from BioStamp's output acceleration data. (**d**) Linear speed obtained from acceleration output using 3-dimensional Pythagorean theorem.

2.6. Comparison Methods

After completing the full steps of the experiment and obtaining the raw data, with the steps outlined in Figure 1, comparisons and correlations between the two systems were determined.

2.6.1. Maximum Angular Displacement Comparison

Maximum angular displacement was calculated to determine the range of motion. For both MoCa and BioStamp, maximum angular displacement values were calculated by averaging the top 5% of the highest angular displacement values. Direct comparisons between averages were made.

2.6.2. Alignment of Trials

To determine agreement between MoCa and BioStamp, each corresponding trial between BioStamp and MoCa must first be aligned to provide corresponding measurements. Resampling using linear interpolation was used to match the sample rate between systems for accurate comparisons [28]. The datasets were offset and trimmed to the same start time; however, MoCa can only give epoch time information to the nearest second of accuracy, whereas the BioStamp has millisecond accuracy, leading to possible misalignment between the two. To account for that, cross correlations were collected to find the highest correlation value offset for each one.

2.6.3. Bland–Altman Analysis

To compare MoCa and BioStamp, Bland–Altman analysis (a form of Tukey mean-difference plot) was utilized to determine agreement as well as systemic and relative bias. We first conducted the Bland–Altman analysis on a motion-by-motion scale to assess relative bias on angular displacement, angular velocity, and linear speed. Secondly, we performed the analysis on the three endpoint metrics across all trials to assess systemic bias. In either case, the premise outlined here for analysis was utilized.

Bland–Altman analysis is typically represented as a scatter plot where the difference between system A and system B are plotted against the mean measurement plotted [29]. The mean difference can then be interpreted as the average bias of system A relative to system B. Limits of agreement are calculated to visually display the typical variation in the differences, with wider limits of agreement indicative of disagreement between systems, and narrower limits of agreement indicative of better alignment. Given a normal distribution of differences, 95% of differences are expected to be within the limits of agreement given by $\overline{d} \pm 1.96 \times \text{SD}$, where $\overline{d}$ is the mean difference and the SD is the standard deviation of the differences [29].

Without a normal distribution of the differences, the limits of agreement become less reliable. In any of the analyses conducted in this experiment, the sample size for any Bland–Altman plot becomes well over 100,000 data points, given the multitude of measurements for any trial. As such, traditional methods for assessing normal distribution become less reliable. Therefore, the distribution of differences was visually inspected for normality.

If the relationship between the differences and the magnitude of the data is complicated, then the difference may be modeled as proportional to the magnitude of the measurement, given such a trend exists [30]. A linear regression line of best fit was modeled for any analysis. The extremely large sample size in any case (>100,000) makes the *p*-value of a linear regression unreliable. Therefore, we predetermined an r-squared value of above 0.5 to signify a significant enough relationship. We then regress the absolute residuals from the first linear regression to the magnitude of the data. For the reasons outlined above, a significant relationship is again determined by an r-squared value above 0.5. In which case, the limits of agreement are determined to incorporate both regressions, $\widehat{D}$ and $\widehat{R}$, as per Formula (1), following established guidelines.

$$\textit{Limits of Agreement} = \widehat{D} \pm 1.96\sqrt{\frac{\pi}{2}}\widehat{R} \quad (1)$$

In the case that the relationship between the absolute residuals and the differences is not significant, then the limits of agreement are determined with the standard deviation, SD, of the residuals of the line of best fit, $\widehat{D}$, as shown in Formula (2), following established guidelines.

$$\textit{limits of Agreement} = \widehat{D} \pm 1.96SD \quad (2)$$

In any case, each trial was aligned as per the steps outlined in Section 2.6.2. Then, the distribution of differences between MoCa and BioStamp were assessed. Given that a distribution of differences was not normal and there was not a significant linear relationship, as determined by the r-squared value, we used nonparametric methods for assessing agreement. Though nonparametric evaluations are not as reliable as parametric evaluations given a small sample size, we circumvent such a limitation given our large sample size in any case. The upper and lower bounds of agreement were given within the 5% percentile and 95% percentile of data, providing 90% of the differences within their bounds.

2.6.4. Relative Limits of Agreements

In order to accurately compare the mean difference and limits of agreement between MoCa and BioStamp, the results of the Bland–Altman analysis had to be normalized to a given movement. Angular displacement limits of agreement would be normalized to the angles typically found for a given movement. Specifically, the upper limit of agreement would be normalized to the typical maximum angle, as both provide a non-negative descriptor for a motion. Moreover, the upper limit of agreement is an equal distance away from the average difference compared to the lower limit of agreement, and as such is the expected case for the maximum angular displacement relative to its minimum angular displacement.

The agreement efficiency for a motion is calculated as the upper limit of agreement relative to the maximum angular displacement, as per Formula (3). By taking the inverse of the ratio of the upper limit of agreement to its maximum angle, a higher value indicates improved agreement efficiency. This transformed allows for a more straightforward understanding of the alignment between MoCa and BioStamp.

$$Agreement\ Efficiency\ (\%) = \left(1 - \frac{Upper\ Limit\ of\ Agreement}{Maximum\ Angle}\right) \times 100 \tag{3}$$

2.6.5. 1-to-1 Correlations

Correlations between MoCa and BioStamp were drawn for several measurements. Angular displacement correlations and angular velocity correlations between the two systems were gathered using similar processes. Resampling and alignment were first conducted as outlined in Section 2.6.2. Pearson correlation coefficients were then calculated for corresponding datasets.

Linear speed correlations required comparing the 2-dimensional MoCa speed and 3-dimensional BioStamp speed. For MoCa, the distance one marker moved in two dimensions, between two frames divided by the time elapsed, produced linear speed. For BioStamp, the linear speed was calculated by dividing the distance traveled by the BioStamp in three dimensions between two sample times by the elapsed time. The two datasets were resampled, trimmed, and offset using the same process as described above. At that point, the linear speed between systems could be accurately correlated.

2.6.6. Aggregate Bar Charts

For each 1-to-1 correlation, a one-line summary was written to a data aggregate file containing the information particular to that file such as the motion, subject, camera angle, trial number, and speed of trial as well as the angular displacement correlation, the angular velocity correlation, and the linear speed correlation. The bar charts were created by grouping the aggregate data by motion and/or speed and then finding the mean of each group. The bar charts created were the average angular displacement correlation per motion, the average angular displacement correlation per motion and speed, the average angular velocity correlation per motion, the average angular velocity correlation per motion and speed, the average linear speed correlation per motion, and the average linear speed correlation per motion and speed.

3. Results

3.1. Motion Tracking

MoCa and BioStamp each demonstrated clear ability and utility to track movements and motion. MoCa tracked movement on a marker basis via position, while BioStamp tracked movement on a stamp basis via gyroscopic tracking. Both MoCa and BioStamp effectively tracked angular displacement in reference to the body angle of the motion displayed. MoCa angular displacement graphs across all motions (Figure 6) showed the pattern of motion reps, demonstrating consistent tracking. The BioStamp system was able to track the defined identical movements (Figure 7) with similar angular displacement patterns.

3.2. Motion Detection by Excursion Size

The six predefined motions were categorized by excursion size (i.e., small, medium, and large). The average maximum angular displacement across all motions is presented in Figure 8. The small motion category consisting of finger pinch resulted in an average maximum angular displacement of 31.05° for MoCa and 37.08° for BioStamp. The medium motion category consisted of shoulder flexion/extension, bicep curl, chest abduction/adduction, and shoulder abduction/adduction. The average maximum angular displacement for shoulder flexion/extension was 103.60° for MoCa and 145.93°

for BioStamp. Bicep curl was 108.97° for MoCa and 107.38° for BioStamp. Chest abduction/adduction was 112.35° for MoCa and 93.71° for BioStamp. Shoulder abduction/adduction was 138.57° for MoCa and 153.20° for BioStamp. The large motion category consisted of body lean. The average maximum angular displacement for body lean was 36.46° for MoCa and 33.78° for BioStamp.

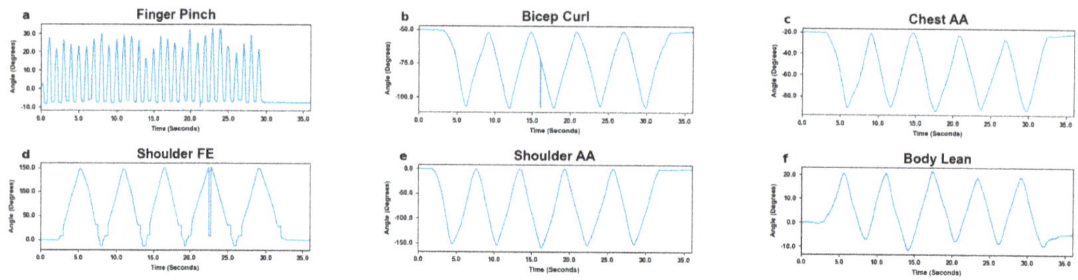

Figure 6. MoCa−captured angular displacement for all six motions: (**a**) finger pinch, (**b**) bicep curl, (**c**) chest abduction/adduction, (**d**) shoulder flexion/extension, (**e**) shoulder abduction/adduction, and (**f**) body lean.

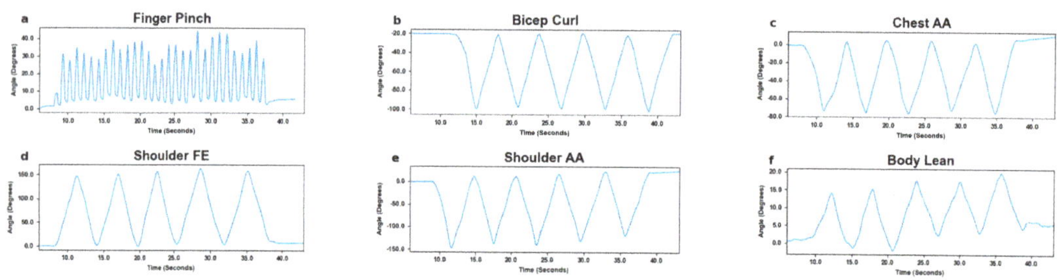

Figure 7. BioStamp−captured angular displacement for all six motions: (**a**) finger pinch, (**b**) bicep curl, (**c**) chest abduction/adduction, (**d**) shoulder flexion/extension, (**e**) shoulder abduction/adduction, and (**f**) body lean.

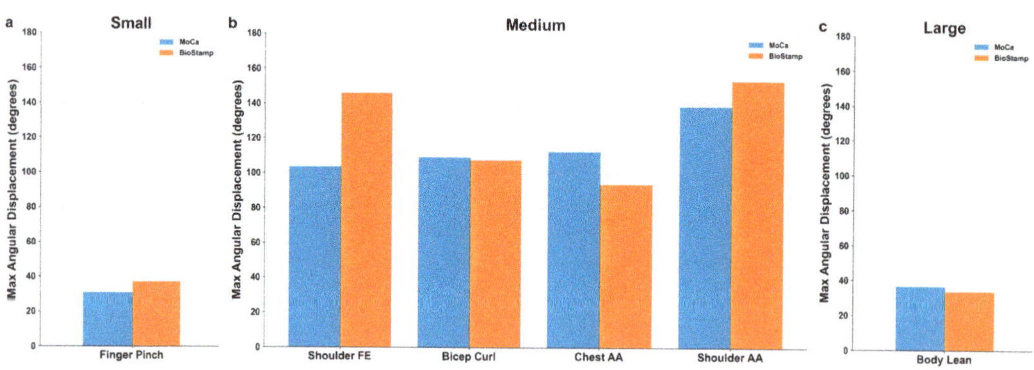

Figure 8. Average maximum angular displacement per motion categorized by motion size: (**a**) small, (**b**) medium, and (**c**) large. MoCa (blue) and BioStamp (orange) are compared side by side.

The Bland–Altman analysis comparing MoCa and BioStamp angular displacement values is presented in Figure 9, organized by motion type. Figure 9a displays the Bland–Altman analysis of the finger pinch motion, the mean difference between MoCa and BioStamp is −5.29 degrees, with 95% limits of agreement ranging from −32.13 to 21.56 degrees. Figure 9b presents the analysis of the bicep curl motion, with a mean difference of 4.58 degrees and the 95% limits of agreement ranging from −19.78 to 28.94 degrees. The chest abduction/adduction motion is represented in Figure 9c, with a mean difference of 8.85 degrees and the 95% limits of agreement ranging from −38.4 to 56.1 degrees. The shoulder flexion/extension motion is analyzed in Figure 9d, with a mean difference of −3.81 degrees and the 95% limits of agreement ranging from −99.6 to 91.98 degrees. Figure 9e focuses on the analysis of the shoulder abduction/adduction motion, with a mean difference of 12.85 degrees and the 95% limits of agreement ranging from −84.46 to 110.16 degrees. Finally, the body lean motion is displayed in Figure 9f, with a mean difference of −2.47 degrees and the 95% limits of agreement ranging from −17.11 to 12.17 degrees.

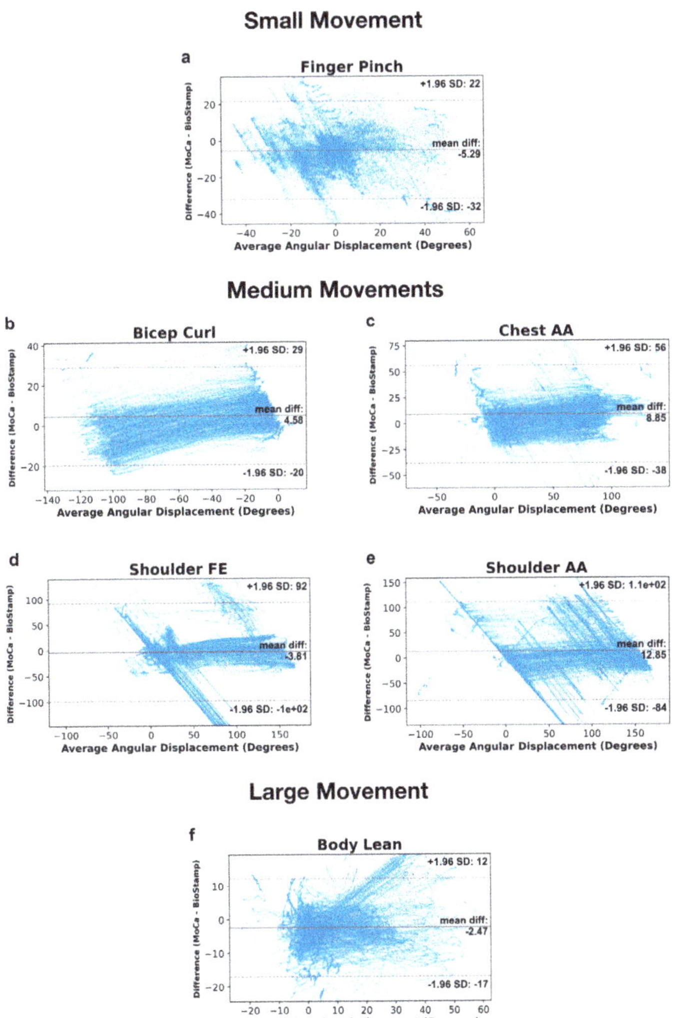

Figure 9. Bland−Altman plots of angular displacement between MoCa and BioStamp per motion categorized by motion size: small, medium, and large. (**a**) Bland−Altman plot of finger pinch movement. (**b**) Bland−Altman plot of bicep curl movement. (**c**) Bland−Altman plot of chest abduction/adduction movement. (**d**) Bland−Altman plot of shoulder flexion/extension movement. (**e**) Bland−Altman plot of shoulder abduction/adduction movement. (**f**) Bland−Altman plot of body lean movement.

The motion-by-motion analysis of angular velocity values between MoCa and BioStamp are presented in Figure 10. Figure 10a displays the Bland–Altman analysis of the finger pinch motion, the range between the fifth percentile and ninety-fifth percentile of differences being between −259.98 degrees per second and 316°/s, respectively. Figure 10b presents the analysis of the bicep curl motion, with the bottom fifth percentile of differences at −33.48°/s and the ninety-fifth percentile of differences at 36.86°/s. The chest abduction/adduction motion is represented in Figure 10c, with the difference represented by a linear relationship having a y-intercept of—0.05°/s, and a slope of 1.52. The 95% limits of agreement are relative to this regression, with y-intercepts at −221.03 and 220.93°/s. The shoulder flexion/extension motion is analyzed in Figure 10d, with the difference represented by a linear relationship having a y-intercept of 21.99°/s and a slope of 1.63. The 95% limits of agreement follow this trend, with y-intercepts at −404.22 and 448.2°/s. Figure 10e focuses on the analysis of the shoulder abduction/adduction motion, with the difference represented by a linear relationship having a y-intercept of 14.34°/s and a slope of 1.38. The 95% limits of agreement align with this trend, with y-intercepts at −392.4 and 421.07°/s. Finally, the body lean motion is displayed in Figure 10f, with the difference represented by a linear relationship having a y-intercept of 1.41°/s and a slope of 1.15. The 95% limits of agreement follow this trend, with y-intercepts at −71.04 and 73.87°/s.

Figure 11 displays the linear speed analysis between MoCa and BioStamp via Bland–Altman plots grouped by motion type. Figure 11a displays the Bland–Altman analysis of the finger pinch motion, with the difference represented by a linear relationship having a y-intercept of −0.07 m/s and a slope of two. The 95% limits of agreement follow the same slope as the linear regression, with y-intercepts at −0.16 and 0.02 m/s. Figure 11b presents the analysis of the bicep curl motion, with the difference represented by a linear relationship having a y-intercept of −0.16 m/s and a slope of 1.84. The 95% limits of agreement are in respect to the linear relationship, with y-intercepts at −0.47 and 0.14 m/s. The chest abduction/adduction motion is represented in Figure 11c, with the difference represented by a linear relationship having a y-intercept of −0.18 m/s and a slope of 1.97. The 95% limits of agreement followthis linear trend, with y-intercepts at −0.48 and 0.12 m/s. The shoulder flexion/extension motion is analyzed in Figure 11d, with the difference represented by a linear relationship having a y-intercept of −0.22 m/s and a slope of 1.99. The 95% limits of agreement follow this linear trend, with y-intercepts at −0.57 and 0.12 m/s. Figure 11e focuses on the analysis of the shoulder abduction/adduction motion, with the difference represented by a linear relationship having a y-intercept of −0.24 m/s and a slope of 1.98. The 95% limits of agreement follow the slope of the linear trend, with y-intercepts at −0.59 and 0.11 m/s. Finally, the body lean motion is displayed in Figure 11f, with the difference represented by a linear relationship having a y-intercept of −0.06 m/s and a slope of 1.92. The 95% limits of agreement follow this linear trend, with y-intercepts at −0.19 and 0.07 m/s.

Figure 12 illustrates the relative limits of agreements for angular displacement between MoCa and BioStamp across the movement sizes. The finger pinch motion is the only motion in the small movement category with an agreement efficiency of 36.71%. In the middle movement category are bicep curl, with an agreement efficiency of 73.24%, chest abduction/adduction, with an agreement efficiency of 45.55%, shoulder abduction/adduction at 24.49%, and shoulder flexion/extension at 26.28%. Body lean is the sole motion in the large movement category, with an agreement efficiency of 65.35%.

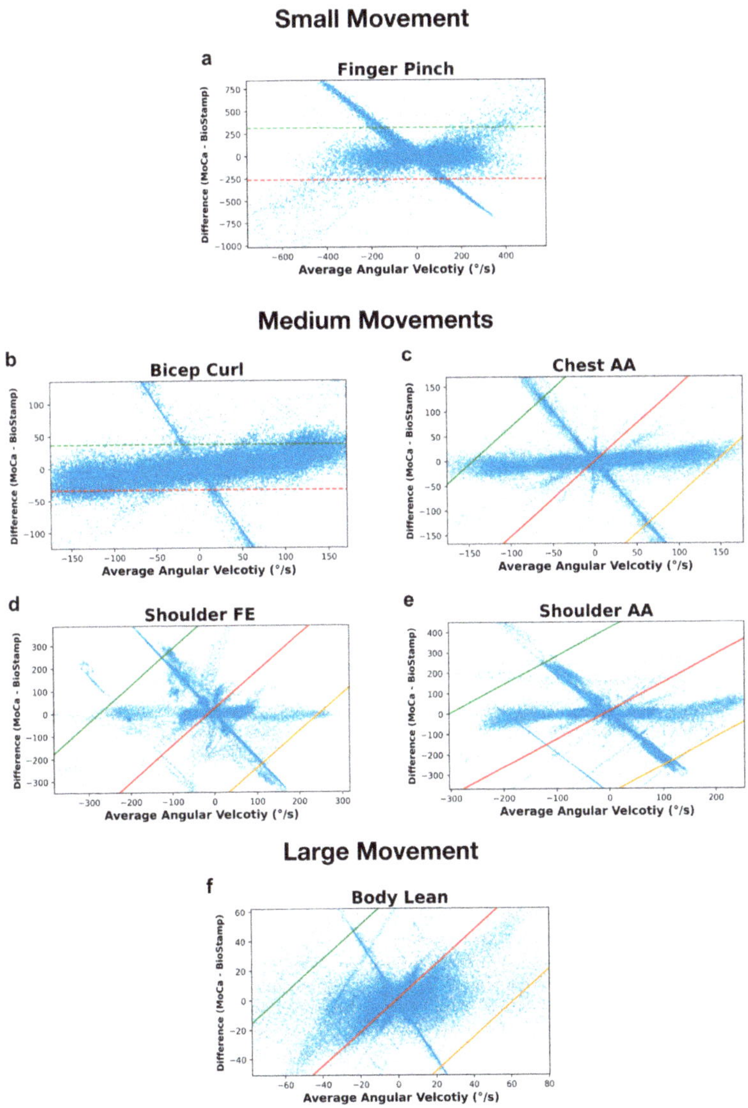

Figure 10. Bland–Altman plots of angular velocity between MoCa and BioStamp per motion categorized by motion size: small, medium, and large. (**a**) Bland–Altman plot of finger pinch movement with the 5% percentile of differences denoted by the red line, and the 95% percentile of differences denoted by green line. (**b**) Bland–Altman plot of bicep curl movement with the 5% percentile of differences denoted by the red line, and the 95% percentile of differences denoted by green line. (**c**) Bland–Altman plot of chest abduction/adduction movement, with the linear regression shown in red, the lower limit of agreement in yellow, and the upper limit of agreement in green. (**d**) Bland–Altman plot of shoulder flexion/extension movement, with the linear regression shown in red, the lower limit of agreement in yellow, and the upper limit of agreement in green. (**e**) Bland–Altman plot of shoulder abduction/adduction movement. (**f**) Bland–Altman plot of body lean movement, with the linear regression shown in red, the lower limit of agreement in yellow, and the upper limit of agreement in green.

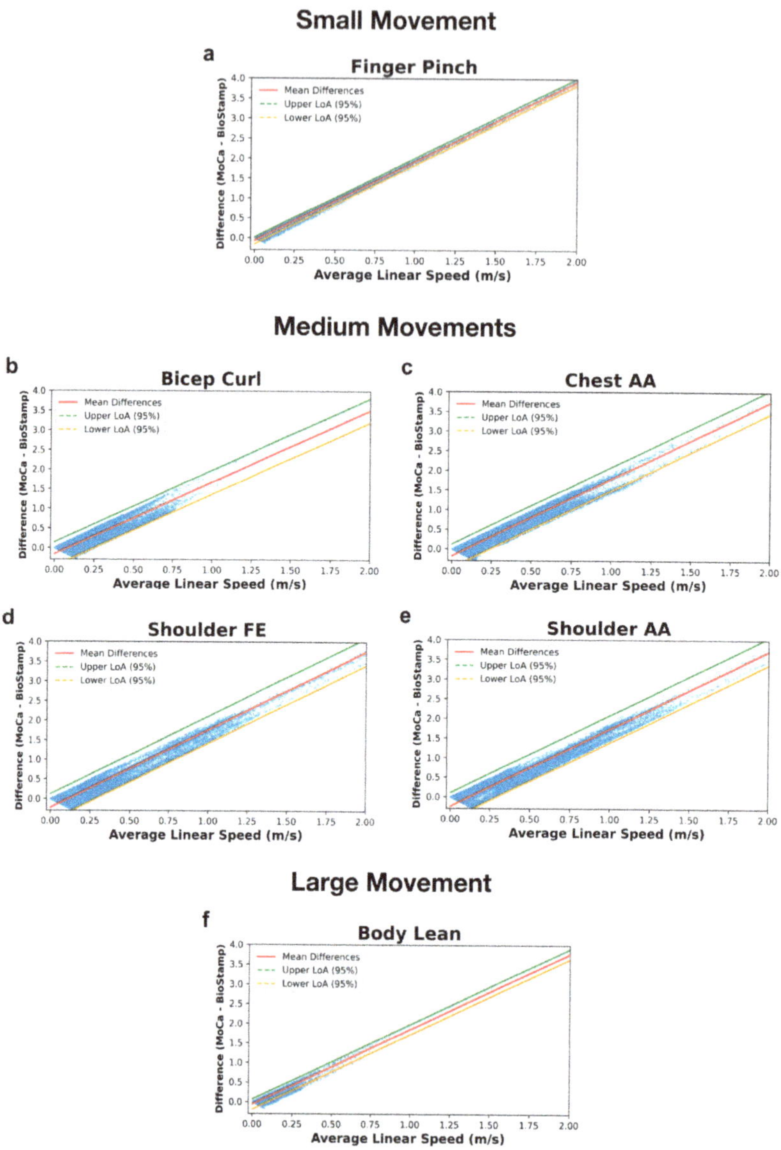

Figure 11. Bland–Altman plots of between MoCa and BioStamp per motion categorized by motion size: small, medium, and large. Blue points indicate single measurement pairs between MoCa and BioStamp. The red line indicates the linear regression, with the lower limit of agreement in yellow, and the upper limit of agreement in green. (**a**) Bland–Altman plot of the finger pinch movement. (**b**) Bland–Altman plot of the bicep curl movement. (**c**) Bland–Altman plot of the chest abduction/adduction movement. (**d**) Bland–Altman plot of the shoulder flexion/extension movement. (**e**) Bland–Altman plot of the shoulder abduction/adduction movement (**f**) Bland–Altman plot of the body lean movement.

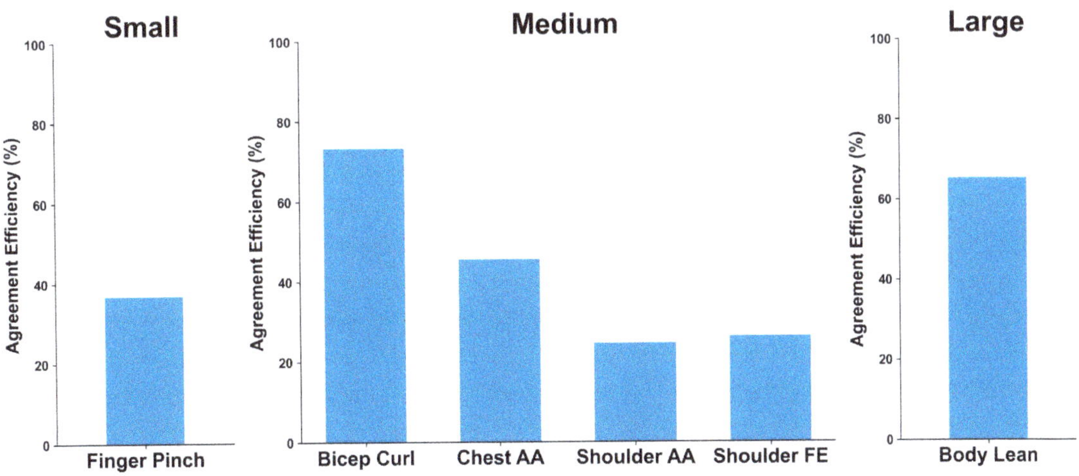

Figure 12. Agreement efficiency (%) for each motion, grouped by motion size categories, small, medium, and large.

3.3. Motion Detection Endpoint Variables

Figure 13 illustrates the Bland–Altman analysis between MoCa and BioStamp across all trials. Figure 13a illustrates the comparison of angular displacement, with a mean difference of −2.89 degrees, and the 95% limits of agreement of −58.3 and 64.08 degrees. Figure 13b demonstrates linear speed between MoCa and BioStamp, with a linear relationship between the meters per second difference and the average meter per second recorded. The slope of the relationship is 1.98 with a y-intercept of −0.16 m/s. The 95% limits of agreement are in respect to this linear trend, with y-intercepts at −0.47 and 0.15 m/s. The comparison of angular velocity is represented in Figure 13c, with a linear regression illustrating the degree per second difference relative to the average angular velocity. The y-intercept of this relationship is 5.3 degrees per second with a slope of 1.31. The 95% limits of agreement are in respect to this linear relationship, with y-intercepts at −332.44 and 333.04 degrees per second.

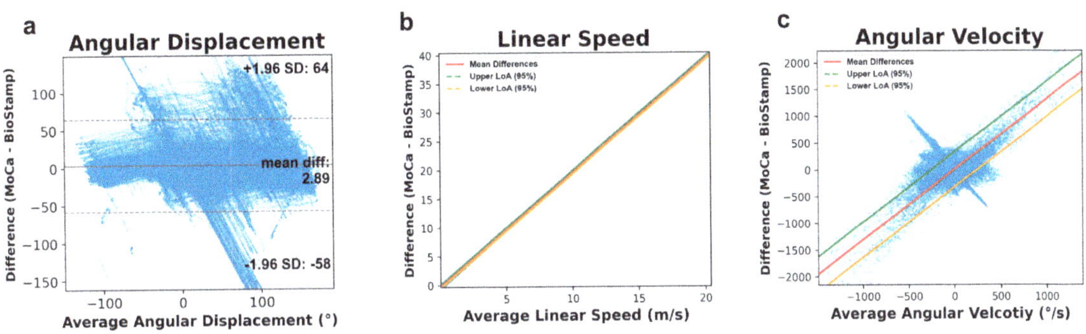

Figure 13. Bland–Altman plot between MoCa and BioStamp across endpoint variables. (**a**) Bland–Altman plot of angular displacement values. (**b**) Bland–Altman plot of linear speed values. (**c**) Bland–Altman plot of angular velocity values.

Figure 14a illustrates the angular displacement correlations between MoCa and BioStamp across all predefined motions. The bicep curl exhibited the highest angular displacement correlation between the two systems at 0.972, followed by chest abduction/adduction at 0.928. Body lean, representing a large movement, had the third-highest correlation at 0.909. Finger pinch, a small movement, showed a correlation of 0.816. Shoulder flexion/extension and shoulder abduction/adduction had correlations of 0.807 and 0.760, respectively. Overall, all motions produced relatively high correlation values when comparing MoCa and BioStamp.

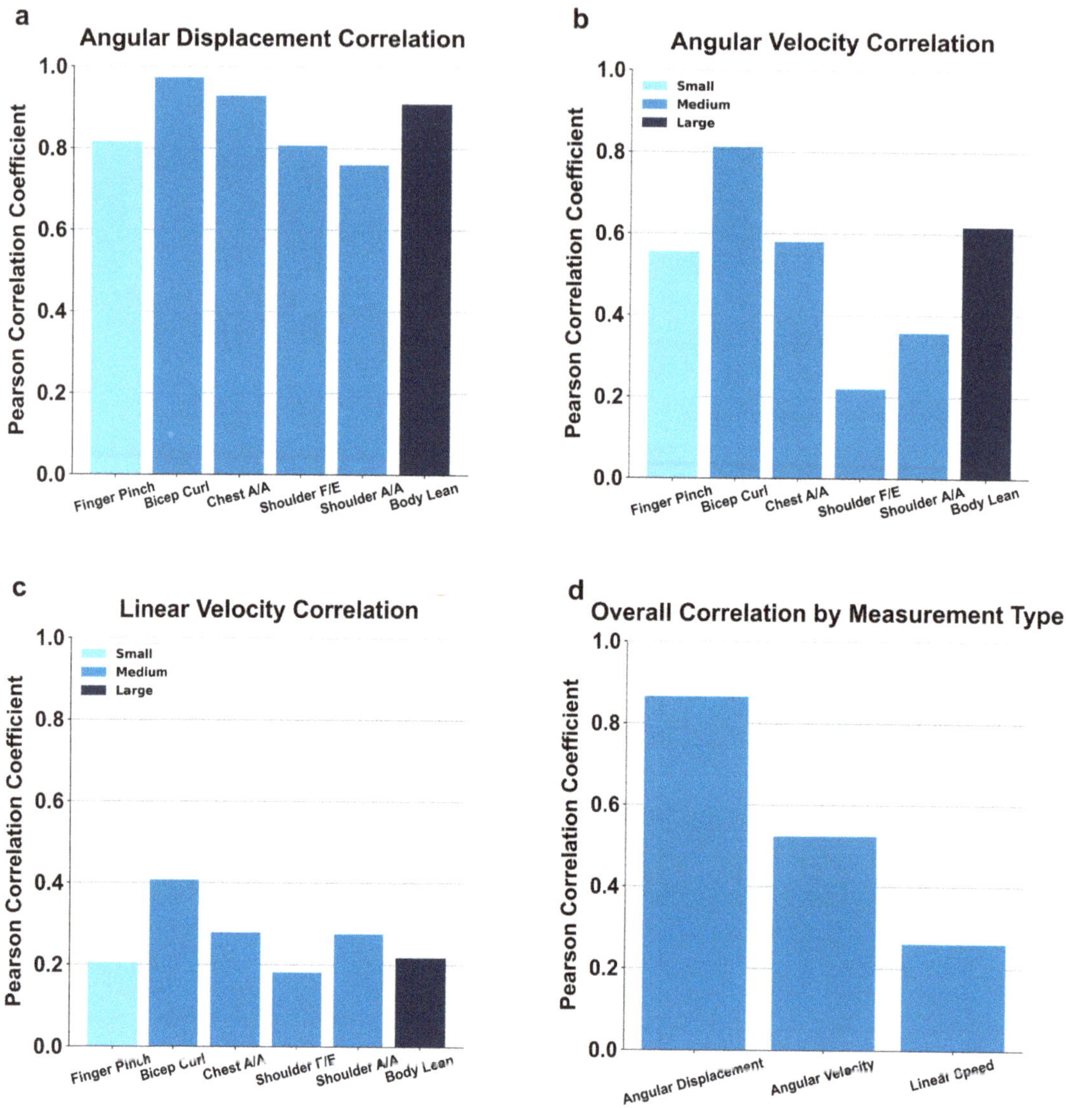

Figure 14. (**a**) Pearson correlation coefficients for angular displacement between MoCa and BioStamp across all predefined motions. (**b**) Pearson correlation coefficients for angular velocity between MoCa and BioStamp across all motions. (**c**) Pearson correlation coefficients for linear speed between MoCa and BioStamp across all motions. (**d**) Average Pearson correlation coefficients for MoCa versus BioStamp across three metrics: angular displacement, angular velocity, and linear speed.

Angular velocity correlations between MoCa and BioStamp are presented in Figure 14b. The highest angular velocity correlation was observed for the bicep curl at 0.812. Body lean and chest abduction/adduction followed with correlations of 0.617 and 0.579, respectively. Finger pinch showed a correlation of 0.556, while shoulder abduction/adduction and shoulder flexion/extension exhibited lower correlations of 0.356 and 0.219, respectively.

Linear speed correlations between MoCa and BioStamp are displayed in Figure 14c. The bicep curl demonstrated the highest average linear speed correlation at 0.406. Other motions showed lower correlations: body lean (0.217), chest abduction/adduction (0.278), finger pinch (0.204), shoulder abduction/adduction (0.275), and shoulder flexion/extension (0.181). The overall average linear speed correlation across all motions was 0.260.

Figure 14d presents the overall correlation metrics between MoCa and BioStamp across three primary measurements. Angular displacement showed the highest correlation at 0.865, followed by angular velocity at 0.523, and linear speed at 0.260.

3.4. Motion Detection by Speed

Figure 15 shows the average angular displacement (a), angular velocity (b), linear speed (c), and average Pearson correlation coefficients delineated by speed (d). The average angular displacement, which includes all motions and recording modes, shows the fast motions with an average 38.038 degrees and the slow motions at 38.523, a 0.485 degree difference between the speeds. The average angular velocity shows the fast motions at 0.017 degrees per second and the slow motions at 0.037 degrees per second, a 0.020 dps difference. The average linear speed records the fast motions at 0.280 m/s and the slow motions at 0.133 m/s, a 0.147 m/s difference. The correlations between three metrics show a slight disparity between speeds, with slower speeds correlating consistently as equal to or higher than the fast speeds. The average angular displacement correlation for fast speeds is 0.835, and for slow speeds is 0.895. The average angular velocity correlation for fast speeds is 0.486, and for slow speeds is 0.560. The average linear speed correlation for fast speeds is 0.253, and for slow speeds is 0.268. On average, slow speeds recorded 9.47% higher correlations than the fast speeds.

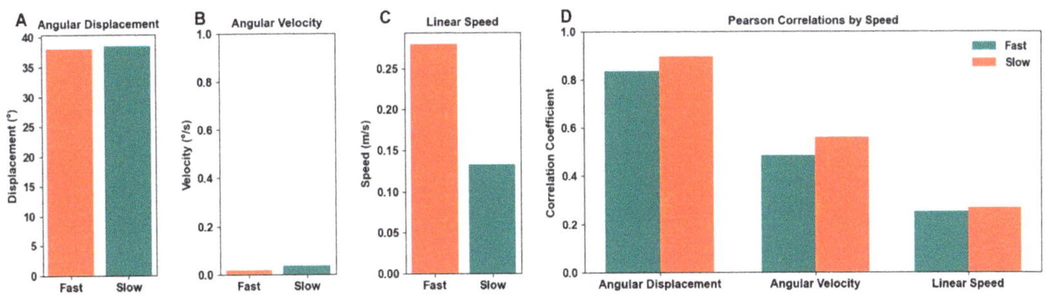

Figure 15. Comparison between slow (orange) and fast (teal) runs. (**A**) Average angular displacement comparison. (**B**) Average angular velocity comparison. (**C**) Average linear speed comparison. (**D**) Pearson correlation coefficients for angular displacement, angular velocity, and linear speed.

4. Discussion

Motion analysis is a critical tool for monitoring body movement as an element of human health, providing important insights as to functional status versus the presence, evolution, or recovery from movement-affecting disease [13,23,31]. The impairment of everyday motions may be an early indicator of changing health [13,25,32]. Motion analysis quantifies movement and is useful to non-invasively identify abnormalities associated with a wide range of diseases [13,17,33,34]. Our study shows that both the MoCa system and the BioStamp allow for a quantitative assessment of a range of human movements of varying excursions. Further, our study shows that each system has its own identifiable differences corresponding to unique advantages and disadvantages.

4.1. Trackability

Six predefined motions were tracked using MoCa and BioStamp to analyze comparable output data for the same identical movements. Maximum angular displacement was calculated for each dataset to analyze the maximum extent of motion exerted in each trial. Figure 8 demonstrates very comparable degrees of maximum angular displacement between systems. Half of the tested motions (bicep curl, chest abduction/adduction, and body lean) had higher averages in MoCa, while the other motions (finger pinch, shoulder flexion/extension, and shoulder abduction/adduction) had higher averages in BioStamp.

Though both systems were being used to track the same motion, the placement of MoCa markers and BioStamps were in slightly different physical locations on the body for each motion, leading to slight differences between MoCa and BioStamp. MoCa markers can be placed anywhere and thus were placed on strategic pivot points and limbs to effectively and optimally capture the fullest motion and discernible angles. BioStamps have placement guidelines per motion (MC10 cloud). The slight placement discrepancy between the BioStamp and MoCa markers may have caused higher maximum angular values in MoCa than in BioStamp.

In our trials, we observed systematic trends where the BioStamp displacement exhibited gradual shifts either upward or downward over time, while the overall range of motion remained constant. BioStamp's angular displacement was derived by integrating the angular velocity measured by the gyroscope. These shifts suggest potential gyroscopic sensor drift, a known issue where error accumulation occurs in the measurement of angular velocity and is thus reflected in the angular displacement trends [35]. Although the system successfully tracked the six predefined motions, additional post-processing corrections are necessary to enhance the accuracy of the displacement data [36].

There was very obvious noise in MoCa's linear speed, as seen in the linear speed Bland–Altman analysis. The proportional bias in any case suggests a systemic issue wherein MoCa generally overestimates at larger linear speeds at any point. MoCa produced angular displacement results that were well aligned to BioStamp, which is supportive evidence that the system does not have trouble tracking motion, but rather the linear speed noise may be indicative of a large sensitivity to movements of the markers.

Overall, the detection of the tested motions was successful using each system. Varying values of angular displacement detected can be attributed to MoCa marker placement or sensor drift inherent to BioStamp. Despite the minor variance, both MoCa and BioStamp effectively captured the motion's extent, shape, and range with good overall correlation, though some movements correlated to a greater degree than others.

4.2. Motion Size Comparison

Size categories were created across the six motions to examine the ability of each system to quantitate motion across differing motion excursion ranges, i.e., sizes, defined in terms of dimensional areas, i.e., as small (<1 sq ft), medium (1–5 sq ft), and large (6–10 sq ft).

4.2.1. Small Motion

Finger pinch was the sole motion in the small motion size category. The small scale of the finger pinch motion did not affect tracking ability and both MoCa and BioStamp were able to track the motion.

The negative mean difference in the angular displacement indicates that MoCa generally produced angles lower than BioStamp. Though the Pearson correlation coefficient was large, the low agreement efficiency indicates that there was a very significant discrepancy between the two systems in terms of angular displacement. Angular velocity between the two systems varied greatly, though it did not exhibit a significant linear relationship between differences and velocity as was the case for other motions. Linear speed had a very strong correlation, with a slope of two. As seen in many examples, it was clear that finger pinch exhibited a large degree of noise in terms of speed. The small motion size may have contributed to the error found within the comparisons. As a suggested use case, twitching and sudden small muscular spasms can arise as signs of chronic kidney disease (CKD) [37]. The finger pinch experiment illustrates that MoCa and BioStamp should go through further accuracy training before being used to assess sudden and small muscular spasms.

4.2.2. Medium Motions

Correlations varied over a spectrum within the medium size motion category, comprising bicep curl, chest abduction/adduction, shoulder abduction/adduction, and shoulder flexion/extension.

Bicep curl had the most aligned angular displacements between systems, indicated by their very high correlation coefficients and agreement efficiencies. The positive mean difference in the angular Bland–Altman analysis indicates that MoCa tended to produce larger angles than BioStamp. It also had the narrowest angular velocity limits of agreement, indicating a greater agreement of velocity than in other motions. The stark slope in the linear Bland–Altman analysis indicates very strong proportional bias.

The chest abduction/adduction movement was aligned between systems better than some motions and worse than others. The angular results indicated that the differences between systems were half that of the observed values, with MoCa having relatively higher angles on average. The stark regressions in both linear speed and angular velocity represent a proportional bias for speed measurements.

Shoulder flexion/extension as well as shoulder abduction/adduction had the lowest agreement between systems compared to all other motions. Both had limits of agreement that were roughly 75% of the total angles for their motions. MoCa tended to produce lower angles than BioStamp for shoulder FE while it tended to produce much larger values for shoulder AA. Both motions had very evident proportional bias in terms of speed, as indicated by the significant linear trends.

As an example of potential use, tracking limb movement in restless leg syndrome (RLS) which is common in chronic kidney disease patients, would be useful in diagnosis and treatment [38]. The medium motion studies demonstrate the ability of both MoCa and BioStamp to track erratic movements in a limb, as occurs in RLS, though addressing systemic noise could benefit the use of either system in such cases.

4.2.3. Large Motion

Body lean was the sole motion in the large size motion category and had alignment between systems second best only to the bicep curl motion. The angular displacement comparisons indicate a large correlation and agreement, with a very slight bias for MoCa to produce lower angles. The speed analysis indicate a proportional bias.

The large size category represents motion tracking for near full-body motions. CKD can cause involuntary movements as well as bodily fatigue that can be apparent on a greater area of the patient's body [39,40]. As such, MoCa's and BioStamp's ability to track body lean's larger size demonstrates the accuracy in large-scale motion abnormality detection for both systems.

4.2.4. Size Definitions

The size definition had seemingly no correlation with how well the motions tracked. Across agreement efficiency, Pearson correlations, and maximum angular displacement, the most observable differences between systems are generally found for the shoulder movements, both belonging to the medium category. Though the bicep curl and body lean motion belonged to different motion size categories, they generally tracked the best and aligned the most between systems. The mean difference bias across motions had no correlation to the size category either, given that three of the medium motions had larger angles for MoCa than BioStamp, with the other three motions having lower angles for MoCa. The speed results indicated a proportional bias for every motion save for the finger pinch and bicep curl angular velocity. Bicep curl's angular velocity Bland–Altman analysis was the only speed analysis that had even remotely comparable differences between MoCa and BioStamp, which makes sense when considering that the angular results were best for the motion.

The agreement efficiency normalizes the differences between systems relative to the typical angles for the motion. That makes the statistic a comparable one, in which case there is a slight trend, with the small motion having the worst agreement, the medium movements having generally better agreement, and the large movement having better agreement. The limitation of analyzing such a trend is the lack of multiple motions in the small and large motion category. Nonetheless, we can estimate that the larger a motion is, as defined by the terms in the paper, the more room for error and thus, the accuracy of the motion. For example, the intricate movements of a finger pinch require the minimal movement of the fingers, whereas the body lean motion requires a full-body tilt. Such disparities in the motions could lend themselves to tracking ability.

It may be worth noting that the difference in agreement between motions in the medium motion category may suggest that motion size alone is not responsible for tracking ability. The motions that had greater MoCa tracking failure were on muscles that have a greater axis of rotation, such as the shoulders. Revisiting Figure 3e shows the markers placed on parts of the arm with a greater chance of twisting away from camera view, such as the shoulder and elbow. The motions may have been more difficult to perform because the subjects did not have an armrest for their arms, which lent itself to more arm swiveling. Additionally, some variance in the orientation of the limb could be explained by the joints' greater range of movement while performing the motion. The motions that performed the best had the best lateral view of all markers. All of the motions tested had the proven ability to have all MoCa markers in view of the camera as MoCa can only track in two dimensions. However, the tendency of the limbs to twist markers out of frame is greater for some motions than others, accounting for some performance reduction.

4.3. Endpoint Variables

We compared the efficacy of each system across motion endpoint variables. The Bland–Altman analysis would thereby display any systemic or relative bias.

The Bland–Altman analysis of angular displacement across all trials displayed a mean difference of 2.89, which indicates a very small systemic bias, where MoCa generally produces angles on average 2.89 degrees larger than BioStamp. This indicates that MoCa tends eto produce angles similar to BioStamp, though the wide limits of agreement indicates variability in differences. This indicates relative bias as opposed to a systemic bias on the behalf of MoCa, given that the mean difference differs from motion to motion. The Pearson correlation coefficient of 86.5% indicates a strong alignment of trends between the systems. Variation in correlation coefficients may be attributed to MoCa's loss of a marker during tracking. When a MoCa marker's position in the video is lost, its coordinates are static until its position can be detected again. When the marker is re-detected, there will be a sudden jump in positional coordinates. The static output of angles during the time of marker loss would reflect as poor correlation, thus attributing to the correlation coefficients between systems, though only slightly. Given a high correlation coefficient, the wide limits of agreement present in the Bland–Altman analysis indicate a difference of absolute values. In any case, the value discrepancies between MoCa and BioStamp may be attributed to sensor drift in BioStamp's gyroscopic output as mentioned previously, which resulted in downward or upward shifts of angles over time.

The Bland–Altman analysis of the angular velocity between systems indicates complex relationships between systems and their output. The general trend is a proportional bias, indicated by the linear regression between the differences and the magnitude of the angular velocity. This indicates that the differences are largely dependent on the average. Visually, there is also an inverse proportional bias, with MoCa overestimating negative angular velocity values and underestimating positive values. The presence of both types of proportional bias indicates high-frequency noise on the behalf of MoCa, wherein for any given velocity value, it will either underestimate or overestimate. Though the sensor drift present in BioStamp's gyroscopic output may also play a part, the noise in MoCa far outweighed the bias effects from BioStamp, as evident by the significance of the linear regression.

The linear speed was the third metric analyzed between the systems. Linear speed correlations were the lowest of the three correlations, and the linear regression present in the Bland–Altman plot indicates a systemic disparity between MoCa and BioStamp. MoCa displayed a large degree of noise, resulting in a great deal of fluctuations in its output, as evident in the low correlation coefficient and large proportional bias in the Bland–Altman analysis. Though MoCa's tendency to lose a marker is attributed in part to the fluctuations in linear speed, it is much more likely that MoCa tends to have a large sensitivity to coordinate tracking and thus produces erratic linear speed data.

4.4. Speed Comparison

In addition to size categorization, another factor we analyzed was the speed of the motion. Both fast and slow paces were performed for each movement. Overall, the speed of the marker and stamps movement had little effect on the trackability of the motion detection systems. In Figure 15, the average angular displacements (a) and velocities (b) of all motions divided into fast and slow paces showed little difference. Linear speed (c) had a much higher value for the fast category, which is expected considering that the fast category is intended to have a faster rate of motion relative to the slow category of motions. The Pearson correlation coefficients of angular displacement, angular velocity, and linear speed between fast and slow are all relatively similar. Slow had slightly higher correlation scores for angular displacement, angular velocity, and linear speed which could be because slower data tracking lends itself to less tracking loss and thus, cleaner data.

4.5. System Comparison

The BioStamp is an FDA-approved device that can track three-dimensional motion and rotational movement. It utilizes a cloud-based system for data storage, which enables instantaneous data upload. MoCa is entirely video-based, capturing motion data in the 2D.

MoCa is an inexpensive and nimble system. It requires several colored stamps and a camera. The BioStamp is currently not easily accessible due to its high cost, limiting its accessibility for patients. The operating costs are almost negligible for MoCa, assuming a camera is available. This makes it readily deployable with a fairly fast setup time in terms of data collection; the subject needs to place the markers per location instruction, set up a camera, and start recording. As it is video-based, qualitative information in the form of video recordings can be reviewed instantly, allowing a researcher or clinician to make small adjustments as needed for data collection.

There exists a very comparable degree of processing required to obtain angular displacement, angular velocity, and linear speed from both MoCa and BioStamp as is; BioStamp requires the processing of acceleration and gyroscope data while MoCa requires the processing of positional data. BioStamp's acceleration data requires normalization according to gravity to obtain accurate data. Static motions may benefit from a simple static normalization, while more dynamic movements may require the dynamic normalization as performed here. BioStamp's angular velocity, like many gyroscopes, is affected by sensor drift and obtaining movement-accurate angular data may require additional processing [36]. MoCa on the other hand does not need to adjust for gravity, given its positional capture of motion. Similarly, sensor drift is inherently not an issue for MoCa. Positional data is recorded in pixels, and obtaining units such as meters requires a measurement of a reference point in the video, such as the subject's arm. BioStamp does not need a reference measurement, given the meters can easily be obtained from its gyroscopic data, given in g's.

Beyond necessary processing components, in advancing these technologies, both systems can benefit from varying degrees of noise-adjustment and smoothing. We examined MoCa's output of angular displacement, angular velocity, and linear speed without any smoothing or filtering applied. Due to the amount of noise present, MoCa's linear speed output can greatly benefit from a high-frequency filtering process to obtain relevant information. As seen by the similarity in the systems' angular displacement, BioStamp benefitted from smoothing on its angular velocity, and by transitivity, its angular displacement as well.

MoCa has visual tracking capabilities that are not inherent to BioStamp. MoCa's positional tracking provides a direct visual indicator of motion, given that it tracked accordingly. The inclusion of the accompanying video from which its data was derived from can also provide substantial qualitative information if need be. BioStamp only provides raw numeric metrics and requires significant processing to create comparable data to that of MoCa's positional data. Therefore, deriving a visual interpretation of a BioStamp recorded motion can be challenging.

Obtaining angular displacement information from MoCa may be more complex than it is for BioStamp, depending on the motion captured. For motions where the angular displacement crosses zero degrees (or 360 degrees), additional calculations are required to account for this transition. Although this was resolved manually in the experiment, alternative methods can automate this process. Additionally, it is vital to clearly delineate the pivot marker from the other markers when calculating the corresponding angle. BioStamp angular displacement was obtained from the sensor that recorded the most motion, and thus has to be selected accordingly.

MoCa is susceptible to color interference. MoCa uses color values to identify and track its markers (HSV values specifically). If there is an object in the frame of a similar color to the marker, the system will not be able to properly track the desired markers. When the subjects' clothing and markers were similar in color, MoCa would interpret the clothing articles as trackable markers, thus causing irreconcilable interference. Lighting variability can greatly affect the success of the marker tracking, causing color distortion that causes the tracking of incorrect positions from its respective video.

The observable advantages and disadvantages of both MoCa and BioStamp are summarized in Table 3.

Table 3. Advantages and disadvantages of MoCa and BioStamp.

MoCa Disadvantages	MoCa Advantages	BioStamp Disadvantages	BioStamp Advantages
Longer processing period post recordings	Tracks angular displacement very well	Greater stamp quantity required for large movement sizes	Tracked consistently across all motions
Rotation in movement causes obscurity	Tracked well on both fast and slow	Suffers from gyroscopic sensor-drift	Tracked well on both fast and slow
Markers easily get obscured	Flexible marker placement	Strict marker placement	Data outputted quickly

4.6. Human Activity Recognition Implications

Human activity recognition (HAR) is a field of computational study that aims to automate the recognition of human activity via the input of a variety of data sources [41]. Relevant to this study, there are modalities of HAR systems that are either based on computer-vision or on inertial measurement unit (IMU) systems. HAR systems based on gyroscopes and accelerometers, such as the BioStamp sensor, have been proven to have substantial efficacy [42]. Pose-estimation, on the other hand, is a form of HAR that utilizes 'keypoints' or essential skeletal features from a video to delineate human motion. OpenPose is an open-source tool that utilizes keypoints extracted from videos in order to produce characteristics on motion [43]. The toolkit currently has over 100 keypoints to extract from a given video. Albeit HAR capabilities are possible via pose-estimation, it is typically effective with a multitude of keyframes; a model designed to be lightweight still required a minimum of 15 keypoints to achieve maximal accuracy [44]. Alternatively, a model designed for low-performing computers required up to 18 keypoints [45].

While HAR is theoretically feasible with MoCa architecture, the current limitation of tracking only three markers significantly affects its adaptability for HAR applications. BioStamp, on the other hand, may perform effectively within HAR contexts, given current implementations on gyroscope and accelerometer sensors.

4.7. Study Limitations

The lack of a ground truth with which to compare both systems is a limitation of the study. Though there was a definition for each trial in terms of the type of motion, the speed, and the recording circumstances, there is still bound to be variance from subject to subject and from trial to trial. Gathering the ground truth of any endpoint in this sense would be difficult, further complicated by the nuances of datapoints at the frequency at which either system captures data. Both MoCa and BioStamp have been tested in terms of statistical error for their respective angular displacements, displaying significantly minimal error [17,22]. This study's accurate representation of real-world data highlights the practical applicability of motion analysis systems such as MoCa and BioStamp.

The subjects that participated in this study were all healthy. Testing on a more diverse population, including those with injury, will be useful to extend and confirm our findings in a more diverse population. Further studies will further define similarities and differences in the population for which these systems were developed for clinical use.

The study as performed was under ambient lighting. Lighting intensity was not controlled here. MoCa trackability may be affected by poor lighting or glare from the camera, which may impact the interpretation of the results [24]. The test mirrored real-world applications; the systems may have to account for a variety of lighting conditions given. This study did not take into account exactly how much light there was at the time of recording nor the type of lighting used. Examining lighting influence will be useful for future experimentation.

This study examined only six predefined motions. While we included a range of excursion sizes, future studies may benefit from other determining factors, be it axis of rotation or specific movements that affect MoCa tracking differently. In future studies, it will be beneficial to include a greater number and variety of motions involving more joints, limbs, mobility, etc., in order to determine on a motion-by-motion basis what the limiting factors are in tracking.

4.8. Current Technology

A comparison study was conducted in 2023 where the extraction of useful body metrics possible from wearable sensors was explored across virtual reality sensors, motion capture, and computer vision [34]. Virtual reality tracking and computer vision gained accuracies of 96% and 100%, respectively, where high accuracy was attributed to the extensive initial calibration for each user equipping the gear and the implementation of neural networks involving significant processing power and high computational complexity (especially in the case of computer vision). Several issues were discussed in the use of these systems in the healthcare system. High-cost equipment and insufficient maintenance posed one issue. Therefore, in response to these concerns, motion capture methods were considered ideal. Motion capture involved fixed sensors on various parts of the body that were able to provide a body 'model' in three-dimensional space and analyze musculoskeletal motion. However, the fixed locations of the sensors to be able to communicate with each other in order to construct the body model limits its use in varying musculoskeletal diseases should the targeted areas of testing not have corresponding sensor locations. Additionally, this system was 'extremely inconvenient' when collecting more than one target point. As such, MoCa is an alternative to the need for non-fixed sensors and low-cost equipment as it functions as a similar motion capture without strict placement options. Unlike the experiments' three-dimensional motion capture, this feature is not yet fully implemented in the data collection process, the next step to improving it to be a high-substance motion capture system.

4.9. Future Improvements

Future improvement of MoCa will address its current limitations. In order to bring MoCa analysis into three-dimensional space, two cameras, or a single stereoscopic camera, may be implemented in combination with three-dimensional markers. Integrating onboard verification of lighting conditions would make the system more concise and viable for real clinical use. To mitigate background color interference, markers could be redesigned to incorporate a unique identifying pattern in place of single-color recognition. Further processing to account for noisy data, a loss of marker tracking, and an automated method for incorporating reference units can all improve the seamlessness of the system, thus making it more applicable for the real world.

The current implementation of MoCa relies entirely on programming scripts that may have to be adjusted for the person and motion at hand. Future implementations should address this and incorporate a graphical user interface (GUI) to provide healthcare providers an intuitive program that is easy to use. The automation of any manual aspect of the data processing may also benefit the usability of the system by eliminating the time needed to set up the post-recording analysis. This may include aspects such as measuring body lengths of the subject for unit estimations and the accessibility to work on motions not tested before.

If MoCa is intended to be used for human activity recognition applications, it may benefit from attaining data from more markers. In its current implementation, MoCa cannot record more than three markers in a single video. The use of dozens of markers would bring the efficacy of MoCa in terms of HAR results to that of other keyframe-based HAR systems [45].

Given the difficulty of establishing a ground-truth when utilizing either system for clinical motion analysis, it may be beneficial to assess whether either system could be used for delineating categories from one another. This may be in the form of testing whether a system can differentiate a healthy control group from a different group, for example. The relative data output between subjects is one method of assessing the applicability of either MoCa or BioStamp.

4.10. Clinical Utility

The findings of this study hold significant implications for healthcare management, disease tracking and rehabilitation. MoCa's simplicity and real-time capabilities position it as an attractive option, especially for telemedicine applications [46]. Patients can undergo motion analysis remotely, reducing the need for clinic visits and potentially alleviating healthcare system over-capacity burdens [47]. Its user-friendly setup and dynamic visualization also facilitates quick adjustments, enhancing data quality and consequent analysis.

MoCa is being studied in disease detection and monitoring, branching beyond simple exercises as studied herein. Pulmonology is currently examining MoCa applicability [48]. Chest conditions exemplified by abnormal chest movements and respiratory fluctuations can be tracked by MoCa sensors detecting variations in the chest rising and falling. Pulmonologists can view the chest fluctuations easily on graph displays outputted by MoCa software version 1.0.

The BioStamp's precision tracking and FDA approval also aligns well with comprehensive clinical assessments. Its potential lies in in-depth analyses that demand accurate motion data, making it a suitable choice for specific research endeavors. However, the challenges of interpreting isolated data highlight the need for a careful consideration of the analysis objectives.

As an example, these systems may be used in monitoring motion abnormalities in patients with chronic kidney disease (CKD). MoCa and BioStamp provide quantifiable and accurate motion analysis that could be performed remotely. CKD has several motion abnormalities that may be indicators of disease status such as restless leg syndrome, tremors, and movement abnormalities arising from bodily fatigue and electrolyte abnormalities [32]. Should any of these signs be detected by MoCa or BioStamp remotely, the patient can be called in for further examination and therapy. Conducting remote motion abnormality detection tests can also accelerate and confirm a diagnosis limiting the need for in-person visits, or increasing the value of a visit via enhanced information gathering in the outpatient setting.

The effectiveness of either system is outlined per movement disorders and body elements in Table 4. The application of MoCa and BioStamp are dependent on the respective motions, given that certain movements lend themselves to poor tracking and others to excellent tracking.

Table 4. Sample applications of MoCa and BioStamp for the assessment of several movement disorders and their respective disease states. Organized based on body elements (whole body, extremity, digit, etc.) and offering commentary on the efficacy of each motion capture modality.

Body Element	Movement Disorders	Disease States	MoCa	BioStamp
Large Whole Body	Limited ROM	Traumatic injury arthritis	Moderate: ROM testing may require tracking over larger distances	Moderate: Should be able to track well but perhaps be wary of motions in the vertical axis
	Chorea	Lesions affecting the striatum Huntington disease Sydenham chorea Levodopa-induced dyskinesia	Poor: Unpredictable large motions may obscure marker placement and be poorly tracked	No issues
	Akathisia	Psychomotor disorder	Moderate: There are multiple manifestations of akathisia. May be appropriate for larger movements, but difficulty tracking smaller motions.	Moderate: Due to BioStamp's difficulty tracking vertical motion, may have some trouble with tracking
	Gait Abnormalities	Parkinson disease Osteoarthritis Traumatic injury Stroke Cerebral palsy	Poor: Due to the unpredictability of ataxic gait, there is a high likelihood of markers on extremities becoming occluded and interfering with tracking	No issues
	Limited ROM	Traumatic injury arthritis	No issues	No issues
	Myoclonus	Uremia Creutzfeldt-Jakob disease Epilepsy syndromes	No issues	No issues
	Restless Leg Syndrome	Low iron stores Uremia Peripheral neuropathy	No issues	No issues

Table 4. *Cont.*

Body Element	Movement Disorders	Disease States	MoCa	BioStamp
Medium Upper and Lower Extremities	Ballismus	Subthalamic nucleus lesion	Moderate: Subjects can present with large involuntary movements and may not be able to prevent marker occlusion	No issues
	Resting Tremor	Parkinson disease Lewy body dementia Multiple system atrophy Progressive supranuclear palsy Wilson disease Dopamine antagonists	No issues	No issues
	Postural Tremor	Essential tremor Orthostatic tremor	No issues	No issues
Small Wrist, Ankle, Hands, Feet, and Digits	Limited ROM	Traumatic injury arthritis	No issues	No issues
	Asterixis	Hepatic encephalopathy Uremic encephalopathy Hypercapnia	No issues	No issues

5. Conclusions

In the realm of motion analysis for healthcare assessment, management, and rehabilitation, MoCa and BioStamp emerge as distinct yet promising tools, each bearing a set of unique advantages and limitations. This study compared and contrasted the motion tracking capabilities of each, defining their respective advantages and limitations. Our findings substantiate our hypotheses that MoCa excels in real-time dynamic two-dimensional visualization and affordability, while BioStamp effectively captures 3D and rotational motion at a higher costs. MoCa and BioStamp correlate well in terms of angular displacement, with lesser correlation in terms of linear speed and angular velocity. The distinct strengths of each system reinforce our hypothesis that MoCa and BioStamp both serve as valuable tools, albeit in different capacities, for motion analysis in rehabilitation and healthcare contexts. MoCa provides more accurate angular data without the need to account for sensor error, making it ideal for tracking range of motion at an affordable price. BioStamp on the other hand excels at providing acceleration data, making it ideal for tracking linear motion at a higher cost.

Author Contributions: Conceptualization, M.J.S.; methodology, M.J.S., G.S.P., Y.A., K.R. and C.H.; software, K.R., C.G., C.H., G.S.P., Y.A. and S.O.; validation, M.J.S.; formal analysis, K.R., C.G., L.D.A., J.R., Z.H. and M.J.S.; investigation, K.R., C.G., C.H., G.S.P., Y.A., and S.O.; resources, M.J.S.; data curation, K.R., C.G., L.D.A., J.R., Z.H., M.L., S.S. and B.T.; writing—original draft preparation, K.R., C.G., L.D.A., J.R., Z.H., G.S.P., M.L., C.H., E.R. and R.C.; writing—review and editing, K.R., C.G., L.D.A., R.C.S. and M.J.S.; visualization, K.R., C.G., L.D.A., J.R., Z.H. and F.A.; supervision, M.J.S.; project administration, M.J.S., G.S.P., K.R. and L.D.A.; funding acquisition, M.J.S. All authors have read and agreed to the published version of the manuscript.

Funding: This work was supported by ACABI—the Arizona Center for Accelerated Biomedical Innovation of the University of Arizona. ACABI had no role in the design of the study, nor in the collection, analysis, and interpretation of data or writing of the manuscript. Support was also provided by NIH NIDDK Grant R25DK128859.

Institutional Review Board Statement: The study was conducted according to the guidelines of the Declaration of Helsinki, and approved by the Institutional Review Board of The University of

Arizona.-protocol code #2107032177 and date of approval. Written informed consent was obtained from all study participants utilizing an IRB-approved consent form.

Informed Consent Statement: Informed consent was obtained from all subjects.

Data Availability Statement: The data that support the findings of this study are available on request from the corresponding author. The data are not publicly available due to privacy.

Conflicts of Interest: The authors declare no conflicts of interest.

References

1. Tintignac, L.A.; Brenner, H.-R.; Rüegg, M.A. Mechanisms Regulating Neuromuscular Junction Development and Function and Causes of Muscle Wasting. *Physiol. Rev.* **2015**, *95*, 809–852. [CrossRef] [PubMed]
2. Visser, M.; Goodpaster, B.H.; Kritchevsky, S.B.; Newman, A.B.; Nevitt, M.; Rubin, S.M.; Simonsick, E.M.; Harris, T.B.; Health ABC Study. Muscle Mass, Muscle Strength, and Muscle Fat Infiltration as Predictors of Incident Mobility Limitations in Well-Functioning Older Persons. *J. Gerontol. Ser. A* **2005**, *60*, 324–333. [CrossRef]
3. Brognara, L.; Luna, O.C.; Traina, F.; Cauli, O. Inflammatory Biomarkers and Gait Impairment in Older Adults: A Systematic Review. *Int. J. Mol. Sci.* **2024**, *25*, 1368. [CrossRef]
4. Anker, S.D.; Chua, T.P.; Ponikowski, P.; Harrington, D.; Swan, J.W.; Kox, W.J.; Poole-Wilson, P.A.; Coats, A.J. Hormonal Changes and Catabolic/Anabolic Imbalance in Chronic Heart Failure and Their Importance for Cardiac Cachexia. *Circulation* **1997**, *96*, 526–534. [CrossRef] [PubMed]
5. Tieland, M.; Trouwborst, I.; Clark, B.C. Skeletal Muscle Performance and Ageing. *J. Cachexia Sarcopenia Muscle* **2018**, *9*, 3–19. [CrossRef] [PubMed]
6. Van Bruggen, H.W.; Van Den Engel-Hoek, L.; Steenks, M.H.; Bronkhorst, E.M.; Creugers, N.H.J.; de Groot, I.J.M.; Kalaykova, S.I. Reduced Mandibular Range of Motion in Duchenne Muscular Dystrophy: Predictive Factors. *J. Oral Rehabil.* **2015**, *42*, 430–438. [CrossRef]
7. Hill, S.; Mong, S.; Vo, Q. Three-Dimensional Motion Analysis for Occupational Therapy Upper Extremity Assessment and Rehabilitation: A Scoping Review. *Open J. Occup. Ther.* **2022**, *10*, 1–14. [CrossRef]
8. Ferreira Dos Santos, L.; Christ, O.; Mate, K.; Schmidt, H.; Krüger, J.; Dohle, C. Movement Visualisation in Virtual Reality Rehabilitation of the Lower Limb: A Systematic Review. *Biomed. Eng. OnLine* **2016**, *15*, 144. [CrossRef]
9. Debnath, B.; O'Brien, M.; Yamaguchi, M.; Behera, A. A Review of Computer Vision-Based Approaches for Physical Rehabilitation and Assessment. *Multimed. Syst.* **2022**, *28*, 209–239. [CrossRef]
10. Colyer, S.L.; Evans, M.; Cosker, D.P.; Salo, A.I.T. A Review of the Evolution of Vision-Based Motion Analysis and the Integration of Advanced Computer Vision Methods Towards Developing a Markerless System. *Sports Med.-Open* **2018**, *4*, 24. [CrossRef]
11. Chander, H.; Burch, R.F.; Talegaonkar, P.; Saucier, D.; Luczak, T.; Ball, J.E.; Turner, A.; Kodithuwakku Arachchige, S.N.K.; Carroll, W.; Smith, B.K.; et al. Wearable Stretch Sensors for Human Movement Monitoring and Fall Detection in Ergonomics. *Int. J. Environ. Res. Public Health* **2020**, *17*, 3554. [CrossRef] [PubMed]
12. Benmessabih, T.; Slama, R.; Havard, V.; Baudry, D. Online Human Motion Analysis in Industrial Context: A Review. *Eng. Appl. Artif. Intell.* **2024**, *131*, 107850. [CrossRef]
13. Breasail, Ó.M.; Biswas, B.; Smith, M.D.; Mazhar, M.K.A.; Tenison, E.; Cullen, A.; Lithander, F.E.; Roudaut, A.; Henderson, E.J. Wearable GPS and Accelerometer Technologies for Monitoring Mobility and Physical Activity in Neurodegenerative Disorders: A Systematic Review. *Sensors* **2021**, *21*, 8261. [CrossRef]
14. Mündermann, L.; Corazza, S.; Andriacchi, T.P. The Evolution of Methods for the Capture of Human Movement Leading to Markerless Motion Capture for Biomechanical Applications. *J. Neuroeng. Rehabil.* **2006**, *3*, 6. [CrossRef] [PubMed]
15. Chinmilli, P.; Redkar, S.; Zhang, W.; Sugar, T. A Review on Wearable Inertial Tracking Based Human Gait Analysis and Control Strategies of Lower-Limb Exoskeletons. *Int. Robot. Autom. J.* **2017**, *3*, 398–415. [CrossRef]
16. Kim, D.-H.; Ghaffari, R.; Lu, N.; Rogers, J.A. Flexible and Stretchable Electronics for Biointegrated Devices. *Annu. Rev. Biomed. Eng.* **2012**, *14*, 113–128. [CrossRef]
17. Vincent, A.C.; Furman, H.; Slepian, R.C.; Ammann, K.R.; Di Maria, C.; Chien, J.H.; Siu, K.-C.; Slepian, M.J. Smart Phone-Based Motion Capture and Analysis: Importance of Operating Envelope Definition and Application to Clinical Use. *Appl. Sci.* **2022**, *12*, 6173. [CrossRef]
18. Wang, L.; Hu, W.; Tan, T. Recent Developments in Human Motion Analysis. *Pattern Recognit.* **2003**, *36*, 585–601. [CrossRef]
19. Pediaditis, M.; Tsiknakis, M.; Leitgeb, N. Vision-Based Motion Detection, Analysis and Recognition of Epileptic Seizures—A Systematic Review. *Comput. Methods Programs Biomed.* **2012**, *108*, 1133–1148. [CrossRef]
20. Ristić-Durrant, D.; Franke, M.; Michels, K. A Review of Vision-Based On-Board Obstacle Detection and Distance Estimation in Railways. *Sensors* **2021**, *21*, 3452. [CrossRef]
21. Randers, M.B.; Mujika, I.; Hewitt, A.; Santisteban, J.; Bischoff, R.; Solano, R.; Zubillaga, A.; Peltola, E.; Krustrup, P.; Mohr, M. Application of Four Different Football Match Analysis Systems: A Comparative Study. *J. Sports Sci.* **2010**, *28*, 171–182. [CrossRef] [PubMed]

22. Ammann, K.R.; Ahamed, T.; Sweedo, A.L.; Ghaffari, R.; Weiner, Y.E.; Slepian, R.C.; Jo, H.; Slepian, M.J. Human Motion Component and Envelope Characterization via Wireless Wearable Sensors. *BMC Biomed. Eng.* **2020**, *2*, 3. [CrossRef]
23. Garlant, J.A.; Ammann, K.R.; Slepian, M.J. Stretchable Electronic Wearable Motion Sensors Delineate Signatures of Human Motion Tasks. *ASAIO J.* **2018**, *64*, 351. [CrossRef] [PubMed]
24. Parks, M.; Chien, J.H.; Siu, K.-C. Development of a Mobile Motion Capture (MO2CA) System for Future Military Application. *Mil. Med.* **2019**, *184* (Suppl. 1), 65–71. [CrossRef]
25. Sun, Y.; He, J.; Lei, S.; Cui, L.; Lu, C.-T. Med-MMHL: A Multi-Modal Dataset for Detecting Human- and LLM-Generated Misinformation in the Medical Domain. *arXiv* **2023**, arXiv:2306.08871.
26. Bourke, A.K.; O'Donovan, K.; Clifford, A.; Ólaighin, G.; Nelson, J. Optimum Gravity Vector and Vertical Acceleration Estimation Using a Tri-Axial Accelerometer for Falls and Normal Activities. In Proceedings of the 2011 Annual International Conference of the IEEE Engineering in Medicine and Biology Society, Boston, MA, USA, 30 August–3 September 2011; pp. 7896–7899. [CrossRef]
27. Yeng, S.; Lin, T.; Lin, Y.-F. The N-Dimensional Pythagorean Theorem. *Linear Multilinear Algebra* **1990**, *26*, 9–13. [CrossRef]
28. Blu, T.; Thévenaz, P.; Unser, M. Linear Interpolation Revitalized. *IEEE J. Mag.* **2004**, *13*, 710–719. [CrossRef]
29. Bland, J.M.; Altman, D.G. Statistical Methods for Assessing Agreement between Two Methods of Clinical Measurement. *Lancet* **1986**, *1*, 307–310.
30. Bland, J.M.; Altman, D.G. Measuring Agreement in Method Comparison Studies. *Stat. Methods Med. Res.* **1999**, *8*, 135–160. [CrossRef]
31. Sun, R.; Moon, Y.; McGinnis, R.S.; Seagers, K.; Motl, R.W.; Sheth, N.; Wright, J.A.; Ghaffari, R.; Patel, S.; Sosnoff, J.J. Assessment of Postural Sway in Individuals with Multiple Sclerosis Using a Novel Wearable Inertial Sensor. *Digit. Biomark.* **2018**, *2*, 1–10. [CrossRef]
32. Mahmood, O.A.; Aliraqi, M.G.; Ali, A.A. Movement Disorders in Chronic Kidney Disease Patients on Hemodialysis in Mosul City. Open Access Maced. *J. Med. Sci.* **2023**, *11*, 145–149. [CrossRef]
33. do Vilas-Boas, M.C.; Cunha, J.P.S. Movement Quantification in Neurological Diseases: Methods and Applications. *IEEE Rev. Biomed. Eng.* **2016**, *9*, 15–31. [CrossRef]
34. Obukhov, A.; Volkov, A.; Pchelintsev, A.; Nazarova, A.; Teselkin, D.; Surkova, E.; Fedorchuk, I. Examination of the Accuracy of Movement Tracking Systems for Monitoring Exercise for Musculoskeletal Rehabilitation. *Sensors* **2023**, *23*, 8058. [CrossRef] [PubMed]
35. Kempe, V. *Inertial MEMS: Principles and Practice*; Cambridge University Press: Cambridge, UK, 2011; ISBN 978-0521766586.
36. Du, J.; Gerdtman, C.; Lindén, M. Signal Quality Improvement Algorithms for MEMS Gyroscope-Based Human Motion Analysis Systems: A Systematic Review. *Sensors* **2018**, *18*, 1123. [CrossRef]
37. Fusagawa, H.; Sato, T.; Yamada, T.; Ashida, Y.; Ichise, N.; Ogon, I.; Teramoto, A.; Yamashita, T.; Tohse, N. Different Metabolic Changes between Fast- and Slow-Twitch Skeletal Muscle Underlie Impaired Muscle Fatigue Resistance in Chronic Kidney Disease. *Biophys. J.* **2022**, *121*, 514a. [CrossRef]
38. Safarpour, Y.; Vaziri, N.D.; Jabbari, B. Movement Disorders in Chronic Kidney Disease—A Descriptive Review. *J. Stroke Cerebrovasc. Dis.* **2021**, *30*, 105408. [CrossRef]
39. Artom, M.; Moss-Morris, R.; Caskey, F.; Chilcot, J. Fatigue in Advanced Kidney Disease. *Kidney Int.* **2014**, *86*, 497–505. [CrossRef] [PubMed]
40. Parker Gregg, L.; Bossola, M.; Ostrosky-Frid, M.S.; Hedayati, S. Fatigue in CKD. *Clin. J. Am. Soc. Nephrol.* **2021**, *16*, 1445–1455. [CrossRef]
41. Dang, L.M.; Min, K.; Wang, H.; Piran, M.J.; Lee, C.H.; Moon, H. Sensor-Based and Vision-Based Human Activity Recognition: A Comprehensive Survey. *Pattern Recognit.* **2020**, *108*, 107561. [CrossRef]
42. Hegde, N.; Bries, M.; Swibas, T.; Melanson, E.; Sazonov, E. Automatic Recognition of Activities of Daily Living Utilizing Insole-Based and Wrist-Worn Wearable Sensors. *IEEE J. Biomed. Health Inform.* **2018**, *22*, 979–988. [CrossRef]
43. Cao, Z.; Simon, T.; Wei, S.-E.; Sheikh, Y. Realtime Multi-Person 2D Pose Estimation Using Part Affinity Fields. *arXiv* **2017**, arXiv:1611.08050. [CrossRef]
44. Zhang, Y.; Wang, Y.; Camps, O.; Sznaier, M. Key Frame Proposal Network for Efficient Pose Estimation in Videos. In *Computer Vision—ECCV 2020*; Vedaldi, A., Bischof, H., Brox, T., Frahm, J.-M., Eds.; Springer International Publishing: Cham, Switzerland, 2020; pp. 609–625. [CrossRef]
45. Osokin, D. Real-Time 2D Multi-Person Pose Estimation on CPU: Lightweight OpenPose. *arXiv* **2018**, arXiv:1811.12004. [CrossRef]
46. Wootton, R. Telemedicine. *BMJ* **2001**, *323*, 557–560. [CrossRef] [PubMed]
47. Kovesdy, C.P. Epidemiology of Chronic Kidney Disease: An Update 2022. *Kidney Int. Suppl.* **2022**, *12*, 7–11. [CrossRef]
48. George, U.Z.; Moon, K.S.; Lee, S.Q. Extraction and Analysis of Respiratory Motion Using a Comprehensive Wearable Health Monitoring System. *Sensors* **2021**, *21*, 1393. [CrossRef]

Disclaimer/Publisher's Note: The statements, opinions and data contained in all publications are solely those of the individual author(s) and contributor(s) and not of MDPI and/or the editor(s). MDPI and/or the editor(s) disclaim responsibility for any injury to people or property resulting from any ideas, methods, instructions or products referred to in the content.

bioengineering

MDPI

Article

Spatiotemporal Gait Asymmetries Remain Unaffected by Increased Load Carriage in Professional Intervention Police Officers

Davor Rožac [1], Mario Kasović [2,3,*] and Damir Knjaz [4]

[1] Department of Kinesiology of Sport, Faculty of Kinesiology, University of Zagreb, 10 000 Zagreb, Croatia; davor.rozac@kif.unizg.hr
[2] Department of General and Applied Kinesiology, Faculty of Kinesiology, University of Zagreb, 10 000 Zagreb, Croatia
[3] Department of Physical Activities and Health Sciences, Faculty of Sport Studies, Masaryk University, 625 00 Brno, Czech Republic
[4] Department of Sports Kinesiology, Faculty of Kinesiology, University of Zagreb, 10 000 Zagreb, Croatia; damir.knjaz@kif.hr
* Correspondence: mario.kasovic@kif.unizg.hr

Abstract: Background: Although evidence indicates that load carriage may have an influence on walking patterns, the specific impacts of progressively increased loads on spatial and temporal gait asymmetries remain underexplored. Therefore, the primary aim of this study was to examine whether an increased load carriage had an effect on spatiotemporal gait asymmetries among intervention police officers. Methods: For the purpose of this study, 96 male intervention police officers were recruited and assessed under four load conditions: (i) "No load", (ii) "a 5 kg load", (iii) "a 25 kg load", and (iv) "a 45 kg load". Spatial and temporal gait parameters were measured using a pedobarographic platform (Zebris FDM). The spatial and temporal gait parameters, along with the ground reaction forces beneath different foot regions, were examined. The gait asymmetry for each parameter was calculated using the formula $(x_{right\,-}\ x_{left})/0.5 \times (x_{right} + x_{left})*100\%$, where "x" represents the numerical value of each parameter for the left and right sides of the body. Results: The findings indicated no statistically significant differences in the spatiotemporal parameters, nor ground reaction force gait asymmetries between the left and right foot, during walking under a progressively increased load carriage. Additionally, the parameter values for both the left and right sides of the body remained consistent, with a high intercorrelation observed across all of the loading conditions. The gait speed and ground reaction forces, which served as covariates, did not significantly change the spatiotemporal gait asymmetries. Conclusions: In summary, this study demonstrates that an increased load carriage did not lead to a progressive rise in spatiotemporal gait asymmetries in professional intervention police officers. However, further examination using an advanced 3-D gait analysis and an assessment of physiological patterns and adaptations is recommended to identify and confirm the key factors influencing gait asymmetry.

Keywords: specialized populations; standardized load carriage; asymmetry index; differences

1. Introduction

Load carriage in specialized populations, such as police officers and their branches, has become a significant factor in ensuring protection and survival in high-risk situations [1,2]. Indeed, carrying an external load can provide the necessary resources for daily combat tasks and missions. Although the load has its benefits, the interaction among the individual, the load, and everyday duties and responsibilities is often associated with overall health and the quality of life [3,4]. Numerous studies have investigated the effects of carrying an external load on physiological and biomechanical changes [5–7]. From a physiological perspective, it is expected that heavier loads increase total and active energy expenditure, heart rate, and breathing characteristics [5] due to the greater forces applied on the musculoskeletal system. On the other hand, when it comes to the biomechanical approach, the literature has consistently reported increased flexion in the trunk, hip, and knee, as well as greater extension moments in the knee and ankle regions of the body [7]. However, there are limited data on spatial and temporal gait characteristics, as well as the differences between the sides of the body, in response to progressively heavier external loads; these have yet to be determined.

During bipedal movements, it is normal to observe a certain level of asymmetry, i.e., the inequality between the left and right sides of the body regarding a given parameter. The term "asymmetry" is one of the key factors and a starting point in defining optimal ergonomic efficiency and load positioning on the body. Thus, it is not surprising that it has gained significant attention over the last two decades [8–10]. Indeed, efforts have been made to determine an optimal level of asymmetry for certain physical performance parameters, indicating that a 15% difference between the sides of the body represents an upper threshold [9]. However, these patterns have rarely been observed in the lower extremities, where the literature indicates an increase of up to 50% when carrying heavier loads [8]. The majority of studies have attempted to examine the effects of uneven load carriage on gait biomechanics [10–15]. When carrying an asymmetrical load, previous kinematic analyses have shown that the body naturally increases extensor moments in the hip and knee of the unloaded leg [12]. While examining joint movement during walking, little is known about the relationship between load carriage and spatiotemporal gait asymmetries [11]. The available studies on this topic have shown an increase in gait asymmetry in the ground reaction forces in the medio-lateral direction when heavier loads (up to roughly 20% of the body's weight) are applied [11]. Most recently, a study by Štefan et al. [16] indicated that a 3.5 kg load significantly increased asymmetries in the gait cycle, particularly during the stance, load response, single-limb support, pre-swing, and swing phases and in the step time, compared to the no-load condition in a large sample of police recruits. However, the limitation of the aforementioned study is its exclusive focus on a 3.5 kg load, while the effects of heavier loads on spatiotemporal gait asymmetries remain unexamined.

As the authors of this study are aware, only a handful of studies have attempted to examine the effects of a gradually increasing load carriage on spatiotemporal gait asymmetries. From a practical standpoint, establishing the potential increases in gait asymmetry may result in the even greater eversion and external rotation of the foot, decreases in the step and stride length, and increases in the step and stride time [17], which could lead to injuries and stress fractures [18–20].

Given the critical role of symmetrical gait in performing daily tasks and assignments, it is reasonable to propose that the addition of weight may alter the gait parameters—both temporally and spatially—and have an immediate impact on gait asymmetries. Such disparities in the values between the left and right sides of the body may lead to an altered posture, a decline in function, and an increased risk of injury. However, analyzing how body asymmetry varies under specific loading conditions may provide valuable insights for rearranging or restructuring the current loads to reduce the risk of harmful biomechanical impacts on the body during walking. Lastly, public health policymakers should gain a better understanding of load safety concerns and the potential applications of the findings.

Therefore, the primary aim of this study was to examine whether an increased load carriage had effects on spatiotemporal gait asymmetries among intervention police officers. We hypothesized that gait asymmetries would gradually increase with the greater load carriage.

2. Materials and Methods

2.1. Study Participants

This observational study was conducted among male officers of the Zagreb Police Department Police Intervention Unit, who were anonymously tested. The sample size was calculated using the G*Power (version 3.1.9.7 GmbH) statistical calculator, with a statistical power of 0.80, $p < 0.05$, and a large effect size (0.40), which resulted in a sufficient sample size of N = 80 participants. Considering the dispersal of the sample during the study's implementation, an additional 20% increase was added to the sample size, resulting in N = 96. All of the subjects recruited for the study had been employees of the Police Intervention Unit for at least three years. All of the participants before and during testing were healthy and had no acute chronic illnesses or disabilities that could prevent their participation in the research or lead to the termination of their participation. Before conducting the study, written informed consent was obtained from all of the participants. The study procedure and the testing protocol were approved by the Ethical Committee of the Faculty of Kinesiology and the Police Intervention Department under the Ministry of Internal Affairs of the Republic of Croatia (Ethical code: 511-01-128-23-1).

2.2. Loading Conditions

Each test subject crossed a platform while bearing one of four standard loads recommended by the Ministry of Internal Affairs for intervention police officers. The first load was body-weight-only (referred to as "No load"); the second was a 5 kg load (referred to as "Load 1"), which consisted of a belt with a pistol that was loaded with a full handgun magazine, an additional full handgun magazine, and handcuffs; the mean weight of all of the participants was ±SD = 4.97 ± 0.25 kg. The third load was a 25 kg load (referred to as "Load 2"), which was upgraded with a helmet, a ballistic vest, and a multipurpose baton. The fourth load was a 45 kg load (referred to as "Load 3"), which was upgraded with additional lower extremity protection and a protective gas mask (or ±SD = 45.10 ± 4.33 kg). The load position in the second loading condition was around the participant's hip; for the third load, the helmet was placed on the head, while a ballistic vest was positioned on the chest region, with a multipurpose baton in front of the trunk; for the final, fourth condition, the protection was placed on the knees and arms and a protective gas mask was put behind the head. The sequence of each load was randomized to reduce the impact of a learning effect [21].

2.3. Spatiotemporal Gait Parameters

In order to determine the spatial and temporal parameters, we used the ZEBRIS FDM 1.12. software, which produced data following each attempt. The laptop and software were connected to the platform and set up on the computer, providing immediate data on the gait biomechanics. Spatial and temporal gait parameters were created and pre-programmed within the software. For example, the software recorded spatial measurements such as foot rotation (°), step length (cm), step width (cm), the length of the gait line from first to final foot contact with the ground (mm), and a single limb support line (mm). The degree of foot rotation was determined by measuring the angle between the foot's position and the line connecting both feet. Step length refers to the distance between the heel of one foot and the heel of the other foot, while stride length combines the distances of both steps. The temporal parameters consisted of step durations (s). Step time was defined as the duration between the heel strikes of both feet upon contact with the ground. Gait speed was presented in km/h. Additionally, other temporal parameters were expressed as a percentage of the gait cycle for each foot: the stance phase, which included the load response; mid-stance; pre-swing; and the swing phase. It should be noted that foot rotation, step length, the length of the gait line from initial to final foot contact, the single support line, step time, and the percentage of the gait cycle were measured for both the left and right feet. The ground reaction forces for both feet beneath the forefoot, midfoot, and hindfoot regions were calculated and are presented in N.

2.4. Testing Procedure

In order to measure the spatiotemporal gait parameters, we utilized a pedobarographic platform from the ZEBRIS company, FDM, GmbH, Munich, Germany, which was equipped with 11,264 sensors that were operating at a sampling rate of 100 Hz and had a sensor area of 149 cm × 54.2 cm. This tool is user-friendly for studying gait characteristics, and we followed a testing procedure similar to that used in previous studies [21]. During one day of measuring all four of the levels of equipment for the members of the intervention police, we demonstrated the operation of the system and data collection to the respondents. The method of walking across the platform was explained to everyone, and it was noted that the selection of standard police equipment in different variants was chosen by random selection. Also, none of the respondents had participated in similar research, and, therefore, the effect of learning or adapting to the measurement process was avoided. Each participant carried a randomly selected load across the platform, after which, the procedure of randomly selecting equipment and walking across the platform was repeated. Two custom-built wooden platforms were positioned before and after the testing area to facilitate normal walking. Upon receiving a signal from the researcher, the participants began to move across the platform. Upon reaching the end of the walkway, the participants stopped, turned around, and headed back to their starting position. After measuring each load by randomly selecting each subject, the raw data were automatically entered into the data matrix. An analysis of cross-correlation across all eight trials demonstrated outstanding reliability ($r > 0.90$).

2.5. Statistical Analysis

To assess data normality, we employed the Kolmogorov–Smirnov test. The variables that followed normal distribution were presented as the mean and the standard deviation (SD), and the variables that were not normally distributed were presented as the median and the interquartile range (25th–75th). Asymmetries between the different loading conditions were tested using a one-way repeated measures ANOVA or the Friedman test. If a significant *p*-value was generated, a Bonferroni *post-hoc* test between the loading conditions was applied. The effect size was presented as the partial eta squared, with the following values: "small" (0.01), "medium" (0.06), and "large" (0.14). The gait asymmetries were calculated using the formula proposed by Robinson et al. [22]: $(x_{right} - x_{left})/0.5*(x_{right} + x_{left})*100\%$, where "x" represents a given parameter being calculated. A score of 0 denotes a perfectly symmetrical gait, while an increasing value in either the positive or negative direction indicates a greater asymmetry. Of note, the right side of the body was chosen habitually, and therefore, the values for the left and right sides of the body were entered into the equation. The statistical significance was set at a priori $p \leq 0.05$. All of the analyses were performed using the Statistical Package for Social Sciences (SPSS Inc., Chicago, IL, USA).

3. Results

Basic descriptive statistics and the changes between the left and right sides of the body under different loading conditions in the spatial gait parameters are presented in Table 1. Carrying heavier loads did not result in significant changes to the spatial gait parameters, indicating that the participants maintained similar gait patterns while carrying these loads. Notably, the intercorrelation between the loading conditions for foot rotation, step length, the length of the gait line, and the single limb support line was $r > 0.90$, with the coefficient of variation (CV) being <1.5% within every loading condition, indicating that the participants exhibited similar spatial values and gait biomechanics. When comparing the sides of the body, the mean difference between the left and right foot was not statistically significant, which was also observed for the symmetry index. Heavier loads did not produce a greater asymmetry in the spatial gait parameters, although more substantial changes in asymmetry were observed for the single limb support line, which approached statistical significance. Foot rotation remained the most stable spatial parameter of gait across the different loading conditions.

Table 1. Changes in the spatial gait parameters under the different loading conditions.

Study Variables	Left Foot	Right Foot	Mean Difference	Symmetry Index	p	η2
Spatial Gait Parameters	**Mean (SD)**	**Mean (SD)**				
Foot rotation (°) *						
No load	8.3 (4.9–11.4)	10.1 (7.4–14.7)	1.8	0.22		
Load 1	7.8 (4.9–11.4)	9.9 (6.1–14.4)	2.1	0.27		
Load 2	8.6 (5.2–11.6)	10.3 (7.7–14.0)	1.7	0.20		
Load 3	8.1 (5.3–10.7)	9.9 (6.7–13.9)	1.8	0.22	0.908	0.002
Step length (cm)						
No load	68.5 (5.6)	67.6 (5.9)	0.9	−0.02		
Load 1	68.7 (6.3)	68.7 (5.8)	0.0	0.00		
Load 2	68.5 (6.3)	68.5 (6.0)	0.0	0.00		
Load 3	68.9 (6.4)	69.0 (6.2)	0.1	0.00	0.424	0.009
Step width (cm)						
No load	15.3 (2.9)		/	/		
Load 1	15.4 (2.7)		/	/		
Load 2	15.6 (2.8)		/	/		
Load 3	15.7 (3.0)		/	/	0.759	0.003
Length of gait line (mm)						
No load	239.1 (26.3)	242.4 (18.2)	3.3	0.01		
Load 1	242.4 (22.1)	239.5 (23.6)	2.9	−0.01		
Load 2	245.1 (17.9)	240.9 (24.9)	4.2	−0.02		
Load 3	242.7 (22.9)	243.3 (19.4)	0.6	0.01	0.160	0.014
Single limb support line (mm)						
No load	121.6 (21.3)	125.7 (13.0)	4.1	0.03		
Load 1	127.1 (20.4)	122.0 (15.4)	5.1	−0.04		
Load 2	124.8 (13.9)	120.6 (17.2)	4.2	−0.03		
Load 3	123.5 (13.8)	120.7 (14.6)	2.8	−0.02	0.090	0.020

* denotes using median and interquartile range (25th–75th percentile); $p < 0.05$.

Changes in the temporal gait parameters are shown in Table 2. Similarly to the spatial gait parameters, no significant changes in any of the measured parameters were observed, irrespective of the side of the body. The intercorrelation coefficient was also extremely high ($r > 0.90$, CV < 2.0%) within each side of the body. When comparing the sides of the body, the mean difference between the left and the right foot was not statistically significant, which was also observed for the symmetry index. Additionally, heavier loads did not produce a greater asymmetry in the temporal gait parameters, although more substantial changes in asymmetry were observed for the stance, load response, and swing phases of the gait.

Table 2. Changes in the temporal gait parameters under the different loading conditions.

Study Variables	Left Foot	Right Foot	Mean Difference	Symmetry Index	*p*	η2
Temporal Gait Parameters	**Mean (SD)**	**Mean (SD)**				
Step time (s)						
No load	0.55 (0.04)	0.55 (0.04)	0.00	0.00		
Load 1	0.54 (0.04)	0.55 (0.06)	−0.01	0.02		
Load 2	0.54 (0.04)	0.55 (0.05)	−0.01	0.02		
Load 3	0.53 (0.04)	0.54 (0.04)	−0.01	0.02	0.576	0.006
Stance phase (%)						
No load	62.1 (2.1)	62.3 (1.7)	0.02	0.00		
Load 1	62.3 (1.9)	61.6 (3.1)	−0.7	−0.01		
Load 2	62.7 (1.8)	62.5 (1.9)	−0.2	0.00		
Load 3	62.8 (1.9)	62.5 (1.9)	−0.3	−0.01	0.140	0.017
Load response (%)						
No load	12.3 (1.5)	12.0 (1.9)	−0.3	−0.02		
Load 1	11.8 (1.6)	12.1 (1.5)	0.3	0.03		
Load 2	12.4 (1.9)	12.7 (2.0)	0.3	0.02		
Load 3	12.6 (1.5)	12.7 (2.2)	0.1	0.01	0.135	0.017
Mid-stance (%)						
No load	37.8 (1.7)	37.5 (3.9)	−0.3	−0.01		
Load 1	38.4 (3.0)	37.5 (2.0)	−0.9	−0.02		
Load 2	37.7 (2.3)	37.2 (2.0)	−0.5	−0.01		
Load 3	37.5 (2.1)	37.2 (2.0)	−0.3	−0.01	0.874	0.002
Pre-swing (%)						
No load	12.1 (1.9)	12.3 (1.5)	0.2	0.02		
Load 1	12.3 (1.6)	12.2 (2.0)	−0.1	−0.01		
Load 2	12.5 (2.0)	12.9 (1.8)	0.4	0.03		
Load 3	12.7 (2.1)	12.7 (1.4)	0.0	0.00	0.318	0.011
Swing phase (%)						
No load	37.9 (2.1)	37.7 (1.7)	−0.2	−0.01		
Load 1	37.6 (1.5)	38.3 (2.9)	0.7	0.02		
Load 2	37.3 (1.8)	37.5 (1.9)	0.2	0.01		
Load 3	37.2 (1.9)	37.5 (1.9)	0.2	0.01	0.161	0.016
Gait speed (km/h)						
No load	4.4 (0.5)		/	/		
Load 1	4.6 (0.5)		/	/		
Load 2	4.6 (0.6)		/	/		
Load 3	4.7 (0.6)		/	/	0.064	0.022

$p < 0.05$.

Table 3 shows changes in the ground reaction force asymmetries following the different loading conditions. The findings indicated no significant changes in the force asymmetries beneath the different foot regions when a gradually heavier load was added. Of note, when each model was adjusted for gait speed and ground reaction force, similar patterns and effect sizes remained.

Table 3. Changes in the ground reaction force asymmetries under the different loading conditions.

Study Variables	Left Foot	Right Foot	Mean Difference	Symmetry Index	p	η2
Temporal Gait Parameters	**Mean (SD)**	**Mean (SD)**				
Forefoot (N)						
No load	852.3 (109.9)	865.6 (113.8)	13.3	0.01		
Load 1	873.0 (166.0)	893.0 (126.7)	20.0	1.79		
Load 2	960.6 (115.1)	967.6 (115.2)	7.0	0.01		
Load 3	978.4 (108.9)	984.4 (114.2)	6.0	0.01	0.151	0.016
Midfoot (N)						
No load	170.6 (70.3)	173.9 (68.7)	3.3	0.08		
Load 1	170.0 (74.2)	178.1 (75.4)	8.1	0.27		
Load 2	187.8 (75.4)	202.1 (81.4)	14.3	0.13		
Load 3	191.9 (82.6)	206.6 (82.0)	14.7	0.17	0.251	0.013
Hindfoot (N)						
No load	588.6 (89.9)	568.1 (84.5)	−20.5	−0.04		
Load 1	609.5 (82.0)	580.5 (94.0)	−29.0	−0.06		
Load 2	651.3 (86.6)	617.4 (87.3)	33.9	−0.06		
Load 3	662.2 (90.4)	636.6 (95.1)	−25.6	−0.03	0.323	0.011

4. Discussion

The main purpose of this study was to examine the effects of an increased load carriage on spatiotemporal gait asymmetries in intervention police officers. The findings of the study indicate no significant differences between the left and right sides of the body, nor any expected increases in the spatial and temporal gait asymmetries following the addition of a gradually heavier load.

To the authors' knowledge, thus far, no studies have explored changes in spatial and temporal gait asymmetries under different loading conditions in intervention police officers. One common approach in detecting gait imbalances typically involves measuring the ground reaction forces between the feet and the ground during a stance position [11,23]. It has been shown that approximately two-thirds of the participants exhibited greater foot asymmetry in the transversal and frontal planes, compared to when carrying no load. However, limited data exist on examining the same patterns during walking. When comparing the sides of the body regarding the ground reaction forces during walking, a study by Zhang et al. [11] found that heavier loads led to a greater asymmetry index, but the same load did not affect both feet equally.

Although we hypothesized that heavier external loads would gradually produce greater spatial and temporal gait asymmetries, we did not observe such findings. One potential mechanism could be attributed to a learning effect and the participants' experience in carrying such loads on a daily basis. For example, of the three loads studied in this research, the first is often carried throughout the day, typically for 8 to 10 h. The second level of equipment is commonly used in urban situations (such as maintaining order at soccer matches, etc.), which require a higher level of risk and an additional level of protection. On average, such equipment is worn two to three times a week for approximately 12 h. The third level of equipment is intended for tasks involving the control of immigrants, terrorist attacks, etc. Intervention police officers wear this equipment for durations of 10 days to 2 weeks, for approximately 10 to 12 h per day. Given the regular use of all of the levels of equipment and the extensive service experience of the intervention police officers, it is reasonable to assume that they have adapted to wearing heavier official gear, which does not significantly alter their walking patterns, particularly in the area of spatial and temporal parameters. Although we did not perform a 3-D analysis of the upper extremities, it is speculated that certain adjustments were made in the inertial patterns of the musculoskeletal system due to the load placement on the body, which may have limited the natural arm swing during walking.

Despite non-significant changes in asymmetry with heavier loads, the evidence implies that the trunk tends to lean away from the side carrying the load, suggesting that motor control responses to external loads may be related to load-carrying strategies and characteristics. Differences in posture between the left and right sides are influenced by the dominant side of the body, which directly affects gait asymmetry throughout the kinetic chain. Although asymmetry often occurs because of variations in stride length or cadence/walking speed [5], the findings of this study did not reveal significant asymmetry changes in these parameters. To overcome this problem, we adjusted for gait speed and ground reaction forces, which may interact with spatial and temporal gait parameters following different loading conditions. However, we found no significant interaction effect of the aforementioned covariates in any of the models, indicating that neither gait speed nor ground reaction forces significantly affected the gait with the heavier loads. The reason for this result may be the relatively homogenous sample of intervention police officers with similar biomechanical gait patterns, constitutions, and load weights, which potentially mimic the possible effect of other habitual factors (like gait speed or ground reaction force) on gait. The second mechanism may be attributed to physiological, rather than biomechanical, responses to heavier loads, as confirmed and highlighted in other studies [24,25]. From a biomechanical perspective, carrying a heavy load near the center of gravity represents the most efficient method, as it minimizes energy consumption [26]. Physiologically, previous studies have shown that an increase in load of 15% may gradually increase both resting and active energy consumption by 5–6%, due to the trunk being positioned more forward compared to the no-load condition [25].

Despite the negative findings, this study is the first to investigate both spatial and temporal gait parameters in a representative sample of intervention police officers. Although the load increments did not affect the gait patterns, the findings of this study may have practical implications for examining the movement patterns of the arms, trunk, hips, and knees, providing more detailed information regarding the various angles and angular velocity properties of the joints. Additionally, the non-significant biomechanical discrepancies in spatial and temporal gait parameters should be interpreted through the lens of physiological mechanisms and 3-D kinematic and kinetic analyses, which would offer better insight into the factors contributing to these patterns.

This study has several limitations. Due to its cross-sectional design, we cannot determine causal relationships regarding the asymmetries, which limits the generalizability of the findings to police recruits, who have not yet gained sufficient experience with police tasks and equipment. Second, we only examined spatiotemporal gait parameters, while 3-D kinematic and electromyography systems would have provided additional insights into the increased gait asymmetries following the application of "a 3.5 kg/7.7 lb load". Third, we did not assess biological and physiological parameters, which may clarify the relationship between the dynamic foot parameters and load carriage. Additionally, we did not gather data regarding injury history or the methods of load carriage, which limits our ability to draw practical implications for repositioning load items and exploring the potential effects of load carriage on injury incidence. Fifth, previous studies have shown different systematic evaluations of the feature encoding techniques of sensory data [27], like codebook-based and deep learning-based approaches. However, the same study confirmed that handcrafted feature-based techniques achieved a high recognition rate of approximately 96.0% for the recognition results of different human movements, showing such approaches to be as relevant as other new and more sophisticated techniques in presenting the data [27]. Finally, the participants walked barefoot over the pressure platform, which may have affected their gait patterns. Therefore, future research that is aimed at examining gait asymmetries during load carriage should focus on longitudinal study designs and comprehensive physiological and biomechanical analyses, as well as load- and injury-related characteristics. These factors may be crucial in limiting the negative effects of load carriage on the gait.

5. Practical Implications

Insignificant differences between the asymmetry of the spatial and temporal parameters of the gait using heavier equipment indicate how the members of the intervention police, as subjects of this research, achieved an established biomechanical pattern of movement in dynamic conditions. Namely, it is to be expected that asymmetries between the right and left side of the body will gradually increase, which was not the case in this study. From a practical point of view, it was determined that the different levels of equipment did not significantly affect asymmetry, which can be explained by learned motor control and ways of carrying the load itself during training or special tasks. However, there is still an unknown regarding the biomechanical differences between the right and left side of the body during long-term walking or running, which we could not confirm in this research. According to Knapik et al. [2] and Boffey et al. [5], the physiological component of carrying an external load can be more influenced than the biomechanical one, especially in populations that are subjected to the same or similar loads on a daily basis. Namely, it has been shown that the consumption of energy and oxygen increases physiologically during a heavy load, and the state of fatigue increases significantly [2,5]. On the other hand, fatigue could also be measured by the time spent walking across the platform with different loads, but due to the nature of the data collection and the daily activities of the emergency police personnel, this was not possible. Nevertheless, walking at a normal and habitual pace with heavier equipment did not affect the biomechanics of the lower extremities, but other components, mentioned in the Discussion Section, need to be further explored.

6. Conclusions

In summary, this study demonstrates that a heavier load carriage did not progressively increase spatial and temporal gait asymmetries in professional intervention police officers. Health and law enforcement personnel can benefit from these findings, as carrying heavy loads does not adversely affect body equilibrium or the disproportion of the gait between the left and the right sides of the body. However, other bodily functions, such as physiological changes during walking with heavier loads, should be examined and integrated into the system to identify the most significant factors influencing gait asymmetry.

Author Contributions: Conceptualization, M.K.; methodology, M.K.; software, D.R.; validation, D.R., M.K., and D.K.; formal analysis, D.R.; investigation, M.K.; resources, M.K.; data curation, D.R.; writing—original draft preparation, D.R., M.K., and D.K.; writing—review and editing, D.R., M.K., and D.K.; visualization, D.R.; supervision, M.K.; project administration, M.K.; funding acquisition, M.K. All authors have read and agreed to the published version of the manuscript.

Funding: This research received no external funding.

Institutional Review Board Statement: This study was approved by the Ethical Committee of the Faculty of Kinesiology and the Police Intervention Department under the Ministry of Internal Affairs of the Republic of Croatia (Ethical code: 511-01-128-23-1).

Informed Consent Statement: All of the subjects gave their informed consent for inclusion before they participated in the study.

Data Availability Statement: The raw data supporting the conclusions of this article will be made available by the authors on request.

Acknowledgments: We would like to thank the Ministry of Internal Affairs and the principal Josip Ćelić (the chairman of the Police School Department) for letting us conduct the study under their Institutional Committee's approval.

Conflicts of Interest: The authors declare no conflicts of interest.

References

1. Knapik, J.; Harman, E.; Reynolds, K. Load carriage using packs: A review of physiological, biomechanical and medical aspects. *Appl. Ergon.* **1996**, *27*, 207–216. [CrossRef] [PubMed]
2. Knapik, J.J.; Reynolds, K.L.; Harman, E. Soldier load carriage: Historical, physiological, biomechanical, and medical aspects. *Mil. Med.* **2004**, *169*, 45–56. [CrossRef] [PubMed]
3. Salvendy, G. *Handbook of Human Factors and Ergonomics*; John Wiley & Sons: Hoboken, NJ, USA, 2012.
4. Larsen, L.B.; Tranberg, R.; Ramstrand, N. Effects of thigh holster use on kinematics and kinetics of active duty police officers. *Clin. Biomech.* **2016**, *37*, 77–82. [CrossRef] [PubMed]
5. Boffey, D.; Harat, I.; Gepner, Y.; Frosti, C.L.; Funk, S.; Hoffman, J.R. The Physiology and Biomechanics of Load Carriage Performance. *Mil. Med.* **2019**, *184*, 83–90. [CrossRef]
6. Faghy, M.A.; Shei, R.J.; Armstrong, N.C.D.; White, M.; Lomax, M. Physiological impact of load carriage exercise: Current understanding and future research directions. *Physiol. Rep.* **2022**, *10*, 15502. [CrossRef]
7. Walsh, G.S.; Low, D.C. Military load carriage effects on the gait of military personnel: A systematic review. *Appl. Ergon.* **2021**, *93*, 103376. [CrossRef]
8. Seeley, M.K.; Umberger, B.R.; Shapiro, R. A test of the functional asymmetry hypothesis in walking. *Gait Posture* **2008**, *28*, 24–28. [CrossRef]
9. Lanshammar, K.; Ribom, E.L. Differences in muscle strength in dominant and non-dominant leg in females aged 20–39 years--a population-based study. *Phys. Ther. Sport* **2011**, *12*, 76–79. [CrossRef]
10. Shi, P.; Fang, Y.; Guo, M.; Yu, H. The effects of asymmetrical loading on gait characteristics. *Biomed. Tech.* **2015**, *60*, 31–37. [CrossRef]
11. Zhang, X.A.; Ye, M.; Wang, C.T. Effect of unilateral load carriage on postures and gait symmetry in ground reaction force during walking. *Comput. Methods Biomech. Biomed. Engin* **2010**, *13*, 339–344. [CrossRef]
12. DeVita, P.; Hong, D.; Hamill, J. Effects of asymmetric load carrying on the biomechanics of walking. *J. Biomech.* **1991**, *24*, 1119–1129, Erratum in *J. Biomech.* **1992**, *25*, 467. [CrossRef]
13. Park, K.; Sy, J.F.; Horn, G.P.; Kesler, R.M.; Petrucci, M.N.; Rosengren, K.S.; Hsiao-Wecksler, E.T. Assessing gait changes in firefighters after firefighting activities and while carrying asymmetric loads. *Appl. Ergon.* **2018**, *70*, 44–50. [CrossRef] [PubMed]
14. Majumdar, D.; Pal, M.S.; Pramanik, A.; Majumdar, D. Kinetic changes in gait during low magnitude military load carriage. *Ergonomics* **2013**, *56*, 1917–1927. [CrossRef] [PubMed]
15. Ozgül, B.; Akalan, N.E.; Kuchimov, S.; Uygur, F.; Temelli, Y.; Polat, M.G. Effects of unilateral backpack carriage on biomechanics of gait in adolescents: A kinematic analysis. *Acta Orthop. Traumatol. Turc.* **2012**, *46*, 269–274. [CrossRef]
16. Štefan, A.; Kasović, M.; Štefan, L. Does a Standardized Load Carriage Increase Spatiotemporal Gait Asymmetries in Police Recruits? A Population-based Study. *Mil. Med.* **2024**, *ahead of print*, usae358. [CrossRef]
17. Kasović, M.; Štefan, L.; Borovec, K.; Zvonař, M.; Cacek, J. Effects of Carrying Police Equipment on Spatiotemporal and Kinetic Gait Parameters in First Year Police Officers. *Int. J. Environ. Res. Public Health* **2020**, *17*, 5750. [CrossRef]
18. Teyhen, D.S.; Shaffer, S.W.; Goffar, S.L.; Kiesel, K.; Butler, R.J.; Rhon, D.I.; Plisky, P.J. Identification of Risk Factors Prospectively Associated with Musculoskeletal Injury in a Warrior Athlete Population. *Sports Health* **2020**, *12*, 564–572. [CrossRef]
19. Yavnai, N.; Bar-Sela, S.; Pantanowitz, M.; Funk, S.; Waddington, G.; Simchas, L.; Svorai-Litvak, S.; Steinberg, N. Incidence of injuries and factors related to injuries in combat soldiers. *BMJ Mil. Health* **2021**, *167*, 418–423. [CrossRef]
20. Sharma, J.; Weston, M.; Batterham, A.M.; Spears, I.R. Gait retraining and incidence of medial tibial stress syndrome in army recruits. *Med. Sci. Sports Exerc.* **2014**, *46*, 1684–1692. [CrossRef]
21. Kasović, M.; Rožac, D.; Štefan, A.; Štefan, L.; Milković, S. Effects of Different Load Carriage on Spatiotemporal Gait Parameters in Elite Intervention Police Officers. *Appl. Sci.* **2024**, *14*, 278. [CrossRef]
22. Robinson, R.O.; Herzog, W.; Nigg, B.M. Use of force platform variables to quantify the effects of chiropractic manipulation on gait symmetry. *J. Manip. Physiol. Ther.* **1987**, *10*, 172–176.
23. Maines, J.M.; Reiser, R.F. Ground reaction force bilateral asymmetries during submaximal sagittal plane lifting from the floor. *Int. J. Industr Ergon.* **2006**, *36*, 109–117. [CrossRef]
24. Stuempfle, K.J.; Drury, D.G.; Wilson, A.L. Effect of load position on physiological and perceptual responses during load carriage with an internal frame backpack. *Ergonomics* **2004**, *47*, 784–789. [CrossRef] [PubMed]

25. Quesada, P.M.; Mengelkoch, L.J.; Hale, R.C.; Simon, S.R. Biomechanical and metabolic effects of varying backpack loading on simulated marching. *Ergonomics* **2000**, *43*, 293–309. [CrossRef]
26. Heglund, N.C.; Willems, P.A.; Penta, M.; Cavagna, G.A. Energy-saving gait mechanics with head-supported loads. *Nature* **1995**, *375*, 52–54. [CrossRef]
27. Fatima, R.; Khan, M.H.; Nisar, M.A.; Doniec, R.; Farid, M.S.; Grzegorzek, M. A Systematic Evaluation of Feature Encoding Techniques for Gait Analysis Using Multimodal Sensory Data. *Sensors* **2024**, *24*, 75. [CrossRef]

Disclaimer/Publisher's Note: The statements, opinions and data contained in all publications are solely those of the individual author(s) and contributor(s) and not of MDPI and/or the editor(s). MDPI and/or the editor(s) disclaim responsibility for any injury to people or property resulting from any ideas, methods, instructions or products referred to in the content.

bioengineering

MDPI

Article

An Assist-as-Needed Control Strategy Based on a Subjective Intention Decline Model

Hao Yan [1,2], Fangcao Zhang [3], Xingao Li [1,2], Chenchen Zhang [1,2], Yunjia Zhang [1,2] and Yongfei Feng [4,*]

1 School of Mechanical and Equipment Engineering, Hebei University of Engineering, Handan 056038, China; yanhao@hebeu.edu.cn (H.Y.); wy2002123@126.com (X.L.); zhang2415198975@163.com (C.Z.); 18631579511@163.com (Y.Z.)
2 Orthopedic Medical Robot Hebei Engineering Research Center, Handan 056038, China
3 School of Mathematics and Physics, Hebei University of Engineering, Handan 056038, China; zhangfangcao@hebeu.edu.cn
4 Faculty of Mechanical Engineering and Mechanics, Ningbo University, Ningbo 315000, China
* Correspondence: fengyongfei@nbu.edu.cn

Abstract: In the rehabilitation training process for stroke patients, the level of excitement in the patient's physiological state has a positive impact on the efficacy of the training. In order to improve patients' initiative during training and prevent dependence on assistive systems, this study proposes an assist-as-needed control strategy based on a subjective intention decline model. The strategy primarily consists of two modules: a subjective intention decline control module and a limb movement assessment module. The subjective intention decline module collects surface electromyography (sEMG) data during patient training and optimizes support vector machine (SVM) using quantum particle swarm optimization (QPSO) algorithms to establish a subjective intention decline model. The limb movement assessment module collects information such as interaction force and position error during training and proposes a method for evaluating the motion state of the affected limb. This model combines traditional impedance control with a method for assessing limb movement and subjective status, automatically adjusting the level of assistive force on the affected limb in real time to enhance its active participation in tasks. Finally, we performed two verification experiments to assess the patient's initiative in participating in the training. The experimental results show that the proposed method effectively reduced the average assist force by 65.66% for the traditional impedance control training system and effectively the average assist force by 35.2% for the control training system using only the assist force module based on force position information. At the same time, the accuracy of the subjective intention attenuation module established in the experiment to identify the fatigue level of the subjects reached 93.41%. Therefore, the proposed method effectively improves the initiative of trainers and also prevents patients from relying on the assist-as-needed control training system.

Keywords: subjective intention attenuation model; quantum particle swarm optimization algorithm; assist-as-needed control strategy

1. Introduction

At present, the application of rehabilitation robots to assist patients in restoring their motor ability has become the main effective way of rehabilitation training, and the application of rehabilitation robots has also made up for the shortage of rehabilitation physicians. Patients' subjective participation is very important to the clinical effect of upper limb rehabilitation [1,2]. Therefore, the robot must have the ability to understand the human motion intention. At present, most rehabilitation robots use a variety of control strategies to integrate the patient's behavior intention into the robot control loop in order to improve the patient's active participation in the training process [3–6]. Current control strategies mainly include admittance control, impedance control, adaptive assist force control, etc. [7,8].

Guo Bingjing proposed an adaptive assist control strategy to quantitatively evaluate the interactive control in the task-oriented space. This method can estimate patients' exercise needs effectively, achieve progressive rehabilitation training, and motivate patients to participate actively and voluntarily in upper limb rehabilitation treatment [9]. Li Huijun proposed an upper limb mirroring control strategy based on an adaptive assist-as-needed strategy [10], which automatically adjusts the assist force of the affected limb in real time to maximize the reduction in the active torque of the affected limb. Guo Yida proposed an assist-as-needed control strategy based on position/force evaluation to stimulate the active participation of subjects in the training process [11]. The outer loop of the control system uses a fuzzy adaptive impedance controller, and the inner loop uses a combination of radial basis functions to control the assist force required by the exoskeleton. Yan Hao proposed a support vector machine fusion QPSO method to assess the degree of patient participation in training tasks [12]. However, this predictive model has certain limitations as it only uses force and position data. The above assist-as-needed force control strategy provides as little assist force as possible according to the patient's real-time state needs to help the patient complete the rehabilitation training task. Thus, during the rehabilitation training process, the system provides an assist force to reach the minimum value, and the patient actively provides the muscle strength to reach the maximum value [13,14], thereby enhancing the patient's initiative and improving the rehabilitation training effect.

Studies have shown that the initiative of stroke patients' subjective intention to participate in training has a great impact on the rehabilitation effect [15,16]. At present, the parameter design and adjustment of the on-demand assistive force control strategy depend on the expert knowledge and previous experience of the therapist, and there is a lack of quantitative control strategy design methods [17]. At the same time, patients who participate in on-demand assistive training many times will have a dependency on the robot's assistive force due to their own inertia, so as to "deceive" the robot into generating greater assistive force or generating inappropriate assistance to reduce the patient's active participation and even miss the opportunity to induce changes in neural plasticity [18]. Therefore, integrating patients' subjective participation into the control strategy is a necessary condition for the robot to provide optimal assistance [19–21].

Therefore, this paper proposes an on-demand assist control strategy based on the subjective intention attenuation model, which adds judgment on the subjective participation level of patients based on previous research on adjusting auxiliary force according to force position data. In this approach, physiological signals are collected from patients during the training process to extract a subjective intention decline control model that evaluate the level of active participation in training. Based on the active participation status, we adjust the auxiliary force required to compensate for the movement of the affected limb in real time. Two comparative experiments were designed to compare the performance differences between the traditional impedance control method, the control training system using only the limb movement assessment module, and the control training system using the proposed method. In the second experiment, the subjects simulated the phenomenon of dependence on the assist force. The subjects were trained using a control training system based on the limb movement assessment module, as well as the control training system proposed in this paper. By analyzing the assist force of the two methods and the task achievement rate after training, the effectiveness of the method in this paper to detect the subjective participation of patients and the effect of reducing the dependence on the assist force were verified.

2. On-Demand Assist Control Strategy of Subjective Intention in the Loop

In this paper, an assist-as-needed control strategy based on a subjective intention attenuation model is proposed. As shown in Figure 1, the on-demand assist control strategy adopts admittance control. In the control strategy, the robot adjusts the auxiliary force in real time based on the force evaluation parameters and subjective intention attenuation model of the patient's training state. Subjects participate in rehabilitation training through man–

machine systems and virtual interfaces, collecting interaction forces, position trajectories, sEMG signals, and subjective fatigue evaluation data of the subjects during the training process. Based on previous research results, a model for limb movement status assessment is designed. The subjective intention attenuation model is trained based on the subjective fatigue evaluation data of the subjects.

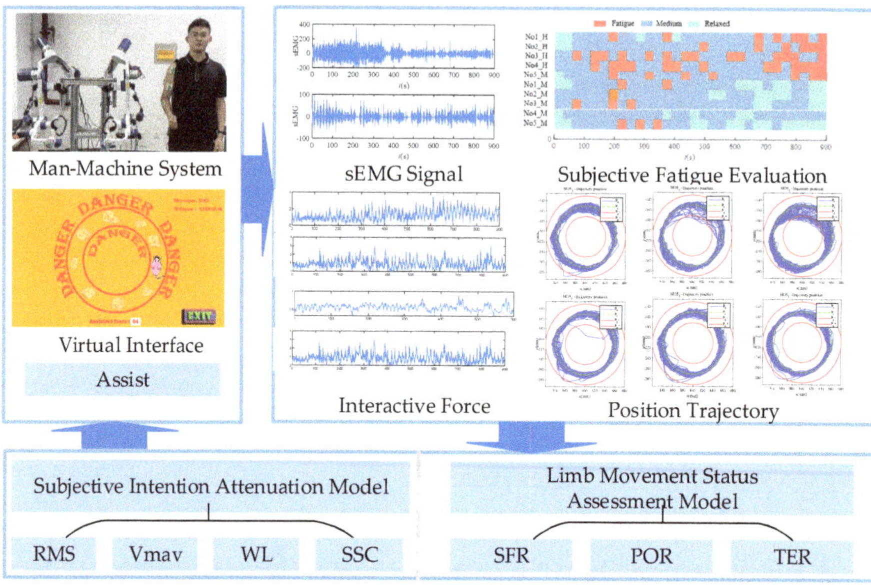

Figure 1. On-demand assist control strategy of subjective intention attenuation model.

2.1. Subjective Intention Attenuation Model

In order to evaluate the degree of patients' subjective participation intention in training, the implicit mathematical relationship between the sEMG signal and the patient's subjective intention is established by a support vector machine algorithm, so as to obtain the attenuation state coefficient α of the patient's subjective intention. The sEMG signal during the training process reflects the patient's subjective intention stimulation. Because of the difference between individual and subjective acceptance ability, the level of stimulation cannot be used as the basis for providing auxiliary force, so the rate of stimulation decline is selected as the attenuation coefficient of subjective intention. The patient's subjective intention attenuation model is established, in which the attenuation coefficient α is mainly determined by the following four characteristics:

The average degree of muscle activation, that is, the sEMG signal amplitude root mean square (RMS), which is determined as follows:

$$RMS = \sqrt{\frac{1}{T_n}\sum_{i=1}^{T_n} sEMG_i^2} \quad (1)$$

Here, T_n is the number of data points of the surface sEMG signal in the subjective intention observation window, and $sEMG_i$ is the data point of the sEMG signal in the observation window. Patients need stronger EMG signals to complete training tasks when they are in a state of fatigue [22], and RMS can reflect this feature well. Therefore, the higher the RMS degree of muscles is, the more excited the muscles are. The lower the RMS degree is, the more relaxed the muscles are.

Muscle waking speed, that is, the mean absolute value (*MAV*), expressed as follows:

$$MAV = \frac{\sum_{i=1}^{T_n} T_i s_i - T_n \overline{T} \cdot \overline{s}}{\sum_{i=1}^{T_n} (T_i)^2 - n(\overline{T})^2} \quad (2)$$

where T_i is discrete-time data, and s_i is the data point of the sEMG signal in the observation window. When the MAV index value is greater than zero, the patient's subjective intention is in the recovery stage. When the index value is less than zero, the patient's subjective intention is declining. When the patient works harder to complete the current task, the higher the level of muscle stimulation, the easier the patient is to experience fatigue, and the smaller the MAV; the range of MAV values is limited to (0, 1) by normalization.

sEMG signal complexity, that is, the Weisfeiler–Lehman (*WL*) value, defined as follows:

$$WL = \sum_{i=1}^{T_n} |sEMG_{i+1} - sEMG_i| \quad (3)$$

In the subjective intention observation window, by adding the waveform length of the sEMG signal, the complexity of the sEMG signal is expressed. The more complex the sEMG signal is, the more muscles the patient has to mobilize to participate in the training. The corresponding waveform length will also increase, and the patient is more likely to experience fatigue. The *WL* index will also increase accordingly; thus, the *WL* value range is limited to (0, 1) by normalization.

Electromyographic signal volatility, that is, the sparse subspace clustering (*SSC*), which is defined as follows:

$$SSC = \frac{1}{T_n} \sum_{i=1}^{T_n - 1} f(i), \text{Among them } f(i) = \begin{cases} 1 & \begin{matrix} s_i > s_{i-1}, s_i > s_{i+1} \; OR \; s_i < s_{i-1}, s_i < s_{i+1} \\ meanwhile |s_i - s_{i+1}| > s_{th} \; OR \; |s_i - s_{i-1}| > s_{th} \end{matrix} \\ 0 & else \end{cases} \quad (4)$$

The data in $f(i)$ are discrete data, where s_{i-1}, s_i, and s_{i+1} are the $i-1$, i, and $i+1$ data in the signal data sequence, respectively. s_{th} is the set noise threshold, and SSC is the number of times the sign of the amplitude change rate changes. When the patient is excited, and the muscle is tense, the muscle signal fluctuates more and the SSC value is larger, which also means that the patient's subjective intention attenuates faster. The range of SSC values is limited to (0, 1) by normalization.

A mathematical model based on support vector classifiers and regression machines was established according to the characteristics of the small sample and non-linear data derived from a small number of patients' training and questionnaire data. The support vector machine is used to determine the classification hyperplane $\omega x + b = 0$ between two different fatigue state evaluation feature data, and then the subjective intention attenuation coefficient function $\alpha_i(x) = \omega^T \cdot \Phi(x_i) + b_i$ is obtained, where $\Phi(x)$ is the kernel function, which is used to transform the sample space dimension. Let the sample dataset $\{(x_i, \alpha_i)\}_{i=1}^{l} \in (R^n \times \alpha)^l$, $x_i \in R^n$ be the input value of the characteristic quantity of the i training data, $\alpha_i \in \alpha = R$ be the output value of the difficulty evaluation of the i training task, and $i = 1, 2, \ldots, l$, l be the total number of samples, and introduce the transformation function $\Phi(x)$ as follows:

$$\Phi : \begin{matrix} R^n \to H \\ x \to X = \Phi(x) \end{matrix} \quad (5)$$

Then, the training sample is $\{(\Phi(x_i), \alpha_i)\}_{i=1}^{l} \in (H \times \alpha)^l$.

Let the decision function, that is,

$$\alpha_i(x) = \omega^T \cdot \Phi(x_i) + b_i, i = 1, 2, \ldots, l \quad (6)$$

In this formula, ω is the weight vector and b is the adjust parameters.

According to the principle of structural risk minimization, the optimization problem is transformed into the problem of finding the minimum value [23]. The radial basis function is selected as the kernel function in the support vector regression (SVR) model. Combined with Lagrange and Karush–Kuhn–Tucker conditions, the dual equation of the optimization function can be derived. Therefore, the estimation function of SVR can be used to predict the degree of active participation of patients using Formula (6).

$$f(x) = \sum_{x_i \in SV} (\alpha_i - \alpha_i^*)(\Phi(x_i) \cdot \Phi(x)) + b \tag{7}$$

The selection of two key parameters C and σ in support vector machine affects the generalization ability and accuracy of learning. In order to eliminate the local optimal problem in parameter selection, the QPSO algorithm is introduced to optimize the parameter selection of the support vector machine, forming the QPSO-SVM hybrid algorithm [24]. The feasible solution updating process of the QPSO algorithm is as follows:

$$\begin{cases} m_{best} = \dfrac{1}{M}\sum\limits_{i=1}^{M} P_i \\ P_{C_{ij}} = \phi P_{ij} + (1-\phi)P_{gj} \\ x_{ij}(t+1) = P_{C_{ij}} \pm \alpha \left| m_{bestj} - x_{ij}(t) \right| \ln\left(\dfrac{1}{u}\right) \end{cases} \tag{8}$$

The particle velocity update formula is as follows:

$$v_{ij}(t+1) = \omega \cdot v_{ij}(t) + c_1 r_{1j}\left[P_{ij}(t) - x_{ij}(t)\right] + c_2 r_{2j}\left[P_{gj}(t) - x_{gj}(t)\right] \tag{9}$$

In this formula, P_{ij} and P_{gj} are the optimal position of the i-th particle and the g-th particle swarm on the j-th dimension, m_{best} is the center point of the current best position on all individuals and dimensions, M is the size of the particle swarm, P_i is the current optimal position of the i-th particle, P_{cij} is the random position between P_{ij} and P_{gj}, α *is* control coefficient, and T_{max} is the maximum number of iterations.

Based on the above theory, the model parameters M and T_{max} of QPSO are initialized, and then the two key parameters C and σ of SVR are optimized by calculating and updating the optimal position and velocity of individual and group particles. The optimization goal is to achieve the minimum value of $fitness(\sigma, \gamma)$. The sample mean square error (MSE) is selected as the particle swarm fitness function, that is,

$$fitness(\sigma, \gamma) = \frac{1}{M}\sum_{i=1}^{M}(\alpha_i - \hat{\alpha}_i)^2 \tag{10}$$

In the above formula, α_i is the actual value, and $\hat{\alpha}_i$ is the predicated value.

2.2. Limb Movement Status Assessment Module

The limb movement state assessment module uses the fluctuations in human–machine interaction force and position information during training tasks to evaluate the movement state of the affected limb. Firstly, multiple specific indicators are extracted from the training information, and then a force position mixed evaluation index β is designed, which is mainly determined by the following three parameters:

The fluctuation rate of limb status, that is,

$$SFR = \frac{1}{T}\int_0^T \sqrt{\left(\frac{d^2F_m^x}{dt^2}\right)^2 + \left(\frac{d^2F_m^y}{dt^2}\right)^2 + \left(\frac{d^2F_m^z}{dt^2}\right)^2}\, dt + \xi \frac{1}{T}\int_0^T \frac{d(F_m - F_d)}{dt} dt \tag{11}$$

where T is the sliding window time parameter, and F_m^x, F_m^y, and F_m^z are the actual interaction forces/moments in the X, Y, and Z directions, calculated by the affected limb and the robot to the end human–computer interaction force F_m in the X, Y, and Z directions. F_d is the expected human–computer interaction force; that is, when the actual human–computer interaction force and the expected human–computer interaction force remain equal during the observation time, the patient's motion state is better; when the actual human–computer interaction force between the affected limb and the robot fluctuates more, it means that the patient's motion state is more unstable, and the *SFR* is larger. The *SFR* value range is limited to (0, 1) by normalization. At the same time, in order to reduce the influence of the weak jitter of the interaction force on the index, a regularization term is added to the *SFR*, and ξ is the regularization coefficient.

Torque efficiency rate (TER), that is,

$$TER = \frac{1}{T}\int_0^T \left(\frac{F_m \cdot F_d}{F_d^{\,2}}\right) dt \tag{12}$$

where F_m is the actual interaction force–torque calculated to the end of the robotic arm, and F_d is the expected human–computer interaction force–torque to complete the training task. The closer the actual interaction force is to the expected assist force direction, and the closer the actual interaction force projection is to the expected assist force, indicating that the greater the effective torque output by the affected limb, that is, the better the motion state of the affected limb, the greater the *TER*. The range of *TER* is (0, 1).

The cumulative rate of robot trajectory offset, that is,

$$POR = \frac{\int_0^T E_p dt}{R \cdot T} \tag{13}$$

where E_p is the geometric distance of the robot end offset task trajectory, R is the radius of the forced boundary designed in the task, and the robot trajectory cannot exceed the forced boundary. The smaller the cumulative offset of the robot's end trajectory is, the better the motion state of the affected limb under the current task intensity, and the smaller the *POR*; the *POR* value range is (0, 1).

β is ultimately determined by the above three parameters, that is,

$$\beta = \frac{1}{b_1 + b_2 + b_3} \cdot [b_1 \cdot POR + b_2 \cdot SFR + b_3 \cdot (1 - TER)] \tag{14}$$

where *POR* is the robot assistance rate in the T time window; *SFR* is the limb state fluctuation rate in the time window; *TER* is the limb torque efficiency in the time window; and b_1, b_2, and b_3 are the weighting factors of the state fluctuation rate and the efficiency, respectively. The better the limb movement state is, the smaller the *SFR*, the greater the *TER*, the smaller the *POR*, and therefore the smaller the β value; that is,β is inversely proportional to the limb state, and the value range is (0, 1).

2.3. On-Demand Assist Control Method

As shown in Figure 2, the on-demand assist control strategy is based on the admittance model. The goal of the rehabilitation training task is to enable patients to overcome their own limb weight and complete the specified trajectory movement; that is, the expected human–computer interaction force is zero during the training period. The virtual human–computer interaction force is obtained by adding the actual human–computer interaction force and the actual auxiliary force applied by the robot on the affected limb. The virtual human–machine interaction force is converted into positional displacement through the admittance model and is then displayed on the task interface.

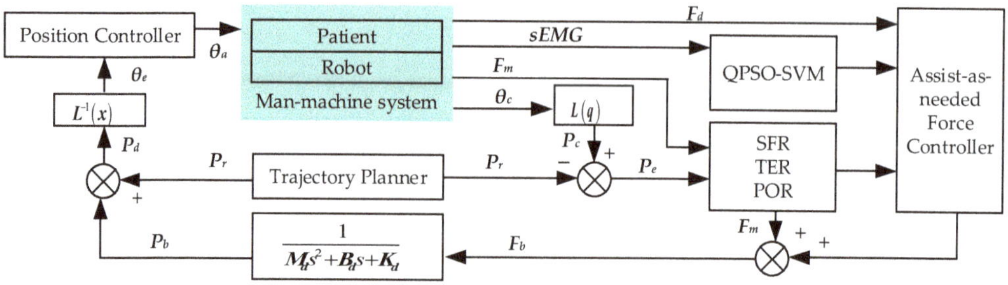

Figure 2. On-demand assist control strategy architecture based on the subjective intent attenuation model.

Since the real human–computer interaction force contains the active motion intention information of each joint of the patient's upper limb and the information of its own weight, the expected assist force provided by the robot is to support the affected limb muscle to complete the corresponding rehabilitation training task under the condition that the affected limb muscle does not work. Therefore, the expected output force–torque of the robot is the human–computer interaction force where the limb weight is converted to the end of the robot arm under the current position of the robot arm, that is,

$$\begin{bmatrix} F_d^x \\ F_d^y \\ F_d^z \end{bmatrix} = L_{3\times 3}(\theta) \cdot C_{3\times 1} \tag{15}$$

Here, F_d^x, F_d^y, and F_d^z are the expected force–torque in the X, Y, and Z directions, respectively. $L_{3\times 3}(\theta)$ is the joint variable term of the manipulator, and $C_{3\times 1}$ is the characteristic parameter term based on the arm length and body weight of different patients.

If the actual output assist force of the robot is the expected assist force, it can be seen from the control block diagram in Figure 2 above that $P_d = P_e$. This indicates that under the condition of ignoring the interference of the environment and the friction occurring in the robot joint, the expected assist force is equal to the human–computer interaction force at the end. Even if there is a structured linear relationship between the actual output assist force and the expected assist force, it easily causes patients to rely on the assistive force system. Therefore, the on-demand assist force control parameter regulator is added. Its input is the robot's expected assist force–torque, the patient's subjective intention attenuation coefficient α, and the limb training state force position evaluation parameter β, and the output is the robot's actual output assist force–torque. The formula is as follows:

$$\begin{aligned} F_a^x &= \left(\alpha - \alpha_{stp} + \beta\alpha_{stp}\right) F_d^x \\ F_a^y &= \left(\alpha - \alpha_{stp} + \beta\alpha_{stp}\right) F_d^y \\ F_a^z &= \left(\alpha - \alpha_{stp} + \beta\alpha_{stp}\right) F_d^z \end{aligned} \tag{16}$$

where F_a^x, F_a^y, and F_a^z are the actual assist force–torque of the robot end in the X, Y, and Z directions, respectively; α is the attenuation coefficient of the patient's subjective intention; α_{stp} is the span of the subjective intention classification; and β is the force position evaluation parameter of the limb training state. The larger the α is, the faster the subjective state of the patient declines, which means that the current task is difficult, and the patient is prone to fatigue. Under the same α coefficient, the smaller the β is, the worse the limb motion state is, and the greater the actual assist force of the robot is. The larger the β is, the better the limb motion state is, and the smaller the actual assist force of the robot is.

3. Experimental Research and Analysis

In this study, four healthy volunteers were recruited, aged 25–27 years old, in good physical condition and without basic diseases. There was no significant difference in the general data of the four healthy volunteers ($p > 0.05$). The experiment was conducted at Henan Xiangyu Medical Equipment Co., Ltd (Anyang City, Henan Province, China). All subjects signed informed consent.

3.1. Experimental System

The experimental interactive system of upper limb rehabilitation on-demand assist control strategy based on the subjective intention attenuation model includes upper limb rehabilitation exoskeleton robot body (ARE-II), sEMG signal acquisition sensor BITalino, control box, virtual scene, and so on. The experimental site is shown in Figure 3. ARE-II has a total of eight degrees of freedom (DOF), which can realize the two-DOF movement of the patient's scapula, the three-DOF movement of the shoulder joint, the one-DOF movement of the elbow joint, and the two-DOF movement of the wrist joint, and can realize the movement of any posture in the patient's space. The designed upper limb rehabilitation robot is arranged with a three-dimensional force sensor at the upper and lower arm constraints, respectively, which can directly obtain the interaction force between the upper limb of the patient and the rehabilitation arm.

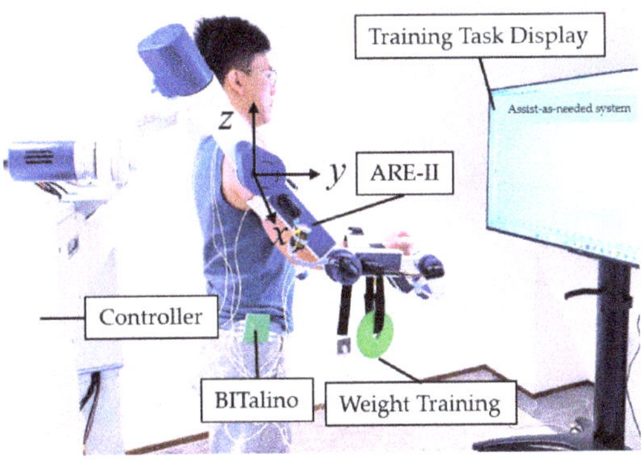

Figure 3. Experimental site.

The upper limb rehabilitation exoskeleton robot (ARE-II) is applied to the rehabilitation training of patients with stroke or spinal cord injury. The left and right are symmetrically arranged. As shown in Figure 4, the length of the mechanical arm is electrically adjustable to meet different sizes of human body. The Z-axis of the three joints of the shoulder intersects at one point to form a ball joint. The Z-axis of the three adjacent joints of joint 3, joint 4, and joint 5 is parallel. The shoulder of the robot is not three-axis perpendicular to each other. The angle between the three rotation axes of the shoulder joint is set as follows: the angle between joint 1 and joint 2 is 60°, the angle between joint 2 and joint 3 is 60°, and the angle between joint 1 and joint 3 is 90°. A fixed coordinate system $O_b - x_b y_b z_b$ is established in the center of the human shoulder joint, and a local fixed coordinate system $O_0 - x_0 y_0 z_0$ is established in the center of the shoulder joint of the upper limb rehabilitation robot. In the initial state, the two coordinate systems coincide. The link coordinate system $O_i - x_i y_i z_i$ $(i = 1, 2, \ldots, 6)$ is added to each joint of the upper limb rehabilitation robot mechanism, where the R_1, R_2, and R_3 motion axes intersect at the axis of the shoulder joint of the robot arm, and the angle between the x_3 and x_4 coordinate axes is 90°. l_1 and l_2 correspond to the length of the upper and lower arms of the human upper limb. The three-dimensional force sensor for detecting the human–computer interaction force is located at the S_1 point on the big arm-connecting rod and the S_2 point on the small arm-connecting rod.

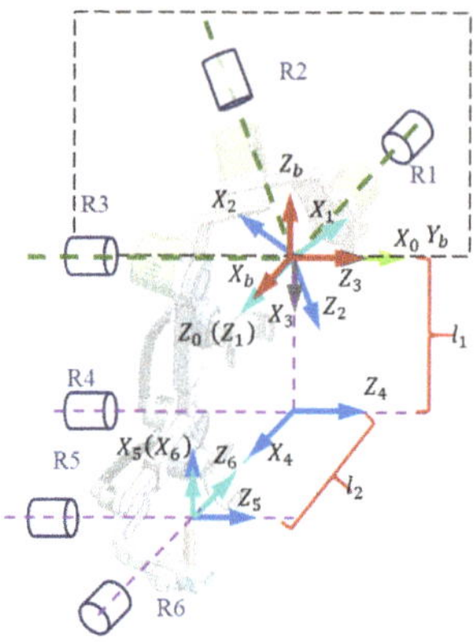

Figure 4. The robot's right-arm coordinate system.

Since the two three-dimensional force sensors are in direct contact with the patient's limbs, the collected data are the actual human–computer interaction force. In order to accurately calculate the expected assist force in the training task, it is necessary to separate the information of the patient's body weight applied to the force sensor. In order to quickly solve the weight of different patients' limbs, the human–computer interaction model is constrained to move in the sagittal plane, and the human–computer interaction model in the sagittal plane is established as shown in Figure 5. In the figure, R_1 and R_2 are the centroid lengths of the affected limbs, respectively. l_1' and l_2' are the distance between the sensor and the joint length at the human–computer interaction constraint; G_1 and G_2 are the weight of each part of the affected limb; and f_{sx}, f_{sy}, f_{ex}, and f_{ey} are human–computer interaction forces, respectively. θ_3 and θ_4 are the joint angles of the manipulator, respectively. In order to facilitate the calculation, two angles θ_3' and θ_4' are defined in the sagittal human–computer interaction model, where $\theta_3' = -(90^\circ + \theta_3)$ and $\theta_4' = 90^\circ - \theta_4$.

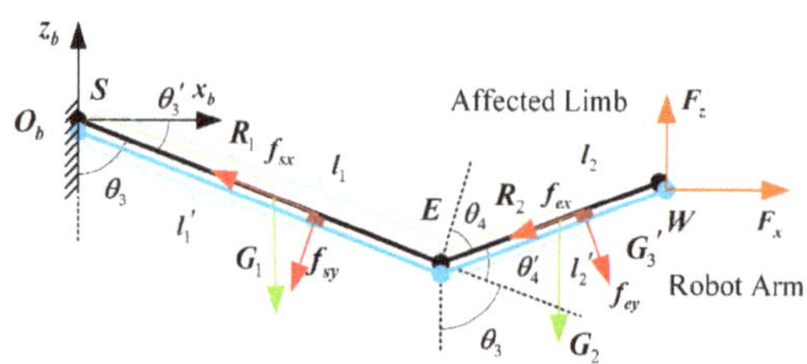

Figure 5. The sagittal in-plane human–computer interaction model.

According to the principle of virtual work, the torque in each joint of the patient's limb is balanced under the action of its own gravity and the support force of the mechanical arm. Through the analysis of the geometric relationship, the human–computer interaction force f_e at the elbow joint is only affected by the weight G_2 of the patient's forearm. The torque M_e at the elbow joint is obtained as follows:

$$M_e = -f_{ey}l_2' = -G_2R_2\cos(\theta_3' + \theta_4') \tag{17}$$

Similarly, the human–computer interaction force at the shoulder joint is analyzed, and the shoulder joint torque M_s is obtained as follows:

$$\begin{aligned} M_s &= -f_{ey}(l_2' + l_1\cos\theta_4') + (-f_{ex}l_1\sin\theta_4') + (-f_{sy}l_1') \\ &= -G_2R_2\cos(\theta_3'+\theta_4') - G_2l_1\cos\theta_3' - G_1R_1\cos\theta_3' \end{aligned} \quad (18)$$

Then, we have

$$\begin{bmatrix} M_s \\ M_e \end{bmatrix} = \begin{bmatrix} -\cos\theta_3' & -\cos(\theta_3'+\theta_4') \\ 0 & -\cos(\theta_3'+\theta_4') \end{bmatrix} \begin{bmatrix} G_1R_1 + G_2l_1 \\ G_2R_2 \end{bmatrix} = L_{2\times2}(\theta)C_{2\times1} \quad (19)$$

The joint variable $L_{2\times2}$ in the above formula is obtained in real time through the joint angles of the robotic arm. The joint torque term $M_{2\times1}$ is obtained by transforming the human–computer interaction force data with the distance between each sensor and the joint force arm. In order to estimate the limb weight of different users as accurately as possible, the robotic arm drives the affected limb to perform random low-speed motion, during which the affected limb remains relaxed. A total of k data are collected in the process, and a more accurate patient characteristic parameter item is obtained as follows:

$$\overline{C}_{2\times1} = \frac{1}{k}\sum_{i=1}^{k} L_{2\times2}(\theta)^{-1}\cdot M_{2\times1} \quad (20)$$

The relationship between the equivalent interaction force at the end of the manipulator and the joint torque is established as follows:

$$\begin{bmatrix} M_s \\ M_e \end{bmatrix} = \begin{bmatrix} -l_2\sin(\theta_3'+\theta_4') - l_1\sin\theta_3' & l_1\cos\theta_3' + l_2\cos(\theta_3'+\theta_4') \\ -l_2\sin(\theta_3'+\theta_4') & l_2\cos(\theta_3'+\theta_4') \end{bmatrix} \begin{bmatrix} F_x \\ F_z \end{bmatrix} = J^T\cdot F \quad (21)$$

In the following, the input parameter of the admittance control strategy of the upper limb rehabilitation robot is the human–computer interaction force–torque signal at the end of the rehabilitation robotic arm. Therefore, the active interaction force of each joint of the rehabilitation robotic arm is transferred to the end of the robotic arm.

$$F = \left(J^{\mathrm{T}}\right)^{-1} M \quad (22)$$

After solving, we have

$$\begin{bmatrix} F_x \\ F_y \end{bmatrix} = \frac{\begin{bmatrix} l_2\cos(\theta_3'+\theta_4') & -(l_1\cos\theta_3' + l_2\cos(\theta_3'+\theta_4')) \\ l_2\sin(\theta_3'+\theta_4') & -(l_2\sin(\theta_3'+\theta_4') + l_1\sin\theta_3') \end{bmatrix} \begin{bmatrix} M_s \\ M_e \end{bmatrix}}{-l_2\cos(\theta_3'+\theta_4')(l_2\sin(\theta_3'+\theta_4') + l_1\sin\theta_3') + l_2\sin(\theta_3'+\theta_4')(l_1\cos\theta_3' + l_2\cos(\theta_3'+\theta_4'))} \quad (23)$$

The expected assist force of the training task is as follows:

$$F_d = J(\theta)^{-1}L_{2\times2}(\theta)\cdot\overline{C}_{2\times1} \quad (24)$$

The electromyographic signal acquisition sensor has five channels, and different electrode attachment points are set according to different experimental schemes. As shown in Figure 6, CH1 was set on the upper end of the trapezius muscle, CH2 was set on the pectoralis major muscle, CH3 was set on the deltoid middle bundle, CH4 was set on the biceps brachii, and CH5 was set on the olecranon as the reference electrode. The subjective intention attenuation rate of the subjects was evaluated by measuring the sEMG signal level of the subjects in real time.

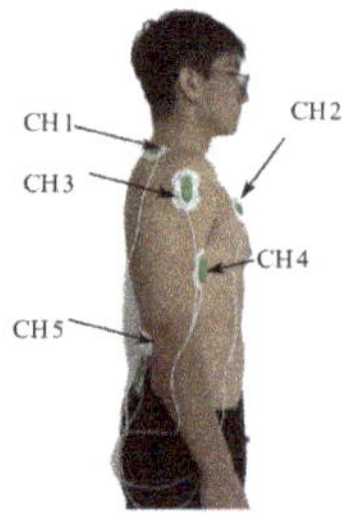

Figure 6. sEMG signal acquisition.

The construction of the virtual scene is completed on the Unity3D platform. The main purpose is to increase the fun and immersion of the subjects during training. At the same time, the real position of the robot's end is displayed on the screen, allowing the subjects to grasp the training situation in real time. The object operated in the designed virtual scene is a mouse, and the patient operates the mouse to walk along an ideal trajectory within a safe area. The coordinates of the mouse and the end of the robotic arm are consistent, setting a task participation scoring mechanism; the closer the value is to the ideal trajectory, the higher the participation score. A 15 min training task was designed, in which participants had to resist the weight of their upper limbs and loads to complete the task. A training score of 60 or above was considered an effective experiment.

3.2. Experimental Scheme

In order to verify the effect of this method on the improvement of patients' initiative, two comparative experiments were set up. In the first experiment, the traditional methods were used, namely, the simple passive training model (M1); the on-demand assist control method (M2) using only the force–position hybrid evaluation index β; and the on-demand assist control method (M3) using the method in this paper. Four subjects participated in the experiment. During the experiment, in order to simulate the patient's state, the subjects loaded a load of 10 pounds on the wrist. The experiment required the subjects' upper limbs to perform circular trajectory motion in the sagittal plane. In the experiment, the subjects needed to try to "deceive" the robot to obtain higher assist force. The specific experimental scheme is shown in Table 1.

Table 1. Experimental scheme.

Subject	Method	Condition	Purpose
A/B	M1: Traditional methods M2: Limb movement assessment method M3: The method of this paper	Complete 15 min trajectory training	Compare the control performance of three methods
C/D	M2: Limb movement assessment method M3: The method of this paper	Try to "deceive" the robot to provide more assistance	Compare two methods to reduce patient dependence

The subjects controlled the upper limb to perform a circular motion trajectory on the sagittal plane. The specific parameters of the experiment were as follows: the center of the circular trajectory $(x_0, z_0) = (400, -210)$ and the radius of motion r = 60 mm. At the same time, the admittance control model parameters were set as follows:

$$M_d = \begin{bmatrix} 0.1 \\ 0.1 \end{bmatrix}, B_d = \begin{bmatrix} 3 \\ 3 \end{bmatrix}, K_d = \begin{bmatrix} 225 \\ 225 \end{bmatrix} \tag{25}$$

At the initial moment of the experiment, the subjective intention attenuation coefficient ($\alpha = 0.2$) and the limb training state force evaluation parameters were set. The moving time window of the subjective intention attenuation was set to 30 s, and the moving speed was 3 s. The moving time window of the training state force evaluation was set to 3 s, and the moving speed was 0.3 s.

During the experiment, the subject's subjective scoring of the current fatigue state was recorded every 30 s. The fatigue state was divided into three grades. A higher score indicates that the subject experienced more fatigue in the 30 s time window, and the actual assist force of the robot was recorded in real time. In order to reduce the influence of accidental factors on the experimental results, the subjects were required to have enough rest time between the two experiments, and extensive simulation training was carried out before participating in the experiment. The experiment duration was set to 15 min to ensure the subjects entered the fatigue state.

3.3. Experimental Results

When the subjects participated in different comparative experiments, the human–robot interaction force between the subjects and the robot, the joint angle of the manipulator, and the surface sEMG signal of the subjects were continuously collected. In experiment 2, the end force data of subject C completing the three training tasks are shown in Figure 7.

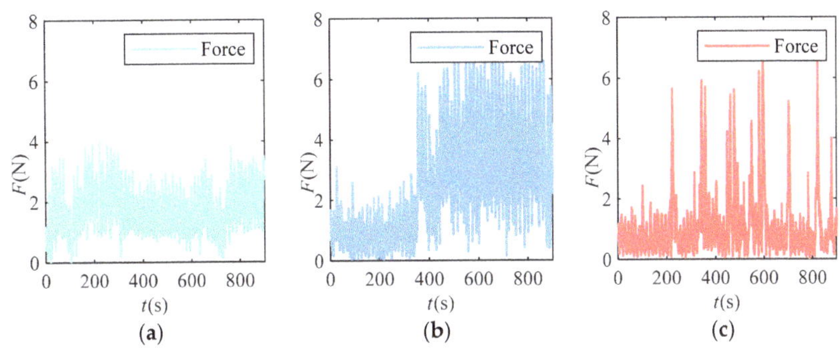

Figure 7. The human–computer interaction force of subject C performing the training task using the three methods: (**a**) eEnd force performance using the M1 traditional control method; (**b**) End force performance using the M2 limb movement assessment method; (**c**) End force performance using the M3 the method of this paper.

From the diagram, it can be seen that in the M1 training task, the subject completely relaxed the limb, and the mechanical arm drove the limb to complete the corresponding training task. In the M2 training task, the level of human–computer interaction remained low for a period of time at the beginning of the training. At 400 s, the subject was too weak to complete the task. At this time, the human–computer interaction force reached its first peak. At 420 s, the subject was challenged again and worked hard to complete the task goal, so the interaction force decreased rapidly. Then, at 500 s, the subject relied on the assist force provided by the robot and deceived the higher assist force by increasing the end force level and fluctuation frequency. In the M3 training task, the subjects constantly attempted to rely on their own strength to complete the training task, so the human–computer interaction force exhibited multiple peaks. From the original data of human–computer interaction force, it can be seen that only relying on the force position information in training to provide the assist force cannot avoid the patient's dependence on the robot assist force. Therefore, it is necessary to extract the attenuation trend of patients' subjective training intention from sEMG signals.

In order to ensure the accuracy of the subjective intention attenuation model and improve the calculation speed of the attenuation coefficient, it was necessary to select three to five features from the existing four-channel sEMG signals as the input of the attenuation model. Therefore, statistical analysis was conducted on these 16 features to obtain the correlation significance and correlation. The average p and F values of the data characteristic quantity compared with each other in the three fatigue states are given in Table 2, where p is the test probability, and F is the influence of random error. When the feature $p < 0.05$ in the table, it means that the feature quantity has a significant difference between different fatigue degrees.

Table 2. Comparison of the significance of characteristic quantities.

Channel Number	Difficulty Comparison	MAV		RMS		WL		SSC	
		p	F	p	F	p	F	p	F
CH1	Tired/Medium	0.001	0.1592	0.0962	0.1587	0.0001	0.2766	3.7×10^{-9}	0.4826
	Tired/Easy	3.24×10^{-7}	0.2281	2.27×10^{-8}	0.2099	2.68×10^{-7}	0.2832	2.17×10^{-7}	0.7296
	Medium/Easy	2.45×10^{-11}	0.0002	0.0962	0.1587	0.0001	0.2766	3.78×10^{-9}	0.4826
CH2	Tired/Medium	0.0134	0.7790	0.2393	0.6471	0.0145	0.8479	0.0033	0.2153
	Tired/Easy	7.59×10^{-13}	0.0214	3.21×10^{-15}	0.9351	1.95×10^{-13}	0.0001	1.26×10^{-18}	0.0041
	Medium/Easy	2.57×10^{-17}	0.0051	2.99×10^{-7}	0.4950	1.34×10^{-11}	2.5×10^{-6}	6.03×10^{-15}	2.5×10^{-7}
CH3	Tired/Medium	9.26×10^{-6}	6.2×10^{-6}	0.0002	2.12×10^{-5}	5.23×10^{-6}	6.83×10^{-7}	0.0011	1.1×10^{-7}
	Tired/Easy	1.08×10^{-9}	0.9632	1.2×10^{-6}	0.0511	1.16×10^{-8}	0.5378	1.49×10^{-18}	0.0008
	Medium/Easy	7.46×10^{-12}	1.8×10^{-8}	7.13×10^{-10}	0.0043	1.35×10^{-11}	2.98×10^{-8}	1.64×10^{-8}	0.0158
CH4	Tired/Medium	0.0497	7.38×10^{-5}	5.44×10^{-5}	0.0058	0.0749	0.0031	0.031274	0.0001
	Tired/Easy	1.8×10^{-21}	3.02×10^{-22}	4.07×10^{-24}	3.59×10^{-18}	1.07×10^{-22}	1.43×10^{-15}	1.4×10^{-20}	0.0046
	Medium/Easy	2.16×10^{-16}	1.94×10^{-16}	1.7×10^{-18}	1.13×10^{-15}	1.33×10^{-16}	1.76×10^{-12}	1.92×10^{-14}	0.3813

According to the data listed in the table, CH1 performs poorly. In the comparison of all features in the three fatigue states, $F > 0.05$ in only *MAV* and *SSC*, but the corresponding $p < 0.05$, meaning that although there were significant differences between features, there were still a large number of overlapping areas in the feature data. In the comparison of all the characteristics of CH2 in the three fatigue states, *MAV*, *WL*, and *SSC* features performed better, and their p values were all less than 0.05, but in the tired/medium comparison, $F > 0.05$, so only *SSC* was selected as the input to avoid overfitting of the model. In the comparison of all the characteristics of CH3 in the three fatigue states, the p-value and F-value of *RMS* and SSC were less than 0.05, which were significant and fatigue-related. As an input, the MAV and *RMS* of CH4 had the same distinguishability. Therefore, the *SSC* of CH2, the *RMS* and *SSC* of CH3, and the *MAV* and *RMS* of CH4 were selected as the input of the subjective intention attenuation model. Figure 8a,b show the change curves of the five features extracted by the sEMG signal with time when subject D performs the M2 and M3 training tasks, respectively, intercepting the moment when the subjective intention attenuates the "fatigue" state. During the "fatigue" period, the five feature quantities have a significant improvement trend. At the same time, it can be seen that in the second half of the M2 training task, although the feature quantity also has a trend of improvement, the amplitude is not large, and the corresponding subjective evaluation of the subjects is also in a "medium" or "relaxed" state.

In order to verify the effectiveness of the active intention attenuation model, the feature quantities of the five training tasks completed by the four subjects were used as the input parameter X_s of the training sample set. At the same time, for subjective fatigue evaluation, data were recorded every 30 s in the training task and were used as the known category information Y_s output of the training set, in which the "fatigue" state was set to "1", the "medium" state was set to "0.6", and the "easy" state set to "0.2". The last experimental data were taken as the prediction sample input X_l and the real output value Y of the prediction sample in the test set. Figure 9 illustrates the actual and predicted values of the fatigue state of the subject Y_l participating in the M3 training task. In this experiment, the difference between the predicted value and the true value of 80.57% of the data was within 0.02. If the tolerance range was extended to 0.05, the accuracy of the subjective intention attenuation model could reach 93.14%, and the average accuracy of the subjective intention attenuation recognition of the four subjects reached 87.62%. In order to further analyze the classification effect of QPSO-MLSSVM on volunteer participation status, the minimum MSE, mean MAE, and minimum RMS were used for evaluation, as shown in Table 3.

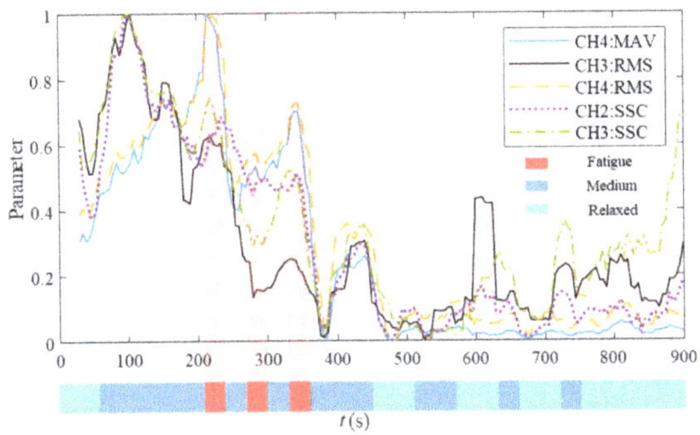

(**a**)

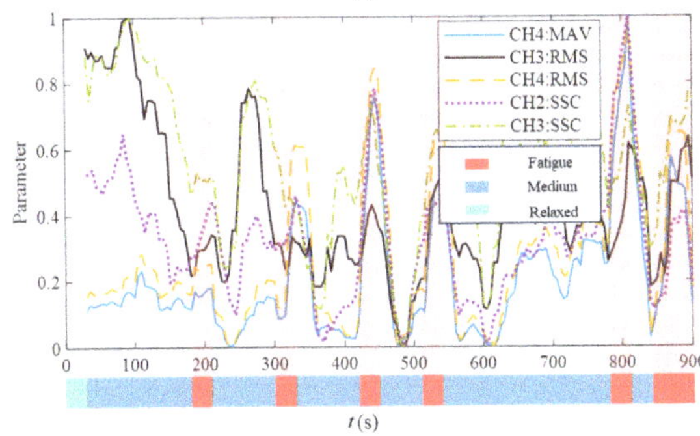

(**b**)

Figure 8. Change curves of sEMG signals' characteristic quantities in training tasks; (**a**) change curve of the characteristic quantity of subject D performing the M2 training task; (**b**) the change curve of the characteristic quantity of subject D performing the M3 training task.

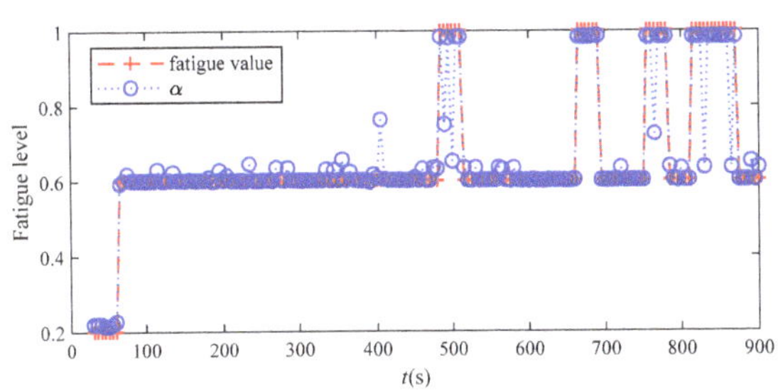

Figure 9. Actual and predicted values of the fatigue state.

Table 3. The error between the predicted and real values of the model.

Title 1	MSE	MAE	RMS
Matching error	1.2104×10^{-4}	0.0191	0.0582

Considering experiment 1, the results of the active verification experiment of subject A are shown in Figure 10. Regarding experiment 2, the results of the fatigue identification and anti-dependence verification experiment of subject C are shown in Figure 11. Table 4 presents the two experimental results, and the data in the table are the average values of all subjects.

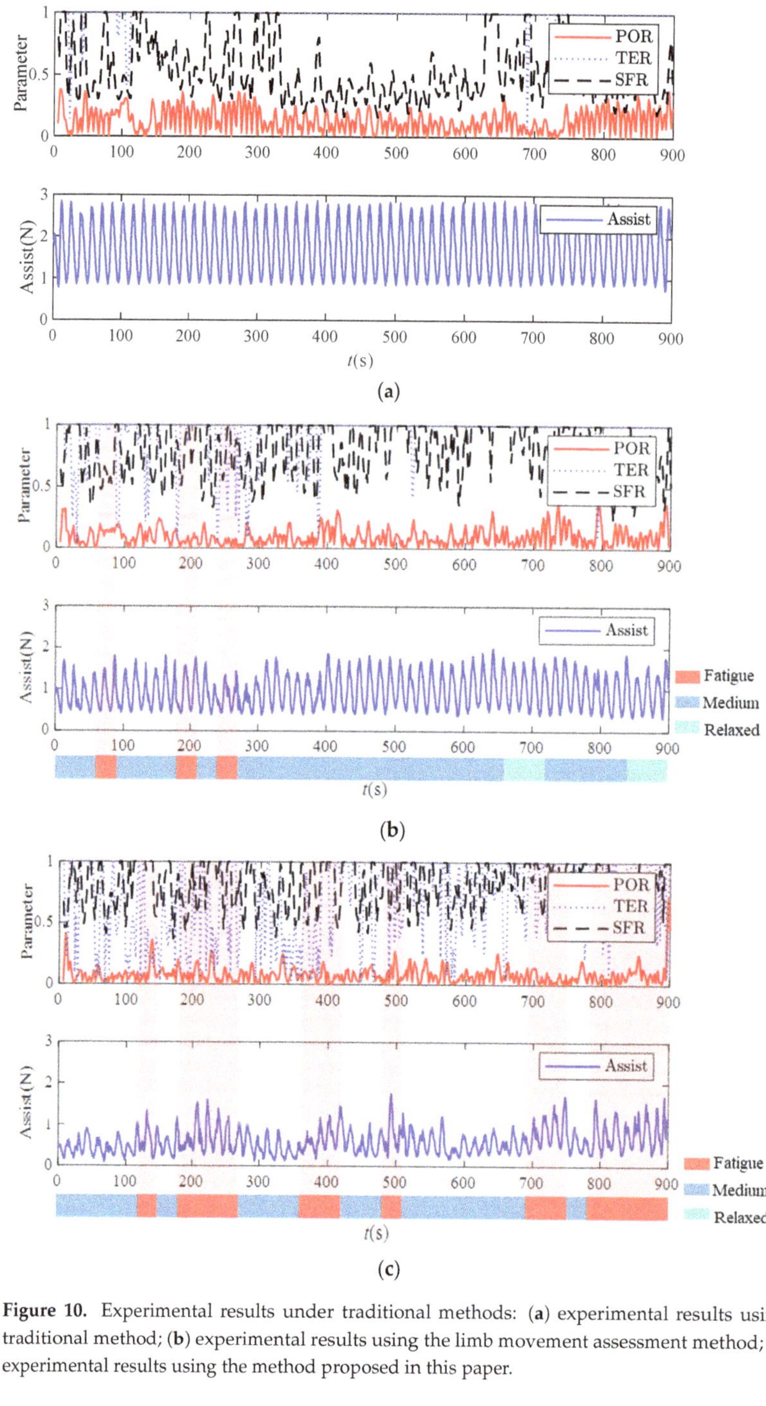

Figure 10. Experimental results under traditional methods: (**a**) experimental results using the traditional method; (**b**) experimental results using the limb movement assessment method; (**c**) the experimental results using the method proposed in this paper.

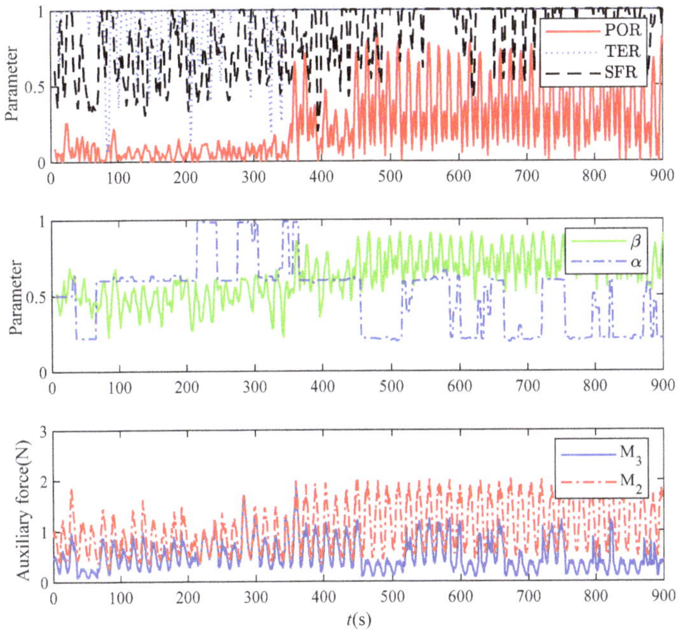

(a)

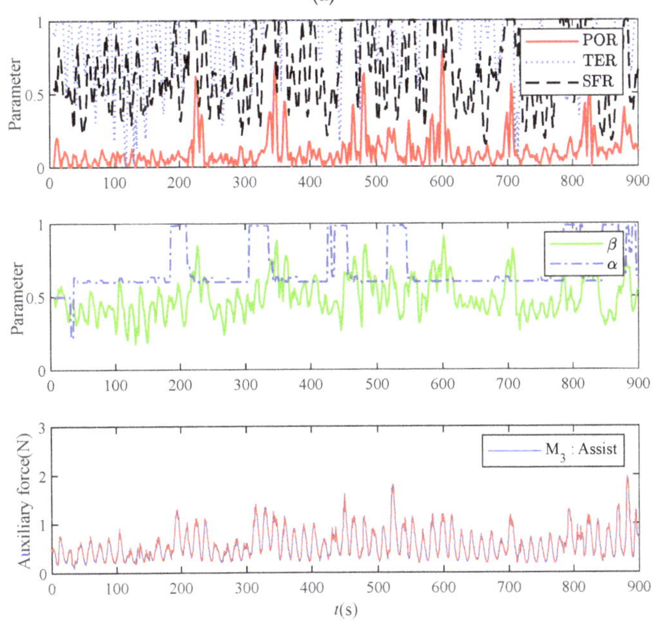

(b)

Figure 11. Subject C's state parameters and robot assist force change curves: (**a**) the experimental results of the M2 training task in experiment 2; (**b**) the experimental results of training tasks using M3.

Table 4. The experimental results of limb initiative verification.

Subject	Method	Average Assist (N)	Reduction Rate of Assist (%)	Fatigue Recognition Rate (%)
A/B	M1: Traditional methods	1.745		
	M2: Limb movement assessment method	0.9247		
	M3: The method of this paper	0.5992	48.8%	93.41%
C/D	M2: Limb movement assessment method.	1.0641		
	M3: The method of this paper	0.5794		

Subject A was selected to analyze the experimental data of three training tasks. In order to eliminate the influence of the assist force dependence phenomenon on the experimental results when subject A performed the M2 experiment, they were required to concentrate as much as possible and rely on their own strength to complete the task when performing the three training tasks.

The analysis chart shows that when the subject's affected limb was unstable and in the fatigue state, the state parameter values increased; at this time, the average assist force of the M1 training task robot was 1.7335 N; the average assist force of the M2 training task robot was 0.97 N; the average assist force of the M3 training task robot was 0.6116 N; and the corresponding training scores were 98, 80.7, and 83.8, respectively. Compared with the traditional method, the average assist force of the overall training task was reduced by 64.72%. Compared with the assist force method based on force position information, the average assist force was reduced by 36.95%, indicating that the effective active torque of the affected limb greatly increased. At the same time, when the state of the affected limb was unstable, and the subject was in the fatigue state, the average assist force of the robot in this method was 1.0341 N, and the average assist force of the robot using M2 was 0.9614 N. Compared with the assist force, the two decreased slightly, but the decrease was not large, indicating that the method in this paper can provide sufficient assist force in the fatigue state.

In experiment 2, which was performed in order to verify the phenomenon of assist force dependence in the M2 training task, subject C had to try to "deceive" the robot to generate more assist force when performing this task. At the same time, in order to verify that the subjective intention attenuation model of M3 can prevent the phenomenon of assist force dependence, the M3 method was used to simulate and compare the data in the M2 training task. Figure 11 shows the performance of subject C in trying to "deceive" the robot to provide more assistive force when performing the M3 training task.

The analysis of the chart shows that when subject C performed the M2 training task. Starting from 450 s, in order to "deceive" the robot to increase the auxiliary force, a deliberately intermittent force was generated to create the phenomenon of unstable motion. The robot increased the average auxiliary force to 1.2313 N. Using M3 to reanalyze the data, the average assist force of the corresponding robot did not increase but rather decreased to 0.6242 N, corresponding to the actual fatigue state of the subject. Therefore, the average assist force was reduced by 49.31% compared with the average assist force of M2. As shown in Figure 11b, although subject C tried to "deceive" the robot several times, the assistive force did not improve.

Considering the results of subjects C/D participating in the M2 and M3 experiments, the average scores of the tasks and the proportion of subjective fatigue state of the subjects throughout the entire training period are shown in Table 5. In order to compare the improvement effect of the on-demand assistive force control strategy on patient initiatives, subjects C/D also underwent five training tasks without the assistive admittance control strategy. By comparison, it can be seen that the average scores of M2 and M3 training tasks were 86.3 and 85.5, respectively, with little difference. However, the proportion of fatigue in M3 was much higher than that in M2. It can be seen that under the same task score, the subjective participation of patients in the M3 task was greater. Comparing the M1 task without assistance and the M3 task, it can be seen that the fatigue rate of M1 without assistance was slightly higher than that of M3, but the average score of M1 without assistance was much lower than that of M3. This is mainly because the subjects had to have more initiative to complete the M1 task without assistance training, and their physical strength decreased faster, which could not support the completion of the training task.

Table 5. The scores of on-demand limb training tasks and proportion of subjective fatigue status.

Subject	Method	Average Score	Proportion of Fatigue State (%)
C/D	M2: Limb movement assessment method	86.3	6
	M3: The method of this paper	85.5	30.67
	M1 without assistance: Traditional methods	48	44.78

4. Discussion

The assist-as-needed rehabilitation training control strategy based on the subjective intention attenuation model in this study aimed to enhance the subjective intention attenuation model and the assist force control model based on the force position information on the traditional admittance model. According to the motion state of the affected limb and the real fatigue state of the patient, the assist force of the robot in the affected limb was adaptively adjusted to improve the initiative of the patient to participate in the training. Through the analysis of two groups of comparative experiments, it can be seen that the average assist force provided by this method was 67% lower than that provided by the traditional method, and the average assist force provided by the on-demand assist training strategy based on the assist force control model using only the force position information was reduced by 16%, thus improving the initiative of the affected limb. We used the method described in this article to avoid situations where patients have not entered the fatigue stage, but the system provides excessive assistance. This method can identify the fatigue state of patients to prevent the occurrence of dependency phenomenon. In experiment 2, the fatigue state recognition rate of M3 reached 93.41%, and the average auxiliary force decreased by 48.8% compared to M2. Therefore, the method in this paper can effectively improve the initiative of the affected limb and meet the requirements of rehabilitation training for the upper limb rehabilitation training system.

Finally, in the study of the method in this paper, two interesting phenomena were found. First, as shown in Figure 8, at the beginning of training, the sEMG signals revealed often relatively high values. If the judgment is based on the subjective intention attenuation model, this indicates a fatigue state. However, due to physical reserve and other reasons, the subjects were not involved in fatigue evaluation in real tasks, so how to determine the emergence of the first fatigue state is the next problem to be solved. Secondly, in the process of processing training data, it was found that the subjects needed a higher assist force and there was a correlation between the trajectory position and speed. Due to space limitations, this work was not carried out here but is planned as a follow-up study.

Author Contributions: Software, writing—original draft preparation, writing—review and editing, H.Y.; methodology, F.Z.; validation, X.L.; conceptualization, formal analysis, C.Z.; investigation, Y.Z.; validation, Y.F. All authors have read and agreed to the published version of the manuscript.

Funding: This work was supported by the Hebei Natural Science Foundation under Grant E2022402059, the Science and Technology Research Project of Hebei Province Higher Education Institutions under Grant QN2023122, the Ningbo International Cooperation Project under Grant 2023H014, the Key Technologies Research and Development Programme under Grant SQ2019YFB130349, and in part by the University–Industry Collaborative Education Programme of the Ministry of Education under Grant 22097118175453.

Institutional Review Board Statement: This study was conducted in accordance with the Declaration of Helsinki and approved by the Biomedical Ethics Committee of Hebei University of Engineering (protocol code BER-YXY-2024001 and date of approval 6 March 2024).

Informed Consent Statement: Informed consent was obtained from all subjects involved in the study. Written informed consent has been obtained from the patient(s) to publish this paper.

Data Availability Statement: The original contributions presented in the study are included in the article, further inquiries can be directed to the corresponding author/s.

Acknowledgments: I would like to thank Henan Xiangyu Medical Equipment Co., Ltd., for providing the experimental site and related experimental equipment for this experiment.

Conflicts of Interest: The authors declare no conflicts of interest.

References

1. Losey, D.P.; Mcdonald, C.G.; Battaglia, E.; O'malley, M.K. A review of intent detection, arbitration, and communication aspects of shared control for physical human-robot interaction. *Appl. Mech. Rev.* **2018**, *70*, 010804. [CrossRef]
2. Yao, Y.; Pei, S.; Guo, J.; Wang, J. Review of Research on Upper-limb Rehabilitation Training Robots. *J. Mech. Eng.* **2024**, *60*, 115–134.
3. Buratti, S.; Deiana, D.; Noccaro, A.; Pinardi, M.; Di, P.G.; Formica, D.; Jarrassé, N. Effect of Vibrotactile Feedback on the Control of the Interaction Force of a Supernumerary Robotic Arm. *Machines* **2023**, *11*, 1085. [CrossRef]
4. Bitikofer, C.K.; Rueda, P.S.; Maura, R.; Wolbrecht, E.T.; Perry, J.C. BLUE SABINO: Development of a BiLateral Upper-Limb Exoskeleton for Simultaneous Assessment of Biomechanical and Neuromuscular Output. *Machines* **2024**, *12*, 617. [CrossRef]
5. Delgado, P.; Gonzalez, N.; Yihun, Y. Integration of sEMG-Based Learning and Adaptive Fuzzy Sliding Mode Control for an Exoskeleton Assist-as-Needed Support System. *Machines* **2023**, *11*, 671. [CrossRef]
6. Lee, H.W.; Lee, K.O.; Kang, I.A.; Kye, J.E.; Park, Y.Y. Design of a Generic Wearable-Robot Monitoring System (GWRMS) for Patients with Lower Limb Paralysis. *Appl. Sci.* **2020**, *10*, 5566. [CrossRef]
7. Laszlo, C.; Munari, D.; Maggioni, S.; Knechtle, D.; Wolf, P.; DeBon, D. Feasibility of an Intelligent Algorithm Based on an Assist-as-Needed Controller for a Robot-Aided Gait Trainer (Lokomat) in Neurological Disorders: A Longitudinal Pilot Study. *Brain Sci.* **2023**, *13*, 612. [CrossRef]
8. Zhang, C.; Yan, H.; Wei, J.; Zhang, F.; Shi, Z.; Li, X. Research on the Safety Design and Trajectory Planning for a New Dual Upper Limb Rehabilitation Robot. *Actuators* **2024**, *13*, 364. [CrossRef]
9. Guo, B.; Li, Z.; Huang, M.; Li, X.; Han, J. Patient's Healthy-Limb Motion Characteristic-Based Assist-As-Needed Control Strategy for Upper-Limb Rehabilitation Robots. *Sensors* **2024**, *24*, 2082. [CrossRef]
10. Li, H.; HU, S.; SONG, A. Adaptive assist-as-needed upper limb mirror control strategy. *Electron. Inf. Technol.* **2022**, *44*, 437–445.
11. Guo, Y.; Wang, H.; Tian, Y.; Xu, J. Position/force evaluation-based assist-as-needed control strategy design for upper limb rehabilitation exoskeleton. *Neural Comput. Appl.* **2022**, *34*, 13075–13090. [CrossRef]
12. Yan, H.; Wang, H.; Vladareanu, L.; Lin, M.; Vladareanu, V.; Li, Y. Detection of participation and training task difficulty applied to the multi-sensor systems of rehabilitation robots. *Sensors* **2019**, *19*, 4681. [CrossRef] [PubMed]
13. Wang, J.; Zuo, G.; Zhang, J.; Shi, C.; Song, T.; Guo, S. Research on assist-as-needed control strategy of wrist function rehabilitation robot. *J. Biomed. Eng.* **2020**, *37*, 129–135. [CrossRef]
14. Yanan, W.; Xihua, L. Correlation and predictive effect of subjective and objective balance function measurements in stroke patients with hemiplegia. *Chin. J. Rehabil. Theory Pract.* **2023**, *29*, 890–895.
15. Hogan, N.; Krebs, H.I.; Rohrer, B.; Palazzolo, J.J.; Dipietro, L.; Fasoli, S.E.; Stein, J.; Hughes, R.; Frontera, W.R.; Lynch, D.; et al. Motions or muscles? Some behavioral factors underlying robotic assistance of motor recovery. *J. Rehabil. Res. Dev.* **2006**, *43*, 605. [CrossRef]
16. Warraich, Z.; Kleim, J.A. Neural plasticity: The biological substrate for neurorehabilitation. *PM R* **2010**, *2*, 208–219. [CrossRef] [PubMed]
17. Fritz, H.; Patzer, D.; Galen, S.S. Robotic exoskeletons for reengaging in everyday activities: Promises, pitfalls, and opportunities. *Disabil. Rehabil.* **2019**, *41*, 560–563. [CrossRef]
18. Casadio, M.; Sanguineti, V. Learning, retention, and slacking: A model of the dynamics of recovery in robot therapy. *IEEE Trans. Neural Syst. Rehabil. Eng.* **2012**, *20*, 286–296. [CrossRef]
19. Zhao, X.; Zhu, J.; Luo, X. Application of ADRC in lower limb rehabilitation training apparatus. *J. Southeast Univ. Nat. Sci.* **2019**, *49*, 1026–1032. [CrossRef]
20. Zhuo, Q.; Shao, C.; Shao, N.; Zhao, Y. Research on one-leg flexibility control of biped robot based on sliding mode impedance. *Transducer Microsyst. Technol.* **2021**, *40*, 26–28. [CrossRef]
21. Zhao, T.; Gong, C.; Zhang, G.; Zhang, S. A safe and high efficiency control strategy of unmanned aerial vehicles partition rendezvous. *J. Electron. Inf. Technol.* **2021**, *43*, 2181–2188.
22. Zhang, X.; Gu, Z. High Accuracy Recognition of Muscle Fatigue Based on sEMG Multifractal and LSTM. *J. Theor. Appl. Mech.* **2024**, *62*, 117–128. [CrossRef]

23. Yan, Z.; Zhi, H. Adaptive admittance control for dual-arm surgical robot using radial basis function neural network. *Chin. J. Med. Phys.* **2024**, *41*, 198–204.
24. Yan, H.; Li, X.; Shi, Z.; Wang, S. Upper limb Movement Prediction Based on Segmented sEMG Signals. *IEEE Access* **2024**, *12*, 119589–119601. [CrossRef]

Disclaimer/Publisher's Note: The statements, opinions and data contained in all publications are solely those of the individual author(s) and contributor(s) and not of MDPI and/or the editor(s). MDPI and/or the editor(s) disclaim responsibility for any injury to people or property resulting from any ideas, methods, instructions or products referred to in the content.

bioengineering

MDPI

Article

Effects of Technique Asymmetry on 500 m Speed Skating Performance

Zimeng Liu [1], Meilin Ding [2], Masen Zhang [3], Bing Yu [4,*] and Hui Liu [5,*]

[1] School of Sport Science, Beijing Sport University, Beijing 100084, China; liuzimeng@bsu.edu.cn
[2] Tianshui Sports Bureau, Tianshui 741000, China; bsudml53@163.com
[3] Department of Physical Education, Northwestern Polytechnical University, Xi'an 710072, China; zhangmasenvip@163.com
[4] Center for Human Movement Science, Division of Physical Therapy, School of Medicine, The University of North Carolina at Chapel Hill, Chapel Hill, NC 27599, USA
[5] China Institute of Sports and Health, Beijing Sport University, Beijing 100084, China
* Correspondence: byu@med.unc.edu (B.Y.); liuhuibupe@163.com (H.L.)

Abstract: This study aimed to determine the effects of technique asymmetry on 500 m straight-track speed skating performance. We analyzed 20 elite skaters, measuring their joint angles, center of mass shift, and times and speeds during the gliding and push-off phases. The technique asymmetry index (ASI) was calculated for each parameter, and paired *t*-tests were used to compare bilateral asymmetry. Spearman correlation coefficients assessed the relationship between the ASI and both the average straight track speed and overall performance. Significant bilateral asymmetries in the knee, push-off, trunk, and hip angles were found in both male and female participants ($p < 0.05$). The male participants demonstrated a higher right push-off speed ($p = 0.029$) and a longer left gliding time ($p = 0.048$). Significant asymmetry was also observed in the lateral shift of the center of mass during each phase of the straight-track skating gait cycle ($p < 0.001$). No significant correlation was found between the ASIs and the overall performance ($p \geq 0.067$). These findings indicate that while elite speed skaters demonstrated significant bilateral technique asymmetry in straight track skating, these asymmetries did not significantly impact their overall performance.

Keywords: technique symmetry; speed skating performance; speed skating training

1. Introduction

Bilateral asymmetries of strength, flexibility, and movements in athletes affect their performance in sports. Running and swimming are sports in which techniques ought to be bilaterally symmetrical. Studies, however, showed that athletes in these sports have bilateral asymmetry in strength and flexibility, which commonly leads to technique asymmetry in these sports [1–3]. In running, technique asymmetry not only reduces performance [4] but also increases the risk of hamstring muscle strain [5] and tibial fatigue fracture [6]. In swimming, technique asymmetry affects the effective propulsion force generated by the left and right limbs, which has a significant negative effect on swimmers' performance [7,8]. The adaptations to asymmetric movements lead to asymmetry in bilateral limb functions [9].

Speed skating is a sport in which skaters show apparent asymmetry in strength. A study demonstrated that the maximum joint torques that professional skaters could generate at the left hip and ankle joints were significantly greater than those generated at the right hip and ankle joints [10]. These hip and ankle strength asymmetries were most likely due to the skaters' adaptations to their skating on the curve track. On the curve track, speed skaters had to push both their legs to the right so they could turn left quickly [11]. Compared to the right leg, the left knee flexion angle is smaller when pushing the ice, so greater strength is needed from the left hip and knee joint extensors [10]. Consequently, the left semitendinosus, rectus femoris, and lateral gastrocnemius have significantly greater strength compared to their right side counterparts [10].

Although bilateral strength and technique asymmetries are necessary for the performance of curve skating, they may have negative effects on the performance of straight track skating and, thus, the overall performance of skating. Studies showed that the average curve speed as well as the average straight track speed of speed skating are significantly correlated with performance [12,13]. Studies also showed that the gliding distance, the trunk flexion angle, the knee flexion angle, the push-off angle, and the shift of center of mass (COM) are important technique factors affecting the average straight track speed [12,14,15]. Understanding the effects of the asymmetry of these technique factors on the performance of speed skating is important for speed skaters to adjust their training programs to maximize their performance.

Technical asymmetry in speed skating not only affects performance on the straight track but is also associated with an increased risk of injury. Studies have shown that a skater's left lower limb is overloaded [16], and significant asymmetry in bilateral gluteus maximus fatigue [17] may increase the risk of lower limb injury [16,17]. Studying asymmetry in speed skating and adjusting training accordingly are important not only for improving performance but also for preventing possible injuries in speed skaters.

The purposes of this study were to determine (1) the bilateral technique asymmetry of elite speed skaters in straight track skating and (2) the effects of bilateral technique asymmetry on skating performance. We hypothesized that in straight track skating, (1) speed skaters could have bilateral asymmetry in their trunk flexion angle, knee flexion angle, and push-off angle; (2) speed skaters could have bilateral asymmetry in the shift of COM; (3) speed skaters may exhibit bilateral asymmetry in speed and time during the gliding and push-off stages; and (4) technique asymmetry could be negatively correlated with the average straight track speed and overall performance of skaters.

2. Methods

2.1. Participants

A total of 10 male and 10 female elite speed skaters were selected and agreed to participate in this study. They were the top 10 finishers in the men's and women's 500 m speed skating competition of the 2020–2021 China National Speed Skating Championships (Harbin, 28 March 2021). For the male participants, the overall performance was 35.99 ± 0.33 s, with the best performance being 35.64 s and the worst performance being 36.42 s. For the female participants, the overall performance was 39.46 ± 0.60 s, with the best performance being 38.34 s and the worst performance being 40.45 s. The best performance of each skater in two 500 m speed skating competitions was used for analyses of performance on the straight track during the first lap.

2.2. Data Collection

Skaters' straight-track skating movements were recorded using 4 time-synchronized video cameras (SONY FDR-AX700, SONY, Tokyo, Japan) with a resolution of 1920 × 1080 at a sampling frequency of 60 frames/s [18]. Considering camera positions relative to movement direction, a shutter speed of 1/500 s was used to obtain videographic images with a blur error of less than 10 mm. The four video cameras were set as two groups with two cameras in each group. One camera was set on the side of the track and the other on the front side of the track in each group. The calibration space of each group of cameras was 14 m long × 6 m wide × 2.5 m high with an overlap area of 4 m long. The total calibrated space was 24 m long × 6 m wide × 2.5 m high. The calibration space was 76 m in front of the starting line.

A suspended calibration system was used to define each calibration space before the competition. The calibration system included four calibration poles with six calibration points suspended on each pole [18]. Five markers were placed in the overlap area of two calibration spaces for defining the reference frame in data processing. The ice surface reference frame was defined with the X-axis pointing in the forward direction of skating, the Y-axis pointing to the left side of the track, and the Z-axis pointing upward. The skaters' skating movements in the calibration space were recorded in the competitions.

2.3. Data Process

The video records of skating were digitized using an artificial intelligence markerless motion capture system (FastMove Inc., Dalian, China) to obtain two-dimensional (2D) coordinates of 21 critical body landmarks [18,19]. Digitized 2D coordinates from two cameras were synchronized using multiple critical events [20,21]. The critical events included blades landing on the ice and blades taking off from the ice. Three-dimensional (3D) coordinates of 21 body landmarks were obtained from synchronized 2D coordinates using the Direct Linear Transformation method [22]. The mean calibration error was less than 0.005 m. The raw 3D coordinates of body landmarks were filtered through the Butterworth low-pass filter with an estimated optimal frequency of 10 Hz [23].

The artificial intelligence markerless motion capture system was used to collect 3D coordinates of body landmarks in this study. The reproducibility of the 3D coordinates of body landmarks collected using this system was rigorously evaluated. The multiple correlation coefficients of repeatedly collected coordinate data were no less than 0.90 [18,19], which indicated that the data obtained using this system were highly reproducible.

2.4. Data Reduction

Displacements and the speeds of whole body COM, movement time, push-off angle, knee and hip flexion angles and range of flexion–extension motions (ROMs), trunk flexion angle, and flexion ROMs were calculated from smoothed 3D coordinates of body landmarks. A speed skating gait cycle on the straight track was defined as the duration between the two consecutive push-offs of the same side and consisted of a gliding phase and a push-off phase for each side (Figure 1). Taking the left side as an example, the left leg gliding phase started when the right blade was taken off the ice and ended when the right blade was placed on the ice. The left leg push-off phase began when the right blade was placed on the ice and ended when the left blade was taken off the ice (Figure 1). We calculated the gliding distance, time, and speed in the gliding phase and push-off phase on each side. We also calculated the COM movement distances in the forward–backward, left–right, and up–down directions during the gliding phase and push-off phase.

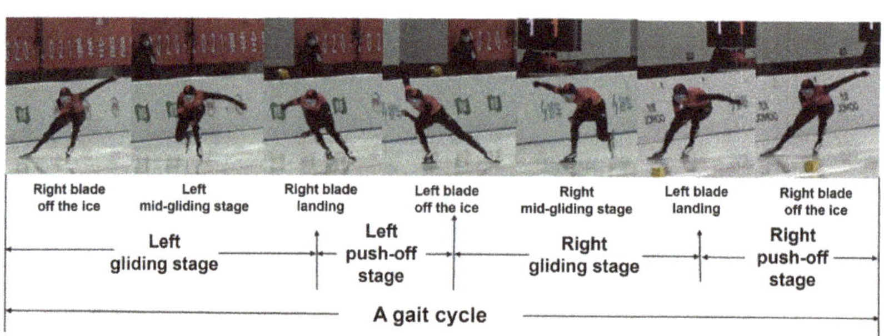

Figure 1. Movement-stage division diagram.

Trunk flexion angle was referred to as the angle between the longitudinal axis of the trunk and the horizontal plane. Hip flexion angle was calculated as the angle between the longitudinal axes of the trunk and the thigh. Knee flexion angle was defined as the angle between the longitudinal axes of the thigh and the calf. Push-off angle was defined as the angle between the longitudinal axis of the calf and the horizontal plane. The range of motion of joints was defined as the difference between the maximum and minimum values of the joint angles in a certain movement phase.

The bilateral asymmetry indexes (ASIs) [24] were calculated as follows:

$$ASI = \frac{|X_R - X_L|}{0.5(X_R + X_L)} \times 100\% \quad (1)$$

where X_R refers to the right leg parameter and X_L refers to the left leg parameter. We calculated the ASIs of joint angles at landing, push-off, and off-ice; ranges of joint motions; COM movement; gliding distance; speed; and time during the push-off phase and gliding phase. The greater the ASI, the greater the bilateral asymmetry of the given technique parameter.

2.5. Data Analyses

To test the first three hypotheses, paired *t*-tests were performed to compare bilateral technique parameters for male and female participants, and there were no multiple comparisons in this study. To test the fourth hypothesis, Spearman correlation coefficients were calculated between the ASIs of the participants' technical parameters and both the average straight track speed and the finishing time of 500 m skating. Statistical testing results with a Type I error rate less than 0.05 were considered statistically significant. All data analyses were performed using SPSS Computer Program Package Version 26.0 (SPSS Science, Chicago, IL, USA). Effect sizes were calculated using Cohen's d. An effect size less than 0.5 was considered small. An effect size greater than 0.5 but not greater than 0.8 was considered medium. An effect size greater than 0.8 was considered large.

3. Results

3.1. Basic Performance Data by Gender

The average straight track speed was 13.53 ± 0.21 m/s for male participants and 12.45 ± 0.25 m/s for female participants. The average straight track speed was significantly correlated to the overall performance for male and female participants (R^2 = 0.442, p = 0.036 for male participants; R^2 = 0.479, p = 0.026 for female participants).

3.2. Asymmetry in Joint Angles and COM Shift

For male participants, the right knee flexion angle at the right blade landing was significantly greater than the left knee flexion angle at the left blade landing (p = 0.004) (Table 1). The trunk flexion angle at the left blade landing was significantly greater than that at the right blade landing (p = 0.028) (Table 1). The left leg push-off angle was significantly greater compared to the right leg push-off angle (takeoff: p = 0.010; opposite-side landing: p = 0.020) (Table 1). No significant differences were observed in other bilateral joint angles and joint ROMs (Tables 1 and 2).

For female participants, the left hip flexion angle at the left blade landing was significantly greater than the right hip flexion angle at the right blade landing (p = 0.040) (Table 1). The trunk flexion angle at the right blade landing was significantly greater than that at the left blade landing (p = 0.009) (Table 1). The trunk flexion angle at the left blade takeoff was significantly greater compared to that at the right blade takeoff (p = 0.048) (Table 1). The right knee flexion angle of the right leg at the right blade takeoff was significantly greater than that at the left blade takeoff (p = 0.032) (Table 1). The range of flexion–extension of the right knee during the right blade push-off phase was significantly greater compared to the left knee during the left blade push-off phase (p = 0.045) (Table 2). No significant differences were observed in other bilateral joint angles and joint ROMs (Tables 1 and 2).

The results of this study also showed that for both male and female speed participants, the left shift of COM during the left gliding phase was significantly greater than the right shift of COM during the right gliding phase (p = 0.001) (Table 3). Similarly, during the right push-off phase, the left shift of COM was significantly greater than the right shift during the left push-off phase (p = 0.001) (Table 3). Figure 2 is a schematic diagram illustrating the asymmetric left–right shift of the participants' COM.

Table 1. Bilateral asymmetry of joint angles at characteristic moments.

Gender	Technique Parameter	Moment	Right Side	Left Side	p-Value	Cohen's d	ASI (%)
Male	Hip flexion angle (°)	Landing	60.5 ± 7.3	63.2 ± 9.9	0.202	0.31	12.17 ± 8.95
		Opposite-side landing	83.2 ± 7.9	84.4 ± 8.0	0.325	0.14	6.43 ± 6.44
		Takeoff	124.6 ± 10.6	126.4 ± 8.3	0.276	0.19	5.89 ± 4.46
	Knee flexion angle (°)	Landing	103.8 ± 8.8	96.2 ± 5.8	**0.004**	0.97	7.53 ± 6.34
		Opposite-side landing	122.9 ± 4.9	124.7 ± 4.7	0.184	0.35	3.59 ± 3.43
		Takeoff	163.0 ± 5.8	160.6 ± 8.6	0.185	0.31	4.02 ± 3.07
	Push-off angle (°)	Opposite-side landing	42.9 ± 3.2	45.9 ± 2.8	**0.020**	0.95	9.31 ± 5.39
		Takeoff	35.1 ± 2.6	37.3 ± 2.8	**0.010**	0.76	7.45 ± 4.82
	Trunk flexion angle (°)	Landing	26.1 ± 3.1	27.6 ± 3.6	**0.028**	0.43	7.87 ± 4.72
		Takeoff	31.9 ± 2.9	31.6 ± 4.6	0.399	0.08	8.86 ± 5.86
Female	Hip flexion angle (°)	Landing	58.4 ± 5.6	63.6 ± 6.5	**0.040**	0.86	12.07 ± 10.15
		Opposite-side landing	91.9 ± 10.8	97.8 ± 9.6	0.066	0.58	10.66 ± 8.28
		Takeoff	128.5 ± 7.1	130.1 ± 9.5	0.278	0.19	4.74 ± 4.27
	Knee flexion angle (°)	Landing	98.7 ± 7.4	100.2 ± 5.5	0.259	0.21	5.24 ± 4.79
		Opposite-side landing	131.8 ± 10.7	134.0 ± 13.5	0.320	0.17	10.08 ± 3.29
		Takeoff	162.4 ± 3.4	155.9 ± 10.5	**0.032**	0.80	6.03 ± 4.45
	Push-off angle (°)	Opposite-side landing	45.2 ± 3.1	46.0 ± 4.1	0.307	0.20	7.17 ± 6.48
		Takeoff	36.4 ± 2.5	36.4 ± 4.2	0.482	0.02	10.84 ± 6.14
	Trunk flexion angle (°)	Landing	28.9 ± 3.1	26.8 ± 4.0	**0.009**	0.57	9.81 ± 7.52
		Takeoff	29.7 ± 2.9	31.7 ± 4.5	**0.048**	0.52	10.05 ± 8.13

The bold in p-Value: Significant difference ($p < 0.05$) between left and right sides.

Table 2. Bilateral asymmetry of joint range of motion.

Gender	Technique Parameter	Stage	Right Side	Left Side	p-Value	Cohen's d	ASI (%)
Male	Hip flexion–extension motion (°)	Gliding	27.3 ± 5.0	27.5 ± 10.4	0.472	0.03	31.45 ± 22.14
		Push-off	41.3 ± 9.5	42.0 ± 9.3	0.417	0.07	19.59 ± 11.37
	Knee flexion–extension motion (°)	Gliding	31.7 ± 6.0	32.5 ± 8.8	0.398	0.10	23.30 ± 16.24
		Push-off	40.4 ± 8.2	36.0 ± 8.6	0.089	0.50	22.75 ± 18.16
	Push-off motion (°)	Push-off	7.8 ± 4.9	8.6 ± 3.8	0.272	0.17	71.36 ± 105.33
	Trunk flexion–extension motion (°)	Gliding	8.7 ± 1.2	8.8 ± 2.7	0.458	0.04	22.77 ± 16.19
		Push-off	4.6 ± 2.0	5.9 ± 3.4	0.165	0.46	53.80 ± 32.89
Female	Hip flexion–extension motion (°)	Gliding	29.8 ± 11.7	37.3 ± 12.2	0.118	0.62	42.93 ± 40.33
		Push-off	36.7 ± 9.2	32.7 ± 12.7	0.116	0.36	24.05 ± 31.13
	Knee flexion–extension motion (°)	Gliding	34.8 ± 16.2	37.8 ± 12.3	0.325	0.20	52.62 ± 30.09
		Push-off	30.8 ± 10.5	25.4 ± 11.0	**0.045**	0.47	33.21 ± 23.95
	Push-off motion (°)	Push-off	8.8 ± 3.6	9.6 ± 3.2	0.284	0.23	40.45 ± 28.35
	Trunk flexion–extension motion (°)	Gliding	7.7 ± 2.7	6.7 ± 1.8	0.102	0.39	29.60 ± 22.80
		Push-off	3.1 ± 1.5	3.7 ± 2.4	0.235	0.26	44.43 ± 27.46

The bold in p-Value: Significant difference ($p < 0.05$) between left and right sides.

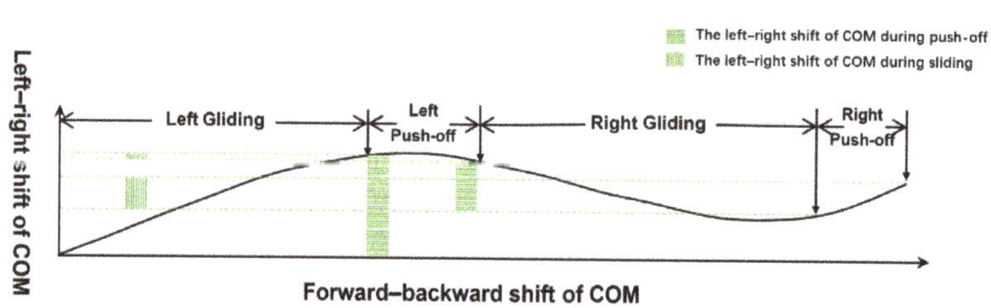

Figure 2. Asymmetry of left–right shift of COM.

Table 3. Bilateral asymmetry of COM movement.

Gender	Stage	COM Movement (m)	Right Side	Left Side	*p*-Value	Cohen's d	ASI (%)
Male	Gliding	Track length	4.923 ± 0.559	5.074 ± 0.325	0.140	0.33	7.85 ± 3.94
		Forward and backward	4.817 ± 0.529	5.009 ± 0.335	0.067	0.43	7.54 ± 3.45
		Left and right	0.181 ± 0.070	0.424 ± 0.081	**<0.001**	3.23	83.20 ± 35.91
		Up and down	0.018 ± 0.012	0.017 ± 0.013	0.456	0.06	90.46 ± 63.20
	Push-off	Track length	1.509 ± 0.254	1.494 ± 0.351	0.452	0.05	20.85 ± 15.29
		Forward and backward	1.500 ± 0.250	1.427 ± 0.387	0.298	0.23	24.35 ± 20.71
		Left and right	0.147 ± 0.068	0.026 ± 0.020	**<0.001**	2.42	133.46 ± 57.20
		Up and down	0.009 ± 0.006	0.009 ± 0.007	0.437	0.07	72.98 ± 67.53
Female	Gliding	Track length	4.435 ± 0.601	4.441 ± 0.392	0.488	0.01	12.21 ± 8.07
		Forward and backward	4.403 ± 0.578	4.380 ± 0.393	0.462	0.04	13.2 ± 38.90
		Left and right	0.128 ± 0.068	0.368 ± 0.083	**<0.001**	3.01	100.77 ± 39.96
		Up and down	0.022 ± 0.014	0.019 ± 0.015	0.344	0.17	80.53 ± 60.65
	Push-off	Track length	1.177 ± 0.297	1.135 ± 0.153	0.326	0.18	19.36 ± 18.10
		Forward and backward	1.168 ± 0.280	1.115 ± 0.137	0.293	0.23	20.37 ± 18.10
		Left and right	0.122 ± 0.042	0.025 ± 0.015	**<0.001**	2.93	123.34 ± 57.35
		Up and down	0.009 ± 0.007	0.010 ± 0.008	0.381	0.16	91.03 ± 64.52

The bold in *p*-Value: Significant difference ($p < 0.05$) between left and right sides.

3.3. Asymmetry in Speed, Distance, and Time

For male participants, their right push-off speed during the right push-off stage was significantly greater than the left push-off speed during the left push-off stage (p = 0.029) (Table 4). The left gliding time was significantly greater than the right gliding time (p = 0.048) (Table 4). No significant differences were observed in bilateral gliding speed, push-off time, push-off distance, and gliding distance.

Table 4. The bilateral asymmetry of speed, distance, and time.

Gender	Technique Parameter	Right Side	Left Side	*p*-Value	Cohen's d	ASI (%)
Male	Gliding speed (m/s)	13.39 ± 0.42	13.29 ± 0.42	0.329	0.22	3.62 ± 3.00
	Push-off speed (m/s)	13.85 ± 0.30	12.64 ± 1.71	**0.029**	0.99	10.35 ± 14.73
	Gliding distance (m)	4.82 ± 0.50	5.01 ± 0.34	0.067	0.43	7.54 ± 3.45
	Push-off distance (m)	1.50 ± 0.24	1.43 ± 0.39	0.298	0.23	24.36 ± 20.71
	Gliding time (s)	0.36 ± 0.04	0.38 ± 0.21	**0.048**	0.53	7.40 ± 5.19
	Push-off time (s)	0.11 ± 0.02	0.11 ± 0.02	0.343	0.16	18.37 ± 13.93
Female	Gliding speed (m/s)	12.52 ± 0.39	12.28 ± 0.37	0.137	0.63	4.50 ± 3.01
	Push-off speed (m/s)	12.74 ± 0.60	12.46 ± 0.95	0.196	0.35	5.21 ± 7.10
	Gliding distance (m)	4.40 ± 0.61	4.38 ± 0.41	0.462	0.04	13.23 ± 8.90
	Push-off distance (m)	1.17 ± 0.30	1.12 ± 0.15	0.293	0.23	20.37 ± 18.10
	Gliding time (s)	0.35 ± 0.05	0.36 ± 0.03	0.377	0.12	10.81 ± 8.81
	Push-off time (s)	0.09 ± 0.02	0.09 ± 0.01	0.406	0.09	17.79 ± 18.37

The bold in *p*-Value: Significant difference ($p < 0.05$) between left and right sides.

For female participants, no significant differences were observed in bilateral speed, distance and time of gliding, or the push-off stage (Table 4).

3.4. Correlation between ASI and Performance

The ASI of knee flexion angles at takeoff was significantly positively correlated with the average straight speed in female skaters (p = 0.044, R^2 = 0.415) (Figure 3). Other ASIs of technical parameters with significant bilateral asymmetry had no significant correlations with average straight speed or overall performance (Figures 3–6).

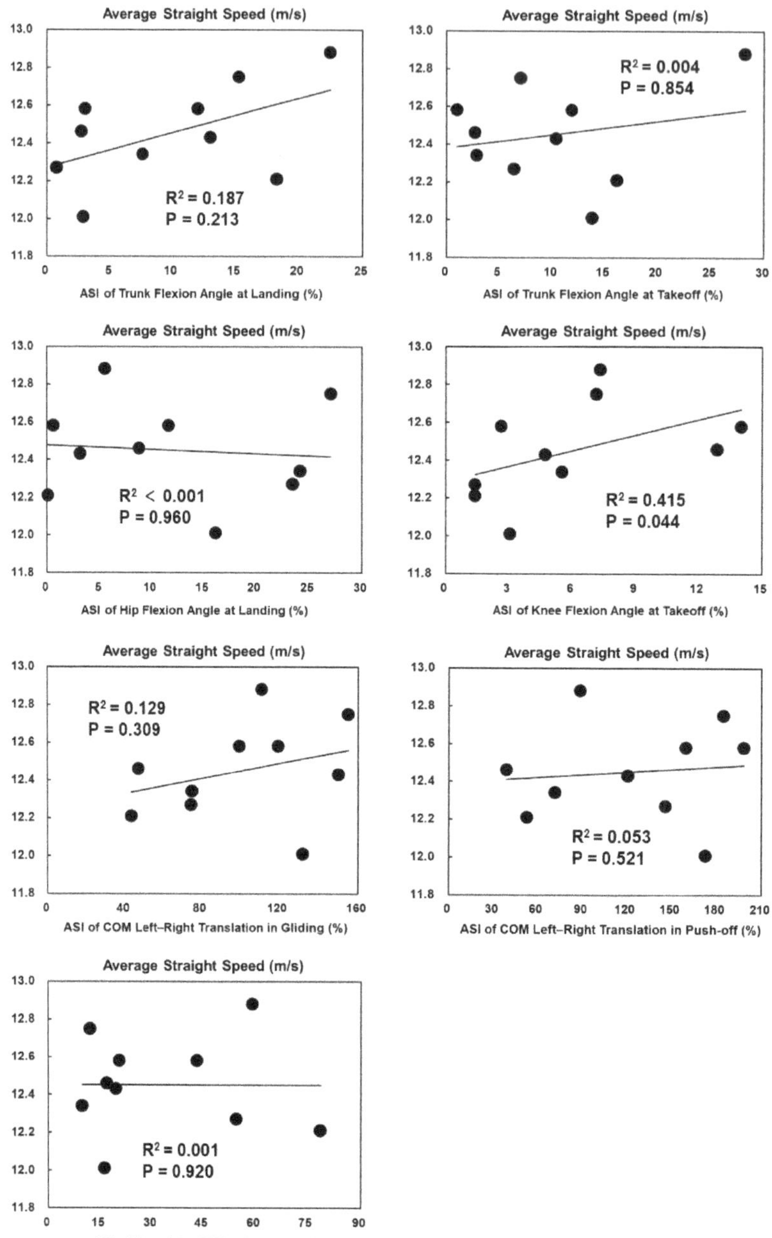

Figure 3. The Spearman correlation coefficient between the ASIs of technical parameters with significant bilateral asymmetry and the average straight speed in females.

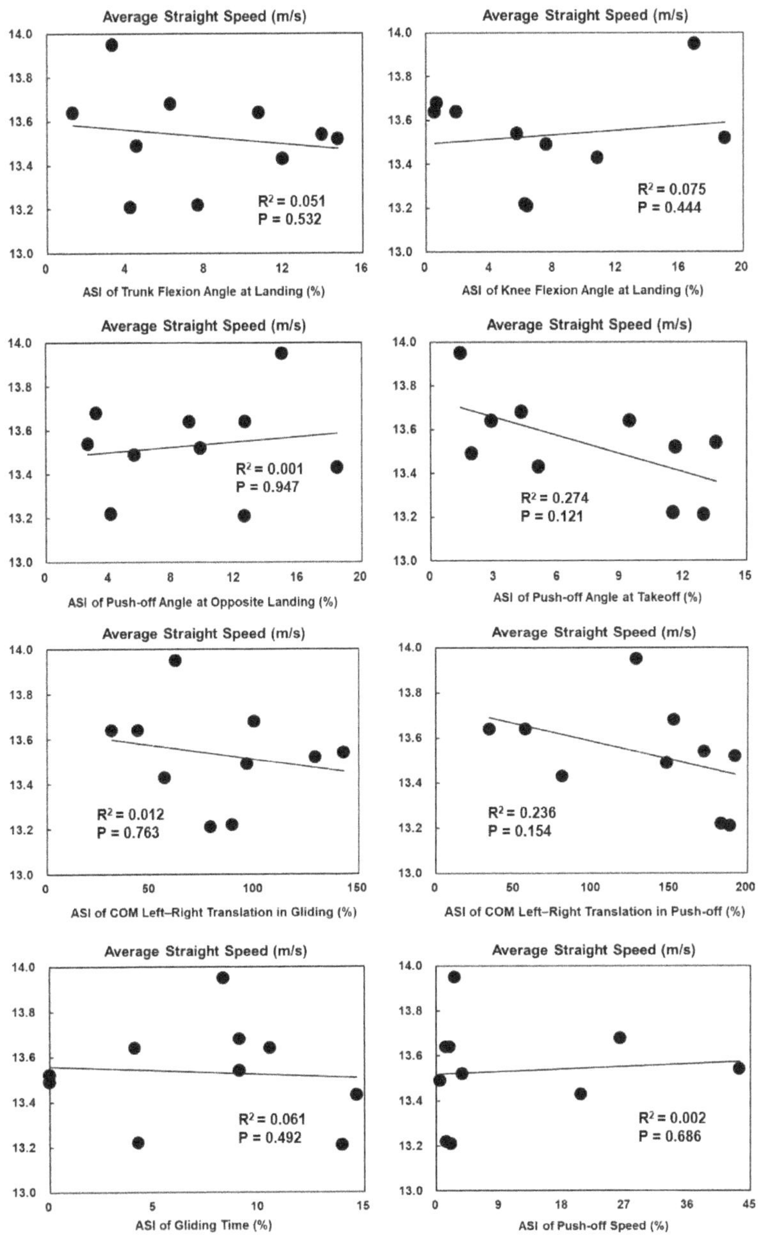

Figure 4. The Spearman correlation coefficient between the ASIs of technical parameters with significant bilateral asymmetry and the average straight speed in males.

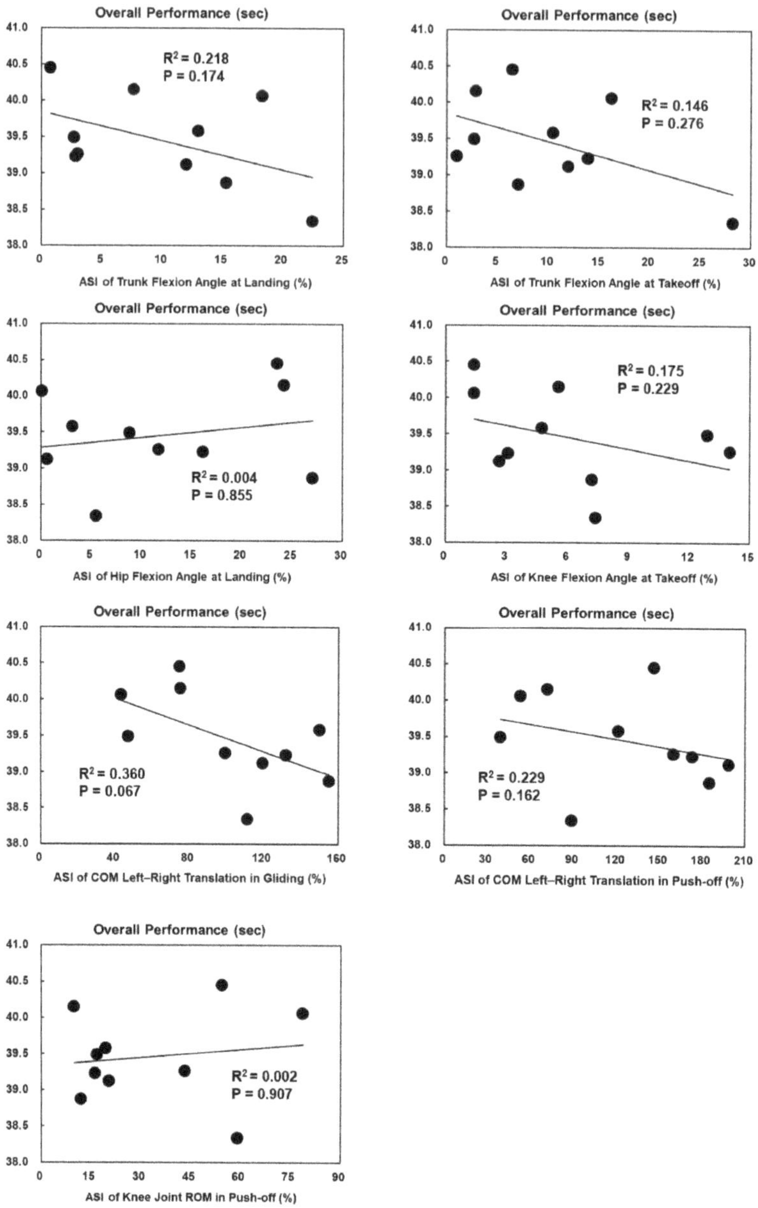

Figure 5. The Spearman correlation coefficient between the ASIs of technical parameters with significant bilateral asymmetry and overall performance in females.

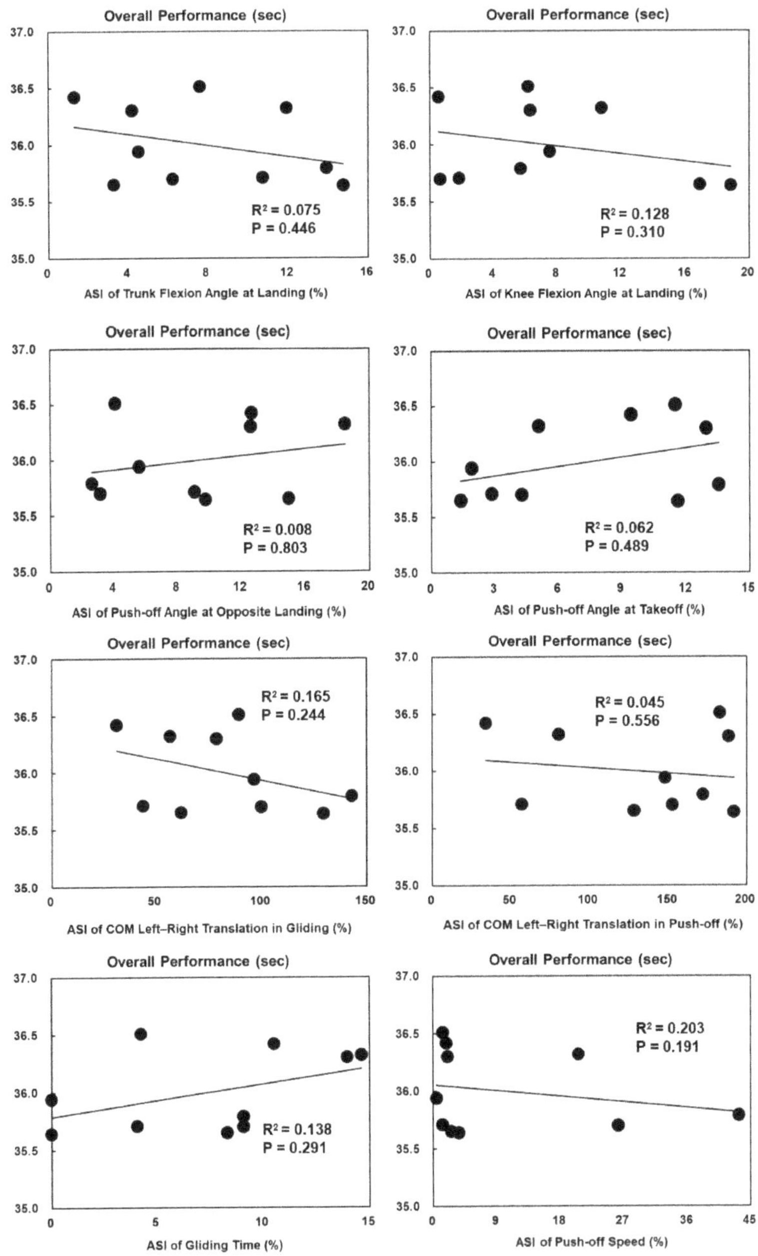

Figure 6. The Spearman correlation coefficient between the ASIs of technical parameters with significant bilateral asymmetry and overall performance in males.

4. Discussion

The results of this study support our first hypothesis that speed skaters would have bilateral asymmetry in trunk flexion angle, knee flexion angle, and push-off angle in straight track skating. The male and female participants in this study showed significant asymmetry in different movements. The results of this study showed that male participants had a significantly smaller trunk flexion angle at the right blade landing compared to that at the left blade landing and significantly greater right knee flexion at the right blade landing compared to the left knee flexion at the left blade landing. The male participants' left push-off angle was also significantly greater than the right push-off angle. These results indicate that, when landing on the right side, male participants' knees exhibited a straighter position, and their trunk leaned more forward. When skaters pushed off with the right side, the angle between their blade and the ice surface was smaller.

These results demonstrated that male participants did indeed have left–right asymmetry in straight track skating. The results also showed that female participants had a significantly smaller trunk flexion angle at the left blade landing compared to that at the right blade landing and a significantly smaller ROM of right knee extension compared to that of the left knee during the push-off phases. Previous studies indicated that trunk flexion angle [25], knee flexion angle [25], and push-off angle [26] may affect speed skaters' power output, which was related to their performance. Smaller trunk flexion angles were advantageous in reducing air friction, so skaters always tried to maintain their trunk in a horizontal position to minimize air friction [25]. Maintaining the trunk in a horizontal position limited the power generated by the hip joint, forcing the skater to rely on knee extension as the primary power generator [25]. Meanwhile, decreasing push-off angles increases lateral push-off force that may increase power output [26]. The technique asymmetries observed in the current study indicate that participants generated more power from their right side than from their left side, which is consistent with the findings of a previous study [27].

The results of this study support our second hypothesis that speed skaters would have bilateral asymmetry in shift of COM. The results of this study demonstrated that, for both male and female participants, the left shift of COM during the left gliding phase was significantly greater than the right shift of COM during the right gliding phase, and the shift of COM during the right push-off phase was significantly greater than that during the left push-off phase. These results demonstrate that the participants of this study had significant bilateral technique asymmetries in the shift of COM in straight track skating. Our study's findings showed a greater shift of COM to the left compared to the shift of COM to the right, which might confirm the greater lower limb extension strength on the participants' right side. Previous research linked skaters' asymmetry in the shift of COM to bilateral push-off time and gliding time [15]. Our study's findings showed that the shift of COM might also be related to skaters' push-off speed. We found that the COM moved more to the left during the right push-off stage, which corresponded with faster right push-off speeds and subsequently longer left gliding times.

The results of this study support our third hypothesis that speed skaters exhibit bilateral asymmetry in speed and time during the gliding and push-off stages. The results of this study showed that male participants had significant bilateral asymmetries in the push-off speed and gliding time. A greater right push-off speed allows for a prolonged duration of gliding on the subsequent left side. For male participants, a greater right push-off speed suggests that the right lower limb could potentially possess greater push-off efficiency. This was consistent with a previous study that found greater extensor strength in the right leg during high-speed movements [28].

The participants of this study all demonstrated significant bilateral asymmetries in the selected technique parameters. The most likely explanation of these technique asymmetries is the long-term training adaptations on curve skating. Speed skaters rely on rapid and full extensions to generate power [29–31]. When speed skaters turn on curves, they tend to shift their COM toward the left leg to maintain balance and mainly use the right leg to provide power to maintain speed, which makes the right leg have more training load compared to the left leg. This long-term increased training load on the right leg results in greater strength in the right leg compared to the left leg, as shown in the literature [28].

The results of this study did not support our fourth hypothesis, which predicted a negative correlation between technique asymmetry and both the average straight track speed and overall performance. Instead, we found a significant positive correlation between the ASI of knee flexion angles at blade takeoff and the average straight track speed in female skaters. Specifically, a greater ASI of knee flexion angle at blade takeoff, with the right side angle being greater than the left, was associated with increased straight track speed. It was hypothesized that a larger right knee angle at takeoff indicated a more active right push-off, compensating for the imbalance caused by the stronger left leg. This asymmetry might have been an adaptation to the imbalance in bilateral force production, benefiting straight track speed but not necessarily affecting overall performance. Overall performance might have been influenced by a variety of other factors. Previous studies repeatedly showed that technique parameters were correlated with the performance of speed skating [12,14,15,25,26]. The results of the current study, combined with the literature, indicate that the effects of left and right leg movements on the performance of speed skating may be proportional. The effects of either leg's movements, therefore, can be predictors of the performance of speed skating, but the difference in movements between the left and right leg are not. Although technique asymmetries do not appear to affect performance in speed skating, the strength asymmetries they cause may still be risk factors for lower extremity injuries [32]. Thus, further research may be needed to find ways to prevent injuries due to technique asymmetries.

The results of this study were limited to a relatively small sample size from the same country in the same speed skating event. The participants of this study were at a similar level. The training programs of these participants have many similarities. These limitations might prevent our study from showing the effects of technique asymmetries on the performance of 500 m speed skating. Further studies with a bigger sample size and in different speed skating events may be needed to confirm the results of the current study. The data of this study were collected in a real competition. The reproducibility of the results cannot be evaluated. Future studies are needed to confirm the results of the current study.

5. Conclusions

Speed skaters have bilateral technique asymmetries in straight track skating that are primarily evident in the knee flexion angle, trunk flexion angle, ROM of the knee joint, push-off angle, shift of COM, push-off speed, and gliding time. Only the asymmetry of the knee joint angle at takeoff has a significant positive effect on the performance of the straight track. Technique asymmetries have no effect on 500 m speed skating overall performance.

Author Contributions: Conceptualization, Z.L. and M.D.; methodology, M.Z.; software, M.D.; formal analysis, Z.L. and M.D.; investigation, M.Z. and M.D.; data curation, Z.L. and M.D.; writing—original draft preparation, Z.L.; writing—review and editing, B.Y. and H.L.; visualization, Z.L.; supervision, B.Y.; funding acquisition, H.L. All authors have read and agreed to the published version of the manuscript.

Funding: This research was funded by a research grant from the National Key Research and Development Program of China (Grant number: 2018YFF0300404).

Institutional Review Board Statement: This study was conducted in accordance with the Declaration of Helsinki and approved by the Sports Science Experiment Ethics Committee of Beijing Sport University (approval number 2020187H).

Informed Consent Statement: Informed consent was obtained from all subjects involved in this study.

Data Availability Statement: Pseudonymized datasets are available to external collaborators subject to agreement on the terms of data use and publication of results. To request the data, please contact Zimeng Liu (liuzimeng@bsu.edu.cn).

Acknowledgments: The authors thank all the skaters and coaches who took part in this study.

Conflicts of Interest: The authors declare no conflicts of interest.

References

1. Evershed, J.; Burkett, B.; Mellifont, R. Musculoskeletal screening to detect asymmetry in swimming. *Phys. Ther. Sport* **2014**, *15*, 33–38. [CrossRef] [PubMed]
2. Meyers, R.W.; Oliver, J.L.; Hughes, M.G.; Lloyd, R.S.; Cronin, J.B. Asymmetry during Maximal Sprint Performance in 11- to 16-Year-Old Boys. *Pediatr. Exerc. Sci.* **2017**, *29*, 94–102. [CrossRef] [PubMed]
3. Rumpf, M.C.; Cronin, J.B.; Mohamad, I.N.; Mohamad, S.; Oliver, J.L.; Hughes, M.G. Kinetic asymmetries during running in male youth. *Phys. Ther. Sport* **2014**, *15*, 53–57. [CrossRef]
4. Blagrove, R.C.; Bishop, C.; Howatson, G.; Hayes, P.R. Inter-limb strength asymmetry in adolescent distance runners: Test-retest reliability and relationships with performance and running economy. *J. Sports Sci.* **2021**, *39*, 312–321. [CrossRef]
5. Ciacci, S.; Di Michele, R.; Fantozzi, S.; Merni, F. Assessment of Kinematic Asymmetry for Reduction of Hamstring Injury Risk. *Int. J. Athl. Ther. Train.* **2013**, *18*, 18–23. [CrossRef]
6. Zifchock, R.A.; Davis, I.; Hamill, J. Kinetic asymmetry in female runners with and without retrospective tibial stress fractures. *J. Biomech.* **2006**, *39*, 2792–2797. [CrossRef] [PubMed]
7. Morouco, P.G.; Marinho, D.A.; Fernandes, R.J.; Marques, M.C. Quantification of upper limb kinetic asymmetries in front crawl swimming. *Hum. Mov. Sci.* **2015**, *40*, 185–192. [CrossRef]
8. dos Santos, K.B.; Pereira, G.; Papoti, M.; Bento, P.C.B.; Rodacki, A. Propulsive Force Asymmetry during Tethered-Swimming. *Int. J. Sports Med.* **2013**, *34*, 606–611. [CrossRef]
9. Danyang, L.; Xu, C.; Yilin, Q.; Lili, N. The Impact of Interlimb Asymmetry on Athletic Performance and Intervention Methods. *J. Wuhan Sports Univ.* **2021**, *55*, 94–100. [CrossRef]
10. de Koning, J.J.; de Groot, G.; Schenau, G.J.v.I. Speed Skating the Curves: A Study of Muscle Coordination and Power Production. *Int. J. Sport Biomech.* **1991**, *7*, 344–358. [CrossRef]
11. de Boer, R.W.; Ettema, G.J.; van Gorkum, H.; de Groot, G.; van Ingen Schenau, G.J. A geometrical model of speed skating the curves. *J. Biomech.* **1988**, *21*, 445–450. [CrossRef] [PubMed]
12. de Boer, R.W.; Nilsen, K.L. The gliding and push-off technique of male and female Olympic speed skaters. *J. Appl. Biomech.* **1989**, *5*, 119–134. [CrossRef]
13. de Boer, R.W.; Nilsen, K.L. Work per stroke and stroke frequency regulation in Olympic speed skating. *J. Appl. Biomech.* **1989**, *5*, 135–150. [CrossRef]
14. van Ingen Schenau, G.J.; de Groot, G. On the origin of differences in performance level between elite male and female speed skaters. *Hum. Mov. Sci.* **1983**, *2*, 151–159. [CrossRef]
15. Burmistrov, A.D.; Chikurov, A.L.; Khudik, S.S.; Radaeva, S.V. Functional Asymmetry of Elite Speed Skaters. *Tomsk State Univ. J.* **2018**, *434*, 143–148. [CrossRef]
16. Konieczny, M.; Skorupska, E.; Domaszewski, P.; Pakosz, P.; Skulska, M.; Herrero, P. Relationship between latent trigger points, lower limb asymmetry and muscle fatigue in elite short-track athletes. *BMC Sports Sci. Med. Rehabil.* **2023**, *15*, 109. [CrossRef]
17. Konieczny, M.; Pakosz, P.; Domaszewski, P.; Skorupska, E. The relationship between asymmetry changes in the slope frequency of bioelectrical activity of the gluteus maximus muscles and experience in short track speed skating athletics. *Isokinet. Exerc. Sci.* **2024**, *preprint*, 1–6. [CrossRef]
18. Liu, H.; Li, H.; Qu, Y.; He, X.; Zhou, Z.; Yu, B. Effectiveness of an Artificial Intelligence System for Automatic Human Motion Capture without Reflection Points. *J. Beijing Sports Univ.* **2021**, *44*, 125–133. [CrossRef]
19. Masen, Z.; Yi, Q.; Jing, C.; Hui, L. Application of motion capture artificial intelligence system in speed skating. *Sci. Technol. Eng.* **2022**, *22*, 5674–5680.
20. Leigh, S.; Gross, M.T.; Li, L.; Yu, B. The relationship between discus throwing performance and combinations of selected technical parameters. *Sports Biomech.* **2008**, *7*, 173–193. [CrossRef]
21. Liu, H.; Leigh, S.; Yu, B. Sequences of upper and lower extremity motions in javelin throwing. *J. Sports Sci.* **2010**, *28*, 1459–1467. [CrossRef] [PubMed]
22. Abdel-Aziz, Y.I.; Karara, H.M. Direct Linear Transformation from Comparator Coordinates into Object Space Coordinates in Close-Range Photogrammetry. *Photogramm. Eng. Remote Sens.* **2015**, *81*, 103–107. [CrossRef]
23. Yu, B.; Andrews, J.G. The Relationship between Free Limb Motions and Performance in the Triple Jump. *J. Appl. Biomech.* **1998**, *14*, 223–237. [CrossRef]
24. Robinson, R.O.; Herzog, W.; Nigg, B.M. Use of force platform variables to quantify the effects of chiropractic manipulation on gait symmetry. *J. Manip. Physiol. Ther.* **1987**, *10*, 172–176.
25. van Ingen Schenau, G.J. The influence of air friction in speed skating. *J. Biomech.* **1982**, *15*, 449–458. [CrossRef]
26. Konings, M.J.; Elferink-Gemser, M.T.; Stoter, I.K.; van der Meer, D.; Otten, E.; Hettinga, F.J. Performance Characteristics of Long-Track Speed Skaters: A Literature Review. *Sports Med.* **2014**, *45*, 505–516. [CrossRef]
27. Qiuping, L. A Comparative Study of Hip Flexor and Extensor Muscle Tension in Speed Skaters. *J. Shenyang Sport Univ.* **2008**, *4*, 67–69.
28. Qiuping, L.; Yongdian, T.; Xiaona, X. A Study on the Quadriceps Characteristics of Chinese Speed Skaters' Knee Joints. *J. Wuhan Sports Univ.* **2006**, *4*, 99–102.
29. Allinger, T.L.; Van den Bogert, A.J. Skating technique for the straights, based on the optimization of a simulation model. *Med. Sci. Sports Exerc.* **1997**, *29*, 279–286. [CrossRef]

30. Houdijk, H.; de Koning, J.J.; de Groot, G.; Bobbert, M.F.; van Ingen Schenau, G.J. Push-off mechanics in speed skating with conventional skates and klapskates. *Med. Sci. Sports Exerc.* **2000**, *32*, 635–641. [CrossRef]
31. de Boer, R.W.; Ettema, G.J.; Faessen, B.G.; Krekels, H.; Hollander, A.P.; de Groot, G.; van Ingen Schenau, G.J. Specific characteristics of speed skating: Implications for summer training. *Med. Sci. Sports Exerc.* **1987**, *19*, 504–510. [CrossRef] [PubMed]
32. Fousekis, K.; Tsepis, E.; Poulmedis, P.; Athanasopoulos, S.; Vagenas, G. Intrinsic risk factors of non-contact quadriceps and hamstring strains in soccer: A prospective study of 100 professional players. *Br. J. Sports Med.* **2011**, *45*, 709–714. [CrossRef] [PubMed]

Disclaimer/Publisher's Note: The statements, opinions and data contained in all publications are solely those of the individual author(s) and contributor(s) and not of MDPI and/or the editor(s). MDPI and/or the editor(s) disclaim responsibility for any injury to people or property resulting from any ideas, methods, instructions or products referred to in the content.

bioengineering

MDPI

Article

Carrying Police Load Increases Gait Asymmetry in Ground Reaction Forces and Plantar Pressures Beneath Different Foot Regions in a Large Sample of Police Recruits

Mario Kasović [1,2,†], Andro Štefan [1,†] and Lovro Štefan [2,3,*]

1 Department of General and Applied Kinesiology, Faculty of Kinesiology, University of Zagreb, 10000 Zagreb, Croatia; mario.kasovic@kif.hr (M.K.); andro.stefan95@gmail.com (A.Š.)
2 Department of Physical Activities and Health Sciences, Faculty of Sports Studies, Masaryk University, 625 00 Brno, Czech Republic
3 Department of Physical Education and Sport, Faculty of Education, Catholic University in Ružomberok, 034 01 Ružomberok, Slovakia
* Correspondence: lovro.stefan1510@gmail.com
† These authors contributed equally to this work.

Abstract: Background: Although carrying external load has negative effects on gait biomechanics, little evidence has been provided regarding its impact on body asymmetry. The main purpose of the present study was to examine, whether standardized equipment produced greater gait asymmetries in ground reaction force and plantar pressure. Methods: For the purpose of this study, we recruited 845 police recruits (609 men and 236 women; 72.1% men and 27.9% women) measured in two conditions: (i) 'no load' and (ii) 'a 3.5 kg load'. Absolute values in ground reaction forces and plantar pressures beneath the different foot regions were assessed with pedobarographic platform (Zebris FDM). Asymmetry was calculated as $(x_{right} - x_{left})/0.5 \times (x_{right} + x_{left}) \times 100\%$, where 'x' represented a given parameter being calculated and a value closer to 0 denoted greater symmetry. Results: Significant differences in ground reaction forces and plantar pressures between the left and right foot were observed, when adding 'a 3.5 kg load'. Compared to the 'no load' condition, carrying 'a 3.5 kg load' significantly increased gait asymmetries for maximal ground reaction forces beneath the forefoot (ES = 0.29), midfoot (ES = 0.20) and hindfoot (ES = 0.19) regions of the foot. For maximal plantar pressures, only the asymmetry beneath the midfoot region of the foot significantly increased (ES = 0.19). Conclusions: Findings of this study indicate that 'a 3.5 kg load' significantly increases ground reaction force and plantar pressure gait asymmetries beneath the forefoot and midfoot regions, compared to 'no load' condition. Due to higher loads, increases in kinetic gait asymmetries may have negative effects on future pain and discomfort in the foot area, possibly causing stress fractures and deviated gait biomechanics in police recruits.

Keywords: special populations; police equipment; load carriage; symmetry; effect size

1. Introduction

Load carriage in special populations, like police officers, is considered a crucial component of everyday physical activity and successful performance of occupational tasks [1,2] Although such load may have beneficial effects for on-duty protection and completing the tasks at maximal level [3,4], previous research has highlighted negative effects of the load on one's health and well-being (Salvendy, 2012), primarily focusing on physiological [3,5] and biomechanical changes [3,4]. In the field of physiology, carrying an external load and gait propulsion may produce higher energy expenditure [3]. On the other hand, from a biomechanical point of view, added mass to body weight may increase moments in the trunk, hip and knee flexion and extension areas, while inconclusive data between the load carriage and ground reaction forces and plantar pressures are detected [4]. Both physiological and biomechanical consequences of carrying heavy loads can also increase the fatigue [6] and the incidence of musculoskeletal injuries [7,8].

Studying gait symmetry has often been a topic of interest for healthcare professionals to detect gait characteristics in normal population [9] and identifying injury risk [10]. A 'perfect symmetry', indicating an equal degree for a given parameter between the left and right foot, has been set to be between 5 and 15% for some motor abilities, like strength [11]; it is reasonable to expect that carrying loads may naturally affect gait asymmetry for up to 50% [12]. With that in line, available studies have shown that carrying an extra load potentially increases hip and knee extensor moments of the unloaded leg [13], changing knee biomechanics [14,15]. Although a common method for assessing the degree of symmetry has been by measuring ground reaction forces [12], the majority of previous studies have investigated the effects of external load on ground reaction force and plantar pressure gait asymmetries during quiet stance [16,17], with limited information for such a phenomenon during gait [12]. A study by Zhang et al. [12] has concluded that carrying a load of 20% body mass increases ground reaction force asymmetries in a mediolateral plane, compared to 0 to 10% conditions. Indeed, an increased gait asymmetry and body compensations following load carriage come from inertial characteristics of the musculoskeletal system [18].

To the best of the authors' knowledge, there has been a lack of studies examining the effects of load carriage on gait asymmetries in terms of ground reaction forces and plantar pressures. Since 'a perfect symmetry' between the sides of the body without carrying a load does not exist, we can speculate that an additional mass added onto the body may even increase gait asymmetry in the aforementioned gait parameters. Indeed, a higher level of ground reaction forces and plantar pressures have been constantly associated with a higher incidence of musculoskeletal injury rate [19,20], which can increase and prolong hospitalization time [21]. Although a load carriage is a necessity for special populations, redistributing load items on the body may be a crucial part for minimizing negative impacts on gait biomechanics.

Therefore, the main purpose of the present study was to examine whether standardized equipment produced greater ground reaction force and plantar pressure gait asymmetries in a large sample of police recruits. We speculated that such loads might increase ground reaction force and plantar pressure asymmetries, especially beneath the hindfoot and forefoot regions.

2. Materials and Methods

2.1. Study Participants

For the purpose of this study, we recruited 900 police recruits, who were part of the Croatian police service at the time. More detailed information about recruitment, sample size characteristics, inclusion and exclusion criteria and data regulations can be found elsewhere [22]. In brief, every year, a police academy recruits and welcomes around 900 healthy men and women, who undertake a special police training program in the duration of one year. In 2023, we were able to recruit all 900 first-year police recruits for our study and 845 of them had eligible data for further analyses (27.9% women). The inclusion criteria included from all participants to be without locomotor and mental acute or chronic diseases, which could prevent them from taking part in the study, and to be in the training program of the police academy on a regular basis. The exclusion criteria included participants suffering from locomotor (injury) or mental (depression or any other disease) and who were ill at the time the study had been conducted. Before the study had been conducted, all participants became familiar with aims, hypotheses, benefits and potential risks of the study and how the findings might translate into practice. Following the Declaration of Helsinki procedure, all analyses were anonymous and all participants gave a written informed consent to participate in the study. This study was approved by the Ministry of Internal Affairs and police academy 'Josip Jović' and the Ethical Committee of the Faculty of Kinesiology, University of Zagreb, Croatia (ethical code number: 511-01-128-23-1).

2.2. Load Equipment

A standardized load equipment being carried by police recruits involved a belt with a gun and a full handgun's magazine, an additional full handgun's magazine, a nightstick and handcuffs, where the final weight was around 3.5 kg (7.7 Ibs) [22,23].

2.3. Ground Reaction Forces and Plantar Pressures

Ground reaction forces and plantar pressures beneath different foot regions were analyzed via an objective method of the Zebris pedobarographic platform (FDM; GmbH, Munich, Germany; number of sensors: 11.264; sampling rate: 100 Hz; sensor area: 149 cm × 54.2 cm). The device uses a multisensory principle which may capture spatiotemporal and kinetic gait characteristics during walking or standing positions. More detailed information of testing the protocols and generating the data can be found elsewhere [22,23]. In brief, each participant walked at a preferred gait speed over the platform eight times, after being instructed not to target the platform or change the patterns of the walk. After completing the first task, the same task was repeated while carrying police equipment. The kinetic gait parameters included generating the data regarding maximal ground reaction forces (N) and plantar pressures (N/cm^2) of the left and right foot of the body for the forefoot, midfoot and hindfoot regions.

2.4. Data Analysis

All procedures were analyzed using Statistical Packages for Social Sciences software version 23 (SPSS Inc., Chicago, IL, USA). First, to test the normality of the study variables, we used the Kolmogorov–Smirnov test. For normally and not normally distributed variables, descriptive statistics are presented as mean and standard deviation (SD) or median and interquartile range (25th and 75th percentile). Student *t*-test for dependent samples or Wilcoxon singed-rank test were used to examine differences between 'no load' vs. 'a 3.5 kg load'. To examine gait asymmetries, we used the formula proposed by Robinson et al. [24]: $(x_{right} - x_{left})/0.5 \times (x_{right} + x_{left}) \times 100\%$, where an 'x' represented a given parameter. A final score closer to 0 denotes a more symmetrical gait, while a score that deviates more from 0 denotes greater asymmetry. Effect size (ES) was used to express the magnitude of the difference between groups and was presented as 'small' (0.2), 'moderate' (0.5), 'large' (0.8) [25]. To test, whether gender had any effects on kinetic gait changes, we used repeated-measures ANOVA with gender as a between-group factor and found no significant interaction between time and gender in any of the studied variables, so we omitted sex-specific presentation of the data. Also, age and body mass index were not significantly correlated to ground reaction force and plantar pressure changes. The significance was set at a priori $p \leq 0.05$.

3. Results

Socio-demographic characteristics of the study participants are presented in Table 1. The data of Table 1 relied on one previous study published by the same authors [22].

Table 1. Basic descriptive statistics of the study participants at baseline.

Variables	Mean (SD)/N (%)	Min–Max	Range
Gender			
Men	609 (72.1%)		
Women	236 (27.9%)		
Age (years)	21.3 ± 2.1	18.7–24.7	6.0
Height (cm)	175.2 ± 14.3	164.3–190.8	26.5
Weight (kg)	74.4 ± 14.5	57.3–100.6	43.3
Body Mass Index (kg/m^2)	24.3 ± 4.8	19.4–28.3	8.9

Changes in ground reaction forces and plantar pressures are presented in Table 2. When carrying 'a 3.5 kg load', significant differences in ground reaction forces for left forefoot (Δ = 2.9%), left midfoot (Δ = 3.6%), right midfoot (Δ = 3.6%) and right hindfoot (Δ = 1.7%) were observed. For plantar pressures, a load of 3.5 kg significantly increased the area beneath the left forefoot (Δ = 2.0%), right forefoot (Δ = 1.2%) and right midfoot (Δ = 0.4%). Finally, the % of time maximal force during stance time was significantly increased beneath the left forefoot (Δ = 0.5%) and right midfoot (Δ = 0.8%), while a significant decrease in left midfoot was shown. Changes in gait asymmetries according to gender showed no significant time* gender interactions for ground reaction forces beneath the forefoot ($F_{1,833}$ = 0.616, p = 0.433), midfoot ($F_{1,833}$ = 0.347, p = 0.556) and hindfoot ($F_{1,833}$ = 0.750, p = 0.387) regions of the foot. Also, when force was applied to a surface as a plantar pressure, we observed no significant time* gender interaction for asymmetries beneath the forefoot ($F_{1,833}$ = 0.743, p = 0.392), midfoot ($F_{1,833}$ = 0.422, p = 0.588) and hindfoot ($F_{1,833}$ = 0.255, p = 0.650) regions of the foot.

Table 2. Gait changes (mean ± SD) in ground reaction forces and plantar pressures beneath different foot regions.

Study Variables	**Load Condition**		***t*-Value**	***p*-Value**
	'No Load'	**'a 3.5 kg Load'**		
Sex, N (%)				
Men/Women	609 (72.1%)/ 236 (27.9%)	609 (72.1%)/ 236 (27.9%)	0.000	1.000
Age (years)	21.3 ± 2.1	21.3 ± 2.1	0.000	1.000
Body Mass Index (kg/m^2)	24.3 ± 4.8	25.4 ± 4.5	−2.176	0.037
Maximal Ground Reaction Forces				
Left Foot				
Forefoot (N)	758.58 (130.70)	780.44 (135.94)	−3.351	< 0.001
Midfoot (N)	145.58 (71.58)	150.83 (78.34)	−2.083	0.037
Hindfoot (N)	513.65 (98.57)	524.38 (98.53)	−1.432	0.152
Right Foot				
Forefoot (N)	766.11 (304.00)	798.78 (336.76)	−1.497	0.135
Midfoot (N)	156.84 (79.10)	162.52 (76.32)	−2.227	0.026
Hindfoot (N)	500.23 (98.86)	508.53 (98.31)	−1.923	0.045
Maximal Plantar Pressures				
Left Foot				
Forefoot (N/cm^2)	44.40 (9.80)	45.28 (9.76)	−1.857	0.049
Midfoot (N/cm^2)	15.01 (7.54)	15.31 (7.60)	−1.088	0.277
Hindfoot (N/cm^2)	33.05 (7.59)	33.69 (7.28)	−0.809	0.419
Right Foot				
Forefoot (N/cm^2)	44.55 (10.07)	45.08 (9.91)	−1.900	0.046
Midfoot (N/cm^2)	15.03 (6.52)	15.64 (6.62)	−1.855	0.049
Hindfoot (N/cm^2)	31.89 (7.07)	32.46 (7.16)	−1.646	0.100

Table 2. *Cont.*

Study Variables	Load Condition		t-Value	p-Value
	'No Load'	'a 3.5 kg Load'		
Time Maximal Force, % of Stance Time				
Left Foot				
Forefoot (%)	74.44 (2.44)	74.79 (2.13)	−3.101	0.002
Midfoot (%)	41.30 (9.62)	41.02 (9.82)	−2.538	0.011
Hindfoot (%)	18.47 (3.69)	18.88 (3.60)	0.570	0.569
Right Foot				
Forefoot (%)	74.16 (3.48)	74.52 (2.28)	−0.596	0.552
Midfoot (%)	39.70 (9.02)	40.00 (9.10)	−2.303	0.021
Hindfoot (%)	18.06 (3.74)	18.27 (4.05)	−1.102	0.271

Table 3 shows asymmetry characteristics in 'no load' and 'a 3.5 kg load' conditions between the left and right foot. Most notably, 'a 3.5 kg load' significantly increased asymmetries in forefoot (ES = 0.29), midfoot (ES = 0.20) and hindfoot (ES = 0.19) regions of the foot for ground reaction forces. For plantar pressures, only the asymmetry beneath the midfoot region of the foot significantly increased (ES = 0.19). Also, the % of time maximal force during stance time significantly increased beneath the hindfoot (ES = 0.17) region of the foot, while other asymmetries were non-significant.

Table 3. Differences in asymmetries between the left and right foot of the body in 'no load' vs. 'a 3.5 kg load' (mean ± SD).

Study Variables	Asymmetry		Mean Diff.	95% Mean Diff.	p-Value
Ground Reaction Forces *	'No Load'	'A 3.5 kg Load'			
Forefoot	0.000 (0.049)	0.014 (0.010)	−0.014	−0.021–0.006	<0.001
Midfoot	0.038 (0.192)	0.076 (0.201)	−0.038	−0.056–−0.019	<0.001
Hindfoot	−0.014 (0.058)	−0.025 (0.058)	0.011	0.005–0.017	<0.001
Plantar Pressures *					
Forefoot	0.001 (0.092)	0.000 (0.089)	0.001	−0.008–0.010	0.779
Midfoot	0.009 (0.171)	0.041 (0.172)	−0.032	−0.049–−0.016	<0.001
Hindfoot	−0.017 (0.085)	−0.019 (0.071)	0.002	−0.005–0.010	0.562
Time Maximal Force, % of Stance Time *					
Forefoot	−0.003 (0.036)	−0.002 (0.017)	−0.001	−0.003–0.002	0.674
Midfoot	−0.018 (0.105)	−0.011 (0.104)	−0.007	−0.017–0.003	0.143
Hindfoot	−0.013 (0.102)	−0.030 (0.101)	0.018	0.008–0.027	<0.001

* All models were adjusted for body mass index.

4. Discussion

This study aimed to investigate the effects of carrying load on ground reaction force and plantar pressure gait asymmetries. The main findings of this study are that (i) 'a 3.5 kg load' significantly increases asymmetries in ground reaction forces, especially in the forefoot and midfoot regions, and (ii) the asymmetry index in plantar pressure also increases, with the largest magnitudes being observed for the forefoot region.

Based on the findings available, this research represents one of the initial examinations of differences in asymmetry under various load conditions among police recruits. As discussed in the Introduction section, previous approaches to defining gait asymmetry between the left and right foot have typically involved measuring ground reaction forces during stance [16,26]. However, there has been limited study on asymmetrical gait analysis during actual gait [12]. Notably, when carrying heavy loads, gait asymmetry in ground reaction forces becomes more pronounced, resulting in differing impacts on the left and right foot. Previous studies have employed asymmetric/unilateral loads to assess the effects of such equipment on kinematic and kinetic gait parameters [12–15,27]. In cases of asymmetric lifting, greater loads are placed on the musculoskeletal system, particularly the trunk, when compared to symmetric lifting techniques [13]. Additionally, the increased asymmetry in ground reaction forces and plantar pressures observed in this study could be attributed to cumulative effects resulting from changes in the inertial patterns of the musculoskeletal system and the restriction of natural arm swing due to load characteristics and lateral trunk position [18]. These findings align with previous research suggesting that deviations in trunk movement away from the loaded side are indicative of motor control actions related to load carriage strategies and characteristics such as weight and shape [12]. Furthermore, it has been observed that compensations between the sides of the body are associated with preferred handedness and alterations in the neuromuscular system. In a study by Alamoudi et al. [27], 20 males carried a load of 10 lbs ($\approx$4.5 kg) in four different modalities of frontal, lateral, bilateral and posterior positions while walking over a Kisler platform (FDM; GmbH, Munich, Germany). Similar to our findings, the compression and shear forces significantly increased with the magnitude of the weight carried, especially in lateral position. This is not surprising, since in our study, a gun with a full handgun's magazine was positioned sideways (left or right side of the body) and might have led to even greater asymmetries. Because of the nature of the load carried, the participants counterbalanced the weight by flexing the trunk, which may have led to an increased distance between the center of mass of the body and weight [28]. Although the latero-flexion of the trunk in the opposite direction prevents from falling and restores body balance, it reduces gait stability [29] and increases gait asymmetry [12]. Also, greater gait asymmetries are often explained by the increased cadence, which occurs to reduce the stress on the joints of the lower limb [30]. Through an exploration of various factors such as load patterns and physiological adaptations [1], policymakers in the healthcare field could potentially revamp existing load structures and adjust their placement on the body. According to a study, the introduction of a '3.5 kg load' was found to have a minor yet noteworthy impact on kinetic gait asymmetry. These alterations were believed to be linked to load placement [31] and increased energy consumption [32].This has been supported previously, where larger individuals classified as 'obese' increase their oxygen and carbon oxide consumption, relative energy expenditure and heart rate [33]. Indeed, obese individuals tend to have higher cardiac stroke volume and a higher mechanical demand on the lungs, which increase inspiratory and expiratory gas volumes and lead to breathing inefficiency [33]. To overcome this problem, we tested the interaction effect of body mass index on gait asymmetries and found non-significant main effects for both men and women, respectively. The cumulative effects of body mass index and 'a 3.5 kg load' carried may not be sufficient to exhibit significant gait changes. First, the participants recruited for this study were a somewhat homogenous group of healthy individuals, with a majority of them being classified as 'normal weight'. Second, a heavier load carried linearly leads to greater gait changes [27] and asymmetries in ground reaction forces and plantar pressures [12], while 'a 3.5 kg load' does not seem to produce such large, but only small effects. Based on the evidence, it is suggested that the safest and most biomechanically appropriate way to carry a load is by using a backpack, keeping the load close to the center of gravity [34]. Although we observed only trivial to small differences between 'no load' vs. 'a 3.5 kg load', there is still an implication of our findings in terms of re-positioning the items of the load. For example, the handgun can be moved to the lateral side of the thigh area to enable the arms to move swiftly during walking. We descriptively observed that the dominant arm often 'freezes' during gait, which increases movements on the opposite side of the body by increasing the lateral flexion of the trunk. In Croatia, the internal policy still dictates that police loads need to be attached around the hips, and future research on this topic are still warranted. Thus, strategies of re-designing police equipment and re-positioning it near the center of body should be implemented within the police system in order to minimize negative effects from the external load on the force and pressure distributions beneath the different foot regions. According to research by Quesada et al. [32], there is a physiological impact of load carriage on the human body. Carrying an additional load equivalent to 15% of the body weight results in a 5–6% increase in metabolic cost. In our own study, we found that a 3.5 kg load, which represents a relative value for our sample, may not significantly increase metabolic cost. However, it can lead to a more pronounced forward lean and distort gait patterns, as indicated by Bobet and Norman [31]. While a 3.5 kg load may not seem substantial enough to induce negative changes in gait, our study revealed that it can lead to increased asymmetries during the gait cycle. Load carriage influences on the anteroposterior and mediolateral planes of the foot, resulting in higher ground reaction forces and plantar pressures, which could lead to discomfort and pain during walking, as noted in previous studies [15,35,36]. Additionally, it may contribute to greater asymmetries between the left and right foot.

Practical implications of our findings can be useful in the field of practice among police officers, because even a small mass of police equipment can lead to a decrease in stability when walking in all planes. On the other hand, in addition to the basic equipment worn by police recruits, the mass of police equipment increases with the difficulty of the task, which can result in even more kinetic asymmetries of gait and increased forces and pressures under certain regions of the feet. One of the mechanisms of prevention of these conditions is the reorganization of police equipment during walking, with the aim of moving the pistol (which is normally carried on the hip) more towards the side of the upper leg, so that the hand on the side of the pistol can have a normal swing while walking. Also, in this way, the position of the torso would move more towards a neutral position (upright stance), which would directly lead to an equal distribution of forces and pressures under the feet on the ground. However, it is important to acknowledge the limitations of our study. The cross-sectional design restricts our ability to establish causal changes in asymmetries and limits the generalizability of our findings to police recruits. Furthermore, our focus on kinetic gait parameters means that we may have missed out on valuable insights provided by 3D kinematic and electromyography systems, which may be served in an inverse dynamic approach for testing torques within each joint. The absence of data pertaining to biological and physiological parameters, injury history and load-carrying techniques further restricts the practical implications of our findings. Finally, the fact that participants walked barefoot over the pressure platform could have impacted the observed gait patterns. Although the nature of the police work strictly dictates wearing appropriate shoes on duty, the methodology of the Zebris platform indicates that all measurements over the platform need to be barefoot-specific, since different types of shoes may mimic true values in ground reaction forces and plantar pressures by absorbing a significant amount of force within the shoe structure. Moving forward, it is essential for subsequent research to adopt a follow-up design and conduct comprehensive physiological and biomechanical analyses. Such studies should also consider load- and injury-related characteristics to mitigate the adverse effects of load carriage on gait.

5. Conclusions

Findings of this study indicate that 'a 3.5 kg load' significantly increases ground reaction force and plantar pressure gait asymmetries beneath the forefoot and midfoot regions, compared to a 'no load' condition. Such asymmetries may have hazardous effects on gait stability and an increased likelihood for musculoskeletal injuries, due to foot pain and discomfort.

These negative changes may impact foot placement on the ground and increase an incidence for future stress fractures and deviated gait biomechanics in police recruits.

Author Contributions: Conceptualization, M.K. and L.Š.; methodology, L.Š.; software, L.Š.; validation, A.Š., M.K. and L.Š.; formal analysis, A.Š. and L.Š.; investigation, M.K.; resources, M.K.; data curation, L.Š.; writing—original draft preparation, A.Š., M.K. and L.Š.; writing—review and editing, A.Š., M.K. and L.Š.; visualization, L.Š.; supervision, M.K.; project administration, M.K.; funding acquisition, M.K. All authors have read and agreed to the published version of the manuscript.

Funding: This research received no external funding.

Institutional Review Board Statement: This study was conducted in accordance with the Declaration of Helsinki, and the protocol was approved by the Ethics Committee of the Ministry of Internal Affairs and police academy 'Josip Jović' and the Ethical Committee of the Faculty of Kinesiology, University of Zagreb, Croatia (ethical code number: 511-01-128-23-1, date: 3 July 2023).

Informed Consent Statement: All subjects gave their informed consent for inclusion before they participated in the study.

Data Availability Statement: The raw data supporting the conclusions of this article will be made available by the authors on request.

Acknowledgments: We would like to thank the Ministry of Internal Affairs and the principal Josip Ćelić (the chairman of the Police School department) for letting us conduct the study under their Institutional Committee approval.

Conflicts of Interest: The authors declare no conflicts of interest.

References

1. Larsen, L.B.; Tranberg, R.; Ramstrand, N. Effects of thigh holster use on kinematics and kinetics of active duty police officers. *Clin. Biomech.* **2016**, *37*, 77–82. [CrossRef] [PubMed]
2. Joseph, A.; Wiley, A.; Orr, R.; Schram, B.; Dawes, J.J. The impact of load carriage on measures of power and agility in tactical occupations: A critical review. *Int. J. Environ. Res. Public Health* **2018**, *15*, 88. [CrossRef] [PubMed]
3. Boffey, D.; Harat, I.; Gepner, Y.; Frosti, C.L.; Funk, S.; Hoffman, J.R. The Physiology and Biomechanics of Load Carriage Performance. *Mil. Med.* **2019**, *184*, 83–90. [CrossRef] [PubMed]
4. Walsh, G.S.; Low, D.C. Military load carriage effects on the gait of military personnel: A systematic review. *Appl. Ergon.* **2021**, *93*, 103376. [CrossRef] [PubMed]
5. Faghy, M.A.; Shei, R.J.; Armstrong, N.C.D.; White, M.; Lomax, M. Physiological impact of load carriage exercise: Current understanding and future research directions. *Physiol. Rep.* **2022**, *10*, 15502. [CrossRef] [PubMed]
6. Fallowfield, J.L.; Blacker, S.D.; Willems, M.E.; Davey, T.; Layden, J. Neuromuscular and cardiovascular responses of Royal Marine recruits to load carriage in the field. *Appl. Ergon.* **2012**, *43*, 1131–1137. [CrossRef]
7. Orr, R.M.; Pope, R. Gender differences in load carriage injuries of Australian army soldiers. *BMC Musculoskelet. Disord.* **2016**, *17*, 488. [CrossRef]
8. Orr, R.M.; Coyle, J.; Johnston, V.; Pope, R. Self-reported load carriage injuries of military soldiers. *Int. J. Inj. Contr. Saf. Promot.* **2017**, *24*, 189–197. [CrossRef]
9. Handžić, I.; Reed, K.B. Perception of gait patterns that deviate from normal and symmetric biped locomotion. *Front. Psychol.* **2015**, *6*, 199. [CrossRef]
10. Helme, M.; Tee, J.; Emmonds, S.; Low, C. Does lower-limb asymmetry increase injury risk in sport? A systematic review. *Phys. Ther. Sport* **2021**, *49*, 204–213. [CrossRef]
11. Lanshammar, K.; Ribom, E.L. Differences in muscle strength in dominant and non-dominant leg in females aged 20-39 years--a population-based study. *Phys. Ther. Sport* **2011**, *12*, 76–79. [CrossRef] [PubMed]
12. Zhang, X.A.; Ye, M.; Wang, C.T. Effect of unilateral load carriage on postures and gait symmetry in ground reaction force during walking. *Comput. Methods Biomech. Biomed. Engin.* **2010**, *13*, 339–344. [CrossRef] [PubMed]
13. DeVita, P.; Hong, D.; Hamill, J. Effects of asymmetric load carrying on the biomechanics of walking. *J. Biomech.* **1991**, *24*, 1119–1129. [CrossRef] [PubMed]
14. Ozgül, B.; Akalan, N.E.; Kuchimov, S.; Uygur, F.; Temelli, Y.; Polat, M.G. Effects of unilateral backpack carriage on biomechanics of gait in adolescents: A kinematic analysis. *Acta Orthop. Traumatol. Turc.* **2012**, *46*, 269–274. [CrossRef] [PubMed]
15. Park, K.; Sy, J.F.; Horn, G.P.; Kesler, R.M.; Petrucci, M.N.; Rosengren, K.S.; Hsiao-Wecksler, E.T. Assessing gait changes in firefighters after firefighting activities and while carrying asymmetric loads. *Appl. Ergon.* **2018**, *70*, 44–50. [CrossRef] [PubMed]
16. Maines, J.M.; Reiser, R.F. Ground reaction force bilateral asymmetries during submaximal sagittal plane lifting from the floor. *Int. J. Industr. Ergon.* **2006**, *36*, 109–117. [CrossRef]

17. Rocheford, E.C.; DeVoe, D.E.; Reiser II, R. FEffect of previous unilateral injuries on ground reaction force bilateral asymmetries during static lifting and standing. *J. Hum. Mov. Stud.* **2006**, *51*, 403–424.
18. Umberger, B.R. Effects of suppressing arm swing on kinematics, kinetics, and energetics of human walking. *J. Biomech.* **2008**, *41*, 2575–2580. [CrossRef]
19. Teyhen, D.S.; Shaffer, S.W.; Goffar, S.L.; Kiesel, K.; Butler, R.J.; Rhon, D.I.; Plisky, P.J. Identification of risk factors prospectively associated with musculoskeletal injury in a warrior athlete population. *Sports Health* **2020**, *12*, 564–572. [CrossRef]
20. Yavnai, N.; Bar-Sela, S.; Pantanowitz, M.; Funk, S.; Waddington, G.; Simchas, L.; Svorai-Litvak, S.; Steinberg, N. Incidence of injuries and factors related to injuries in combat soldiers. *BMJ Mil. Health* **2021**, *167*, 418–423. [CrossRef]
21. Canham-Chervak, M.; Rappole, C.; Grier, T.; Jones, B.H. Injury mechanisms, activities, and limited work days in US army infantry units. *U.S. Army Med. Dep. J.* **2018**, *2-18*, 6–13.
22. Štefan, A.; Kasović, M.; Štefan, L. Does a standardized load carriage increase spatiotemporal gait asymmetries in police recruits? A population-based study. *Mil. Med.* **2024**, usae358. [CrossRef] [PubMed]
23. Štefan, A.; Kasović, M.; Štefan, L. Load carriage and changes in spatiotemporal and kinetic biomechanical foot parameters during quiet stance in a large sample of police recruits. *Appl. Sci.* **2024**, *14*, 3274. [CrossRef]
24. Robinson, R.O.; Herzog, W.; Nigg, B.M. Use of force platform variables to quantify the effects of chiropractic manipulation on gait symmetry. *J. Manip. Physiol. Ther.* **1987**, *10*, 172–176.
25. Sullivan, G.M.; Feinn, R. Using effect size-or why the *p*-value is not enough. *J. Grad. Med. Educ.* **2012**, *4*, 279–282. [CrossRef]
26. Chavet, P.; Lafortune, M.A.; Gray, J.R. Asymmetry of lower extremity responses to external impact loading. *Hum. Mov. Sci.* **1997**, *16*, 391–406. [CrossRef]
27. Alamoudi, M.; Travascio, F.; Onar-Thomas, A.; Eltoukhy, M.; Asfour, S. The effects of different carrying methods on locomotion stability, gait spatio-temporal parameters and spinal stresses. *Int. J. Ind. Ergon.* **2018**, *67*, 81–88. [CrossRef]
28. Holbein, M.; Redfern, M. Postural Stability While Walking and Carrying Loads in Various Postures. *Proc. Hum. Factors Ergon. Soc. Annu. Meet.* **1994**, *38*, 564–567. [CrossRef]
29. Fowler, N.E.; Rodacki, A.L.; Rodacki, C.D. Changes in stature and spine kinematics during a loaded walking task. *Gait Posture* **2006**, *23*, 133–141. [CrossRef]
30. Singh, T.; Koh, M. Effects of backpack load position on spatiotemporal parameters and trunk forward lean. *Gait Posture* **2009**, *29*, 49–53. [CrossRef]
31. Bobet, J.; Norman, R.W. Effects of load placement on back muscle activity in load carriage. *Eur. J. Appl. Physiol. Occup. Physiol.* **1984**, *53*, 71–75. [CrossRef] [PubMed]
32. Quesada, P.M.; Mengelkoch, L.J.; Hale, R.C.; Simon, S.R. Biomechanical and metabolic effects of varying backpack loading on simulated marching. *Ergonomics* **2000**, *43*, 293–309. [CrossRef] [PubMed]
33. Lemus, S.A.; Volz, M.; Tiozzo, E.; Perry, A.; Best, T.M.; Travascio, F. The effect of clinically elevated body mass index on physiological stress during manual lifting activities. *PLoS ONE* **2022**, *17*, e0278858. [CrossRef] [PubMed]
34. Heglund, N.C.; Willems, P.A.; Penta, M.; Cavagna, G.A. Energy-saving gait mechanics with head-supported loads. *Nature* **1995**, *375*, 52–54. [CrossRef] [PubMed]
35. Goffar, S.L.; Reber, R.J.; Christiansen, B.C.; Miller, R.B.; Naylor, J.A.; Rodriguez, B.M.; Walker, M.J.; Teyhen, D.S. Changes in dynamic plantar pressure during loaded gait. *Phys. Ther.* **2013**, *93*, 1175–1184. [CrossRef]
36. Majumdar, D.; Pal, M.S.; Pramanik, A.; Majumdar, D. Kinetic changes in gait during low magnitude military load carriage. *Ergonomics* **2013**, *56*, 1917–1927. [CrossRef] [PubMed]

Disclaimer/Publisher's Note: The statements, opinions and data contained in all publications are solely those of the individual author(s) and contributor(s) and not of MDPI and/or the editor(s). MDPI and/or the editor(s) disclaim responsibility for any injury to people or property resulting from any ideas, methods, instructions or products referred to in the content.

bioengineering

MDPI

Article

Deep-Learning-Based Recovery of Missing Optical Marker Trajectories in 3D Motion Capture Systems

Oleksandr Yuhai [1,†], Ahnryul Choi [2,†], Yubin Cho [1], Hyunggun Kim [1,*] and Joung Hwan Mun [1,*]

[1] Department of Bio-Mechatronic Engineering, College of Biotechnology and Bioengineering, Sungkyunkwan University, Suwon 16419, Republic of Korea; oleksandr@g.skku.edu (O.Y.); yubinc@g.skku.edu (Y.C.)

[2] Department of Biomedical Engineering, College of Medical Convergence, Catholic Kwandong University, Gangneung 25601, Republic of Korea; achoi@cku.ac.kr

[*] Correspondence: hkim.bme@skku.edu (H.K.); jmun@skku.edu (J.H.M.); Tel.: +82-31-290-7827 (J.H.M.)

[†] These authors contributed equally to this work.

Abstract: Motion capture (MoCap) technology, essential for biomechanics and motion analysis, faces challenges from data loss due to occlusions and technical issues. Traditional recovery methods, based on inter-marker relationships or independent marker treatment, have limitations. This study introduces a novel U-net-inspired bi-directional long short-term memory (U-Bi-LSTM) autoencoder-based technique for recovering missing MoCap data across multi-camera setups. Leveraging multi-camera and triangulated 3D data, this method employs a sophisticated U-shaped deep learning structure with an adaptive Huber regression layer, enhancing outlier robustness and minimizing reconstruction errors, proving particularly beneficial for long-term data loss scenarios. Our approach surpasses traditional piecewise cubic spline and state-of-the-art sparse low rank methods, demonstrating statistically significant improvements in reconstruction error across various gap lengths and numbers. This research not only advances the technical capabilities of MoCap systems but also enriches the analytical tools available for biomechanical research, offering new possibilities for enhancing athletic performance, optimizing rehabilitation protocols, and developing personalized treatment plans based on precise biomechanical data.

Keywords: motion capture and analysis; long-term missing data; multi-camera data integration; artificial intelligence; adaptive Huber loss; data augmentation

1. Introduction

Motion capture (MoCap) technology, which is a linchpin in the realm of dynamic movement analysis, has become indispensable across a wide range of applications, from artistically focused applications, where it is used to create enchanting visuals in cinema and animation, to precision-dependent fields, where it is used in biomechanics and surgical navigation [1–3]. In particular, optical-marker-based MoCap systems offer unparalleled spatial and temporal accuracy, as they capture the intricacies of human motion by triangulating the three-dimensional (3D) positions of markers from multiple two-dimensional (2D) perspectives [4]. The advent of optical-marker-based MoCap has galvanized the creative and scientific communities in a wide-ranging manner, with example applications including its use in enhancing the creation of lifelike animations, the analysis of athletic performance, the study of intricate biomechanical processes, and advancements in surgical techniques through enhanced navigational aids [3–5]. In entertainment, MoCap serves as the backbone for creating compelling and immersive experiences; in clinical settings, it aids in the diagnosis and rehabilitation of gait abnormalities; and in the athletic arena, it provides critical insights into performance optimization and injury prevention [6–8].

Despite these profound impacts, MoCap technology is not without its challenges. One such challenge is the phenomenon of data loss, which is a significant obstacle to the seamless application of MoCap. Such data loss typically arises from occlusions, i.e., cases in which a marker becomes obscured from the view of the cameras due to the natural movement of limbs, interactions with props, or environmental constraints [9]. Other factors that contribute to data loss include marker detachment, technical malfunctions, and limitations in the camera's field of vision [5,9]. Such disruptions result in incomplete datasets, which compromise the integrity of the motion capture process and can lead to inaccurate analyses and interpretations [9,10]. In this context, various data recovery methods for MoCap have been proposed, each of which is tailored to overcome the challenges of data loss. These methods can be broadly categorized into two distinct groups based on their dependency on inter-marker relationships and predefined motion models.

Group 1 encompasses methods that utilize specific inter-marker relations and motion models. Although data-driven methods like local coordinate system interpolation, principal component analysis (PCA), and low rank matrix completion [11–15] are efficient, they may overfit, and they fail to capture the complexity of dynamic movements. Model-based methods, such as Kalman filter or the inverse-kinematics-based gap filling method [16–18], ensure physical consistency, but they are limited by rigid assumptions and struggle when faced with unexpected occlusions. While machine-learning-based methods show promise, particularly when using neural networks [19–22], they are hampered by their reliance on extensive training data and focus on skeletal data, indicating the inherited limitations tied to human body constraints. Recently, deep-learning-based methods, specifically leveraging LSTM architectures [20,21], have attracted attention for use in the recovery of missing data. LSTMs are favored for their proficiency in learning temporal dependencies, which is crucial for accurately predicting the sequence of movements in MoCap data. Despite their advantages, such models often require the use of substantial training datasets and may not effectively capture complex spatial relationships or sufficiently generalize across different movement types. Hybrid methods like linear dynamical systems (LDS) with constraints, low-dimensional Kalman smoothing, group-sparse low-rank (GS-LR), and probabilistic model averaging (PMA) [23–28] attempt to integrate the advantages of other approaches, but these all involve high computational complexity and require intensive parameter tuning.

These methods are fundamentally dependent on precise inter-marker relationships, meaning they require at least two markers with accurately known connections between them to be used, as well as specific predefined motion models [11,17,24,28]. While this dependency enhances data recovery accuracy in certain specialized scenarios, it simultaneously imposes significant limitations on the broader applicability of such methods. Specifically, these methods demand considerable effort, time, and computational resources [11,22] to define and maintain these exact inter-marker relationships and pre-defined motion models. Consequently, a model that has been calibrated for a particular skeletal structure or movement pattern may not yield accurate results when it is applied to different marker configurations or different types of motion [28]. This limitation becomes particularly pronounced in diverse applications where it is essential to use adaptable models, as well as when opportunities for training data for specific scenarios are either not readily available or are too constrained.

Meanwhile, Group 2 includes methods that treat the recovery of each marker's data independently. This group includes techniques like cubic and Hermite interpolation [29], which provide quick fixes for short-term data gaps. However, they are also constrained by the quality of input data, and they may struggle with longer gaps or more complex motions. The sparse low-rank method [28] is adept at reconstructing data from highly incomplete datasets, but its sensitivity to the specific context of data loss may cause it to struggle with extended data loss periods [14,22].

Although the methods in Group 2 address the primary limitation of Group 1's dependency on specific relationships and models, they also face their own set of challenges. For example, cubic spline interpolations, despite being independent of inter-marker constraints, may not effectively restore long-term missing MoCap data gaps [17] due to their inability to handle non-linearities and complex motion patterns that fall outside of their training data. As another example, although sparse low-rank methods are powerful for incomplete datasets, they may also falter when faced with extended data loss, thus necessitating a context-sensitive approach to reconstruction. Long-term missing MoCap data gaps represent a critical problem due to the associated loss of information, which can lead to significant inaccuracies in movement analysis [22]. This leads to difficulties arising from the need to infer data over extended periods, where traditional methods typically fail to capture the inherent dynamics of motion or the unique characteristics of individual markers.

With this background, the main purpose of the current research is to address the pervasive challenge of long-term data loss in multi-camera motion capture systems by using a novel recovery algorithm. The proposed U-net-inspired bi-directional long short-term memory (U-Bi-LSTM) autoencoder-based method is engineered to operate independently of marker relationships, thus making it versatile for various applications, including biomechanical analysis and surgical navigation. The methodological contributions of this paper are threefold: First, a preliminary stage is initiated in which multi-camera tracking data is newly augmented, missing data gaps are created, and initial imputation is conducted to refine the dataset. Next, the U-Bi-LSTM framework intricately processes the temporal and spatial complexities of MoCap data, and the final validation phase rigorously assesses the model's accuracy and robustness across various motion capture scenarios. The main contributions of this paper are elaborated upon in the following:

1. Advanced data recovery deep learning model. At the core of this research is the newly proposed U-Bi-LSTM model, which is a sophisticated deep learning structure that is inspired by U-net and enhanced with bidirectional LSTM networks. This model is notable for its ability to intricately capture the temporal dependencies and spatial nuances that are inherent in MoCap data, thus representing a significant leap from traditional linear prediction models. A notable feature of this model is its integration of an adaptive Huber regression layer, which replaces classical regression approaches. This layer is specifically chosen for its robustness against outliers and effectiveness in minimizing reconstruction errors, particularly in scenarios involving long-term data loss. Complementing this advanced architecture, the proposed method begins with a preliminary phase utilizing piecewise cubic spline (PCS) interpolation or sparse low rank (SLR) matrix completion. This preliminary phase is critical in refining the integrity of the dataset, thereby setting a solid foundation for the deep learning process and ultimately ensuring enhanced accuracy in the reconstructed data.
2. Holistic multi-camera data synthesis and augmentation. The proposed algorithm uniquely integrates available multi-camera UV data as well as triangulated 3D (X, Y, Z) data, ultimately allowing for an all-encompassing reconstruction that meticulously considers inter-camera relationships. This holistic approach not only guarantees the fidelity of the recovered data but also establishes the U-Bi-LSTM as an all-encompassing solution for MoCap data recovery challenges. The algorithm also features a novel multi-camera approach to data augmentation: It meticulously augments UV tracking data from multi-camera systems, thus preserving the spatio-temporal relationships while adapting the augmentation process to align with specific camera resolutions. This method applies transformations such as translation, rotation, scaling, and noise addition in a systematic manner that maintains data uniformity and adherence to camera resolution constraints.
3. Rigorous validation. Lastly, the effectiveness of the proposed deep-learning-based method is thoroughly validated against datasets characterized by extensive missing data. In these validation scenarios, the model consistently demonstrates superior accuracy compared to reconstructions prepared using only PCS or the state-of-the-art SLR missing data recovery method. This superior performance underscores the model's capability to significantly enhance traditional data imputation techniques. The algorithm was rigorously tested in various dynamic scenarios, including cases involving the recovery of lost data with diverse lengths and frequencies. These scenarios encompassed movements such as manipulating a calibration wand with varying

speeds and patterns, performing arm abduction and adduction, hip flexion of different intensities, and movements occurring during surface registration using a surgical navigation probe. The robustness and versatility demonstrated in these tests underscore the algorithm's applicability and potential impact across a wide range of MoCap applications.

2. Materials and Methods

This section details the multi-faceted approach used in the present study to recover motion capture data that has been lost in multi-camera systems, including the data collection with precise calibration, experimentation capturing diverse movements, extensive data augmentation for robust training datasets, and simulation of realistic missing data for effective algorithm training and testing. This methodology integrates the traditional imputation methods—PCS and SLR—with an advanced U-Bi-LSTM network, which is an autoencoder that is designed for intricate data pattern recognition. The efficacy of the recovery process is scrutinized using reconstruction error by utilizing root mean square error (RMSE) metrics and wand length error. Figure 1 visualizes the detailed workflow, which encapsulates the entire process from the initial data capture to the final performance assessment, thus showcasing a cohesive strategy for data recovery.

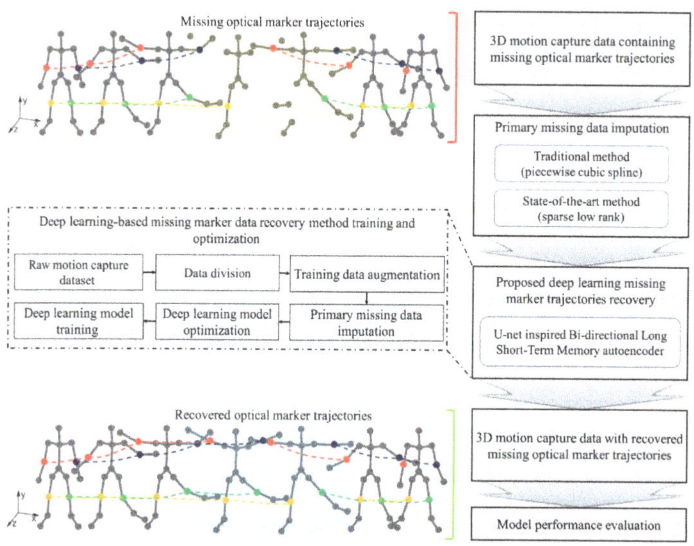

Figure 1. Comprehensive workflow for proposed deep-learning-enhanced multi-camera missing tracking data recovery method. The figure illustrates the process of capturing human movements and the occurrence of missing optical marker trajectories, demonstrated in the area highlighted in light yellow. Using the proposed deep learning method, these missing trajectories are accurately reconstructed, as shown in the area highlighted in light blue. The red and blue markers represent the RFLB and LFLB markers, respectively, while the yellow and green markers represent the RKNE and LKNE markers.

2.1. Experiments

A strategic data collection setup was established to effectively capture and recover lost multi-camera MoCap tracking data. This setup included four synchronized CMOS cameras (OptiTrack FLEX: V100; Natural Point, Corvallis, OR, USA), each configured with a resolution of 640 × 480 and a frame rate of 100 Hz. These cameras were strategically positioned at intervals of 5 m to create an extensive field of view, as depicted in Figure 2a, to ensure maximal coverage for tracking. The data collection commenced with a meticulous multi-camera calibration process involving a three-axis frame and a calibration wand with known marker 3D coordinates and distances, along with the direct linear transformation (DLT)-based algorithm proposed by Shin et al. [4]. This setup guaranteed the precision required for the proposed method. After calibration, two male volunteers were recruited in generating ten distinct datasets. The first volunteer, aged 25 years old, had a height of 166 cm and a weight of 98 kg. The second volunteer, aged 26 years old, had a height of 173 cm and a weight of 68 kg. Before the experiment, subjects were informed about how to properly perform activities like wanding and surgical navigation, as well as exercises like arm abduction, adduction, and hip flexion, with a demonstration provided. During the exercises, each subject alternated between the right and left limbs for abduction, adduction, and hip flexion. The subjects gradually increased the exercise speed every 10 s, from the slowest to the fastest possible speed, according to their perceptions [30]. Each volunteer performed random movements with the calibration wand that were recorded for 50 s (equating to 5000 frames) within the carefully defined zone corresponding to the collective field of view of all cameras, as illustrated in Figure 2a. The accuracy of this data collection method was validated by comparing the triangulated distances between the markers on the calibration wand against their known distances, and this process yielded an average error margin of about 0.5 mm. This precision demonstrates the reliability of the multi-camera setup and the data collection process. Four of the five datasets that were randomly chosen from each of the two subjects were used as the training data for the deep-learning algorithm, while the remaining datasets were reserved for testing.

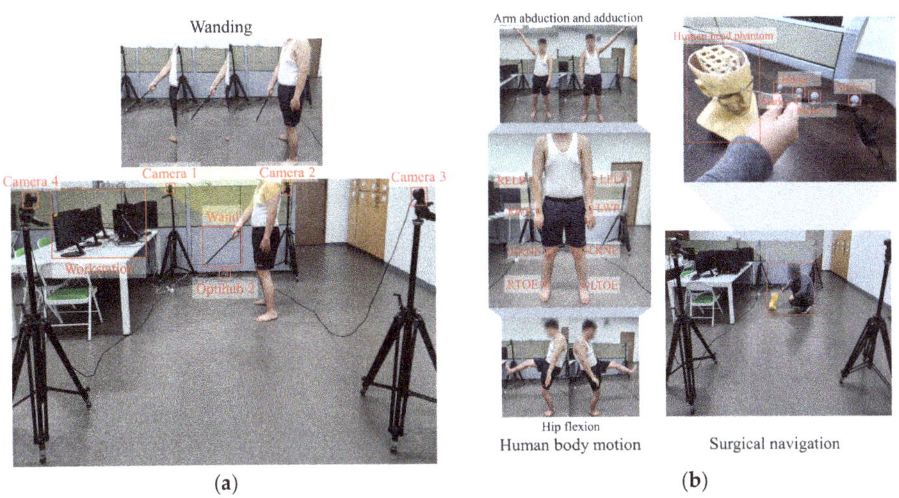

Figure 2. Experimental setup: (**a**) Schematics of the experimental multi-camera setup for MoCap data collection. (**b**) Marker placement for human body motion and surgical navigation validation experiments.

To further validate the proposed method's performance and robustness, additional experiments involving human body motion tracking were conducted, such as arm abduction and adduction, hip flexion, and surgical navigation by performing surface registration.

1. Human body motion tracking. In total, four markers were attached to the bodies of two subjects, as shown in Figure 2b. Each subject performed arm abduction and adduction, and hip flexion exercises for 50 s, twice at varying intensities. During arm abduction and adduction, the markers on the right and left elbows and wrists (RELB, RWR, LELB, LWR) were tracked and used for validation. Meanwhile, during hip flexion, the markers on the knees and toes (RKNE, RTOE, LKNE, LTOE) were tracked and used for validation.

2. Surgical navigation experiment. Using a human head phantom [3] and a passive probe (NDI, Waterloo, ON, Canada), as depicted in Figure 2b, each subject carried out

surface registration by tracing the probe over the phantom's face for 50 s, twice at different intensities. Markers 1, 2, 3, and 4 on the probe, as demonstrated in Figure 2b, were used for validation in these surgical navigation exercises.

All experimental procedures were conducted while following the approved ethical guidelines set by the Ethics Committee of Sungkyunkwan University.

2.2. Data Augmentation

The data augmentation process is a pivotal phase in preparing our training dataset, which is instrumental for the effective application of the proposed deep learning algorithm. Augmentation was meticulously applied to the multi-camera UV tracking data of the calibration wand in the manner described in the Experiments section herein. This process was designed not only to enhance the dataset with realistic variations but also to ensure that the necessary spatio-temporal fidelity for multi-camera MoCap systems would be achieved. As shown in Figure 3, the augmentation method was executed following an automated and systematic approach. Starting with synchronized and preprocessed UV data from each camera, the algorithm introduced transformations—translation, rotation, scaling, and noise addition—in a consistent manner across all frames and cameras. The transformation parameters were dynamically generated for each dataset iteration, involving small random translations (±0.05 units), rotations (±5 degrees), scaling factors (1 ± 0.02), and noise levels (±0.01 units) to simulate realistic and subtle variations in the camera capture conditions. These transformations were mathematically formulated to both respect the camera's resolution boundaries and preserve the original data's spatial and temporal relationships.

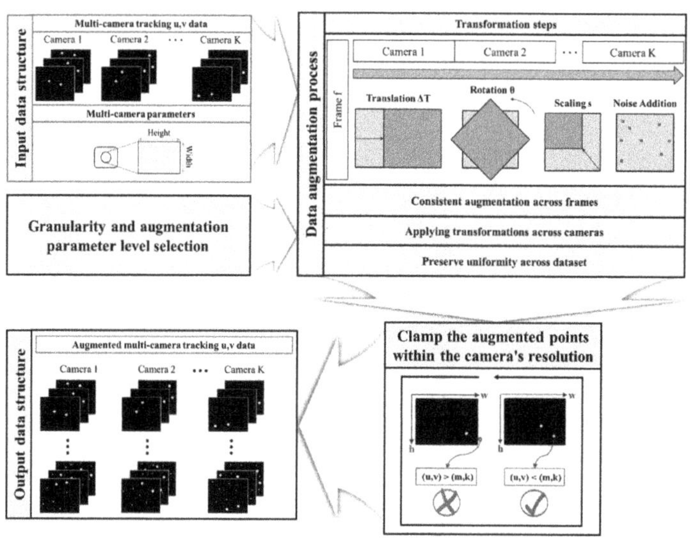

Figure 3. Schematic of the proposed data augmentation process for multi-camera motion tracking. First, collection of synchronized and preprocessed UV data from each camera occurs. Using the collected UV data and camera system information, such as resolution, determination of the augmentation parameters and their granularity is performed. The data is then augmented by applying transformations (translation, rotation, scaling, and noise addition) consistently across all frames and cameras. The augmented points are clamped within the camera's resolution, considering the maximum width (m) and height (k). Any marker UV data that exceeds the camera's field of view limits is eliminated. Finally, the remaining augmented UV data that stays within the entire camera's field of view is used to generate augmented datasets ready for training the deep learning model.

It was critical to adhere to the resolution limits to ensure that the augmented points did not fall outside of the camera's field of view. As an example, a point $P_{original}$ translated by a vector $\Delta T = (\Delta u,\ \Delta v)$ would be given by

$$P_{new} = P_{original} + \Delta T \tag{1}$$

This would then be rotated around the origin by an angle θ, using the rotation matrix R, which is defined as

$$R = \begin{bmatrix} \cos(\theta) & -\sin(\theta) \\ \sin(\theta) & \cos(\theta) \end{bmatrix} \tag{2}$$

The rotated point $P_{rotated}$ is then scaled by a factor s. The scaling transformation, effectively altering the magnification of data points, was applied as

$$P_{scaled} = P_{rotated} \times s \tag{3}$$

where the s was randomly selected within the range of 0.98 to 1.02, representing a $\pm 2\%$ change from the original size. Then, random Gaussian noise $N = (N_u,\ N_v)$ is added to introduce variability. Finally, the augmented point $P_{augmented}$ is clamped within the camera resolution $C = (C_u,\ C_v)$ as follows:

$$P_{augmented} = \min\Big(\max\Big(P_{final},\ (0,\ 0)\Big),\ C\Big) \tag{4}$$

Granularity—a measure of the fineness with which the transformation parameter space is sampled—was one of the key considerations in automatic augmentation parameter selection. It was used to determine the diversity of the augmentation by specifying the number of discrete levels within the permissible range for each transformation. Carefully calibrating the granularity allowed us to generate a spectrum of variations that enriched the training datasets while preserving the integrity of the motion data. In this study, the granularity was set at 10, meaning each transformation parameter (translation, rotation, scale, and noise) was selected 10 times randomly within their defined ranges.

By applying this rigorous augmentation method to our initial training datasets, we were able to increase the number of datasets that we could use for training by a factor of 100. This significant enhancement in the quantity and variety of training data is expected to directly contribute to increasing the proposed deep learning algorithm's ability to learn and generalize across a comprehensive range of data loss conditions, thereby enhancing its performance in the recovery of lost tracking data.

2.3. Missing Data Simulation

To establish a robust foundation for evaluating the proposed deep-learning-based data recovery method, it was imperative to simulate realistic scenarios involving a loss of tracking data within a multi-camera MoCap system. This simulation process is critical for developing and testing the effectiveness of data recovery algorithms under conditions that closely mimic those that lead to real-world data loss due to occlusions, camera malfunctions, or environmental interferences. The simulation algorithm commenced with the initialization of parameters to dictate the number and duration of gaps within the tracking data. This was done to introduce data loss across the datasets in a uniform manner to ensure comprehensive training and testing of the recovery algorithm. A systematic approach was used to simulate gaps or missing data points in the UV tracking data captured by multiple cameras. The algorithm was designed to ensure that the object remains detectable at all times, preserving the basic level of data integrity necessary for successful recovery. Specifically, in this study, the fixed base level refers to the minimum visibility threshold across the camera network, maintained within a tracking volume defined by an intersection of the visible zones of all cameras, approximately measuring 4 m (length) × 3 m (width) × 2 m (height). This arrangement guarantees the minimal visibility of the object by at least one camera at all times, pivotal for robust multi-camera tracking and data recovery. For each simulated gap, the algorithm randomly selected a subset of cameras and a starting frame within the sequence, while taking care not to exceed the data bounds. A crucial validation step was executed to ensure that the object remained visible to at least one camera during the gap period. If these conditions were satisfied, the algorithm introduced missing values to represent missing data in the UV coordinates for the selected frames. This simulation was then extended to the corresponding XYZ data to align the 3D spatial information with the 2D planar gaps. The integrity of the 3D spatial data was adjusted based on the simulated 2D planar data, thus ensuring consistency across dimensions. This adjustment was considered to be vital for maintaining a long-term missing data scenario for data recovery testing, as the loss in UV data must be accurately reflected in the XYZ data to simulate real-world conditions under which it is not possible for 3D data to be reliably triangulated. For the purposes of the current study, which seeks to develop a method that is adept at recovering tracking data with long-term gaps, five gaps were randomly introduced in each training dataset. These gaps varied in duration, ranging from 100 to 900 frames, to ensure a proportional representation of different gap lengths. The simulation covered both markers on the calibration wand used during data collection, thus reflecting the diversity of the data loss scenarios involved. Approximately equal numbers of training datasets contained five gaps of each duration, thus indicating that a balanced environment for the proposed deep learning algorithm's training and validation has been successfully established. This meticulous simulation process has allowed us to generate a comprehensive set of datasets that replicate the complexities of close to real-world data loss in MoCap systems, thus providing a solid foundation for the development and evaluation of advanced data recovery methods.

2.4. Missing Data Recovery Model

Our approach for recovering missing tracking data in a multi-camera system follows a sequential methodology, starting with traditional data imputation methods before advancing to a sophisticated deep learning architecture. The entire process is depicted in Figure 4, which showcases the intricate U-Bi-LSTM network design.

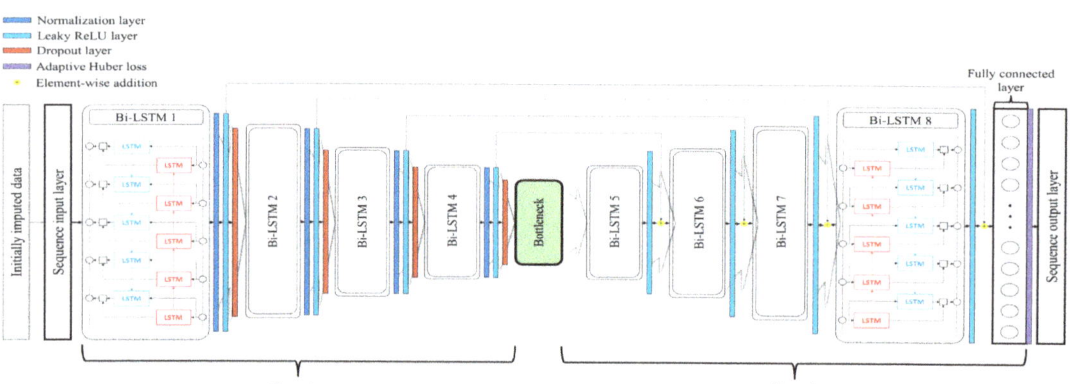

Figure 4. Schematic workflow of the proposed U-Bi-LSTM network.

2.4.1. Primary Missing Data Imputation Methods

To begin, we employ general imputation methods to approximate the missing data points. This stage uses either the PCS method or SLR imputation according to the nature of the specific dataset.

Piecewise cubic spline missing data imputation method. The MATLAB (R2023a, MathWorks corp., USA) function *fillmissing* [31] is used here. This function applies spline interpolation column-wise, first across the u and v coordinates of each camera and then on the X, Y, and Z positions. The spline function can be mathematically expressed as

$$S(x) = a_n(x - x_i)^2 + b_n(x - x_i)^2 + c_n(x - x_i)^2 + d_n \quad (5)$$

where $S(x)$ represents the spline function, and where a_n, b_n, c_n, and d_n are spline coefficients for the i-th interval. This method is particularly effective for non-linear data, as it ensures smooth continuity in the imputed data.

Sparse low-rank missing data imputation method. The SLR missing data imputation method proposed by Kamali et al. [28] employs an optimization framework to recover missing MoCap data. This technique separates multi-camera UV data and triangulated XYZ data, and it addresses them through a SLR matrix completion approach. The objective is to find matrices L and S that minimize the nuclear norm $||L||_*$ of L, which is the sum of its singular values to promote low-rank solutions, and the L_1 norm $||S||_1$ of S, the sum of the absolute values of its entries to encourage sparsity in the data matrix D. The regularization parameter λ, which is set within the range from 10^4 to 10^5, dictates the sparsity level of the solution, which affects both the accuracy and robustness of the reconstruction [28]. The SLR method is formulated as an optimization problem as follows:

$$minimize \ ||L||_* + \lambda||S||_1, \ subject \ to \ D = L + S \quad (6)$$

Here, $||L||_*$ represents the nuclear norm of the matrix L. $||S||_1$ denotes the L_1 norm of the matrix S. Meanwhile, the parameter λ is a regularization parameter that controls the trade-off between these priorities of low-rank and sparsity.

2.4.2. Deep-Learning-Based Missing Data Recovery Method

U-Bi-LSTM network. The proposed U-Bi-LSTM network, which is shown in Figure 4, is designed as an autoencoder, and it is specifically tailored for the recovery of missing data in multi-camera tracking systems. Initially, the dataset containing imputed missing data, which has been processed using traditional PCS or state-of-the-art SLR method, is transformed into an appropriate sequential format suitable for the U-Bi-LSTM network. For a single input dataset, this format is represented as (minimum sequence length) × (UV coordinates for each camera, and X, Y, Z coordinates). The core of the network consists of multiple bidirectional LSTM (Bi-LSTM) layers, each with varying numbers of hidden units (256, 128, 64, 32), ultimately leading to a bottleneck layer of size 16. This design enables the network to learn complex patterns in the data at different levels of abstraction [32]. The Bi-LSTM layers are formulated as follows:

$$\overrightarrow{H_t} = LSTM(\overrightarrow{X_t}, \overrightarrow{H}_{t-1}; \overrightarrow{\Theta}) \quad (7)$$

$$\overleftarrow{H_t} = LSTM(\overleftarrow{X_t}, \overleftarrow{H}_{t+1}; \overleftarrow{\Theta}) \quad (8)$$

$$H_t = [\overrightarrow{H_t}, \overleftarrow{H_t}] \quad (9)$$

Here, $\overrightarrow{H_t}$ and $\overleftarrow{H_t}$ are the hidden states at time t for the forward and backward passes, respectively; $\overrightarrow{X_t}$ and $\overleftarrow{X_t}$ are the inputs at time t for the forward and backward passes, respectively; and $\overrightarrow{\Theta}$ and $\overleftarrow{\Theta}$ are the parameters of the LSTM layers for the forward and backward directions, respectively. Each Bi-LSTM layer is followed by a layer normalization and a leaky ReLU activation function. The layer normalization ensures that the network's internal features have a mean of zero and a standard deviation of one, thus enhancing the training stability [33]. The leaky ReLU function introduces non-linearity and allows for small gradients when the unit is not active, which enhances the network's ability to learn complex patterns [34,35]. Dropout layers are interspersed throughout the architecture with a fixed rate of 0.5. These layers randomly deactivate some fraction of the neurons during training, thus preventing overfitting and enhancing the network's generalization ability [36]. L2 regularization—consistently set to 0.001 across the network—is used to penalize large weights, with the aim of encouraging the development of simpler models that can generalize better to new data [37]. The architecture features a bottleneck layer of size 16 that acts as a compressed representation of the input data. The decoder part mirrors the encoder, with ascending numbers of hidden units (32, 64, 128, 256). It progressively reconstructs the data from the compressed representation provided by the bottleneck layer, with this reconstruction facilitated by the information that has been retained and carried over by the skip connections. The skip connections in the U-Bi-LSTM network are structurally akin to those found in U-net, which is known for its U-shaped architecture. This similarity is particularly evident in the way these connections bridge the gap between the encoder and decoder components of the autoencoder. The U-shaped architecture ensures a seamless flow of information, as it provides a pathway for context and details from the input layers to be directly funneled into the deeper layers of the network [38]. In the U-Bi-LSTM network, long skip connections are strategically placed to connect corresponding layers of the encoder and decoder. These connections bypass one or more intermediate layers to directly transmit information across the network. They are essential for preserving fine-grained details that might otherwise be lost in deeper layers. These skip connections are implemented through element-wise addition [39]. This method involves the direct summation of feature maps from an encoder layer to the corresponding feature maps in a decoder layer. The element-wise addition ensures that the essential features are retained and emphasized during the data reconstruction process. The final layer of the network is a fully connected the fully connected layer that integrates all the learned high-level features by performing a weighted sum across all nodes of the previous layer and then subsequently mapping this integration back to the original input dimensionality [37]. This process is essential for reconstructing the missing data by applying the learned transformations to the compressed feature representation from the bottleneck layer. The weights and biases of the fully connected layer are optimized through training to effectively translate the learned temporal patterns into a meaningful reconstruction of the original input sequence.

Adaptive Huber loss. The adaptive Huber loss function is a crucial aspect of the U-Bi-LSTM network due to its robust approach to handling prediction errors, particularly in the presence of outliers. This function adapts the traditional Huber loss [40], which is defined as a piecewise function transitioning from a quadratic to a linear form based on a predefined threshold in order to balance its sensitivity to errors of different magnitudes. For a set of predictions Y and targets T, the adaptive Huber loss L can be mathematically represented as

$$L(Y,\ T) = \frac{1}{N}\sum_{j=1}^{n} L_j\left(Y_j,\ T_j\right) \quad (10)$$

where L_j indicates the individual loss for each prediction, computed by

$$L_j\left(Y_j,\ T_j\right) = \begin{cases} 0.5 \times \left(Y_j - T_j\right)^2, if\ \left|Y_j - T_j\right| \le \delta_j \\ \delta \times \left(\left|Y_j - T_j\right| - 0.5 \times \delta_j^2\right), otherwise \end{cases} \quad (11)$$

where $\left|Y_j - T_j\right|$ is the absolute error for each element, δ_j is the adaptively determined transition point that dictates the shift from quadratic to linear behavior in the loss function, and N represents the count of predictions. Crucially, δ_j, which is the adaptive transition point for each prediction, is dynamically calculated utilizing the median absolute deviation (MAD) from the prediction errors. MAD is a robust statistic that provides an estimate of variability, and it is less influenced by outliers compared to standard deviation [41]. It is defined as the median of the absolute deviations from the data set's median:

$$MAD = median(|X_i - median(X)|) \quad (12)$$

where X_i are individual observations of the dataset X. MAD is particularly useful in datasets that may contain significant outliers, such as those obtained by multi-camera motion tracking systems. Consequently, the adaptive transition point δ_j can be determined as

$$\delta_j = max(\alpha \times MAD(|T - Y|), \epsilon) \tag{13}$$

Here, α is a scaling parameter influencing the loss function's sensitivity to outliers with the aim of ensuring it remains robust against extreme errors, and ϵ is a small constant guaranteeing the transition point does not reach zero, which maintains the stability and responsiveness of the loss function.

This adaptability of the Huber loss is particularly advantageous for datasets with notable outliers, as it offers a measured approach to penalizing errors. It allows the U-Bi-LSTM network to train in a stable manner and not be overly influenced by dataset deviations. This feature is pivotal in complex multi-camera tracking systems that are marked by various levels of noise and discrepancies. The integration of MAD into the adaptive Huber loss calculation ensures that the U-Bi-LSTM network accurately captures data trends and maintains high predictive accuracy, which is critical for achieving robust and generalizable performance in practical multi-camera tracking applications.

Ablation analysis. To investigate the individual and combined effects of various components of the U-Bi-LSTM network on the recovery of missing MoCap data, we conducted an ablation study [42] using wanding activity data. This study focused on comparing the following four network configurations: (1) Bi-LSTM with U-net components using adaptive Huber loss, (2) Bi-LSTM with U-net components using RMSE regression loss, (3) Bi-LSTM alone with adaptive Huber loss, and (4) Bi-LSTM alone with RMSE regression loss. This design allowed us to isolate the impact of each component and loss function on the overall performance of the network. Each variant was subjected to the same multi-camera missing data imputation process and trained under identical conditions to ensure a fair comparison. We then measured the model's ability to reconstruct missing data points in the MoCap sequences. The data used in this study comprised sequences featuring artificially introduced gaps of various lengths and frequencies to simulate real-world data loss scenarios in multi-camera tracking systems. For each configuration, we recorded the missing data reconstruction error using root mean square error (RMSE), which quantitatively measures the average magnitude of the error between the predicted and actual values. A lower RMSE value indicates better performance in reconstructing the original data.

Hyperparameter optimization. In this study, we implemented a grid search methodology to systematically navigate through a predefined hyperparameter space to optimize the U-Bi-LSTM model's performance. Grid search is an exhaustive method of searching through a manually specified subset of the hyperparameter space of a learning algorithm [43]. A grid search algorithm must be guided by some performance metric, such as missing data reconstruction RMSE, which is typically measured by cross-validation on the training set or evaluation on a held-out validation set. The hyperparameters we evaluated include input normalization techniques, the length of input sequences, the adaptive Huber alpha value, the maximum number of training epochs, mini-batch sizes, choice of optimizer, and the learning rate schedule. Mathematically, the grid search can be represented as

$$Optimal\ hyperparameters = argmin_{h \in H}\, CV(f(D_{train}, h)) \tag{14}$$

where H is the hyperparameter space, CV denotes the cross-validation function, f represents the learning algorithm, D_{train} is the training dataset, and h are the hyperparameters. For each hyperparameter set h, the performance metric CV was calculated. This metric is often calculated as the average of the validation scores obtained from the cross-validation process.

2.4.3. Performance Measure

To objectively assess the performance of the proposed data recovery algorithms, i.e., PCS, SLR, PCS U-Bi-LSTM, and SLR U-Bi-LSTM, we implemented a rigorous validation framework. Tracking data were systematically occluded to simulate missing gaps across a variety of tool-based and human body-based MoCap activities. This simulation was applied to the datasets, each of which comprised 5000 frames collected from two volunteers and was intended to reflect a realistic spectrum of motion intensities and spatial trajectories. One of the main goals of this research is to develop a method that can be used to efficiently recover long-term missing data gaps, which typically have a length of more than 0.5 s, and which significantly increase the complexity of data recovery as they grow in length and number [44]. Specifically, missing data gaps were generated at intervals of 1 to 9 s (100 to 900 frames), representing different lengths of data absence. These intervals were introduced in each dataset with a frequency ranging from one to five non-overlapping gaps to evaluate the algorithms' performance against both the length and the frequency of missing data. This strategy ensured that gaps would not be created at the dataset's extremities to avoid the inherent limitations of the PCS method, which struggles with edge-located data loss. This procedure was iteratively conducted five times to calculate the missing data reconstruction error for each method, and an average was obtained from these calculations to minimize any variability introduced by differences in the nature of the tracking data in terms of gap location, outliers, or anomalies. The performance measure using the missing data reconstruction error for each method was determined based on the RMSE, which was calculated solely over the intervals of simulated data loss. This metric served as a standardized method for quantifying the accuracy of the data recovery process, and it can be expressed as follows:

$$RMSE = \sqrt{\frac{1}{N}\sum_{i=1}^{N}(O_i - R_i)^2} \tag{15}$$

where O_i represents the original data points, R_i denotes the data points reconstructed using the evaluated method, and N is the number of data points within the missing data gaps.

For additional validation of the proposed method, wand length error, denoted as $L_{\text{wand error}}$, was calculated to measure the accuracy of the distance between two markers on the calibration wand. Upon reconstructing the 3D positions of the markers, the wand length error was computed as the absolute difference between the calculated Euclidean distance and the original known length, L_{original}, between the markers. The wand length error over all n frames containing the recovered markers' data can be expressed according to the following formula:

$$L_{\text{wand error}} = \sum_{i=1}^{n}\left|\sqrt{(x_{2,i} - x_{1,i})^2 + (y_{2,i} - y_{1,i})^2 + (z_{2,i} - z_{1,i})^2} - L_{\text{original}}\right|_2 \tag{16}$$

Here, $|\cdot|_2$ represents the Euclidean norm, and $(x_{1,i}, y_{1,i}, z_{1,i})$ and $(x_{2,i}, y_{2,i}, z_{2,i})$ denote the 3D coordinates of the first and second markers, respectively, for each i-th data point within the missing data gaps. This metric is particularly relevant because it directly reflects the physical accuracy of the motion capture system's data recovery process, which is an approach that is often utilized to assess performance in related research due to its straightforward representation of spatial recovery accuracy [4]. The bone length between adjacent joints was not used as an additional performance measure due to the well-documented phenomenon of soft tissue artifact (STA), where markers affixed to the skin may not accurately reflect the motion of the underlying bone, thereby potentially introducing errors affecting the interpretation of skeletal movements [12]. This issue is particularly pronounced in high-mobility areas, where the relative movement of the skin to the bone can significantly affect the accuracy of joint angle calculations, and by extension, the inferred bone lengths. Consequently, focusing on wand length error allows for a more direct and unaffected measure of the recovery method's accuracy while sidestepping the complexities introduced by STA.

To further substantiate the efficacy of the methods, we employed a paired *t*-test for comparative analysis. This statistical test was chosen to validate the significance of the performance improvements observed with the U-Bi-LSTM-enhanced methods compared to their traditional counterparts. A *p*-value of less than 0.05 was considered to be indicative of statistically significant differences, with such findings bolstering the assertion that the advanced algorithms provide a notable enhancement in data recovery, particularly in the context of long-term gap restoration. The entire methodology, including augmentation, data loss simulation, and model training and optimization, was executed using MATLAB while IBM SPSS Statistics (SPSS 29.0, IBM corp., USA) was used for performance evaluation and statistical analysis; all calculations were conducted on a computing machine equipped with an AMD Ryzen 7 3700X 8-Core CPU @ 3.60 GHz, an NVIDIA GeForce RTX 2080 Ti GPU 11 GB, and 48 GB RAM, running on the Windows 10 operating system.

3. Results and Discussion

Results of ablation analysis. The ablation analysis, which was meticulously conducted over five iterations, unveiled significant insights into the performance enhancements afforded by each configuration. The detailed results are presented in Table S1 and visualized in Figure 5, which delineates the average results and the standard deviation (reconstruction error ± SD) for the restoration of the lost 3D coordinates of markers on the calibration wand for each of the four architectures evaluated in this study.

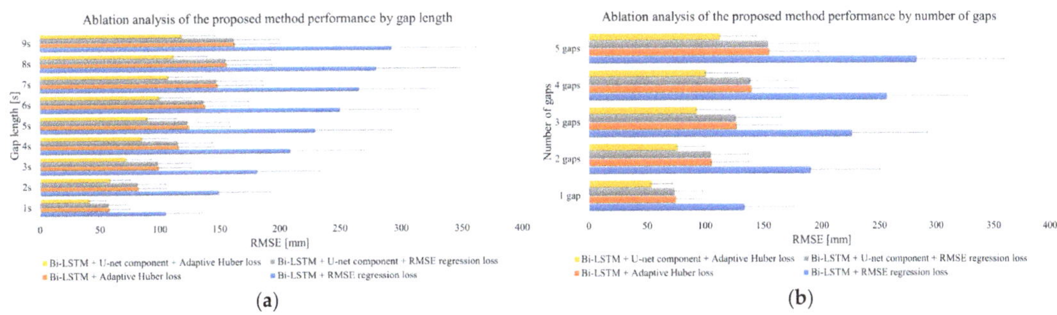

Figure 5. Ablation analysis of proposed method: (**a**) depending on the gap length; (**b**) depending on the number of gaps.

Notably, the results obtained from the ablation study, as extracted from the RMSE values, distinctly show that the architecture integrating Bi-LSTM with both U-net-inspired skip connections and an adaptive Huber loss function significantly outperformed the other examined architectures. It is imperative to mention that, in this rigorous examination, the input data for the proposed architecture did not undergo preliminary recovery with classical methods such as PCS or SLR. This was a deliberate methodological choice to ensure that the proposed model's raw corrective capacity was authentically evaluated. The Bi-LSTM autoencoder was chosen as the foundational model for this investigation based on its adeptness at leveraging both preceding and subsequent data points within a sequence, which is pivotal for accurate prediction in sequential data analysis. Compared to the conventional unidirectional LSTM, the Bi-LSTM's dual-directional learning framework enables the model to encapsulate a comprehensive temporal context, thereby enhancing its predictive accuracy for sequential data recovery tasks. References substantiating this preference include seminal works that highlight the superiority of Bi-LSTMs over single-direction LSTMs in various sequential data processing tasks [45,46]. Upon scrutinizing the outcomes presented in Figure 5, the effective impact of the U-net-inspired skip connections and the adaptive Huber loss function in the proposed Bi-LSTM autoencoder is evident.

The U-net component introduces an innovative mechanism for feature retention across the depth of the network, which is particularly beneficial for complex patterns inherent in MoCap data. The adaptive Huber loss function—with its dynamic error sensitivity adjustment—enhances the robustness of the network, particularly when used with datasets characterized by anomalies or significant outliers. The results obtained herein necessitate a thorough, scientifically sound explanation of the contributions of the adaptive Huber loss and the U-net component to the model's performance. The adaptive Huber loss amalgamates the advantages of L1 and L2 loss functions, thus introducing a conditional approach that is less sensitive to outliers and ultimately improving model reliability when faced with aberrant data. The U-net-inspired skip connections effectively facilitate the flow of gradient and information through the network, countering the vanishing gradient issue and aiding in the accurate reconstruction of the lost data. The deployment of these advanced architectural components results in a substantial increase in the model's efficacy in reconstructing missing data.

Results of hyperparameter optimization. Upon completion of the grid search with fivefold cross-validation, we selected the optimal hyperparameters that minimized the reconstruction error of missing data in the MoCap sequences for the proposed U-Bi-LSTM-enhanced models. Table 1 presents the results of this optimization process while outlining the best-performing hyperparameters for each of the PCS U-Bi-LSTM and SLR U-Bi-LSTM models.

Table 1. Optimized hyperparameters of the PCS U-Bi-LSTM and SLR U-Bi-LSTM.

	Training Option	Range of Parameters	PCS U-Bi-LSTM Selected Parameters	SLR U-Bi-LSTM Selected Parameters
1	Input normalization	[zero-center, zscore, rescale-symmetric, rescale-zero-one]	zscore	rescale-zero-one
2	Input length	[10, 50, 100, 1000]	10	10
3	Adaptive Huber alpha	[0.0001, 0.001, 0.01, 1, 1.345]	0.01	0.01
4	Maximum epoch	[5, 10, 20, 30, 40, 50]	5	5
5	Mini batch size	[8, 16, 32, 64]	32	64
6	Optimizer	[sgdm, rmsprop, adam]	adam	adam
7	Initial learning rate	$[1 \times 10^{-6}, 1 \times 10^{-5}, 1 \times 10^{-4}, 1 \times 10^{-3}, 1 \times 10^{-2}]$	0.001	0.001
8	Learning rate drop period	-	10	10
9	Learning rate drop factor	-	0.2	0.2

The results showed that z-score normalization was the most effective input normalization method for PCS U-Bi-LSTM, which is likely due to its ability to standardize feature scales and thus facilitate more stable and faster convergence during the training process. Similarly, rescale-zero-one normalization was considered to be optimal for SLR U-Bi-LSTM, possibly due to its effect on preserving the proportionate scaling of features. The chosen shorter input length (10) allowed for faster processing times while retaining sufficient temporal dynamics, balancing computational efficiency and model performance. An adaptive Huber alpha value of 0.01 was chosen for both models to maintain error sensitivity while reducing the influence of outliers. The mini-batch size was set to 32 for PCS U-Bi-LSTM and 64 for SLR U Bi LSTM, catering to the models' computational requirements and balancing training speed. The optimization favored a moderate number of epochs (5), which suggests that the model was able to learn the essential patterns within a relatively small number of iterations without overfitting to the training data. The adam optimizer was preferred due to its adaptive learning rate capabilities, which is supported by the results of previous research, indicating its effectiveness in various deep learning scenarios [39]. The learning rate drop period of 10 and drop factor of 0.2 ensured that the learning rate decayed in a controlled manner, fine-tuning the model's weights and biases. Overall, the results of the hyperparameter optimization underscore the importance of careful tuning when developing robust deep learning models, as the chosen parameters significantly impact model performance.

In this study, we empirically evaluated our MoCap data reconstruction methods under rigorous iterative testing. Each of the four methods—PCS, SLR, PCS U-Bi-LSTM, and SLR U-Bi-LSTM—was subjected to five iterations of validation to ensure the reliability and reproducibility of results. The missing data reconstruction RMSE for each method was calculated over each iteration, thus culminating in an aggregate analysis that was used in the plotting of Figures 6 and 7.

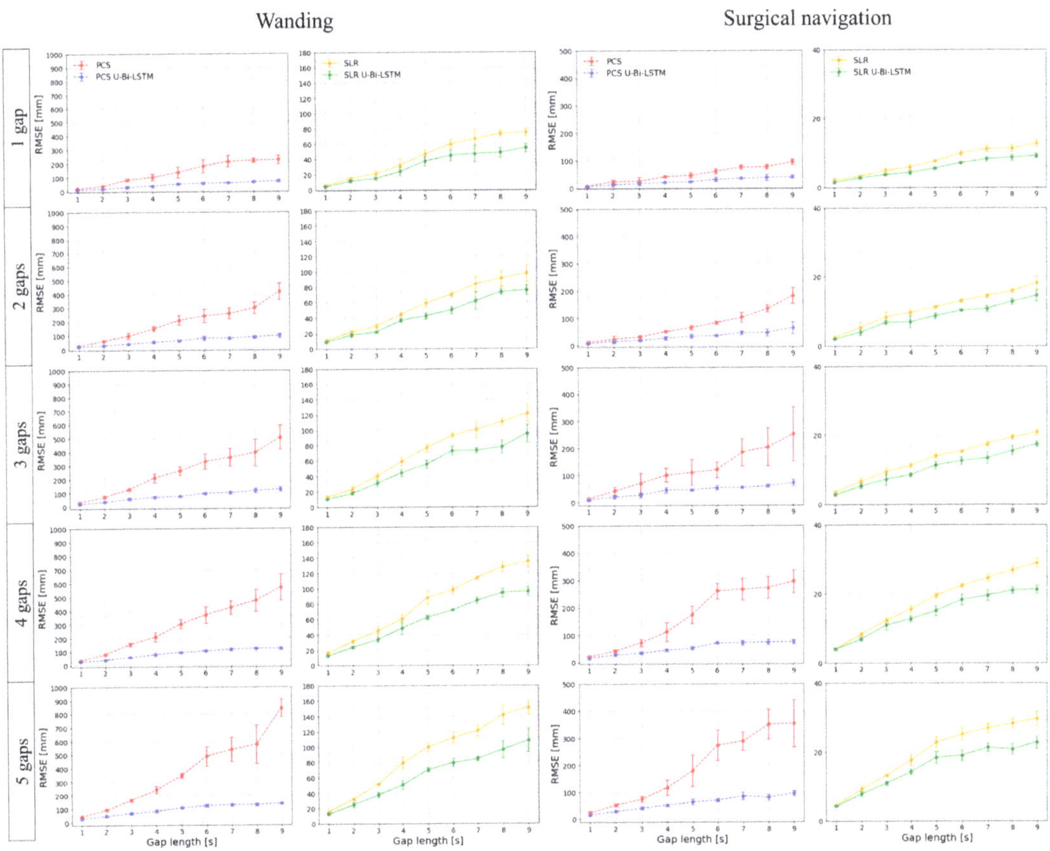

Figure 6. Multi-trial performance assessment of missing data recovery methods by gap length and frequency in tool-based MoCap activities.

For the tool-based MoCap activities (i.e., wanding and surgical navigation), our results—as depicted in Figure 6—demonstrate that both PCS U-Bi-LSTM and SLR U-Bi-LSTM outperformed their counterparts, regardless of the length or number of the missing data gaps. The proposed PCS U-Bi-LSTM showed a consistently lower missing data reconstruction RMSE compared to the conventional PCS, while the proposed SLR U-Bi-LSTM was superior to the state-of-the-art SLR method. Figure 7 extends the analysis described above to human-body-based MoCap activities (arm abduction and adduction, and hip flexion). The advanced U-Bi-LSTM models maintained a consistent trend of reduced RMSE values, thus indicating that our improvements were not confined to tool-based scenarios, as they also extended to complex human movements. The iterative approach and subsequent RMSE calculations provided a comprehensive view of the models' capabilities, ultimately reinforcing the notion that the proposed U-Bi-LSTM-enhanced methods achieved strong performance under varying conditions and movement intensities.

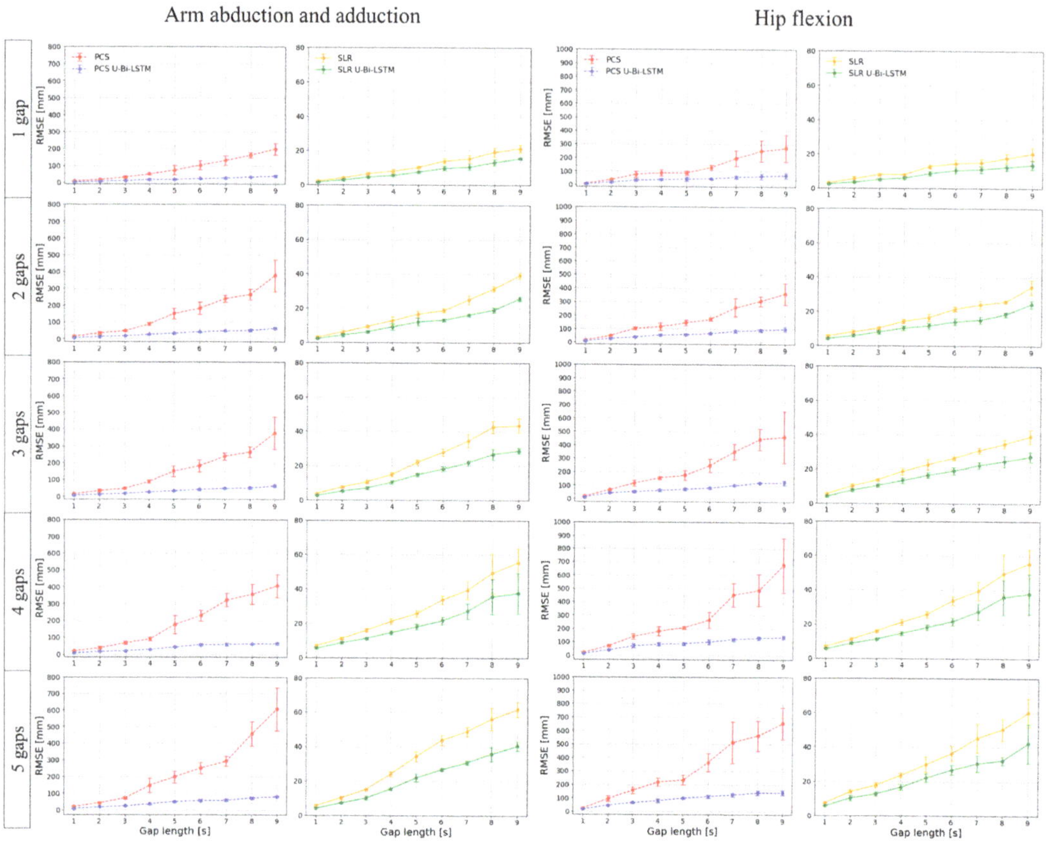

Figure 7. Multi-trial performance assessment of missing data recovery methods by gap length and frequency in human-body-based MoCap activities.

Figures 8 and 9 provide a visual representation of the performance of the different methods across all activities and gap metrics. The RMSE values were meticulously calculated for each gap length and gap number, where the PCS and SLR methods served as benchmarks against their advanced U-Bi-LSTM-enhanced counterparts.

By scrutinizing the results in Figure 8, it can be seen that in tool-based activities such as wanding, the PCS method exhibited a missing data reconstruction RMSE of 30.5584 ± 8.8504 mm for a 1 s gap, and that this was significantly reduced to 19.3654 ± 6.5213 mm with the application of the PCS U-Bi-LSTM method. Meanwhile, the SLR method, which showed an RMSE of 12.1592 ± 4.1677 mm for the same 1 s gap, demonstrated a decrease to 9.4656 ± 3.4081 mm with the application of the SLR U-Bi-LSTM method. As the gap length increased to 9 s, the RMSE for PCS rose sharply to 512.2272 ± 225.5896 mm, while the PCS U-Bi-LSTM method exhibited a more restrained increase, showing an RMSE of 110.6526 ± 26.7792 mm. The SLR method's RMSE at a 9 s gap was 115.7212 ± 30.3819 mm, which was also outperformed by the SLR U-Bi-LSTM method's RMSE of 86.0258 ± 21.1674 mm. Similar improvements were noted in the context of human-body-based activities. For example, during arm abduction and adduction exercises, the PCS method's RMSE for a 1 s gap was 15.602 ± 4.5177 mm, compared to the PCS U-Bi-LSTM's improved RMSE of

7.303 ± 1.9384 mm. Meanwhile, the SLR method's RMSE was 3.9112 ± 1.3355 mm, which was further reduced to 2.848 ± 1.0633 mm with the SLR U-Bi-LSTM method. By similarly scrutinizing the results in Figure 9, it can be seen that with just one gap, in the same tool-based activities such as wanding, the PCS's RMSE was 134.1418 ± 80.3905 mm, which was significantly higher than the PCS U-Bi-LSTM's RMSE of 42.532 ± 21.3899 mm. Meanwhile, the SLR method's RMSE at one gap was 43.6169 ± 26.2159 mm, and this was decreased to 31.6491 ± 18.598 mm with the SLR U-Bi-LSTM. As the number of gaps increased to five, the PCS method's RMSE surged to 369.5683 ± 263.0945 mm, whereas the RMSE of the PCS U-Bi-LSTM method managed to remain at a more reasonable level of 92.8601 ± 40.3424 mm. Similarly, the SLR method's RMSE for five gaps was 89.3563 ± 47.9494 mm, which was reduced in the SLR U-Bi-LSTM method to 62.7153 ± 33.2244 mm. Moreover, the bar graphs in Figures 8 and 9 display the results of the paired *t*-test comparative analyses by gap length and gap number for all MoCap activities, where it can clearly be seen that both the PCS U-Bi-LSTM and SLR U-Bi-LSTM methods achieved significantly reduced RMSEs and standard deviations across all gap lengths and gap numbers. Altogether, the results revealed that PCS U-Bi-LSTM and SLR U-Bi-LSTM achieved statistically significant improvements ($p < 0.05$) over their general counterparts across all activities, gap lengths, and gap numbers.

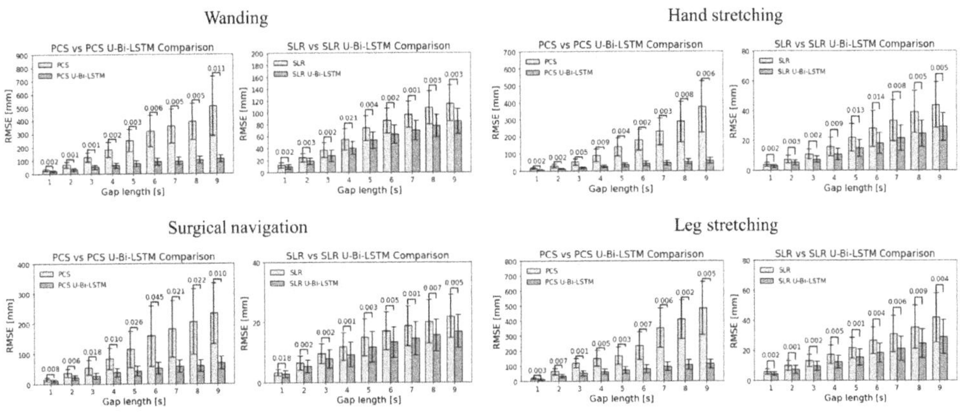

Figure 8. Paired *t*-test comparative analyses of MoCap data recovery methods performance by gap length.

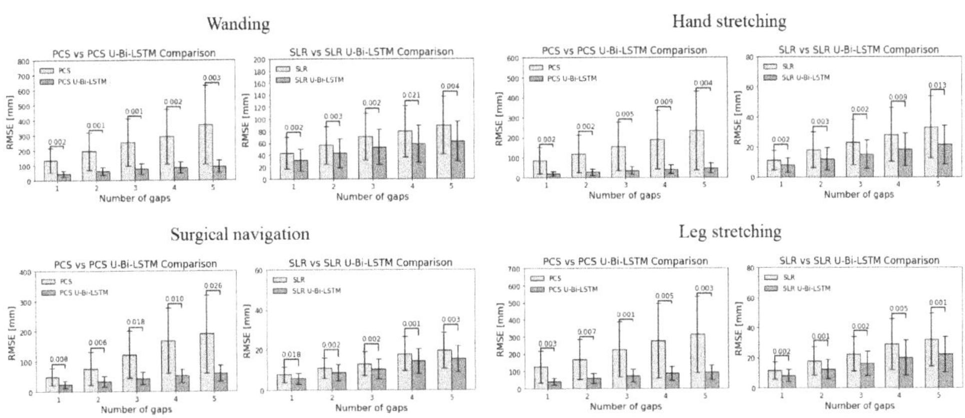

Figure 9. Paired *t*-test comparative analyses of MoCap data recovery methods performance by number of gaps.

An additional performance validation was conducted using the wand length error, and the results of this validation highlighted distinct differences in data recovery capabilities between the conventional and U-Bi-LSTM-enhanced methods, visually represented in Figure 10. In Figure 10, a direct comparison of the four data recovery methods—PCS, PCS U-Bi-LSTM, SLR, and SLR U-Bi-LSTM—is presented for tracking a missing data gap of 100 frames (Figure 10a) and 900 frames (Figure 10b) in wand length tracking.

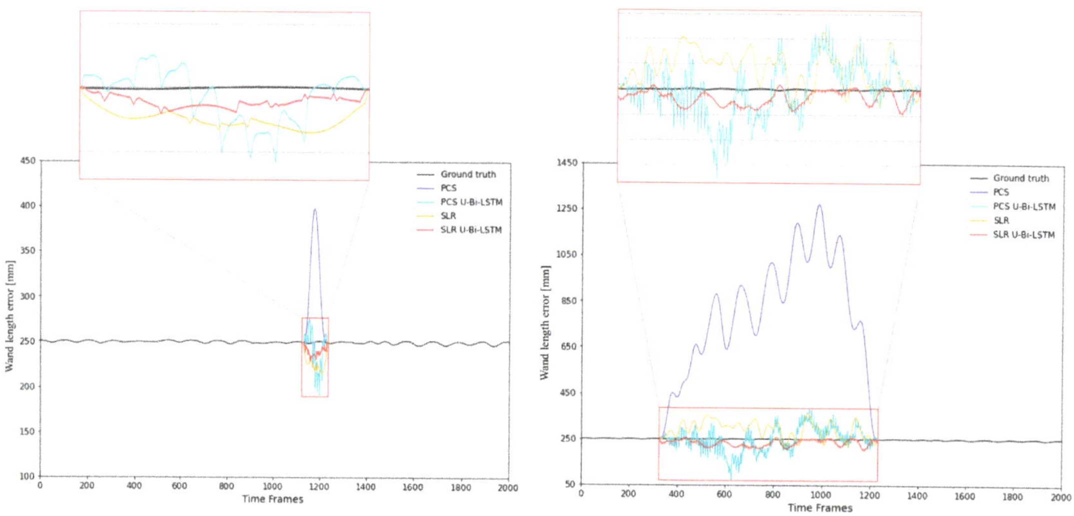

(a) (b)

Figure 10. Comparison of the PCS, PCS U-Bi-LSTM, SLR, and SLR U-Bi-LSTM methods for the recovery of missing motion capture data in wand length tracking: analysis over (**a**) 100 frame and (**b**) 900 frame gaps.

In Figure 10a, which illustrates the recovery performance for a missing data gap of 100 frames, the U-Bi-LSTM-enhanced models (both PCS U-Bi-LSTM and SLR U-Bi-LSTM) delivered superior results compared to their conventional counterparts. While the PCS method showed a prominent spike far from the ground truth baseline and significant noise, PCS U-Bi-LSTM managed to reduce noise and maintains a closer trend. Similarly, SLR U-Bi-LSTM demonstrated a consistent recovery pattern with fewer fluctuations than SLR alone. Notably, the hybrid SLR U-Bi-LSTM model remained closest to the ground truth, indicating its effective management of long-range dependencies. In Figure 10b, the gap extended to 900 frames, which further tests the robustness of these models. PCS continued to struggle, with sustained deviations throughout the interval. PCS U-Bi-LSTM demonstrated a more accurate trend but still showed high noise levels. SLR performed relatively better than PCS, but SLR U-Bi-LSTM offered the most controlled pattern with minimal fluctuations. This demonstrates that the proposed U-Bi-LSTM-enhanced models are significantly more effective for extended gaps, especially in minimizing errors and aligning closely to the original data pattern.

More detailed results of comparative analyses of traditional data recovery methods such as PCS and state-of-the-art SLR, as well as U-Bi-LSTM-enhanced models, are summarized in Table S2. This table illustrates that the U-Bi-LSTM-enhanced methods, PCS U-Bi-LSTM and SLR U-Bi-LSTM, consistently demonstrated significantly lower wand length error values than the basic PCS and SLR methods across various conditions of gap length and number of gaps. To further assess the performance of the proposed enhancement in a comparative framework, the PCS U-Bi-LSTM and SLR U-Bi-LSTM methods were also evaluated against several state-of-the-art deep learning methods, specifically the bidirectional attention network (BAN) [20] and the attention-based LSTM with least squares constraint (A-LSTM+LS) [21].

The wand length error presented in Figure 11 reveals distinct performance differentials between the four methods—BAN, A-LSTM+LS, PCS U-Bi-LSTM, and SLR U-Bi-LSTM—across varying gap lengths and numbers of gaps. The PCS U-Bi-LSTM and SLR U-Bi-LSTM methods consistently demonstrated superior performance in reducing wand length error compared to BAN and A-LSTM+LS. This superiority is quantitatively significant, with RMSE values markedly lower for the U-Bi-LSTM enhanced models across all tested conditions. As the gap length increased from 1 s to 9 s and the number of gaps from 1 to 5, wand length error showed an increasing trend in all methods, but the proposed U-Bi-LSTM methods demonstrated a smaller increase in wand length error as the gap length and number of gaps increased compared to the state-of-the-art deep learning methods (BAN and A-LSTM+LS). Statistical analysis conducted through paired t-tests confirms that the differences in RMSEs between each pair of methods were statistically significant ($p < 0.05$). This not only suggests a genuine performance enhancement by the U-Bi-LSTM architectures but also reinforces the reliability of these findings under the varied experimental conditions. The narrower standard deviation ranges for the PCS U-Bi-LSTM and SLR U-Bi-LSTM methods further underscore their robustness and consistency in performance, a crucial attribute for practical deployment in MoCap applications where variability can greatly affect the fidelity of motion capture reconstructions. The enhanced performance of the U-Bi-LSTM models can be attributed to their architectural features. The integration of Bi-LSTM layers enables effective learning of dependencies in time-series data both forward and backward in time, a feature that is critical in accurately bridging lengthy data gaps. The U-net-inspired skip connections facilitate the preservation and integration of feature information across the network, enhancing the model's ability to reconstruct complex motion patterns from fragmented inputs. The adaptive Huber loss function further refines the model's error sensitivity, balancing the treatment of outliers and reducing the influence of large errors, which is particularly beneficial in scenarios with significant data gaps. In comparison, while A-LSTM+LS and BAN incorporate sophisticated learning mechanisms, their lesser performance relative to the U-Bi-LSTM models might stem from their potential limitations in effectively handling extensive and diverse data gaps. A-LSTM+LS, despite its attention mechanisms and least squares constraint, which typically aid in stabilizing the learning process, still falls short against the proposed U-Bi-LSTM-enhanced methods. This indicates that while attention mechanisms provide a focused learning capability, without the structural and loss function optimizations in the U-Bi-LSTM models, their efficacy is limited in long-term missing MoCap data recovery tasks. BAN's performance lagging behind A-LSTM+LS could be attributed to its reliance on bidirectional attention without the regularization benefits provided by the least squares constraints, making it more susceptible to variations in data with extensive missing segments. The strong dependence of BAN and A-LSTM+LS on inter-marker relations and predefined motion models is possibly one of the main reasons for their relatively large wand length error (where there was only one reference marker) compared to the proposed U-Bi-LSTM-enhanced methods. These state-of-the-art deep learning methods often rely heavily on correlations between markers to predict missing data, which can falter in scenarios where data are available only from a single marker or where marker interactions are complex. In contrast, the PCS U-Bi-LSTM and SLR U-Bi-LSTM methods are specifically designed to effectively and independently recover long-term lost data by utilizing available multi-camera UV data in combination with XYZ marker tracking data. This approach leverages the fundamental motion capture process where UV coordinates from multiple camera views are used to triangulate the XYZ positions in 3D space. Even when complete triangulation is hindered due to missing data, the integration of available UV data from at least one camera can significantly enhance the accuracy of reconstructing lost tracking data. This method capitalizes on any available data to infer missing information more robustly than the methods relying solely on inter-marker relational models or available XYZ data, providing a resilient framework against scenarios with incomplete data. This is particularly advantageous in complex MoCap environments where precise tracking is critical and long-term data loss may frequently occur.

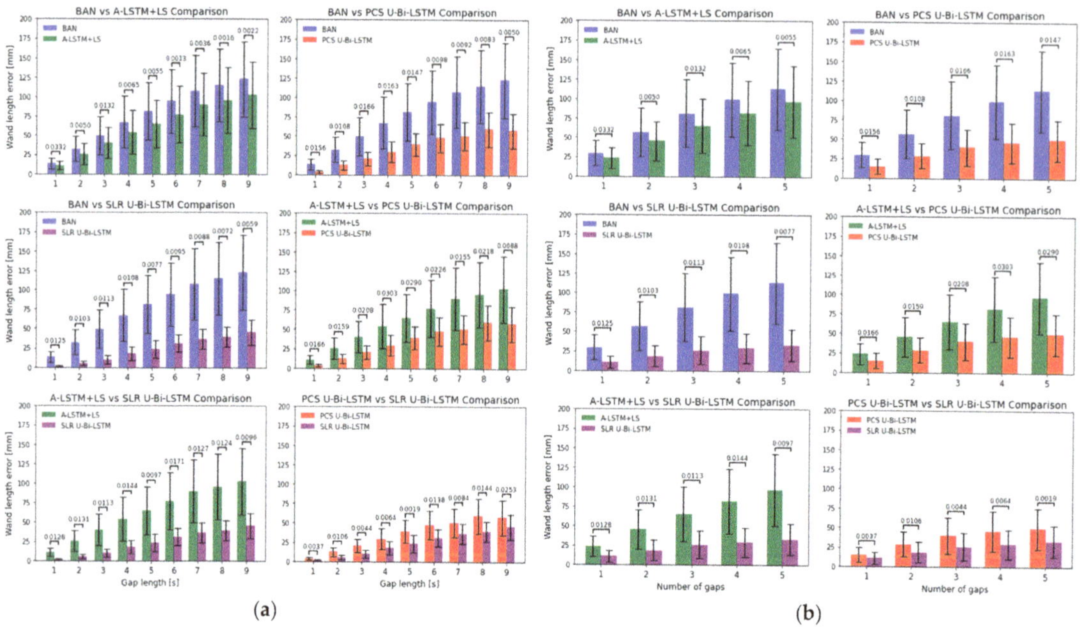

Figure 11. Comparative analyses of wand length error reduction by the U-Bi-LSTM enhanced and state-of-the-art MoCap data recovery deep learning methods across varied missing data gap conditions. (**a**) Wand length error comparison by gap length, and (**b**) by number of gaps.

Therefore, the proposed methods not only show lower mean reconstruction errors but also show reduced variability, as evidenced by the narrower confidence intervals. The results of the statistical analyses reinforce these observations, confirming that the performance enhancement is not sporadic but consistently substantial across all experimental motions and recovery scenarios. In essence, the integration of U-net-inspired skip connections, adaptive Huber loss, and bidirectional learning into the U-Bi-LSTM framework results in a methodologically solid and empirically robust approach. This novel framework has proven its efficacy through rigorous testing, and its effects are validated by substantial reductions in error metrics, thus affirming its capacity for precise and dependable MoCap data recovery across the board.

While the enhanced methods demonstrated remarkable performance, certain limitations were also identified:

- Camera layout and positioning sensitivity. The efficacy of the proposed methods relies heavily on precise multicamera UV data as well as triangulated X, Y, Z data, making it highly sensitive to nuances in camera positioning and layout. The high accuracy in recovering lost tracking data demonstrated by the method proposed in this study presupposes an environment where cameras are correctly positioned, thus enabling rigorous multi-camera calibration and reliable object tracking. Any deviation from the recommended setup [4,5] would necessitate a recalibration of the system and potentially retraining of the algorithm, which may pose challenges when applied in practice in varied environments that differ from the initial configuration. Moreover, real-world applications might encounter physical or logistical constraints that preclude ideal camera placements. Consequently, future research could focus on devising more flexible models that can autonomously adapt to camera layout changes.

This could be achieved by using advanced machine learning techniques that learn to discern and adjust to the most effective configurations based on feedback from the environment [47].

- Impact of environmental changes on model performance. Environmental factors such as lighting variations and obstructions pose significant challenges to the consistency of MoCap data quality. The proposed model was developed in controlled laboratory conditions with carefully curated datasets, enabling us to isolate and focus on recovering lost tracking data. This does not yet account for more nuanced disturbances like noise or marker mismatches. Hence, the model's resilience to environmental perturbations must be comprehensively evaluated before it can be successfully implemented in real-world applications. Future research directions could include the integration of pre-processing layers capable of identifying and compensating for such environmental influences, thus enhancing the model's overall robustness [48,49].
- Dependence on extensive training data. This model's reliance on a large volume of high-quality training data remains a notable limitation. While data augmentation strategies are employed in an attempt to mitigate this issue, the collection of diverse and comprehensive datasets is crucial for the continued success and improvement of these models. In future research, exploring generative models for synthesizing MoCap data under varied conditions [50,51] could significantly alleviate the constraints imposed by the need for large training datasets.

4. Conclusions

In conclusion, the present work has empirically validated that introducing U-Bi-LSTM to traditional PCS and state-of-the-art SLR methods leads to significant advancements for independent long-term missing data recovery in motion capture. Compared to previous approaches, our model tackles inherent challenges by adapting to varying conditions through its bidirectional nature, U-net-inspired skip connections, and adaptive Huber loss. These features, among others, allow the model to handle long-term gaps and maintain data integrity. Quantitative analyses demonstrated marked improvements in missing data recovery error values across various types and intensities of motion, gap lengths, and numbers of gaps, with statistical analyses confirming the statistical significance of these results. These findings not only encourage the use of PCS U-Bi-LSTM and SLR U-Bi-LSTM as robust solutions for motion capture data integrity, but they also pave the way for further research to continue refining and adapting these deep-learning-based techniques for broader applications in motion analysis.

Supplementary Materials: The following supporting information can be downloaded at https://www.mdpi.com/article/10.3390/bioengineering11060560/s1. Table S1: Results of an ablation study of the proposed U-Bi-LSTM architecture on motion capture missing data reconstruction error across various gap lengths and numbers. The results of the architecture with the smallest reconstruction error are highlighted in bold; Table S2: Comparative analysis of wand length error (RMSE+SD) [mm] using the traditional PCS, state-of-the-art SLR, and the proposed PCS U-Bi-LSTM and SLR U-Bi-LSTM with different gaps lengths and numbers. The results of the method with the smallest wand length error are highlighted in bold.

Author Contributions: Conceptualization, O.Y. and A.C.; methodology, O.Y.; validation, O.Y.; formal analysis, O.Y.; resources, Y.C., H.K. and J.H.M.; data curation, O.Y.; writing—original draft preparation, O.Y. and A.C.; writing—review and editing, O.Y., A.C. and J.H.M.; supervision, J.H.M.; project administration, H.K. and J.H.M.; funding acquisition, J.H.M. All authors have read and agreed to the published version of the manuscript.

Funding: This research was funded by the Technology Innovation Program (project no: 20016285) funded by the Ministry of Trade, Industry and Energy (MOTIE, Korea), and this work was in part supported by National Research Foundation of Korea (NRF), Korea Government (MSIT), grant number 2021R1A2C1009951.

Institutional Review Board Statement: The study was approved by the Ethics Committee of Sungkyunkwan University (IRB-2024-05-026).

Informed Consent Statement: Informed consent was obtained from all subjects involved in the study.

Data Availability Statement: The data that support the findings of this study are available on request from the corresponding author. The data are not publicly available due to privacy or ethical restrictions.

Conflicts of Interest: The authors declare no conflicts of interest.

References

1. Nagymáté, G.; Kiss, R.M. Application of OptiTrack motion capture systems in human movement analysis: A systematic literature review. *Recent Innov. Mechatron.* **2018**, *5*, 1–9. [CrossRef] [PubMed]
2. Zubova, S.P.; Svetlana, P.; Raetskiy, K.A. Modeling the trajectory of motion of a linear dynamic system with multi-point conditions. *Math. Biosci. Eng.* **2021**, *29*, 7861–7876. [CrossRef] [PubMed]
3. Yoo, H.; Choi, A.; Mun, J.H. Acquisition of point cloud in CT image space to improve accuracy of surface registration: Application to neurosurgical navigation system. *J. Mech. Sci. Technol.* **2020**, *34*, 2667–2677. [CrossRef]
4. Shin, K.Y.; Mun, J.H. A multi-camera calibration method using a 3-axis frame and wand. *Int. J. Precis. Eng. Manuf.* **2012**, *13*, 283–289. [CrossRef]
5. Chatzitofis, A.; Zarpalas, D.; Daras, P.; Kollias, S. DeMoCap: Low-cost marker-based motion capture. *Int. J. Comput. Vis.* **2021**, *129*, 3338–3366. [CrossRef]
6. Cuadrado, J.; Michaud, F.; Lugrís, U.; Pérez Soto, M. Using accelerometer data to tune the parameters of an extended kalman filter for optical motion capture: Preliminary application to gait analysis. *Sensors* **2021**, *21*, 427. [CrossRef] [PubMed]
7. Onal, S.; Leefers, M.; Smith, B.; Cho, S. Predicting running injury using kinematic and kinetic parameters generated by an optical motion capture system. *SN Appl. Sci.* **2019**, *1*, 675. [CrossRef]
8. Rodríguez, J.; Marín, J.; Royo, A.C.; Padrón, L.; Pérez-Soto, M.; Marín, J.J. KeepRunning: A MoCap-Based Rapid Test to Prevent Musculoskeletal Running Injuries. *Sensors* **2023**, *23*, 9336. [CrossRef] [PubMed]
9. Islam, A.; Asikuzzaman, M.; Khyam, M.O.; Noor-A-Rahim, M.; Pickering, M.R. Stereo vision-based 3D positioning and tracking. *IEEE Access* **2020**, *8*, 138771–138787. [CrossRef]
10. Begon, M.; Wieber, P.-B.; Yeadon, M.R. Kinematics estimation of straddled movements on high bar from a limited number of skin markers using a chain model. *J. Biomech.* **2008**, *41*, 581–586. [CrossRef]
11. Liu, G.; McMillan, L. Estimation of missing markers in human motion capture. *Visual Comput.* **2006**, *22*, 721–728. [CrossRef]
12. Howarth, S.J.; Callaghan, J.P. Quantitative assessment of the accuracy for three interpolation techniques in kinematic analysis of human movement. *Comput. Methods Biomech. Biomed. Eng.* **2010**, *13*, 847–855. [CrossRef] [PubMed]
13. Tan, C.H.; Hou, J.; Chau, L.P. Human motion capture data recovery using trajectory-based matrix completion. *Electron. Lett.* **2013**, *49*, 752–754. [CrossRef]
14. Feng, Y.; Xiao, J.; Zhuang, Y.; Yang, X.; Zhang, J.J.; Song, R. Exploiting temporal stability and low-rank structure for motion capture data refinement. *Inf. Sci.* **2014**, *277*, 777–793. [CrossRef]
15. Gløersen, Ø.; Federolf, P. Predicting missing marker trajectories in human motion data using marker intercorrelations. *PLoS ONE* **2016**, *11*, e0152616. [CrossRef] [PubMed]
16. Wu, Q.; Boulanger, P. Real-time estimation of missing markers for reconstruction of human motion. In Proceedings of the Symposium on Virtual Reality, Uberlandia, Brazil, 23–26 May 2011; pp. 161–168. [CrossRef]
17. Federolf, P.A. A novel approach to solve the "missing marker problem" in marker-based motion analysis that exploits the segment coordination patterns in multi-limb motion data. *PLoS ONE* **2013**, *8*, e78689. [CrossRef] [PubMed]
18. Camargo, J.; Ramanathan, A.; Csomay-Shanklin, N.; Young, A. Automated gap-filling for marker-based biomechanical motion capture data. *Comput. Methods Biomech. Biomed. Eng.* **2020**, *23*, 1180–1189. [CrossRef] [PubMed]
19. Holden, D.; Saito, J.; Komura, T. A deep learning framework for character motion synthesis and editing. *ACM Trans. Graph.* **2016**, *35*, 1–11. [CrossRef]
20. Cui, Q.; Sun, H.; Li, Y.; Kong, Y. A deep bi-directional attention network for human motion recovery. In Proceedings of the International Joint Conference on Artificial Intelligence, Macao, China, 10–16 August 2019; pp. 701–707. [CrossRef]
21. Ji, L.; Liu, R.; Zhou, D.; Zhang, Q.; Wei, X. Missing data recovery for human mocap data based on a-lstm and ls constraint. In Proceedings of the IEEE International Conference on Signal and Image Processing, Nanjing, China, 23–25 October 2020; pp. 729–734. [CrossRef]
22. Zheng, C.; Zhuang, Q.; Peng, S.J. Efficient motion capture data recovery via relationship-aggregated graph network and temporal pattern reasoning. *Math. Biosci. Eng.* **2023**, *20*, 11313–11327. [CrossRef]
23. Li, L.; McCann, J.; Pollard, N.; Faloutsos, C. Bolero: A principled technique for including bone length constraints in motion capture occlusion filling. In Proceedings of the 2010 ACM SIGGRAPH/Eurographics Symposium on Computer Animation, Madrid, Spain, 2–4 July 2010; pp. 179–188. [CrossRef]

24. Aristidou, A.; Lasenby, J. Real-time marker prediction and CoR estimation in optical motion capture. *Vis. Comput.* **2013**, *29*, 7–26. [CrossRef]
25. Burke, M.; Lasenby, J. Estimating missing marker positions using low dimensional Kalman smoothing. *J. Biomech.* **2016**, *49*, 1854–1858. [CrossRef] [PubMed]
26. Tits, M.; Tilmanne, J.; Dutoit, T. Robust and automatic motion-capture data recovery using soft skeleton constraints and model averaging. *PLoS ONE* **2018**, *13*, e0199744. [CrossRef] [PubMed]
27. Yang, J.; Guo, X.; Li, K.; Wang, M.; Lai, Y.K.; Wu, F. Spatio-temporal reconstruction for 3D motion recovery. *IEEE Trans. Circuits Syst. Video Technol.* **2019**, *30*, 1583–1596. [CrossRef]
28. Kamali, K.; Akbari, A.A.; Desrosiers, C.; Akbarzadeh, A.; Otis, M.J.; Ayena, J.C. Low-Rank and sparse recovery of human gait data. *Sensors* **2020**, *20*, 4525. [CrossRef] [PubMed]
29. Coburn, J.; Crisco, J.J. Interpolating three-dimensional kinematic data using quaternion splines and Hermite curves. *J. Biomech. Eng.* **2004**, *127*, 311–317. [CrossRef] [PubMed]
30. Naruse, K.; Sakuma, H.; Hirai, T. Properties of internal speed control and psychophysiological response during continuous forearm rotation movement. *Percept. Mot. Skills* **2001**, *93*, 387–396. [CrossRef] [PubMed]
31. The MathWorks Inc. *MATLAB*, version: 9.13.0 (R2022b); The MathWorks Inc.: Natick, MA, USA, 2022.
32. Mun, F.; Choi, A. Deep learning approach to estimate foot pressure distribution in walking with application for a cost-effective insole system. *J. Neuroeng. Rehabil.* **2022**, *19*, 4. [CrossRef] [PubMed]
33. Ba, J.L.; Kiros, J.R.; Hinton, G.E. Layer normalization. *arXiv* **2016**, arXiv:1607.06450. [CrossRef]
34. Zhang, Y.D.; Pan, C.; Sun, J.; Tang, C. Multiple sclerosis identification by convolutional neural network with dropout and parametric ReLU. *J. Comput. Sci.* **2018**, *28*, 1–10. [CrossRef]
35. Choi, A.; Park, E.; Kim, T.H.; Im, G.J.; Mun, J.H. A novel optimization-based convolution neural network to estimate the contribution of sensory inputs to postural stability during quiet standing. *IEEE J. Biomed. Health Inform.* **2022**, *26*, 4414–4425. [CrossRef]
36. Salehin, I.; Kang, D.K. A review on dropout regularization approaches for deep neural networks within the scholarly domain. *Electronics* **2023**, *12*, 3106. [CrossRef]
37. Hou, B.; Yang, J.; Wang, P.; Yan, R. LSTM-based auto-encoder model for ECG arrhythmias classification. *IEEE Trans. Instrum. Meas.* **2020**, *69*, 1232–1240. [CrossRef]
38. Xiang, T.; Zhang, C.; Wang, X.; Song, Y.; Liu, D.; Huang, H. Towards bidirectional skip connections in encoder-decoder architectures and beyond. *Med. Image Anal.* **2022**, *78*, 102420. [CrossRef]
39. Choi, A.; Kim, T.H.; Yuhai, O.; Jeong, S.; Kim, K.; Kim, H.; Mun, J.H. Deep learning-based near-fall detection algorithm for fall risk monitoring system using a single inertial measurement unit. *IEEE Trans. Neural Syst. Rehabil. Eng.* **2022**, *30*, 2385–2394. [CrossRef]
40. Yang, Y.; Zhou, H.; Wu, J.; Ding, Z.; Wang, Y.G. Robustified extreme learning machine regression with applications in outlier-blended wind-speed forecasting. *Appl. Soft Comput.* **2022**, *122*, 108814. [CrossRef]
41. Leys, C.; Ley, C.; Klein, O.; Bernard, P.; Licata, L. Detecting outliers: Do not use standard deviation around the mean, use absolute deviation around the median. *J. Exp. Social Psychol.* **2013**, *49*, 764–766. [CrossRef]
42. Mustaqeem, S.M.; Kwon, S. CLSTM: Deep feature-based speech emotion recognition using the hierarchical convlstm network. *Mathematics* **2020**, *8*, 2133. [CrossRef]
43. Ali, Y.A.; Awwad, E.M.; Al-Razgan, M.; Maarouf, A. Hyperparameter search for machine learning algorithms for optimizing the computational complexity. *Processes* **2023**, *11*, 349. [CrossRef]
44. Li, Z.; Yu, H.; Kieu, H.D.; Vuong, T.L.; Zhang, J.J. PCA-Based Robust Motion Data Recovery. *IEEE Access* **2020**, *8*, 76980–76990. [CrossRef]
45. Shahid, F.; Zameer, A.; Muneeb, M. Predictions for COVID-19 with deep learning models of LSTM, GRU and Bi-LSTM. *Chaos Solitons Fractals* **2020**, *140*, 110212. [CrossRef]
46. da Silva, D.G.; Meneses, A.A. de Moura. Comparing Long Short-Term Memory (LSTM) and bidirectional LSTM deep neural networks for power consumption prediction. *Energy Rep.* **2023**, *10*, 3315–3334. [CrossRef]
47. Aissaoui, A.; Ouafi, A.; Pudlo, P.; Gillet, C.; Baarir, Z.E.; Taleb-Ahmed, A. Designing a camera placement assistance system for human motion capture based on a guided genetic algorithm. *Virtual Real.* **2018**, *22*, 13–23. [CrossRef]
48. Holden, D. Robust solving of optical motion capture data by denoising. *ACM Trans. Graph.* **2018**, *37*, 1–12. [CrossRef]
49. Sedmidubsky, J.; Zezula, P. Similarity-Based Processing of Motion Capture Data. In Proceedings of the 26th ACM International Conference on Multimedia, Seoul, Republic of Korea, 22–26 October 2018; pp. 2087–2089. [CrossRef]
50. Ma, J.; Bai, S.; Zhou, C. Pretrained diffusion models for unified human motion synthesis. *arXiv* **2022**, arXiv:2212.02837. [CrossRef]
51. Li, W.; Chen, X.; Li, P.; Sorkine-Hornung, O.; Chen, B. Example-based motion synthesis via generative motion matching. *ACM Trans. Graph.* **2023**, *42*, 1–12. [CrossRef]

Disclaimer/Publisher's Note: The statements, opinions and data contained in all publications are solely those of the individual author(s) and contributor(s) and not of MDPI and/or the editor(s). MDPI and/or the editor(s) disclaim responsibility for any injury to people or property resulting from any ideas, methods, instructions or products referred to in the content.

bioengineering

MDPI

Review

Could Novel Spinal Braces with Flexibility, Robotic Components, and Individualized Design Generate Sufficient Biomechanical Treatment Efficacy in Patients with Scoliosis?

Chen He [1], Jinkun Xie [1], Rong Pang [1], Bingshan Hu [1] and Christina Zong-Hao Ma [2,3,*]

1 School of Health Science and Engineering, University of Shanghai for Science and Technology, Shanghai 200093, China; hechen@usst.edu.cn (C.H.); 18567285086@163.com (J.X.); pangrong23@163.com (R.P.); hbs922@163.com (B.H.)

2 Department of Biomedical Engineering, The Hong Kong Polytechnic University, Hong Kong SAR 999077, China

3 Research Institute for Smart Ageing, The Hong Kong Polytechnic University, Hong Kong SAR 999077, China

* Correspondence: czh.ma@polyu.edu.hk; Tel.: +852-2766-7671; Fax: +852-2334-2429

Abstract: Background: Patients with adolescent idiopathic scoliosis (AIS) require effective bracing to control curve progression. However, most traditional spinal braces commonly pose challenges in terms of undesired bulkiness and restricted mobility. Recent advancements have focused on innovative brace designs, utilizing novel materials and structural configurations to improve wearability and functionality. However, it remains unclear how effective these next-generation braces are biomechanically compared to traditional braces. Objectives: This review aimed to analyze the design features of next-generation AIS braces and assess their biomechanical effectiveness via reviewing contemporary studies. Methods: Studies on newly designed scoliosis braces over the past decade were searched in databases, including Web of Science, PubMed, ScienceDirect, Wiley, EBCOHost and SpringerLink. The Joanna Briggs Institute Critical Appraisal Checklist for Cohort Studies was adopted to evaluate the quality of the included studies. The data extracted for biomechanical effect analysis included brace components/materials, design principle, interfacial pressure, morphological changes, and intercomparison parameters. Results: A total of 19 studies encompassing 12 different kinds of braces met the inclusion/exclusion criteria. Clinical effectiveness was reported in 14 studies, with an average short-term Cobb angle correction of 25.4% (range: 12.41–34.3%) and long-term correction of 18.22% (range: 15.79–19.3%). This result aligned broadly with the previously reported efficacy of the traditional braces in short-term cases (range: 12.36–31.33%), but was lower than the long-term ones (range: 23.02–33.6%). Two included studies reported an interface pressure range between 6.0 kPa and 24.4 kPa for novel braces, which was comparable to that of the traditional braces (4.8–30.0 kPa). Additionally, five of six studies reported the trunk asymmetric parameters and demonstrated improvement in trunk alignment. Conclusions: This study demonstrates that most newly designed scoliosis braces could achieve comparable biomechanical efficacy to the conventional designs, particularly in interface pressure management and Cobb angle correction. However, future clinical adoption of these novel braces requires further improvements of ergonomic design and three-dimensional correction, as well as more investigation and rigorous evidence on the long-term treatment outcomes and cost-effectiveness.

Keywords: scoliosis; spinal brace; smart brace; spinal orthosis; biomechanical effect; treatment efficacy

1. Introduction

Scoliosis is a three-dimensional (3D) spinal deformity that primarily occurred in adolescents who are in the process of rapid growth [1,2]. Severe scoliosis may lead to some musculoskeletal, respiratory, and neurological problems [3,4]. Among all the treatment options, the spinal brace (or orthosis) intervention has been regarded as an effective conservative treatment for scoliosis, especially for the moderate curvatures [5,6].

Scoliosis braces, such as Milwaukee brace [7], Boston brace [8], Cheneau brace [9], Lyon brace [10], and Wilmington brace [11], have been used clinically for decades. These braces applied the three-point pressure principle: a correction force at the level of apical vertebrae and the counterforce at the upper end and lower end level of the scoliotic curve, via some correction pads and the shell of spinal braces [12]. These spinal braces have been proven effective in treating scoliosis, with over 18 h of wearing time every day [13]. The night-time braces, such as Charleston brace [14] and Providence brace [15], were developed for patients with mild scoliosis to wear only at night. However, these rigid spinal braces have the limitations of restraining trunk motion and producing discomfort during wearing, leading to poor compliance rate in patients with scoliosis [16].

To improve the compliance rate, some flexible braces, such as SpineCor brace [17] and TriaC brace [18], were developed in the 2000s to facilitate trunk movement and improve patients' wearing comfort. Some previous studies have also reported higher compliance of the flexible braces than that of the rigid ones [19,20]. Nevertheless, a critical trade-off has emerged, as the corrective efficacy of these flexible braces has remained controversial and often less predictable [17].

In recent years, some novel scoliosis braces with new materials, structures, or functionality have been developed. These braces combined the elastic and rigid materials and were reported to be capable of correcting spinal deformity while allowing body movement [21]. Some more complexed electronic scoliosis robots, which were composed of three corrective platforms aligned with three-point pressure planes, were also developed to correct spinal curvature in three levels independently [22,23]. Proponents suggested that this design allowed the trunk to be maintained in a corrected position, potentially achieving the necessary correction while addressing the mobility limitations [24].

The developments of novel scoliosis brace imply potential effects in key biomechanical parameters—interface pressure distribution and morphological correction—compared to traditional braces. These parameters are critical, as interface pressure directly influences brace effectiveness and comfort, while morphological correction, as measured by Cobb angle reduction and body symmetry, reflects clinical success. Regarding interface pressure, previous studies reported that the overall interface pressure of the traditional braces ranged from 4.80 to 30.00 kPa, including the Boston brace (4.80–30.00 kPa) [25,26], Chêneau brace (7.34–9.45 kPa) [27], Milwaukee brace (7.53–9.31 kPa) [28,29], TLSO brace (7.09 kPa) [30], and Charleston brace (8.93–18.53 kPa) [31]. For morphological outcomes, evidence demonstrated that traditional braces achieved short-term (<6 months) Cobb angle reductions of 12.36% to 31.33%, across the SpineCor brace (17.36–21.35%) [32,33], Cheneau brace (15.50–31.33%) [34,35], Boston brace (19.4%) [34], and TLSO brace (12.36–15.90%) [32,33]. Meanwhile, the long-term (>6 months) treatment outcomes showed a further enhanced efficacy of 23.02–33.6%, based on the results of the SpineCor brace (31.34%) [36], Cheneau brace (25.6–30.89%) [34,35,37], and Boston brace (23.02–33.6%) [34,36,37]. Beyond the curvature correction, the patient's body symmetry [38] would also be crucial, as it reflects trunk balance and alignment, which are vital for achieving effective scoliosis correction [39,40]. Although the interface pressure ranges and the short/long-term morphological outcomes were documented for traditional braces, there is an absence of evidence evaluating whether the novel brace designs could also achieve comparable biomechanical effectiveness or not, in terms of the pressure distribution, Cobb correction, and body symmetry parameters.

Most published review papers and meta-analysis studies have predominantly focused on synthesizing the Cobb angle progression prevention/correction of traditional brace [41–43], or comparing different traditional braces [44]. Some reviews have summarized the general ranges of the measured interface pressure across various traditional braces [45,46]. Some other reviews have focused on the impact of patient compliance or quality of life on the brace treatment efficacy [47,48]. However, there is a notable lack of reviews analyzing the innovative design features of more novel braces and critically evaluating the emerging evidence regarding their biomechanical performance and underlying treatment mechanisms. With the potential application of novel and smart scoliosis braces, it is necessary to systematically conduct a review and synthesis of the latest evidence on the biomechanical effect and clinical efficacy of the novel scoliosis braces, to guide future clinical practice and research directions.

To address the above-mentioned issues, the objectives of this review are (1) to identify the novel design features and trends of the reported novel scoliosis braces; and (2) to evaluate the evidence concerning the novel scoliosis braces' biomechanical effects on interface pressure and morphological changes. It is expected that the findings of this study can offer synthesized evidence regarding the implementation of the newly developed scoliosis braces in clinical practice and inspire future brace designs for patients with scoliosis.

2. Materials and Methods

2.1. Search Strategy

Published studies were searched using a three-step search strategy. An initial search at MeSH browser was first undertaken to analyze the keywords contained in the titles and abstracts, and the index terms used to describe the article. The keywords that were identified for literature search were "AIS", "scoliosis", "spine deformity", "brace/braces", "orthotic device", "orthosis/orthoses", "biomechanical effect", and "biomechanics". A second search across databases of Web of Science, PubMed, ScienceDirect, Wiley, EBCOHost and SpringerLink was undertaken using all identified keywords and index terms. An example of the literature search results from Web of Science is provided in Table 1. Thirdly, the reference lists of the identified reports and studies were searched for additional studies.

Table 1. Literature search from Web of Science.

Search	Query	Results
Web of science	Search:(((TS = (scoliosis)) OR TS = (Spine deformity)) OR TS = (AIS)) AND (((((((TS = (orthosis*)) OR TS = (Orthotic Devices)) OR TS = (Orthosis)) OR TS = (Orthose*)) OR TS = (Parapodium*)) OR TS = (Conservative Treatment)) OR TS = (Conservative Management)) OR TS = (Conservative Therapy)) AND (((((((((((((TS = (Biomechanical Phenomena)) OR TS = (Biomechanics)) OR TS = (Biomechanic*)) OR TS = (Biomechanic Phenomena)) OR TS = (Kinematics)) OR TS = (Invention*)) OR TS = (Technological Innovations)) OR TS = (design)) OR TS = (new)) OR TS = (devise*)) OR TS = (exploitation)) OR TS = (develop)) OR TS = (development)) OR TS = (exploiting))	668

Note: This search strategy employed the asterisk (*) as a truncation wildcard to retrieve plurals forms and variant endings (e.g., Orthosis* to capture Orthosis, Orthoses, Orthotic), thereby enhancing search sensitivity.

The inclusion criteria were studies that (1) focused on a novel scoliosis brace; (2) provided a clear description of the brace's design and components; (3) reported quantitative biomechanical outcomes; and (4) were published in English between 2014 and 2024. The exclusion criteria were studies that (1) focused on traditional scoliosis brace or minor modifications of traditional designs; (2) focused on spinal brace for non-scoliotic conditions; and (3) lacked essential design details or biomechanical data. Scoliosis braces were identified as traditional or novel based on their fundamental design philosophy and date of conception. Traditional braces were defined as clinically established, widely adopted designs validated through decades of use—including but not limited to the Milwaukee, Boston, Chêneau, Lyon, and SpineCor braces. Novel braces, by contrast, were developed and documented within the past decade (2014–2024) and incorporated substantial innovations in one or more domains: materials (use of non-traditional materials beyond conventional polyethylene plastics or elastic straps), structure (introduction of new structural concepts), or functionality (integration of novel capabilities). It is important to note that minor iterative adjustments or customizations of conventional braces did not qualify as a novel brace.

All identified studies were collated and uploaded into EndNote for removal of duplicate articles. Titles and abstracts were screened by two independent reviewers (J.X. and R.P.). The full text of the screened studies was assessed in detail to determine the compliance with the inclusion criteria by two independent reviewers (J.X. and R.P.). Exclusion of full-text sources that did not meet the inclusion criteria was documented along with the specific reasons. Any disagreements that arose between the two reviewers at each stage of the screening process were resolved through discussion, or with an additional reviewer (C.H.). This literature review was conducted and reported in accordance with the Preferred Reporting Items for Systematic Reviews and Meta-Analyses (PRISMA) guidelines and was registered with PROSPERO (Registration ID: CRD420251130681).

2.2. Assessment of Methodological Quality

Studies selected for retrieval were assessed by two independent reviewers for quality evaluation (J.X. and R.P.). The Joanna Briggs Institute (JBI) Critical Appraisal Checklist for Cohort Studies was adopted to assess the quality of the included studies. Any disagreements that arose between reviewers were resolved through discussion, or with a third reviewer (C.H.).

2.3. Extraction and Analysis

Data were extracted using a self-developed data extraction tool. The extracted data included brace components/materials, interface pressure, design principle, morphological changes, and intercomparison parameters. The draft data extraction tool was modified and revised as necessary during the process of extracting data from each included study.

3. Results

3.1. Search Results

Full details of the search results are illustrated in a PRISMA flow diagram (Figure 1). A systematic search across the above-reported databases yielded 2503 records initially. After removing 1484 duplicates, 1019 records were further screened for title/abstract, with 992 additional studies excluded. Full-text retrieval was then sought for the remaining 27 articles, with 3 articles inaccessible. The remaining 24 articles were assessed in full text, resulting in 5 exclusions. Finally, a total of 19 studies were included in this literature review.

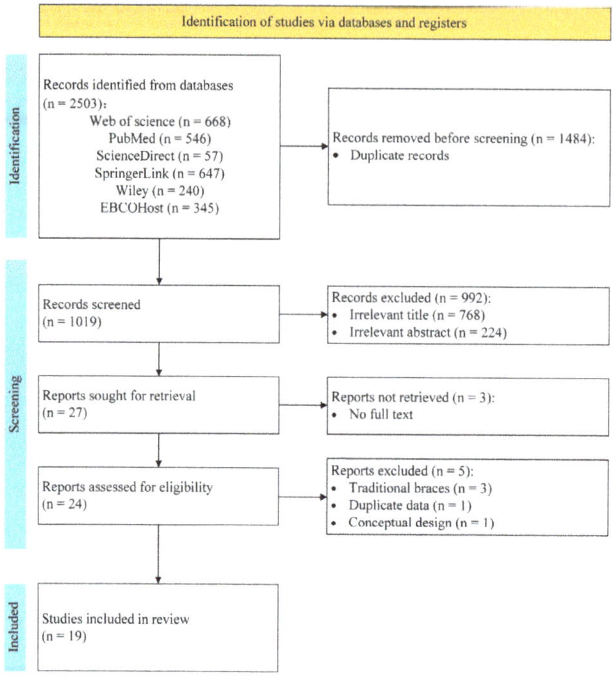

Figure 1. Prisma flow diagram.

3.2. Methodological Quality

The methodological quality of the included studies is presented in Table 2. Twelve articles were scored 5 points or above. Two articles were scored below 5 points, primarily attributed to the lack of control group, absence of follow-up or insufficient follow-up duration. Five articles were scored 0 points, because they were not clinical trials and thus did not meet the checklist criteria.

Table 2. Methodological quality of the included studies (n = 19).

No.	Author	1	2	3	4	5	6	7	8	9	10	11	Total
1	Liu et al. (2014) [49]	N	Y	Y	N	N	Y	Y	N	N	N	N	4/11
2	Liu et al. (2015) [50]	N	Y	Y	N	N	Y	Y	N	N	N	Y	5/11
3	Yip et al. (2016) [51]	N	Y	Y	N	N	Y	Y	Y	N	N	Y	6/11
4	Fok et al. (2018) [52]	N	N	Y	N	N	Y	Y	Y	N	N	Y	5/11
5	Liu et al. (2022) [53]	N	Y	Y	N	N	Y	Y	N	N	N	Y	5/11
6	Chan et al. (2018) [54]	Y	Y	Y	Y	Y	Y	Y	N	N	N	N	7/11
7	Ye et al. (2023) [55]	N	Y	Y	N	N	Y	Y	N	N	N	Y	5/11
8	Wang and Zing. (2017) [21]	N	Y	Y	Y	Y	Y	Y	Y	Y	Y	Y	10/11
9	Wong et al. (2020) [56]	N	Y	Y	N	N	Y	Y	N	N	N	Y	5/11
10	Wong et al. (2021) [57]	N	Y	Y	N	N	Y	Y	N	N	N	Y	5/11
11	Fok et al. (2022) [58]	N	N	Y	N	N	N	Y	N	N	N	Y	3/11
12	Fung et al. (2020) [5]	N	Y	Y	N	N	Y	Y	N	N	N	Y	5/11
13	Ali et al. (2021) [3]	N	N	N	N	N	N	N	N	N	N	N	0/11
14	Nakamura et al. (2014) [59]	N	Y	Y	N	N	Y	Y	Y	Y	Y	Y	8/11

Table 2. *Cont.*

No.	Author	1	2	3	4	5	6	7	8	9	10	11	Total
15	Kajiura et al. (2019) [60]	N	Y	Y	N	N	Y	Y	Y	Y	N	Y	7/11
16	Ring and Kim. (2016) [61]	N	N	N	N	N	N	N	N	N	N	N	0/11
17	Nijssen et al. (2017) [62]	N	N	N	N	N	N	N	N	N	N	N	0/11
18	Park et al. (2015) [63]	N	N	N	N	N	N	N	N	N	N	N	0/11
19	Park et al. (2018) [23]	N	N	N	N	N	N	N	N	N	N	N	0/11

Y: Yes; N: No.

While the five articles that were scored 0 points were excluded from the subsequent biomechanical analysis due to the lack of clinical data/outcomes, these five articles were retained for inclusion in the novel design analysis section, as these studies provided essential, detailed descriptions of the novel features and concepts under investigation. Such information offered insights into the engineering rationale and technical specifications that cannot be derived solely from most clinical cohort studies. Furthermore, these conceptual and design-focused studies contributed to the understanding of the developmental history/trajectory of these novel technologies, facilitating a comprehensive review and synthesis of the brace design innovations.

3.3. Characteristics of the Included Studies

The brace components, correction principles, and experimental data extracted in each article are tabulated (Table 3), in which data from different articles of the same brace were merged together. Two studies [61,62] did not specify the names of their newly developed braces, which was designated as a Soft Brace (1st/2nd edition) in this review.

Table 3. Characteristics of the included studies.

NO.	Authors	Brace Design			Clinical Outcomes		
		Brace Name/Type	Brace Components	Correction Principle	Subjects	Study Duration	Results
1.	Liu et al. (2014) [49]				N = 7; 11.43 ± 0.98 ys; Cobb = 10–20°	3 h	• Shoulder height difference: 1.27 to 0.16 cm; • Front bending: 30 to 15 cm; • Lateral bending: 45 to 42.5 cm (Left), 45.5 to 39.5 cm (Right)
2.	Liu et al. (2015) [50]				N = 9; 11.33 ± 1.00 ys; Cobb = 12.33° ± 4.99°	8 h/d for 3 m	• Cobb increases: 18.29° ± 3.82°; • Shoulder tilt decrease: 2.91° ± 1.30° to 2.15° ± 0.91°
3.	Yip et al. (2016) [51]	Posture correction girdle (1st edition)	Resin bones; Elastic straps; Pads.	Elastic stretch; Corrective point pressure force	N = 7; 11.14 ± 0.90 ys; Cobb = 9.43° ± 6.11° (T); 10.57° ± 4.79° (L)	8 h/d for 6 m	Rotation angle decrease: 2.78° to 1.16°
4.	Fok et al. (2018) [52]				N = 10; 13.5 ± 1.4 ys; Cobb = 19.0° ± 6.4°	8 h/d for 6 m	• Cobb decrease: 16.0° ± 7.7° • Less cobb correction than that of SpineCor brace [33]
5.	Liu et al. (2022) [53]				N = 4; 12.25 ± 0.50 ys; Cobb = 15.78° ± 2.63°	2 h	Cobb decrease: 11° ± 4.55°
6.	Chan et al. (2018) [54]	Posture correction girdle (2nd edition)	Shape Memory Alloy (SMA); Elastic straps; Semi-rigid Pads.	Elastic stretch; Corrective point pressure	Study Group (2nd edition): N = 1; 14 ys; Cobb = 34° (T)/24° (L); Control Group (1nd edition): N = 1; 14 ys; Cobb = 28.9°	2 h	• Cobb angle decrease: Study Group: 22.7° (T)/23.8° (L); Control Group: 21.4°
7.	Ye et al. (2023) [55]	Posture correction girdle (3rd edition)	Resin bones; Elastic straps; Smart air cushion system	Dynamic pressure control via airbag; Three-point pressure	N = 3; 12.33 ± 0.47 ys; Cobb = 13.60° ± 3.45°	2 h	• Shoulder tilt decreases 53.8% (average 0.89° to 0.17°); • pelvic tilt decreases 36.8% (average 1.14° to 0.72°); • shoulder–pelvic rotation decreases 56.6% (average 1.22° to 0.53°)

Table 3. *Cont.*

NO.	Authors	Brace Design			Clinical Outcomes		
		Brace Name/Type	Brace Components	Correction Principle	Subjects	Study Duration	Results
8.	Wang and Zing. (2017) [21]	FLEXpine	Soft frame; Elastic bands.	Three-point pressure;	Study Group: N = 10; wear FLEXpine or traditional brace; Cobb: 16.45° ± 0.98° Control Group: N = 8; wear FLEXpine brace With FLEXpine Exercise program; Cobb: 7.65° ± 2.5°	3 m	• Cobb angle decrease: Study Group: 13.23° ± 3.24°; Control Group: 4.55° ± 2.32°
9.	Wong et al. (2020) [56]	Anisotropic textile brace	Elastic textile material; Hinged artificial backbone; Pads.	Three-point pressure	N = 1; 12 ys; Cobb = 21°	2 h	Cobb angle decrease: 15.4°
10.	Wong et al. (2021) [57]				N = 1; 11 ys; Cobb: 23.1° (T)/27.8° (L); Study Group (Boston); Control Group (Anisotropic textile brace)	2 h	• Cobb angle decrease: Study Group: 14.6° (T)/25.2° (L); SVA (−21.2 to −8.2) Control Group: 14.8° (T)/22.6° (L) SVA (−21.2° to −26°)
11.	Fok et al. (2022) [58]				N = 5; 12.2 ± 0.45 ys; Cobb: 20.7° ± 4.13° (T) 20.2° ± 2.13° (L)	2 h	• POTSI decrease: 22.1–38.6% to 14.1–43.2%; • Cobb angle decrease: 11.9° ± 9.22° (T); 20.1° ± 5.39° (L) • Interfacial pressure: 6.0–24.4 kPa(T)/6.1–9.7 kPa (L) (Comparable to rigid brace [26,30])
12.	Fung et al. (2020) [5]	Textile-based scoliosis brace	Pads; Rigid straps; BOA lancing system; Resin Bones.	Three-point pressure	N = 1; 21 ys; Cobb: 11.1° (T)/24.8° (L)	2 h	• Interface pressure: 17.62–20.98 kPa (comparable to rigid brace [27,31,64])

Table 3. *Cont.*

NO.	Authors	Brace Design			Clinical Outcomes		
		Brace Name/Type	Brace Components	Correction Principle	Subjects	Study Duration	Results
13.	Ali et al. (2021) [3]	Soft Active Dynamic Brace	Twisted String Actuation (TSA); Corrective band.	Three-point pressure correction; Trunk rotation with lateral flexion	No subject	Not applicable	Not Applicable
14.	Nakamura et al. (2014) [59]	Dynamic Spinal Brace (DSB) (1st edition)	Rigid shell; Polycarbonate strut; Corrective band.	Posture control Three-point pressure	N = 52; 10 ys; Cobb: 41.9° ± 16.91° SPO: 9.4° ± 7.01°	20.8 m (6.8–35.7 m)	• Cobb angle decrease: 36.7° ± 16.21° (1 h); 49.4° ± 25.4° (long term) • SPO decrease: 7.4° ± 5.71° (1 h); 10.6° ± 9.01° (long term)
15.	Kajiura et al. (2019) [60]	Dynamic Spinal Brace (DSB) (2nd edition)	Elastic ring-shaped support	Posture control Three-point pressure	N = 219; 13.4 ys; Cobb ≥ 20°	6 y (3–9 y)	• Cobb angle decrease: 34.3% (1 h); 19.3% (long term) • Comparable cobb correction to TLSO [65]
16.	Ring and kim (2016) [61]	Soft brace (1st edition)	Corrective rings	Spine displacement control	No subject	Not applicable	Not applicable
17.	Nijssen et al. (2017) [62]	Soft brace (2nd edition)	Shell mechanisms; Force generators.	Two-fold force-controlled correction method	No subject	Not applicable	Not applicable
18.	Park et al. (2015) [63]	Robotic Spine Exoskeleton (RoSE)	Corrective rings; Stewart platforms; UPS configuration; Force and position sensor.	Displacement control; 3D dynamic adjustable correction	No subject	Not applicable	Not applicable
19.	Park et al. (2018) [23]	Robotic Spine Exoskeleton (RoSE)	Corrective rings; Stewart platforms; UPS configuration; Force and position sensor.	Displacement control; 3D dynamic adjustable correction	No subject	Not applicable	Not applicable

T—thoracic curve, L—lumbar curve, POTSI—posterior trunk asymmetry index, m—month, N—number, ys—years, SVA—sagittal vertical axis, SPO—spinal pelvic obliquity, UPS—universal prismatic and spherical joint. Notes: In this table, different colors represent distinct brace designs. Variations in shade within a single color represent different clinical evaluations or design stages of the same brace design.

3.4. Novel Designs Features

The novel braces identified from 19 included studies could be categorized as flexible garment-style braces [5,49–58], angular braces [23,61–63], and modular braces [3,21,59,60] according to the structural design. The innovative features of novel braces are presented in Figure 2

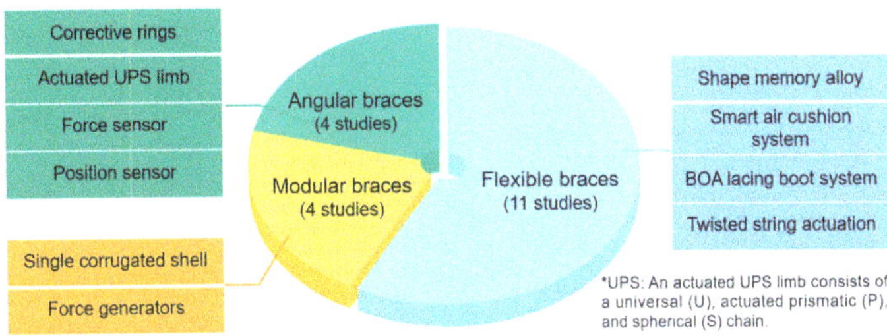

Figure 2. Novel design features of scoliosis braces.

Flexible garment-style braces included six braces named Posture Correction Girdle (1st–3rd editions), Anisotropic Textile Brace, Textile-based Scoliosis Brace, and Soft Active Dynamic Brace. Braces with flexibility emphasized flexible characteristics in materials or structures, aiming to reduce movement restrictions and improve comfort. These designs featured full-coverage vests enveloping patients' shoulders, torso, and hips with flexible components. Angular braces included three braces named Soft Brace (1st–2nd edition) and RoSE Brace. These devices shared a common structure—three parallel rings positioned at the thoracic, lumbar, and pelvic regions, respectively—to provide spinal support and correction forces. Some angular braces incorporated robotic components of perceivable or controllable functional units, including but not limited to active or semi-active mechanical adjustment, sensing, monitoring, or automatic regulation devices, in the brace design.

Modular braces included two braces named FLEXpine and DSB (2nd edition). These braces covered the specific trunk segments with adjustable components to apply force. Such individualized designs can adapt according to changes in the body shape, curvature, or growth dynamics through modular, segment-replaceable, or adjustable elements.

For brace components, paddings were applied in four braces (i.e., Posture Correction Girdle [1st–2nd editions], Anisotropic Textile Brace, and Textile-based Scoliosis Brace) [5,49–54,56–58]. Some smart control systems, such as the smart airbag system, twisted string actuation (TSA), and actuated UPS (Universal joint, actuated Prismatic chain, Spherical joint) limb and sensor, were implemented in three braces (i.e., Posture Correction Girdle [3rd edition], Soft Active Dynamic Brace, and RoSE) [3,23,55,63]. Novel materials of shape memory alloy and SMA were applied in the Posture Correction Girdle (2nd edition) [50].

3.5. Analysis of Correction Principles

Nine studies mentioned the three-point pressure principle in their brace designs [3,5,21,55–60], whereas four studies introduced the displacement control as a methodological approach for achieving the three-dimensional spinal correction [23,61–63]. In addition to coronal correction, the Soft Active Dynamic Brace claimed an anti-rotational mechanism in the brace design [3], and the Posture Correction Girdle (3rd edition) reported an anti-rotational efficacy (shoulder–pelvic rotation decreased 56.6%) in their study [55].

3.6. Interface Pressure Measurement

Two studies quantified the interface pressure for novel braces [5,58]. Anisotropic Textile Brace demonstrated higher pressure range in thoracic region (6.0–24.4 kPa) than that of the lumbar region (6.1–9.7 kPa) [58]. Textile-based Scoliosis Brace exhibited a narrower pressure range of 17.62–20.98 kPa [5] in comparison with that of Charleston night-time braces (8.93–18.53 kPa) [31]. The overall pressure range of both thoracic and lumbar region reached 6.0–24.4 kPa.

3.7. Outcomes of Morphological Evaluation

Fourteen studies reported morphological changes of the spine and trunk upon or after wearing the brace, among which ten studies [21,50,52–54,56–60] reported the Cobb angle change, with a short-term correction averaging 25.4% (12.41–34.3%) in six studies and a long-term correction averaging 18.22% (15.79–19.3%) in three studies. Data from Liu et al. [50] (reporting an increase in Cobb angle after wearing brace) was excluded from the pooled analysis, due to the inconsistent tools adopted for curvature assessment before and after using the brace (radiograph versus motion capture assessment) in the study. The intercomparison among different braces showed that the Posture Correction Girdle (1st edition) demonstrated marginally inferior Cobb angle correction as compared to the SpineCor brace (16% vs. 21.3%) [33,52], and the Dynamic Spinal Brace (2nd edition) exhibited a comparable efficacy to TLSO in Cobb angle improvement (immediate: 34.3% vs. 38.1%; final: 19.3% vs. 22.65%) [60,65].

Beyond Cobb angle correction, the trunk asymmetry parameters were reported in six studies, including the reduced shoulder height difference from 1.27 to 0.16 cm [49], reduced shoulder tilt from 2.91° to 2.15° [50] and from 0.89° to 0.17° [55] in two sides, reduced pelvic tilt angle from 1.14° to 0.72° [55], changed sagittal vertical axis (SVA) angle from −21.2° to −26° [57], changed posterior trunk asymmetry index (POTSI) from 22.1 to 38.6% to 14.1–43.2% [58], and increased spinal pelvic obliquity (SPO) from 9.4° to 10.6° [51,55,59]. Additionally, the rotation correction was reported in two studies, including reduced shoulder–pelvic rotation from 1.22° to 0.53° [55] and reduced rotation angle in horizontal plane from 2.78° to 1.16° [51].

The duration of brace intervention varied considerably across different studies, ranging from 2 h [5,53–58] and 3 h [49] to 3 months [21,50] and 6 months [51,52,59,60]. The relevant assessments were primarily short-term, with eight studies evaluating the effects within 24 h and two studies conducting evaluations exceeding 1 year.

The participant recruitment also differed: three studies enrolled larger cohorts (with 18 [21], 52 [59], and 219 [60] participants), while the remaining twelve studies included smaller groups (5 ± 3 participants). Control groups were recruited in three studies [21,54,57].

4. Discussion

The potential application of novel scoliosis braces requires a systematic synthesis of current evidence concerning their biomechanical performance and therapeutic efficacy. This review aims to characterize emerging design innovations and evaluate the biomechanical evidence base. The synthesized findings demonstrates that the majority of recently developed brace designs achieve biomechanical performance comparable to conventional braces, particularly in managing interface pressure distributions and reducing Cobb angle magnitude.

4.1. Novel Designs

There are generally three different novel brace designs, including the flexible garment-based braces, angular braces, and modular braces. Each design has its pros and conc that need to be considered when selecting the appropriate prescription for patients with scoliosis. Further optimization is also needed for each of these novel brace designs. More details can be found below.

By integrating the elastic correction components within the fabric structure to deliver corrective forces, the flexible garment-based braces offered advantages in improving comfort, esthetics, and concealability [66]. This led to improved patient compliance, which was a critical factor in achieving sustained biomechanical efficacy [67,68]. Some flexible braces incorporated specialized material compositions and functional elements, to ensure consistent correction. For instance, the use of SMA has replaced the conventional resin-based support structures, to enhance durability and elasticity. Some more advanced functional modules, such as the Smart Air Cushion System, BOA Lacing Boot System and TSA, were employed to improve the adjustability and enable intelligent control of correction. However, the inherent flexibility of these braces may provide less restriction as compared to rigid braces [5,49–58]. Consequently, the successful correction relied partly on the patient's active participation and conscious effort towards maintaining a proper posture [32].

Angular braces adopted an innovative design paradigm by utilizing three parallel rings (thoracic, lumbar, pelvic) to deliver targeted, adjustable three-dimensional forces [69]. The robotic Spine Exoskeleton (RoSE) integrated an actuated UPS limb as a programmable force generator, complemented by force and position sensors. The sensor array enabled real-time closed-loop monitoring and adjustment of both correction force vectors and patient trunk displacement within the brace. The independent control of each correction ring demonstrated enhanced capacity to address complex three-dimensional spinal deformities. However, the substantial weight and bulk might compromise patient compliance as compared to the conventional braces [70]. This dichotomy underscored the need for continued innovation to balance precise biomechanical control with the acceptable ergonomic practicality in spinal correction technologies. In contrast, the Soft Brace (2nd edition) utilized a corrugated geometric configuration to achieve multi-directional compliance. Concurrently, its force generators maintained a constant correction force (40–77.5 N) within a predefined displacement range based on the zero-stiffness principle [62]. This design optimized correction efficiency through force–displacement coupling.

Modular braces usually combined individual segments with elastic materials in the brace structure, ensuring effective correction of spinal deformities while minimizing the coverage of patient's torso. The Soft Active Dynamic Brace exemplified this principle through four adjustable elastic bands controlled by lightweight twisted string actuators (TSAs), allowing for precise force modulation [3]. The DSB (2nd edition) adopted segmented architecture to accommodate diverse body shapes and discrete contact points. While this design exhibited insufficient pelvic support compared to the rigid brace incorporating rigid pelvic bases, further improvement was required on reinforcing the pelvic structure to enhance stability. The FLEXpine brace utilized a modular structure comprising curved, interlocking segments contoured to the torso. This configuration allowed localized adjustments and adaptation to spinal curvature changes over time. Nevertheless, its reliance on elastic components probably compromised the sustained pressure delivery. Integration of more rigid elements could be prioritized to improve pressure maintenance without sacrificing adaptability in future developments [21].

To sum up, the flexible brace systems prioritized comfort and compliance, angular designs maximized correction precision, and modular architectures leveraged the manufacturing advancements to balance adaptability and longevity. Future work could explore synergies between these different approaches, such as integrating sensor-driven feedback into modular frameworks or enhancing angular systems with flexible interfaces, to optimize the treatment outcomes in patients with scoliosis.

4.2. Correction Principles

Two fundamental correction mechanisms, including the force-controlled approach and displacement-controlled approach, were mentioned in the novel scoliosis braces. The force-controlled approach extended the traditional three-point force system (i.e., a primary convex force with two counterforces) in the coronal plane, by incorporating multi-planar force vectors, as seen in the Soft Active Dynamic Brace and the Posture Correction Girdle [3,49]. In contrast, the ring-shaped braces employed a displacement-controlled correction approach, where three corrective rings were positioned at different anatomical levels (corresponding to the three force application points in traditional three-point systems) to deliver correction force through electrodynamic actuators [63]. While optimal three-dimensional biomechanical correction was achievable from a mechanical perspective, the more complex interactions with the human torso's musculoskeletal system rendered its practical application significantly [71]. Further efforts shall be made to improve the appearance, ergonomics, and application potential of such robotic designs, as well as the patient's compliance while maintaining the biomechanical correction.

4.3. Interface Pressure

The interface pressure between the brace and the trunk served as a critical parameter for evaluating the biomechanical effects of spinal braces. The overall interface pressure range of novel braces (6.0–24.4 kPa) has been on par with that of traditional rigid braces (4.80–30.00 kPa) [25–31]. Specifically, the Anisotropic Textile Brace demonstrated a pressure range that closely aligned with traditional rigid braces [26,30], supporting the textile-based flexible designs as viable alternatives in interface pressure management in the future. Lower interface pressure was observed in the lumbar region than that of thoracic region, which likely stemmed from the anatomical and material factors. This is because the pliable soft tissues of the lumbar region, combined with the reduced correction capacity of flexible brace components in this area, may limit the force transmission efficiency [50,55,66]. Similarly, a Textile-based Scoliosis Brace demonstrated a narrower and higher range of interface pressure as compared to that of the Charleston night-time braces [27,31,64], indicating improved interface pressure consistency. This may have resulted from the replacement of elastic textile materials or the design of resin bones/hinged backbone, enabling targeted force application while reducing variability.

Notably, higher interface pressure did not necessarily translate to better correction outcomes. The correlation between interface pressure and Cobb angle reduction becomes non-linear beyond some specific force thresholds, suggesting diminished returns on spinal correction with uncontrolled pressure escalation [55,68]. Therefore, the focus in future clinical practice should be on achieving the optimal curve correction while maximizing the interface pressure within an appropriate range.

4.4. Morphological Evaluation

This review demonstrated that novel spinal braces achieved overall comparable Cobb angle correction to the traditional braces. The pooled short-term correction of 25.4% and long-term correction of 18.22% aligned with the expected range of brace management and broadly matched the reported traditional brace efficacy in short-term treatments (12.36% to 31.33%) [32–35]. However, the long-term correction efficacy is lower than in the traditional braces (23.02–33.6%) [34–37]. The inter-study comparisons also supported this finding. Specifically, two included studies reported that the Posture Correction Girdle was slightly less effective than SpineCor, and the DSB (2nd edition) performed equivalently to TLSO in both immediate and final correction [60,65]. The observed decrease in correction magnitude from short-term to long-term, alongside the reports of diminishing garment-style brace efficacy over time [5,60], suggests a potential challenge for achieving sustained effectiveness. This attenuation might be attributable to the fabric degradation in Soft Braces, compromising the elasticity, structural support, and correction forces that are necessary for long-term maintenance of correction. Meanwhile, the effectiveness of angular braces in correcting Cobb angles lacked clinical evidence, primarily due to the fabrication complexities and the relatively new emergence, making the long-term assessment challenging. Establishing these braces' value required further study of underlying mechanisms, conducting iterative clinical trials, and tracking the Cobb angle changes to assess the short-term and long-term effectiveness.

The three-dimensional trunk asymmetric parameters showed a generally positive trend in improving the appearance of patients with scoliosis upon wearing the developed braces with novel designs. The reductions that occurred in shoulder height and tilt and pelvic tilt indicated improved coronal trunk alignment and symmetry [49,55]. The rotational deformities, including shoulder–pelvic rotation [55] and horizontal plane rotation [51], also showed substantial correction upon wearing the brace. The changes in SVA suggested a beneficial shift in sagittal alignment [57], though the response in POTSI varied across different individuals [58]. Overall, these results indicated the brace's efficacy in reducing the shoulder imbalance, pelvic tilt, and rotational deformities of patients with scoliosis.

Although the reviewed braces with novel designs generally demonstrated biomechanical efficacy comparable to traditional braces, it shall be noted that limited previous studies have evaluated the cost-effectiveness of these novel braces. The braces incorporating advanced components (e.g., sensors, actuators) tended to have higher costs, which may not be an affordable option and may lead to limited access for patients, especially in resource-constrained settings. Future research should extend beyond the existing biomechanical validation to evaluate the cost-effectiveness of novel scoliosis braces, generating evidence for future clinical decision-making. For clinicians, this underscores the necessity of balancing treatment efficacy with affordability when making a clinical prescription, particularly in low- and middle-income countries. It shall be noted that when the treatment outcomes are similar, cost-efficient options should be prioritized over more expensive ones.

4.5. Limitations

This literature review has some limitations. Firstly, some included studies focused more on the design concept with less quantitative biomechanical evaluation of the scoliosis braces, making the synthesis of relevant clinical evidence unavailable in this review. Future studies need to move beyond the conceptual brace descriptions to conducting instrumented evaluations on patients, such as the radiographic analysis, pressure mapping, and 3D motion capture, to quantify the biomechanical effects. Secondly, the inhomogeneous data for evaluating the biomechanical effects of scoliosis brace in the included studies rendered it challenging to conduct a systematic comparison. It is critical to adopt standardized biomechanical parameters in future studies, to enable cross-study comparisons in future literature reviews/meta-analyses. Thirdly, while this review has adopted a systematic searching strategy to identify the qualified studies, papers not published in English were not included in this review. This may exclude some studies with the same focus.

5. Conclusions

This study demonstrates that most newly designed scoliosis braces could achieve comparable biomechanical efficacy to the conventional designs, particularly in interface pressure management and Cobb angle correction. However, future clinical adoption of these novel braces requires further improvements of ergonomic design and three-dimensional correction, as well as more investigation and rigorous evidence on the long-term treatment outcomes and cost-effectiveness.

Author Contributions: Conceptualization, C.H., J.X., R.P., B.H. and C.Z.-H.M.; methodology, C.H., J.X., R.P., B.H. and C.Z.-H.M.; Software, C.H., J.X., R.P. and B.H.; data curation, C.H., J.X., R.P., B.H. and C.Z.-H.M.; writing—original draft preparation, C.H. and J.X.; writing—review and editing, R.P., B.H. and C.Z.-H.M.; funding acquisition, C.H. and B.H. All authors have read and agreed to the published version of the manuscript.

Funding: This research was funded by the Research and Innovation Team Project from Shidong hospital, grant number 2024KYCX2403; National Key Research and Development Program of China, grant number 2022YFC3601400.

Institutional Review Board Statement: Not applicable.

Informed Consent Statement: Not applicable.

Data Availability Statement: All data generated or analyzed in this study are included in this published article.

Conflicts of Interest: The authors declare no conflicts of interest.

Abbreviations

The following abbreviations are used in this manuscript:

AIS	Adolescent Idiopathic Scoliosis
ATSI	Anterior Trunk Symmetry Index
DSB	Dynamic Spinal Brace
L/T curve	Lumbar curve/Thoracic curve
m	month
No.	Number
POTSI	Posterior Trunk Asymmetry Index
PRISMA	The Preferred Reporting Items for Systematic Reviews and Meta-Analyses
SMA	Shape Memory Alloy
SPO	Spinal Pelvic Obliquity
SVA	Sagittal Vertical Axis
TLSO	Thoracic Lumbosacral Orthosis
TSA	Twisted String Actuation
UPS	The Universal Prismatic and Spherical joint
ys	years

References

1. Niu, X.; Yang, C.; Tian, B.; Li, X.; Zheng, S.; Cong, D.; Han, J.; Agrawal, S.K. Investigation of robotic braces for patients with idiopathic scoliosis (IS)—Review of the literature and description of a novel brace. *J. Mech. Med. Biol.* **2018**, *18*, 180038. [CrossRef]
2. Stokes, I.A.; Bigalow, L.C.; Moreland, M.S. Three-dimensional spinal curvature in idiopathic scoliosis. *J. Orthop. Res.* **1987**, *5*, 102–113. [CrossRef]
3. Ali, A.; Fontanari, V.; Fontana, M.; Schmoelz, W. Soft Active Dynamic Brace for Spinal Deformities. In Proceedings of the 14th International Joint Conference on Biomedical Engineering Systems and Technologies, Vienna, Austria, 11–13 February 2021; Volume 1, pp. 169–174.

4. Weinstein, S.L.; Dolan, L.A.; Cheng, J.C.Y.; Danielsson, A.; Morcuende, J.A. Adolescent idiopathic scoliosis. *Lancet* **2008**, *371*, 1527–1537. [CrossRef]
5. Fung, O.H.-Y.; Yip, J.; Cheung, M.-C.; Yick, K.-L.; Kwan, K.Y.-H.; Cheung, K.M.-C.; Cheung, J.P.-Y.; Tse, C.-Y. Exploring mass customization and textile application in medical products: Re-designing scoliosis brace for shorter production lead time and better quality of life. *Text. Res. J.* **2020**, *90*, 2304–2321. [CrossRef]
6. Negrini, S.; Aulisa, A.G.; Aulisa, L.; Circo, A.B.; de Mauroy, J.C.; Durmala, J.; Grivas, T.B.; Knott, P.; Kotwicki, T.; Maruyama, T.; et al. 2011 SOSORT guidelines: Orthopaedic and Rehabilitation treatment of idiopathic scoliosis during growth. *Scoliosis* **2012**, *7*, 3. [CrossRef]
7. Keim, H.A. The Milwaukee brace for treatment of scoliosis. *J. Pediatr.* **1971**, *78*, 864–866. [CrossRef] [PubMed]
8. Watts, H.G.; Hall, J.E.; Stanish, W. The Boston brace system for the treatment of low thoracic and lumbar scoliosis by the use of a girdle without superstructure. *Clin. Orthop. Relat. Res.* **1977**, *126*, 87–92. [CrossRef]
9. De Giorgi, S.; Piazzolla, A.; Tafuri, S.; Borracci, C.; Martucci, A.; De Giorgi, G. Chneau brace for adolescent idiopathic scoliosis: Long-term results. Can it prevent surgery? *Eur. Spine J.* **2013**, *22*, S815–S822. [CrossRef]
10. de Mauroy, J.C.; Lecante, C.; Barral, F.; Daureu, D.; Gualerzi, S.; Gagliano, R. The Lyon brace. *Disabil. Rehabil. Assist. Technol.* **2008**, *3*, 139–145. [CrossRef]
11. Bassett, G.S.; Bunnell, W.P.; MacEwen, G.D. Treatment of idiopathic scoliosis with the Wilmington brace. Results in patients with a twenty to thirty-nine-degree curve. *J. Bone Joint Surg. Am.* **1986**, *68*, 602–605. [CrossRef]
12. Grivas, T.B.; Kaspiris, A. *European Braces Widely Used for Conservative Scoliosis Treatment*; Studies in Health Technology and Informatics; IOS Press: Amsterdam, The Netherlands, 2010; Volume 158, pp. 157–166. [CrossRef]
13. Weinstein, S.L.; Dolan, L.A.; Wright, J.G.; Dobbs, M.B. Effects of bracing in adolescents with idiopathic scoliosis. *N. Engl. J. Med.* **2013**, *369*, 1512–1521. [CrossRef]
14. Lee, C.S.; Hwang, C.J.; Kim, D.J.; Kim, J.H.; Kim, Y.T.; Lee, M.Y.; Yoon, S.J.; Lee, D.H. Effectiveness of the Charleston Night-time Bending Brace in the Treatment of Adolescent Idiopathic Scoliosis. *J. Pediatr. Orthoped.* **2012**, *32*, 368–372. [CrossRef]
15. Wiemann, J.M.; Shah, S.A.; Price, C.T. Nighttime Bracing Versus Observation for Early Adolescent Idiopathic Scoliosis. *J. Pediatr. Orthoped.* **2014**, *34*, 603–606. [CrossRef]
16. Karol, L.A.; Virostek, D.; Felton, K.; Wheeler, L. Effect of Compliance Counseling on Brace Use and Success in Patients with Adolescent Idiopathic Scoliosis. *J. Bone Joint Surg. Am.* **2016**, *98*, 9–14. [CrossRef]
17. Coillard, C.; Leroux, M.A.; Zabjek, K.F.; Rivard, C.H. SpineCor--a non-rigid brace for the treatment of idiopathic scoliosis: Post-treatment results. *Eur. Spine J.* **2003**, *12*, 141–148. [CrossRef]
18. Veldhuizen, A.G.; Cheung, J.; Bulthuis, G.J.; Nijenbanning, G. A new orthotic device in the non-operative treatment of idiopathic scoliosis. *Med. Eng. Phys.* **2002**, *24*, 209–218. [CrossRef]
19. Gonzalez Vicente, L.; Jimenez Barrios, M.; Gonzalez-Santos, J.; Santamaria-Pelaez, M.; Soto-Camara, R.; Mielgo-Ayuso, J.; Fernandez-Lazaro, D.; Gonzalez-Bernal, J.J. The ISJ 3D Brace, a Providence Brace Evolution, as a Surgery Prevention Method in Idiopathic Scoliosis. *J. Clin. Med.* **2021**, *10*, 3915. [CrossRef]
20. Capek, V.; Baranto, A.; Brisby, H.; Westin, O. Nighttime versus Fulltime Brace Treatment for Adolescent Idiopathic Scoliosis: Which Brace to Choose? A Retrospective Study on 358 Patients. *J. Clin. Med.* **2023**, *12*, 7684. [CrossRef] [PubMed]
21. Wang, S.V.; Zing, S. Bracing Effects of the Flexpine in Scoliosis Patients. *Am. Sci. Res. J. Eng. Technol. Sci.* **2017**, *34*, 261–268.
22. Niu, X.; Yang, C.; Han, J.; Agrawal, S.K. Concept design of a novel robotic spinal brace for the treatment of scoliosis. *Proc. Inst. Mech. Eng. Part H-J. Eng. Med.* **2018**, *232*, 1230–1244. [CrossRef]
23. Park, J.H.; Stegall, P.R.; Roye, D.P.; Agrawal, S.K. Robotic Spine Exoskeleton (RoSE): Characterizing the 3-D Stiffness of the Human Torso in the Treatment of Spine Deformity. *IEEE Trans. Neural Syst. Rehabil. Eng.* **2018**, *26*, 1026–1035. [CrossRef] [PubMed]
24. Ray, R.; Nouaille, L.; Colobert, B.; Calistri, L.; Poisson, G. Design and position control of a robotic brace dedicated to the treatment of scoliosis. *Robotica* **2023**, *41*, 1466–1482. [CrossRef]
25. Mac-Thiong, J.M.; Petit, Y.; Aubin, C.E.; Delorme, S.; Dansereau, J.; Labelle, H. Biomechanical evaluation of the Boston brace system for the treatment of adolescent idiopathic scoliosis: Relationship between strap tension and brace interface forces. *Spine* **2004**, *29*, 26–32. [CrossRef]
26. van den Hout, J.A.; van Rhijn, L.W.; van den Munckhof, R.J.; van Ooy, A. Interface corrective force measurements in Boston brace treatment. *Eur. Spine J.* **2002**, *11*, 332–335. [CrossRef]
27. Pham, V.M.; Houilliez, A.; Schill, A.; Carpentier, A.; Herbaux, B.; Thevenon, A. Study of the pressures applied by a Cheneau brace for correction of adolescent idiopathic scoliosis. *Prosthet. Orthot. Int.* **2008**, *32*, 345–355. [CrossRef]
28. Babaee, T.; Kamyab, M.; Ahmadi, A.; Sanjari, M.A.; Ganjavian, M.S. Measurement of Milwaukee Brace Pad Pressure in Adolescent Round Back Deformity Treatment. *Asian Spine J.* **2017**, *11*, 627–633. [CrossRef] [PubMed]
29. Wong, M.S.; Evans, J.H. Biomechanical evaluation of the Milwaukee brace. *Prosthet. Orthot. Int.* **1998**, *22*, 54–67. [CrossRef]

30. Wong, M.S.; Mak, A.F.; Luk, K.D.; Evans, J.H.; Brown, B. Effectiveness and biomechanics of spinal orthoses in the treatment of adolescent idiopathic scoliosis (AIS). *Prosthet. Orthot. Int.* **2000**, *24*, 148–162. [CrossRef]
31. Lou, E.; Durdle, N.G.; Raso, V.J.; Hill, D.L. A system for measuring pressures exerted by braces in the treatment of scoliosis. *IEEE Trans. Instrum. Meas.* **1994**, *43*, 661–664. [CrossRef]
32. Wong, M.S.; Cheng, J.C.Y.; Lam, T.P.; Ng, B.K.W.; Sin, S.W.; Lee-Shum, S.L.F.; Chow, D.H.K.; Tam, S.Y.P. The effect of rigid versus flexible spinal orthosis on the clinical efficacy and acceptance of the patients with adolescent idiopathic scoliosis. *Spine* **2008**, *33*, 1360–1365. [CrossRef]
33. Guo, J.; Lam, T.P.; Wong, M.S.; Ng, B.K.W.; Lee, K.M.; Liu, K.L.; Hung, L.H.; Lau, A.H.Y.; Sin, S.W.; Kwok, W.K.; et al. A prospective randomized controlled study on the treatment outcome of SpineCor brace versus rigid brace for adolescent idiopathic scoliosis with follow-up according to the SRS standardized criteria. *Eur. Spine J.* **2014**, *23*, 2650–2657. [CrossRef] [PubMed]
34. Karimi, M.; Nadi, A. Comparative analysis of Boston and Cheneau braces in treating scoliosis: A 2-year follow-up study on curve reduction. *N. Am. Spine Soc. J.* **2024**, *19*, 100337. [CrossRef]
35. Korovessis, P.; Syrimpeis, V.; Tsekouras, V.; Vardakastanis, K.; Fennema, P. Effect of the Cheneau Brace in the Natural History of Moderate Adolescent Idiopathic Scoliosis in Girls: Cohort Analysis of a Selected Homogenous Population of 100 Consecutive Skeletally Immature Patients. *Spine Deform.* **2018**, *6*, 514–522. [CrossRef]
36. Gutman, G.; Benoit, M.; Joncas, J.; Beauséjour, M.; Barchi, S.; Labelle, H.; Parent, S.; Mac-Thiong, J.M. The effectiveness of the SpineCor brace for the conservative treatment of adolescent idiopathic scoliosis. Comparison with the Boston brace. *Spine J.* **2016**, *16*, 626–631. [CrossRef] [PubMed]
37. Minsk, M.K.; Venuti, K.D.; Daumit, G.L.; Sponseller, P.D. Effectiveness of the Rigo Cheneau versus Boston-style orthoses for adolescent idiopathic scoliosis: A retrospective study. *Scoliosis Spinal Disord.* **2017**, *12*, 7. [CrossRef]
38. Zaina, F.; Negrini, S.; Atanasio, S. TRACE (Trunk Aesthetic Clinical Evaluation), a routine clinical tool to evaluate aesthetics in scoliosis patients: Development from the Aesthetic Index (AI) and repeatability. *Scoliosis* **2009**, *4*, 3. [CrossRef]
39. Han, K.-S.; Kim, G.-W.; Kang, S.-R.; Ko, M.-H.; Seo, J.-H. Clinical evaluation of the effectiveness of a new orthotic device for the non-operative treatment of scoliosis. *Technol. Health Care* **2020**, *28*, S229–S236. [CrossRef]
40. Drummond, D.; Breed, A.L.; Narechania, R. Relationship of spine deformity and pelvic obliquity on sitting pressure distributions and decubitus ulceration. *J. Pediatr. Orthop.* **1985**, *5*, 396–402. [CrossRef]
41. Ruffilli, A.; Fiore, M.; Barile, F.; Pasini, S.; Faldini, C. Evaluation of night-time bracing efficacy in the treatment of adolescent idiopathic scoliosis: A systematic review. *Spine Deform.* **2021**, *9*, 671–678. [CrossRef]
42. Angelliaume, A.; Pfirrmann, C.; Alhada, T.; Sales de Gauzy, J. Non-operative treatment of adolescent idiopathic scoliosis. *Orthop. Traumatol. Surg. Res. OTSR* **2025**, *111*, 104078. [CrossRef] [PubMed]
43. Karavidas, N. Bracing In The Treatment Of Adolescent Idiopathic Scoliosis: Evidence To Date. *Adolesc. Health Med. Ther.* **2019**, *10*, 153–172. [CrossRef]
44. Lee, Y.J.; Wang, W.J.; Mohamad, S.M.; Chandren, J.R.; Abd Gani, S.M.; Chung, W.H.; Chiu, C.K.; Chan, C.Y.W. A comparison between Boston brace and European braces in the treatment of adolescent idiopathic scoliosis (AIS) patients: A systematic review based on the standardised Scoliosis Research Society (SRS) inclusion criteria for brace treatment. *Eur. Spine J.* **2024**, *33*, 93–102. [CrossRef]
45. Luo, C.; Wu, H.; Liu, W.; Luo, Y.; Jie, Y.; Ma, C.Z.; Wong, M. The Biomechanics of Spinal Orthoses for Adolescent Idiopathic Scoliosis: A Systematic Review of the Controlling Forces. *Bioengineering* **2024**, *11*, 1242. [CrossRef] [PubMed]
46. Nie, W.Z.; Ye, M.; Wang, Z.Y. Infinite models in scoliosis: A review of the literature and analysis of personal experience. *Biomed. Tech.* **2008**, *53*, 174–180. [CrossRef] [PubMed]
47. Rahimi, S.; Kiaghadi, A.; Fallahian, N. Effective factors on brace compliance in idiopathic scoliosis: A literature review. *Disabil. Rehabil. Assist. Technol.* **2020**, *15*, 917–923. [CrossRef]
48. Wang, H.; Tetteroo, D.; Arts, J.J.C.; Markopoulos, P.; Ito, K. Quality of life of adolescent idiopathic scoliosis patients under brace treatment: A brief communication of literature review. *Qual. Life Res.* **2021**, *30*, 703–711. [CrossRef]
49. Liu, P.; Yip, J.; Yick, K.; Yuen, C.; Law, D. An Ergonomic Flexible Girdle Design for Preteen and Teenage Girls with Early Scoliosis. *J. Fiber Bioeng. Inform.* **2014**, *7*, 233–246. [CrossRef]
50. Liu, P.-Y.; Yip, J.; Yick, K.-L.; Yuen, C.-W.; Tse, C.-Y.; Ng, Z.; Law, D. Effects of a tailor-made girdle on posture of adolescents with early scoliosis. *Text. Res. J.* **2015**, *85*, 1234–1246. [CrossRef]
51. Yip, J.; Liu, P.-Y.; Yick, K.-L.; Cheung, M.-C.; Tse, C.-Y.; Ng, Z. Effect of a Functional Garment on Postural Control for Adolescents with Early Scoliosis: A Six-Month Wear Trial Study. In *Advances in Physical Ergonomics and Human Factors, Proceedings of the AHFE 2016 International Conference on Physical Ergonomics and Human Factors, Orlando, FL, USA, 27–31 July 2016*; Springer International Publishing: Cham, Switzerland, 2016; Volume 489, pp. 143–154.
52. Fok, Q.; Yip, J.; Yick, K.L.; Ng, S.P.; Tse, C.Y. Effectiveness of Posture Correction Girdle as Conservative Treatment for Adolescent Idiopathic Scoliosis: A Preliminary Study. *Orthop. Res. Online J.* **2018**, *1*, 91–93. [CrossRef]

53. Liu, P.; Yip, J.; Chen, B.; He, L.; Cheung, J.; Yick, K.; Ng, Z. Immediate Effects of Posture Correction Girdle on Adolescents with Early Scoliosis. In *Healthcare and Medical Devices*; AHFE International: Orlando, FL, USA, 2022; Volume 51, pp. 100–107. [CrossRef]
54. Chan, W.Y.; Yip, J.; Yick, K.L.; Ng, S.P.; Lu, L.; Cheung, K.M.; Kwan, K.Y.; Cheung, J.P.; Yeung, K.W.; Tse, C.Y. Mechanical and Clinical Evaluation of a Shape Memory Alloy and Conventional Struts in a Flexible Scoliotic Brace. *Ann. Biomed. Eng.* **2018**, *46*, 1194–1205. [CrossRef]
55. Ye, Z.; Yip, J.; Cheung, J.P.Y.; Liang, R.; Zhang, J.; Li, X.; Tong, R.K.-Y. Posture correction girdle with intelligent padding system to dynamically adjust the pressure distribution and correct the scoliotic spine. In *Healthcare and Medical Devices*; AHFE International: Orlando, FL, USA, 2023; Volume 79, pp. 12–20. [CrossRef]
56. Wong, S.-H.; Yip, J.; Yick, K.; Ng, Z. Preliminary wear trial of anisotropic textile brace for adolescent idiopathic scoliosis. In Proceedings of the ISERD International Conference, Zurich, Switzerland, 16–17 February 2020.
57. Wong, C.S.; Yip, J.; Yick, K.; Ng, Z.S. A Case Study of Initial In-Brace Spinal Correction of Anisotropic Textile Brace and Boston Brace. In Proceedings of the AHFE Virtual Conference on Human Factors and Ergonomics in Healthcare and Medical Devices, Electr Network, Virtual, 25–29 July 2021; pp. 109–115.
58. Fok, Q.; Yip, J.; Yick, K.; Ng, S. Design and fabrication of anisotropic textile brace for exerting corrective forces on spinal curvature. *J. Ind. Text.* **2022**, *51*, 1682S–1702S. [CrossRef]
59. Nakamura, N.; Uesugi, M.; Inaba, Y.; Machida, J.; Okuzumi, S.; Saito, T. Use of dynamic spinal brace in the management of neuromuscular scoliosis: A preliminary report. *J. Pediatr. Orthop. B* **2014**, *23*, 291–298. [CrossRef]
60. Kajiura, I.; Kawabata, H.; Okawa, A.; Minobe, Y.; Matsuyama, M.; Yoshida, K.; Suzuki, T. Concept and treatment outcomes of dynamic spinal brace for scoliosis in cerebral palsy. *J. Pediatr. Orthop. B* **2019**, *28*, 351–355. [CrossRef]
61. Ring, J.B.; Kim, C. A passive brace to improve activities of daily living utilizing compliant parallel mechanisms. In Proceedings of the ASME International Design Engineering Technical Conferences and Computers and Information in Engineering Conference (IDETC/CIE), Charlotte, NC, USA, 21–24 August 2016.
62. Nijssen, J.P.A.; Radaelli, G.; Herder, J.L.; Kim, C.J.; Ring, J.B. Design and Analysis of a Shell Mechanism Based Two-Fold Force Controlled Scoliosis Brace. In Proceedings of the ASME International Design Engineering Technical Conferences and Computers and Information in Engineering Conference, Cleveland, OH, USA, 6–9 August 2017.
63. Park, J.-H.; Stegall, P.; Agrawal, S.K. Dynamic Brace for Correction of Abnormal Postures of the Human Spine. In Proceedings of the IEEE International Conference on Robotics and Automation (ICRA), Seattle, WA, USA, 26–30 May 2015; pp. 5922–5927.
64. Périé, D.; Aubin, C.E.; Petit, Y.; Beauséjour, M.; Dansereau, J.; Labelle, H. Boston brace correction in idiopathic scoliosis: A biomechanical study. *Spine* **2003**, *28*, 1672–1677. [CrossRef] [PubMed]
65. Terjesen, T.; Lange, J.E.; Steen, H. Treatment of scoliosis with spinal bracing in quadriplegic cerebral palsy. *Dev. Med. Child. Neurol.* **2000**, *42*, 448–454. [CrossRef] [PubMed]
66. Hui, C.-L.; Piao, J.; Wong, M.S.; Chen, Z. Study of Textile Fabric Materials used in Spinal Braces for Scoliosis. *J. Med. Biol. Eng.* **2020**, *40*, 356–371. [CrossRef]
67. Aulisa, A.G.; Giordano, M.; Falciglia, F.; Marzetti, E.; Poscia, A.; Guzzanti, V. Correlation between compliance and brace treatment in juvenile and adolescent idiopathic scoliosis: SOSORT 2014 award winner. *Scoliosis* **2014**, *9*, 6. [CrossRef]
68. Haleem, S.; Nnadi, C. Scoliosis: A review. *Paediatr. Child Health* **2018**, *28*, 209–217. [CrossRef]
69. Guo, X.; Zhou, Z.; Mai, J.; Wang, Q. Kinematic and Kinetic Analysis of 3-RPR Based Robotic Lumbar Brace. In Proceedings of the IEEE/ASME International Conference on Advanced Intelligent Mechatronics (AIM), Electr Network, Boston, MA, USA, 6–9 July 2020; pp. 1828–1833.
70. Herget, G.W.; Patermann, S.; Strohm, P.C.; Zwingmann, J.; Eichelberger, P.; SÜDkamp, N.P.; HirschmÜLler, A. Spinal Orthoses: The Crucial Role of Comfort on Compliance of Wearing—Monocentric Prospective Pilot Study of Randomized Cross-Over Design. *Acta Chir. Orthop. et Traumatol. Cechoslov.* **2017**, *84*, 91–96. [CrossRef]
71. Niu, X.; Yang, C.; Tian, B.; Li, X.; Han, J. Modal Decoupled Dynamics Feed-Forward Active Force Control of Spatial Multi-DOF Parallel Robotic Manipulator. *Math. Probl. Eng.* **2019**, *2019*, 1835308. [CrossRef]

Disclaimer/Publisher's Note: The statements, opinions and data contained in all publications are solely those of the individual author(s) and contributor(s) and not of MDPI and/or the editor(s). MDPI and/or the editor(s) disclaim responsibility for any injury to people or property resulting from any ideas, methods, instructions or products referred to in the content.

bioengineering

Review

Contractile and Mechanical Properties of Quadriceps Muscles Measured by the Method of Tensiomyography (TMG) in Professional Soccer Players: A Systematic Review, Meta-Analysis, and Meta-Regression

Daniel Fernández-Baeza *, Germán Díaz-Ureña and Cristina González-Millán

Faculty of Health, Universidad Francisco de Vitoria, 28223 Madrid, Spain; german.diaz@ufv.es (G.D.-U.); 24crgonzalez9@gmail.com (C.G.-M.)
* Correspondence: d.fbaeza.prof@ufv.es

Abstract: Tensiomyography (TMG) is a non-invasive tool used to assess contractile properties. This systematic review aimed to accomplish the following: (1) Analyze quadriceps TMG parameters in professional football players during the season and compare them with reference values. (2) Assess the differences in TMG parameters between quadriceps muscles. A PRISMA-guided search in PubMed, Web of Science, and Sport Discus (up to March 2024) identified 139 studies. Twelve in-season professional soccer players (20–29 years old) and quadriceps tensiomyography parameters were included (muscle displacement, delay time, and contraction time). All the studies were assessed using the Newcastle–Ottawa scale, scoring 7/9 to 8/9, indicating good quality. The findings of this study were that of the nine parameters analyzed, three variables were found to differ significantly. The weighted mean values were as follows: rectus femoris (contraction time 30.11 ms, muscle displacement 8.88 mL, delay time, 24.68 ms), vastus medialis (contraction time 25.29 ms, muscle displacement 7.45 mL, delay time, 21.27 ms), and vastus lateralis (contraction time 23.21 ms, muscle displacement 5.31 mL, delay time, 21.89 Â ms). Furthermore, significant differences were observed in muscle displacement between the rectus femoris and vastus medialis, and between the rectus femoris and vastus lateralis. The TMG can serve as a valuable device for assessing neuromuscular function in soccer players.

Keywords: tensiomyography; thigh; soccer; knee; quadriceps; rectus femoris

1. Introduction

Evaluating muscle function is essential for designing programs aimed at improving sports performance and preventing injuries [1]. In this context, tensiomyography (TMG) has emerged as a well-established, noninvasive, and objective method for assessing the mechanical and contractile properties of muscles over the past two decades [2,3]. TMG applies electrical stimulation to the superficial muscles, generating parameters that provide insights into muscle contraction time (Tc) measured in milliseconds, muscle displacement (Dm) measured in millimeters, which indicates muscle tone, and the following variables related to fatigue: relaxation time (Tr) measured in milliseconds, delay time (Td) measured in milliseconds, and maintenance time of contraction (Ts) measured in milliseconds [4,5]. Additionally, TMG provides data that enable the identification of lateral asymmetries (between both legs) and functional imbalances, such as those between agonist and antagonist muscles (e.g., hamstrings and quadriceps) [6].

The contraction time measures the time it takes for a muscle to reach its peak contraction after receiving an electrical or neural stimulus. It is an indicator of the muscle response speed. It has been observed that this parameter is a good indicator of the prevalence of fast-twitch fibers [7]. Shorter Tc is considered to reflect a higher rate of force production [8]. A player with a low Tc in the quadriceps has the advantages of powerful shots and acceleration. Conversely, a high Tc in certain stabilizing muscles may help sustain a prolonged effort.

Muscle displacement measures the extent to which a muscle deforms or displaces itself during contraction. It is considered to reflect muscle belly stiffness [9] and has been shown to be altered by muscle fatigue and ageing [8,10]. Dm and Tr have also been shown to increase with increasing muscle fatigue [11]. Different training states also reflect variations in TMG, with athletes with a prevalence of strength and power training having shorter Tc and smaller Dm [12–14]. Furthermore, it has been observed that Dm increases when atrophy occurs in the muscle architecture [15,16]. Players with an optimal Dm exhibit better muscle recovery and efficiency in repetitive actions such as running or passing. If a player shows low Dm in the leg muscles, they might experience issues such as early fatigue or limited mobility.

The delay time was defined as the interval between the stimulus and the start of the muscle contraction. This indicates neuromuscular efficiency and muscle readiness. A short Td is critical for actions such as sharp accelerations, quick directional changes, and fast reactions to dynamic game situations. A long Td can hinder a player's ability to react swiftly, particularly under the physical and mental stress of an intense match. The relaxation time measures the time it takes for a muscle to return to its resting state after contraction. This reflects the muscle's ability to recover and prepare for subsequent actions. In football, a short Tr in muscles such as the hamstrings or quadriceps allows players to perform repeated high-intensity efforts, such as sprints and tackles. A prolonged Tr can reduce effectiveness during prolonged play, increasing the risk of errors or injuries, particularly in the later stages of a match. The maintenance time of contraction measures how long a muscle can sustain contraction under load, reflecting muscular endurance and resistance to fatigue. Players with long Ts values in the core and leg muscles maintain strength and stability throughout the match, which is vital for midfielders and defenders. Short Ts may lead to reduced effectiveness in critical moments, such as holding defensive positions or sustaining pace during extended runs.

Muscle injuries are among the most prevalent types of injuries in football [17]. In total, 92% of all muscle injuries affect the four major muscle groups of the lower limbs: hamstrings (37%), adductors (23%), quadriceps (19%), and calf muscles (13%) [17]. Quadriceps injuries result in more missed games than hamstring and groin injuries, with a reinjury rate of 17% [17]. Quadriceps muscle strains are particularly common in sports involving repeated kicking and sprinting, making them a frequent occurrence in various forms of football worldwide [18].

Numerous studies have used TMG to assess soccer players [19–26]. However, it was not until this year that an interesting study conducted a systematic review of the literature to comprehensively synthesize existing studies reporting TMG-derived lower limb parameters in soccer players [27]. Regarding the use of TMG in injury prevention, to date, there is only one experimental study in which the number of hamstring injuries was reduced after implementing an individualized training program for each player-based TMG datum [20]. Another issue is that there is no consensus regarding appropriate values for professional football players. The TMG software provides specific reference values for all parameters, which represent the asverages of the values most frequently encountered in assessments performed by software developers (TMG-BMC Ltd., Ljubljana, Slovenia). Therefore, the aims of this study were twofold: (1) to analyze TMG parameters in the quadriceps of professional football players during the competitive season to determine the most frequent values and compare them with TMG software reference values. (2) To assess the differences in TMG parameters among the quadriceps muscles.

2. Materials and Methods

A systematic review was conducted from 10 November to 22 December 2023, to search for published scientific evidence on the contractile and mechanical properties of healthy professional soccer players during the competitive season. The reporting flow diagram of this systematic review was based on the Preferred Reporting Items for Systematic Reviews and Meta-Analyses (PRISMA) guidelines [28] (Figure 1). This review was registered in PROSPERO (CRD42024506270).

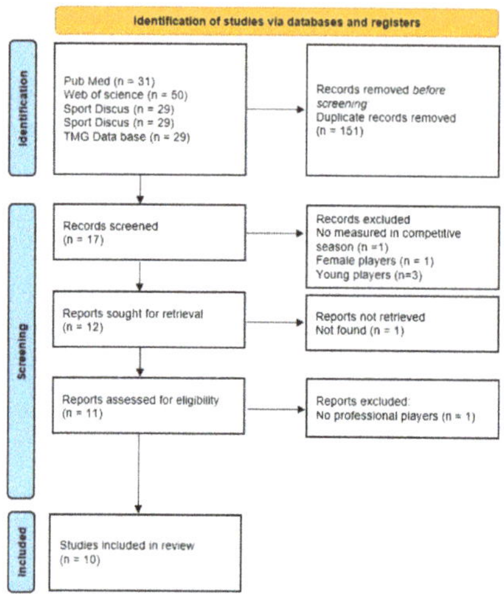

Figure 1. PRISMA flow diagram of the included studies.

2.1. Search Strategy

The authors independently performed a literature search of PubMed, Web of Science, and Sport Discus electronic databases. In addition, the authors conducted a thorough search of the TMG-BMC website (TMG-BMC Ltd., Ljubljana, Slovenia, 2022) to identify additional articles. The following terms and their combinations were used as a search strategy string: (a) target population: "soccer" or "football" and "player," or "; (b) intervention: "tensiomyography," or "TMG"; (c) outcome corresponded to tensiomyography assessment. The inclusion criteria consisted of samples of professional male soccer players measured during the competitive season. The authors consulted other experts in the field to identify additional published studies.

2.2. Eligibility Criteria

Eligible studies were selected based on the criteria of healthy soccer or football players and the use of TMG, and all types of studies were included in this review, except case studies and reviews. Overall, the selected studies focused on changes in TMG-derived parameters.

The inclusion criteria were male sex, age between 20 and 29 years, and professional soccer players measured during the competitive season. Younger and female football players were not included because of the significant differences in physical, physiological, and biomechanical characteristics between male and female football players [29]. The focus of this study was on homogenizing the sample to more precisely analyze the impact of these variables on male football players, including women, which could introduce biases that would compromise the internal validity of the findings.

Studies reporting inappropriate populations for this review were excluded. Studies on teenagers and players aged > 29 years were excluded.

2.3. Study Selection and Data Extraction

Titles and abstracts from electronic searches were independently screened by the authors. The authors (D-F and G-D) then checked the full texts of the selected articles to consider the fit with eligibility criteria. In case of any disagreement between the authors, a third reviewer (C-G) was consulted to make the final decision. The authors (D-F and G-D) extracted the data separately. In case of disagreement, the third author cross-examined doubtful data. The following data were extracted: authors, year of publication, study population (sample size and age), and TMG parameters of the biceps femoris and semitendinosus knee flexors. These two muscles provide a more specific and relevant assessment of the contractile and mechanical properties that directly affect athletic performance and injury prevention. Three TMG variables were extracted: contraction time (Tc), which is fundamental for analyzing how quickly a muscle can generate force and directly influence its performance. Delay time (Td) is crucial for understanding muscle activation speed, which is essential in sports in which reaction time is key. Muscle displacement is a key indicator of muscle contraction and recovery capacity and is relevant for monitoring muscle fatigue and assessing the risk of injury. These three parameters (Td, Tc, and Dm) allow for a comprehensive evaluation of muscle performance and injury prevention, aligned directly with the objectives of the study in elite athletes. The relaxation time and sustain time variables were not extracted because, while complementary, they are not crucial for evaluating the central aspects of muscle performance that are of the greatest interest in this study. In case of missing data, the authors of the publications were contacted. We used the data for the dominant leg (kicking) for analysis. The TMG 3.6 software (TMG-BMC d.o.o., Ljubljana, Slovenia) calculated the average values with the specific muscle contractile and mechanical properties based on sex, age, and sport/position, regardless of laterality or dominant side. A weighted averaging technique was used to obtain the pooled averages and standard deviations of Tc, Dm, and Td.

2.4. Statistical Analyses

To enhance the reproducibility of the results, the weighted mean and standard deviation were calculated using the sample size for each study. Specifically, the mean value and standard deviation of the control group were derived from the weighted mean value and standard deviation based on the sample size of the three subgroups using the TMG software. The standard deviation for the control group was provided by software developers at our request. The standardized mean difference was used as the outcome measure, with data fitted to a random-effects model to account for the variability between studies.

Heterogeneity analysis involved estimating tau^2 using the restricted maximum-likelihood estimator. Additionally, the Q test and I^2 statistics were reported. To assess potential outliers and influential studies, studentized residuals and Cook's distances were applied within the context of the model. Funnel plot asymmetry was examined using the rank correlation test (Begg and Mazumdar correlation test) and regression test (Egger regression), using the standard error of the observed outcomes as a predictor.

Cohen's kappa (κ) was calculated to measure the inter-rater reliability for the two authors who selected the studies. The normalized reaction velocity (Vrn) was calculated using the formula 0.8/Tc [19]. To minimize the risk of overfitting, meta-regression was performed using age as a covariate. A scatter plot was created to display the original data points.

A linear mixed model (LMM) was used to compare the differences among muscles, with the sample size included as a random effect. To further investigate the differences between muscle groups, multiple comparisons were performed using Tukey's test. Statistical analyses were conducted using the RStudio v. 2023.09.1+494, the Meta package v.6.5, the lme4 package v.1.1-35.5, and the ggplot2 package v.3.5.1 for graphical results.

2.5. Methodological Quality Assessment

The quality of the selected studies was assessed using the Newcastle–Ottawa scale (NOS). Articles with an NOS score of less than 7 were excluded. Subsequently, the risk of bias of the selected articles was reviewed by the authors (D-F and G-D). Any discrepancies between the authors were resolved through consultation with a third reviewer (C-G) for the final decision.

3. Results

The NOS score [30] varied from 7 to 8 in all studies, suggesting that all the articles were of good quality.

Table 1 lists the results for all combinations used in this review.

Table 1. Specific search equation results.

	PubMed	Sport Discus	Web of Science
Soccer and TMG	20	20	34
Soccer and tensiomyography	28	27	52
Football and TMG	8	12	16
Football and Tensiomyography	10	15	24
(((Soccer)) OR (football)) AND ((TMG)))	22	16	36
(((Soccer)) OR (football)) AND ((tensiomyography)))	31	16	55
(((Soccer players)) OR (football players)) AND ((tensiomyography)))	31	10	50
(((Soccer players)) OR (football players)) AND ((TMG)))	22	10	32
(((soccer players)) OR (football players)) AND ((TMG) OR (tensiomyography)))	31	29	50

A flowchart of the study selection process is presented in Figure 1.

Table 2 shows the Egger regression, Begg and Mazumdar correlation tests, and Rosenthal Fail-Safe Number. The results indicated no substantial publication bias for most TMG variables across the muscles, as shown by the non-significant Egger regression and Begg–Mazumdar correlation tests. However, the significant R-F-S-N values suggest strong effect sizes for all the variables. The significant Begg–Mazumdar correlation for Dm in the VM muscle indicated a potential publication bias for this specific variable.

Table 2. Egger regression, Begg-and-Mazumdar correlation test, and Rosenthal's Fail-Safe Number.

Muscle	TMG Variable	Egger Regression Value (p-Value)	B-M Correlation Value (p-Value)	R-F-S-N Value (p-Value)
VM	Tc	0.541 (0.59)	0.07 (0.90)	142 (<0.001)
	Dm	−1.479 (0.14)	−0.64 (0.03)	219 (<0.001)
	Td	1.30 (0.19)	0.14 (0.77)	383 (<0.001)
RF	Tc	−0.332 (0.74)	−0.08 (0.69)	77 (<0.001)
	Dm	−0.44 (0.66)	0.00 (1)	147 (<0.001)
	Td	−0.20 (0.84)	0.16 (0.61)	16 (0.003)
VL	Tc	0.436 (0.66)	0.00 (1)	637 (<0.001)
	Dm	−0.783 (0.43)	−0.50 (0.11)	74 (<0.001)
	Td	0.887 (0.37)	−0.14 (0.77)	66 (<0.001)

Note: B-M correlation = Begg-and-Mazundar correlation test, R-F-S-N = Rosenthal's Fail-Safe Number.

Table 3 presents the heterogeneity statistics of each variable. The results indicated significant heterogeneity across all the TMG variables and muscles, as evidenced by the high I^2 and H^2 values and significant Q statistics (p-values < 0.001).

Table 4 shows the values of the random effects model. Regarding the average outcome ($\hat{\mu} - value$), in VM and VL, most of the variables were negative values. However, in the RF group, most were positive. The higher the positive values ($\hat{\mu} - value$), the higher the values in the studies related to TMG. In the VM, both the Dm and Td showed significant differences. In the VL, only Tc showed significant differences. No significant differences were observed in the RF.

Table 3. Heterogeneity statistics.

Muscle	TMG Variable	I^2	H^2	Q	p-Value
VM	Tc	97.92	48.18	514.57	<0.001
	Dm	92.45	13.24	65.99	<0.001
	Td	83.77	6.16	28.54	<0.001
RF	Tc	90.62	10.66	175.48	<0.001
	Dm	91.17	11.32	210.361	<0.001
	Td	75.19	4.03	34.57	<0.001
VL	Tc	99.06	106.04	1193.98	<0.001
	Dm	95.07	20.29	84.44	<0.001
	Td	95.67	23.09	267.00	<0.001

Table 4. Random-effects model.

TMG Parameters	k	$\hat{\mu}$	CI (95%) Lower Bound	CI (95%) Upper Bound	Z	p
Tc VM	8	0.641	−0.145	1.426	1.60	0.11
Dm VM	8	−0.588	−1.003	−0.173	−2.77	<0.01 *
Td VM	7	−0.663	−0.965	−0.361	−4.30	<0.001 *
Tc RF	16	−0.241	−0.586	0.104	−1.37	0.17
Dm RF	16	0.232	−0.124	0.588	1.28	0.20
Td RF	9	0.186	−0.092	0.465	1.31	0.19
Tc VL	8	1.20	0.031	2.368	2.01	0.04 *
Dm VL	8	−0.342	−0.853	0.169	−1.31	0.19
Td VL	7	0.547	−0.025	1.119	1.87	0.06

Note: k = number of articles, $\hat{\mu}$ = Tau^2 estimator: restricted maximum likelihood, CI = confidence interval, * = significant differences.

Table 5 shows the values of the meta-regression mixed-effects model using age as a covariable. No significant effects were observed, except for Tc in RF and VL. Although Tc in VM has no significant effect ($p = 0.06$), it has been considered. Figure 2 shows the results of the meta-regression analysis of the three variables. Each point represents the number of participants in a group. To illustrate the predictions of the REML model, a regression line was added to show the expected response time based on age. The confidence interval is based on the estimated variance of the predictions derived from the REML model.

Table 5. Mixed-effects model.

TMG Parameters	k	$\hat{\mu}$	CI (95%) Lower Bound	CI (95%) Upper Bound	Z	p
Tc VM	8	0.405	−0.03	0.84	1.823	0.07
Dm VM	8	−0.002	−0.288	0.283	−0.017	0.99
Td VM	7	−0.093	−0.274	0.088	−1.001	0.31
Tc RF	16	0.239	0.068	0.411	2.734	<0.01
Dm RF	16	0.035	−0.181	0.252	0.32	0.75
Td RF	9	0.016	−0.183	0.214	0.155	0.88
Tc VL	8	0.652	0.031	1.274	2.057	0.04
Dm VL	8	−0.009	−0.363	0.345	−0.052	0.96
Td VL	7	0.279	−0.007	0.566	1.909	0.06

Note: k = number of articles, $\hat{\mu}$ = Tau^2 estimator: restricted maximum likelihood, CI = confidence interval.

Figures 3–5 show the forest plot of the meta-regression results, including the model fitting weights, standardized mean differences (SMD), 95% confidence intervals (CI), and effect sizes for each included study. Each horizontal line represents the confidence interval for a specific study, and the size of the square indicates the weight of the study in the meta-analysis. The central vertical line represents the null effect (standardized mean difference (SMD) = 0). Negative values located on the central vertical line in Figures 3–5 indicate lower values than those indicated by the TMG as normal values, whereas positive values located to the right of the central line indicate higher values than those indicated by the TMG as normal values. In Dm VM, most of the values included in the studies were lower than the TMG values. In addition, as shown in Table 4, this model was significantly different from the TMG values. All the included studies had similar weights in the fitting model. For both Td VM and Tc VL, most of the included studies were estimated to be positive, but one study was negative [31].

(A)
(B)
(C)

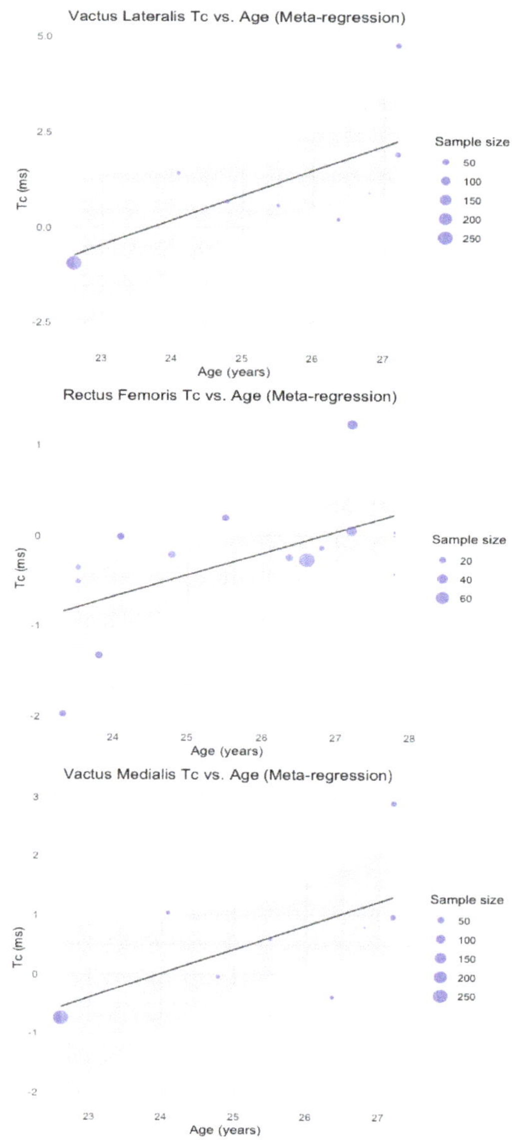

Figure 2. Results of the meta-regression analysis investigating the moderating effect of age on the time of contraction of the vastus lateralis (**A**), rectus femoris (**B**), and vastus medialis (**C**) muscles in soccer players. Blue dots represent primary studies, solid lines denote meta-regression prediction lines, and the gray area indicates the 95% confidence intervals around the mean.

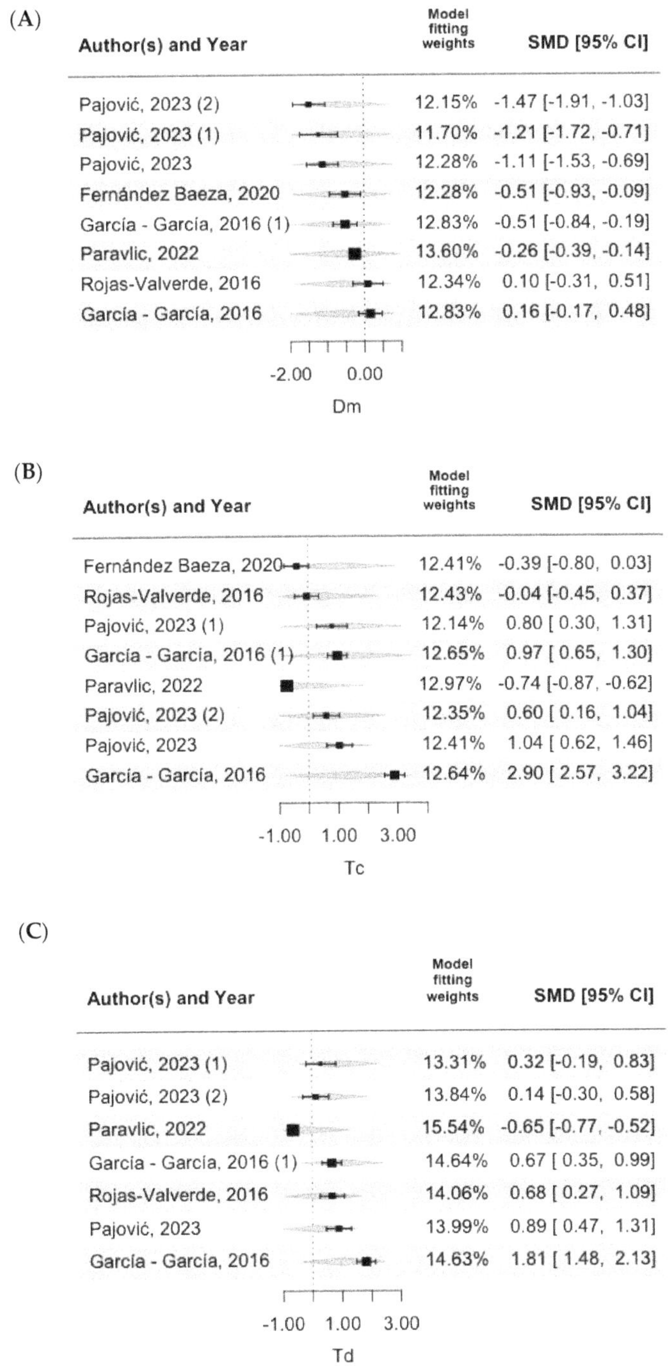

Figure 3. VM forest plot. Note: (**A**) Dm (muscle displacement), (**B**) Tc (contraction time), (**C**) Td (delay time) [26,32–35].

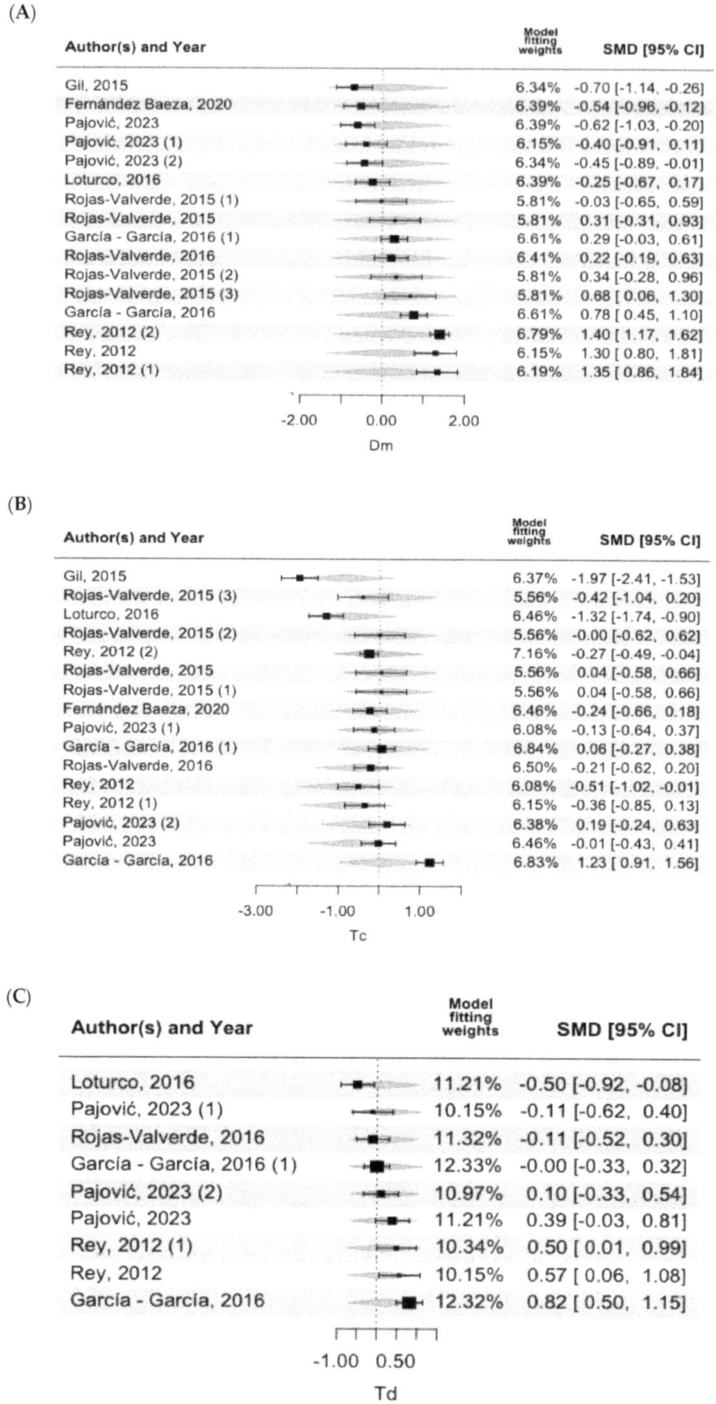

Figure 4. RF forest plot. Note: (**A**) Dm (muscle displacement), (**B**) Tc (contraction time), (**C**) Td (delay time) [19,20,22–24,26,33–35].

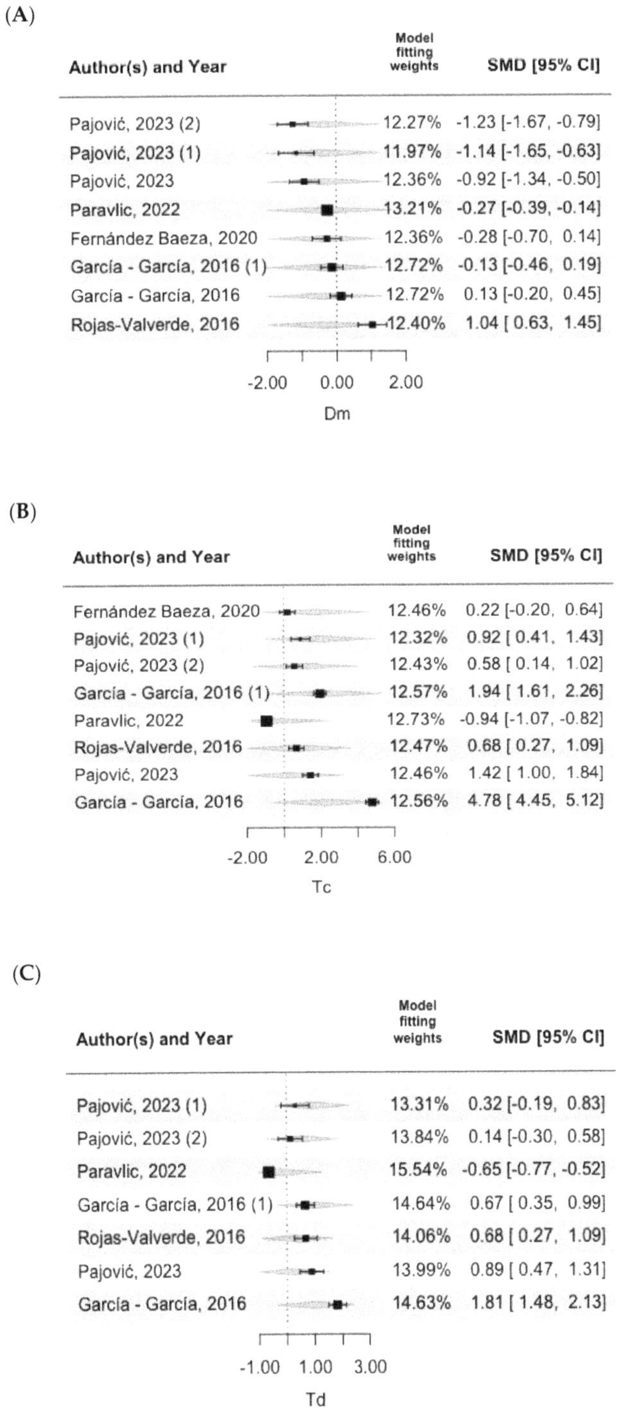

Figure 5. VL forest plot. Note: (**A**) Dm (muscle displacement), (**B**) Tc (contraction time), (**C**) Td (delay time) [26,32–35].

According to the studentized residuals and Cook's distances, although some of the studies showed high values in both analyses due to sample size, the number of studies included in each variable, and their weights in the model fitting, none of the studies were excluded and considered to be overly influential on any of the variables.

Table 5 shows the descriptive values of the muscles measured in each study. All the measurements were performed on the dominant leg. The authors who selected the studies to be included in this meta-analysis had an excellent inter-rater reliability (κ = 1).

Table 6 shows the studies selected in this review, the study code to identify it in the forest plot, and the TMG parameter data for each muscle.

Table 6. Studies selected.

CODE	REFERENCES	AGE	SAMPLE	VM	RF	VL	TMG
Rey, 2012	Rey et al., 2012 [24]	23.5 (3.4)	15		28.2 (2.6)		Tc (ms)
					11.1 (3.9)		Dm (mm)
					25.7 (1.8)		Td (ms)
Rey, 2012 (1)	Rey et al., 2012 [24]	23.5 (3.4)	16		29.1 (4)		Tc (ms)
					11.2 (2.3)		Dm (mm)
					25.5 (1.8)		Td (ms)
Rey, 2012 (2)	Rey et al., 2012 [23]	26.6 (4.4)	78		29.63 (3.99)		Tc (ms)
					11.34 (3.09)		Dm (mm)
					25.91 (2.02)		Td (ms)
Loturco, 2016	Loturco et al., 2016 [19]	23.8 (4.2)	22		23.5 (3.9)		Tc (ms)
					7.28 (3.27)		Dm (mm)
					22.7 (2.7)		Td (ms)
Paravlic, 2022	Paravlic et al., 2022 [32]	22.59 (3.91)	57	22.92 (2.38)		19.91 (2.24)	Tc (ms)
				7.65 (1.32)		5.3 (1.43)	Dm (mm)
				21.21 (1.84)		20.63 (1.57)	Td (ms)
Fernández-Baeza 2020	Fernández et al., 2020 [33]	26.36 (4.68)	22	24.09 (2.57)	29.77 (9.5)	23.33 (3.07)	Tc (ms)
				7.2 (1.81)	6.56 (2.92)	5.28 (1.17)	Dm (mm)
Pajovic, 2023	Pajović et al., 2023 [26]	24.09 (5.1)	22	28.9 (6.3)	31.1 (6.2)	26.9 (5.76)	Tc (ms)
				6.13 (1.68)	6.37 (3)	4.31 (1.64)	Dm (mm)
				22.3 (1.46)	25.2 (4.66)	24.1 (3.72)	Td (ms)
Pajovic, 2023 (1)	Pajović et al., 2023 [26]	26.8 (3.7)	15	28.1 (6.03)	30.4 (5)	25.4 (5.71)	Tc (ms)
				5.95 (1.52)	6.9 (2.45)	3.97 (1.13)	Dm (mm)
				21.9 (1.56)	23.8 (1.91)	22.8 (1.83)	Td (ms)
Pajovic, 2023 (2)	Pajović et al., 2023 [26]	25.5 (5.7)	20	27.4 (4.15)	32.3 (7.92)	24.4 (3.67)	Tc (ms)
				5.48 (2.04)	6.79 (2.48)	3.83 (1.33)	Dm (mm)
				22.07 (1.66)	24.4 (2.77)	22.4 (1.39)	Td (ms)

Table 6. *Cont.*

CODE	REFERENCES	AGE	SAMPLE	VM	RF	VL	TMG
Gil, 2015	Gil et al., 2015 [20]	23.3 (4.8)	20	19.74 (3.16)			Tc (ms)
				6.16 (1.9)			Dm (mm)
Rojas Valverde, 2015	Rojas-Valverde et al., 2015 [22]	27.78 (2.87)	10	31.39 (4.58)			Tc (ms)
				8.64 (2.63)			Dm (mm)
Rojas Valverde, 2015 (1)	Rojas-Valverde et al., 2015 [22]	27.78 (2.87)	10	31.4 (4.4)			Tc (ms)
				7.81 (2.06)			Dm (mm)
Rojas Valverde, 2015 (2)	Rojas Valverde et al., 2015 [22]	27.78 (2.87)	10	31.16 (4.49)			Tc (ms)
				8.73 (2.33)			Dm (mm)
Rojas Valverde, 2015 (3)	Rojas-Valverde et al., 2015 [22]	27.78 (2.87)	10	28.73 (4.28)			Tc (ms)
				9.57 (2.18)			Dm (mm)
García-García, 2016	García et al., 2016 [34]	27.2 (3.3)	37	35.2 (5.4)	38.3 (3.3)	36.9 (4.4)	Tc (ms)
				8.4 (1.4)	9.8 (2.4)	5.9 (1.5)	Dm (mm)
				20.7 (1.3)	26.4 (1.6)	26.2 (4)	Td (ms)
García-García, 2016 (1)	García et al., 2016 [34]	27.2 (3.3)	37	28.7 (6.7)	31.5 (5.8)	28.5 (7.2)	Tc (ms)
				7.2 (1.1)	8.6 (2.4)	5.5 (1.8)	Dm (mm)
				20.2 (1.4)	24.1 (2.1)	23.6 (3)	Td (ms)
Rojas-Valverde, 2016	Rojas-Valverde et al., 2016 [35]	24.78 (3.9)	23	(25.25) (2.95)	29.95 (2.32)	24.68 (4)	Tc (ms)
				8.29 (1.49)	8.42 (3.15)	7.29 (2.47)	Dm (mm)
				22.44 (1.56)	23,8 (1.27)	23.62 (1.38)	Td (ms)

Each group in each study was considered an individual group to compare their values with the TMG values. The weighted average values are listed in Table 7.

Table 7. Weighted average values in the studies analyzed and the TMG software of TMG parameters.

	VM_RA	VM_SOFT	RF_RA	RF_SOFT	VL_RA	VL_SOFT
Tc (ms)	25.29 (3.43)	25.39 (3.37)	30.11 (4.66)	31.17 (5.80)	23.21 (3.33)	22.67 (2.96)
n	442	5120	367	5552	442	5117
Dm (mm)	7.45 (1.4)	8.12 (1.79)	8.88 (2.74)	7.89 (2.46)	5.31 (1.5)	5.71 (1.52)
n	442	5120	367	5552	442	5117
Td (ms)	21.27 (1.70)	22.90 (2.12)	24.68 (2.26)	24.11 (2.79)	21.89 (2.01)	22.08 (2.27)
n	420	5120	207	5552	420	5117
Vrn (mm/ms)	0.0322	0.0315	0.0271	0.0257	0.0358	0.0353
n	442	5120	367	5552	442	5117

Note: VM_RA = vastus medialis research article; VM _SOFT = vastus medialis software TMG; RF_RA = rectus femoris research article; RF _SOFT = rectus femoris software TMG; VL_RA = vastus lateralis research article; VL _SOFT = vastus lateralis software TMG.

Table 8 shows the values of the multiple comparisons related to the differences among the VL, VM, and RF.

Table 8. Multiple comparisons of means: Tukey's contrasts.

TMG Variable	Parameter	Estimate	Std. Error	t Value/z Value	*p*-Value	95% CI (Lower)	95% CI (Upper)
Dm	VL-RF	−3.08	0.49	−6.29	<0.001	−4.22	−1.93
	VM-RF	−1.21	0.49	−2.48	0.035	−2.36	−0.07
	VM-VL	1.87	0.52	3.61	<0.001	0.65	3.08
Tc	VL-RF	−3.39	1.51	−2.24	0.065	−6.94	0.16
	VM-RF	−2.07	1.51	−1.37	0.358	−5.62	1.48
	VM-VL	1.32	1.64	0.81	0.700	−2.52	5.15
Td	VL-RF	−1.29	0.64	−2.00	0.112	−2.80	0.22
	VM-RF	−3.08	0.64	−4.78	<0.001	−4.59	−1.57
	VM-VL	−1.79	0.68	−2.62	0.024	−3.39	−0.19

Note: Std. Error = standard error, CI = confidence interval.

There were significant differences between all the comparisons for DM. Regarding Td, there were significant differences in both VM–RF and VM–VL. No significant differences were observed in Tc.

4. Discussion

The objectives of this review were twofold: (1) to examine scientific evidence on TMG parameters in the quadriceps muscles of professional soccer players during the competitive season, comparing these findings with reference values provided by the software, and (2) to assess whether differences exist in the TMG parameters across different quadriceps muscles. Additionally, the most frequently recorded values represent the most repeated measurements of the contractile and mechanical properties in these athletes; however, the most frequently repeated values are not necessarily the optimal ones.

(1) Evidence on TMG parameters

The main findings of this study reveal that of the nine parameters analyzed, three variables differed significantly from the most frequently reported values by the TMG software, and from the scientific literature reviewed. Significant differences were identified in the vastus medialis for two variables. The first was Td ($p < 0.001$), a variable associated with fatigue [36]. The studies reported a lower Td than the software (21.27 ms vs. 22.90 ms, respectively) (Table 7), due to the players' skill level. The software data included well-trained soccer players, whereas the participants in the studies were professional players. In elite players, fatigue induced by a soccer match appears less pronounced and recovery is more rapid than in lower-level players [37].

The other variable was muscle displacement (Dm) ($p < 0.01$), with lower Dm values in the studies (7.45 mm) than in the software (8.12 mm). This difference may also reflect discrepancies in the participant levels. Previous research has observed that playing level influences VM Dm, with elite players showing lower Dm (7.26 mm) than highly trained players (7.94 mm) [27].

Another significant difference was found in the contraction time (Tc) of the vastus lateralis (VL) ($p < 0.04$), with a higher Tc reported in the literature (23.21 ms) than in the software data (22.67 ms). This may be attributed to the timing of the measurements in the articles, which were taken during the competitive season, while the software measurements were taken during the preseason. It is well known that the cumulative load from training and matches can lead to fatigue, which is reflected in prolonged contraction time [11,36].

However, no significant differences were observed in any rectus femoris (RF) parameters (Table 4) between the TMG software data and the studies analyzed. This finding indicates that both the subjects in the studies and those in the software exhibited similar values because of the inherent physical demands of soccer, which shape the RF characteristics.

Age has a significant influence on tensiomyography (TMG)-derived parameters, reflecting broader trends in muscle mechanics and functionality. The meta-regression analysis revealed that the contraction time (Tc) increased with age across the quadriceps muscles, notably in the rectus femoris (RF) and vastus lateralis (VL), suggesting slower muscle responses, probably due to age-associated declines in the properties of type II (fast-twitch) muscle fibers and reductions in muscle elasticity. Although the changes in Tc for the vastus medialis (VM) did not reach statistical significance ($p = 0.06$), the confidence interval (−0.03 to 0.84) indicated a high probability (96.6%) that age-related modulation also affects this muscle. This suggests that contraction time increases with age, which is consistent with the findings of Paravlic [27]. These findings align with established evidence of age-related neuromuscular changes, including reduced activation efficiency, decreased mitochondrial density, increased muscle stiffness, and sarcopenia. This highlights the need to integrate age-specific approaches into training and rehabilitation programs to address the decline in muscle performance and mitigate the associated risk of injury.

(2) Differences across quadriceps muscles

When analyzing the differences between the rectus femoris (RF) and both vastus muscles, significant differences were observed in Dm between the RF and vastus medialis (VM) ($p < 0.0351$) and between the RF and vastus lateralis (VL) ($p < 0.001$). Dm was greater in the RF (8.88 mm) than in the VM (7.45 mm) and VL (5.31 mm), indicating that the rectus femoris exhibits a lower muscle tone. Dm is a parameter that reflects muscle tone and stiffness. A large displacement in the stimulated muscle suggests reduced muscle tone, whereas minimal displacement implies increased stiffness. Conversely, an optimal Dm level (depending on age, player level, and sport characteristics, among other variables) reflects adequate muscle tone [23]. In terms of contraction time measured in milliseconds in our study, the TMG measurements revealed that the contraction time (Tc) of the rectus femoris was slower (30.11 ms) than that of the vastus muscles, both the medialis (25.29 ms) and lateralis (23.21 ms). The contraction time reflects muscle contraction speed: a low contraction time indicates a high contraction speed, while a high contraction time suggests a slower muscle [38]. Thus, our findings suggest that the RF has a lower muscle tone and is slower than the vastus medialis and lateralis muscles. These differences in the quadriceps muscles were also noted in Paravlic's 2024 study [27], specifically between the VL and RF, which found that the RF showed poorer Dm and Tc values than the VL at different competition levels.

These highly imbalanced TMG values between the RF and the vastus muscles could potentially increase the risk of injury to the rectus femoris. This could be because the rectus femoris is highly prone to injury due to its biarticular role as a knee extensor and hip flexor. Its dual-joint function is subject to combined stresses, especially during actions such as sprinting or kicking, when simultaneous hip flexion and knee extension increase the mechanical loads. Its susceptibility is heightened by its longer length and reduced cross-sectional area, limiting its ability to dissipate force. Additionally, overextension during extreme motion or fatigue-induced imbalances with other quadriceps muscles amplify the risk of strain, particularly at the musculotendinous junction. This is an important factor to be considered in injury prevention and rehabilitation.

It is important to note that the rectus femoris is the most frequently injured quadriceps muscle [39]. The rectus femoris extends the knee, flexes the hip, and stabilizes the pelvis over the femur during weight-bearing activities [40]. Muscle strain injuries typically occur during eccentric muscle actions. In soccer, both sprinting and kicking require eccentric action of the rectus femoris, and its biarticular nature contributes to vulnerability to injuries [18]. Furthermore, in Scurr et al.'s 2011 [41] study measuring electromyographic activity in the quadriceps group during the contact phase of a kick, the vastus lateralis was found to be the most active muscle during the contact phase (89%), followed by the vastus medialis (83%), and the rectus femoris as found to be the least active (77%). This imbalance among the quadriceps muscles, due to the biomechanical and anatomical characteristics of the RF, as well as its lower involvement in certain actions, may pose an injury risk.

The present review was limited by the number of studies analyzed. There were parameters that demonstrated significant differences between the software and the studies analyzed; however, the number of players measured with the TMG software was greater than that in the studies analyzed. To conclude, an additional limitation of the present study is the potential bias in the selection of the TMG parameters. The analysis prioritized Dm and Tc, as these are the most frequently reported parameters in the scientific literature, facilitating their interpretation and comparison with previous studies. However, this selection may have excluded relevant information provided by Tr and Ts, which are parameters that, although they are less studied and potentially more sensitive to fatigue or sensor positioning, offer a complementary perspective on muscle dynamics. This limitation could also have been influenced by the lower consistency with which the latter parameters were measured. Future research should consider a more comprehensive approach that incorporates all parameters to provide a more thorough assessment of muscle behavior. Finally, the reference data provided by the software did not differentiate between the playing levels of football players, such as professionals and amateurs.

5. Conclusions

The software values described the contractile properties of the quadriceps in football players, as there was no significant difference between the studies analyzed. The rectus femoris exhibited the lowest muscle tone and muscle strength compared to the other quadriceps muscles. Its values demonstrate a significant imbalance when compared to the vastus muscles, indicating vulnerability in its function and potential for injury. This imbalance may contribute to an increased risk during high-intensity movements, in which proper muscle coordination and strength are crucial for injury prevention. Addressing this discrepancy through targeted rehabilitation and training interventions could potentially improve muscle balance, enhance overall knee and hip function, and reduce the risk of strain and injury. Future research should focus on strategies to correct these imbalances and improve the performance of the rectus femoris considering its biarticular role in both knee extension and hip flexion.

Author Contributions: Conceptualization, D.F.-B. and C.G.-M.; methodology, G.D.-U.; software, G.D.-U.; validation, D.F.-B., C.G.-M. and G.D.-U.; formal analysis, G.D.-U.; investigation, D.F.-B.; resources, D.F.-B.; data curation, C.G.-M.; writing—original draft preparation, D.F.-B.; writing—review and editing, C.G.-M.; visualization, G.D.-U.; supervision, C.G.-M. All authors have read and agreed to the published version of the manuscript.

Funding: This study received funding from the Francisco de Vitoria University (UFV2024-15).

Conflicts of Interest: The authors declare no conflicts of interest.

References

1. Maffiuletti, N.A.; Aagaard, P.; Blazevich, A.J.; Folland, J.; Tillin, N.; Duchateau, J. Rate of Force Development: Physiological and Methodological Considerations. *Eur. J. Appl. Physiol.* **2016**, *116*, 1091–1116. [CrossRef] [PubMed]
2. Rusu, L.; Călina, M.L.; Avramescu, E.T.; Păun, E.; Vasilescu, M.; Gorelick, M.L.; Brown, J.M.M.; Dahmane, R.; Valenčič, V.; Knez, N.N.; et al. Medicina Del Deporte. *J. Electromyogr. Kinesiol.* **2011**, *21*, 98–102.
3. Dahmane, R.; Djordjevič, S.; Smerdu, V. Adaptive Potential of Human Biceps Femoris Muscle Demonstrated by Histochemical, Immunohistochemical and Mechanomyographical Methods. *Med. Biol. Eng. Comput.* **2006**, *44*, 999–1006. [CrossRef]
4. Gimeno, E.M.; Campa, F.; Badicu, G.; Castizo-Olier, J.; Palomera-Fanegas, E.; Sebio-Garcia, R. Changes in Muscle Contractile Properties after Cold-or Warm-Water Immersion Using Tensiomyography: A Cross-over Randomised Trial. *Sensors* **2020**, *20*, 3193. [CrossRef] [PubMed]
5. Rodríguez-Matoso, D.; Silva-Grigoletto, D.; García-Manso, J.; Rodríguez-Matoso, D.; Rodríguez-Ruiz, D.; Sarmiento, S.; Vaamonde, D.; Da Silva-Grigoletto, M. Reproducibility of Muscle Response Measurements Using Tensiomyography in a Range of Positions. *Rev. Andal. Med. Deporte* **2010**, *3*, 81–86.
6. García-García, O.; Cuba-Dorado, A.; Álvarez-Yates, T.; Carballo-López, J.; Iglesias-Caamaño, M. Clinical Utility of Tensiomyography for Muscle Function Analysis in Athletes. *Open Access J. Sports Med.* **2019**, *10*, 49–69. [CrossRef] [PubMed]
7. Dahmane, R.; Djordjevič, S.; Šimunič, B.; Valenčič, V. Spatial Fiber Type Distribution in Normal Human Muscle: Histochemical and Tensiomyographical Evaluation. *J. Biomech.* **2005**, *38*, 2451–2459. [CrossRef] [PubMed]
8. Rusu, L.D.; Cosma, G.G.; Cernaianu, S.M.; Marin, M.N.; Rusu, P.F.A.; Ciocănescu, D.P.; Neferu, F.N. Tensiomyography Method Used for Neuromuscular Assessment of Muscle Training. *J. Neuroeng. Rehabil.* **2013**, *10*, 67. [CrossRef] [PubMed]
9. Whitehead, N.P.; Weerakkody, N.S.; Gregory, J. Changes in Passive Tension of Muscle in Humans and Animals after Eccentric Exercise. *J. Physiol.* **2001**, *2*, 593–604. [CrossRef]

10. Macgregor, L.J.; Ditroilo, M.; Smith, I.J.; Fairweather, M.M.; Hunter, A.M. Reduced Radial Displacement of the Gastrocnemius Medialis Muscle After Electrically Elicited Fatigue. *J. Sport. Rehabil.* **2016**, *25*, 241–247. [CrossRef] [PubMed]
11. García-Manso, J.M.J.M.; Rodríguez-Ruiz, D.; Rodríguez-Matoso, D.; de Yves, S.; Sarmiento, S.; Quiroga, M. Assessment of Muscle Fatigue after an Ultra-Endurance Triathlon Using Tensiomyography (TMG). *J. Sports Sci.* **2011**, *29*, 619–625. [CrossRef]
12. Šimuni, B.; Pišot, R.; Rittweger, J.; Degens, H. Age-Related Slowing of Contractile Properties Differs between Power, Endurance, and Nonathletes: A Tensiomyographic Assessment. *J. Gerontol. Ser. A Biol. Sci. Med. Sci.* **2018**, *73*, 1602–1608. [CrossRef] [PubMed]
13. de Paula Simola, R.Á.; Raeder, C.; Wiewelhove, T.; Kellmann, M.; Meyer, T.; Pfeiffer, M.; Ferrauti, A. Muscle Mechanical Properties of Strength and Endurance Athletes and Changes after One Week of Intensive Training. *J. Electromyogr. Kinesiol.* **2016**, *30*, 73–80. [CrossRef] [PubMed]
14. Loturco, I.; Gil, S.; Laurino, C.F.D.S.; Roschel, H.; Kobal, R.; Cal Abad, C.C.; Nakamura, F.Y. Differences in Muscle Mechanical Properties between Elite Power and Endurance Athletes: A Comparative Study. *J. Strength. Cond. Res.* **2015**, *29*, 1723–1728. [CrossRef] [PubMed]
15. Pišot, R.; Narici, M.V.; Šimunič, B.; De Boer, M.; Seynnes, O.; Jurdana, M.; Biolo, G.; Mekjavič, I.B. Whole Muscle Contractile Parameters and Thickness Loss during 35-Day Bed Rest. *Eur. J. Appl. Physiol.* **2008**, *104*, 409–414. [CrossRef]
16. Šimunič, B.; Koren, K.; Rittweger, J.; Lazzer, S.; Reggiani, C.; Rejc, E.; Pišot, R.; Narici, M.; Degens, H. Tensiomyography Detects Early Hallmarks of Bed-Rest-Induced Atrophy before Changes in Muscle Architecture. *J. Appl. Physiol.* **2019**, *126*, 815–822. [CrossRef] [PubMed]
17. Ekstrand, J.; Hägglund, M.; Waldén, M. Epidemiology of Muscle Injuries in Professional Football (Soccer). *Am. J. Sports Med.* **2011**, *39*, 1226–1232. [CrossRef]
18. Ekstrand, J.; Hägglund, M.; Waldén, M. Injury Incidence and Injury Patterns in Professional Football: The UEFA Injury Study. *Br. J. Sports Med.* **2011**, *45*, 553–558. [CrossRef] [PubMed]
19. Loturco, I.; Pereira, L.A.; Kobal, R.; Kitamura, K.; Ramírez-Campillo, R.; Zanetti, V.; Cal Abad, C.C.; Nakamura, F.Y. Muscle Contraction Velocity: A Suitable Approach to Analyze the Functional Adaptations in Elite Soccer Players. *J. Sports Sci. Med.* **2016**, *15*, 483–491. [PubMed]
20. Gil, S.; Loturco, I.; Tricoli, V.; Ugrinowitsch, C.; Kobal, R.; Cal Abad, C.C.; Roschel, H. Tensiomyography Parameters and Jumping and Sprinting Performance in Brazilian Elite Soccer Players. *Sports Biomech.* **2015**, *14*, 340–350. [CrossRef]
21. Loturco, I.; Pereira, L.A.; Kobal, R.; Abad, C.C.C.; Komatsu, W.; Cunha, R.; Arliani, G.; Ejnisman, B.; Pochini, A.D.C.; Nakamura, F.Y.; et al. Functional Screening Tests: Interrelationships and Ability to Predict Vertical Jump Performance. *Int. J. Sports Med.* **2018**, *39*, 189–197. [CrossRef]
22. Rojas-Valverde, D.F.; Gutiérrez-Vargas, R.; Sánchez-Ureña, B.A.; Gutiérrez-Vargas, J.C.; Cruz-Fuentes, I.; Salas-Cabrera, J. Comportamiento Neuromuscular Posterior a La Competencia En Jugadores Profesionales de Fútbol de Costa Rica: Un Seguimiento Tensiomiográfico. *Pensar En Mov. Rev. De Cienc. Del Ejerc. Y La Salud* **2015**, *13*, 1–15. [CrossRef]
23. Rey, E.; Lago-Peñas, C.; Lago-Ballesteros, J. Tensiomyography of Selected Lower-Limb Muscles in Professional Soccer Players. *J. Electromyogr. Kinesiol.* **2012**, *22*, 866–872. [CrossRef] [PubMed]
24. Rey, E.; Lago-Peñas, C.; Lago-Ballesteros, J.; Casais, L. The Effect of Recovery Strategies on Contractile Properties Using Tensiomyography and Perceived Muscle Soreness in Professional Soccer Players. *J. Strength. Cond. Res.* **2012**, *26*, 3081–3088. [CrossRef]
25. Beato, M.; Madruga-Parera, M.; Piqueras-Sanchiz, F.; Moreno-Pérez, V.; Romero-Rodriguez, D. Acute Effect of Eccentric Overload Exercises on Change of Direction Performance and Lower-Limb Muscle Contractile Function. *J. Strength Cond. Res.* **2021**, *35*, 3327–3333. [CrossRef]
26. Pajović, L.; Toskić, L.; Stanković, V.; Lilić, L.; Cicović, B. Muscle Contractile Properties Measured by the Tensiomyography (TMG) Method in Top-Level Football Players of Different Playing Positions: The Case of Serbian Super League. *Int. J. Environ. Res. Public Health* **2023**, *20*, 924. [CrossRef]
27. Paravlic, A.H. Establishing Reference Values for Tensiomyography-Derived in Soccer Players: Insights from a Systematic Review, Meta-Analysis and Meta-Regression. *Biol. Sport* **2025**, *42*, 171–192. [CrossRef]
28. Page, M.J.; McKenzie, J.E.; Bossuyt, P.M.; Boutron, I.; Hoffmann, T.C.; Mulrow, C.D.; Shamseer, L.; Tetzlaff, J.M.; Akl, E.A.; Brennan, S.E.; et al. The PRISMA 2020 Statement: An Updated Guideline for Reporting Systematic Reviews. *BMJ* **2021**, *372*, n71. [CrossRef] [PubMed]
29. Haizlip, K.M.; Harrison, B.C.; Leinwand, L.A. Sex-Based Differences in Skeletal Muscle Kinetics and Fiber-Type Composition. *Physiology* **2015**, *30*, 30–39. [CrossRef] [PubMed]
30. Lok, C.K.; Mertz, D.; Loeb, M. Newcastle-Ottawa Scale: Comparing Reviewers' to Authors' Assessments. *BMC Med. Res. Methodol.* **2014**, *14*, 45. [CrossRef]
31. Paravlic, A.H.; Milanović, Z.; Abazović, E.; Vučković, G.; Spudić, D.; Rošker, Z.M.; Pajek, M.; Vodičar, J. The Muscle Contractile Properties in Female Soccer Players: Inter-Limb Comparison Using Tensiomyography. *J. Musculoskelet. Neuronal Interact.* **2022**, *22*, 179–192. [PubMed]
32. Paravlic, A.H.; Simunic, B.; Pisot, S.; Kleva, M.; Teraz, K.; Vogrin, M.; Marusic, U.; Pisot, R. Lower-Limb Muscle Contractile Properties, Explosive Power and the Subjective Response of Elite Soccer Players to the COVID-19 Lockdown. *Int. J. Environ. Res. Public Health* **2022**, *19*, 474. [CrossRef] [PubMed]

33. Fernádez-Baeza, D.; González-Millán, C. Estudio descriptivo de las propiedades contráctiles de los músculos flexo-extensores de rodilla en futbolistas profesionales y aficionados. *J Sport Health Res* **2020**, *12*, 458–471.
34. García-García, O.; Serrano-Gómez, V.; Hernández-Mendo, A.; Tapia-Flores, A. Assessment of the In-Season Changes in Mechanical and Neuromuscular Characteristics in Professional Soccer Players. *J. Sports Med. Phys. Fit.* **2016**, *56*, 714–723.
35. Rojas-Valverde, D.; Gutiérrez-Vargas, R.; Sánchez-Ureña, B.; Vargas, J.C.G.; Hernández-Castro, A.; Salas-Cabrera, J. Estado Del Balance Neuromuscular y Masa Magra de Extremidades Inferiores de Jugadores Profesionales de Fútbol de La Primera División de Costa Rica. *Apunts. Educ. Fis. Y Deportes* **2016**, *3*, 63–70. [CrossRef]
36. Muñoz-Pérez, I.; Varela-Sanz, A.; Lago-Fuentes, C.; Navarro-Patón, R.; Mecías-Calvo, M. Central and Peripheral Fatigue in Recreational Trail Runners: A Pilot Study. *Int. J. Environ. Res. Public Health* **2023**, *20*, 402. [CrossRef] [PubMed]
37. Rampinini, E.; Bosio, A.; Ferraresi, I.; Petruolo, A.; Morelli, A.; Sassi, A. Match-Related Fatigue in Soccer Players. *Med. Sci. Sports Exerc.* **2011**, *43*, 2161–2170. [CrossRef]
38. Rodríguez-Matoso, D.; Rodríguez-Ruiz, D.; Quiroga, M.E.; Sarmiento, S.; De Saa, Y.; García-Manso, J.M. Tensiomygraphy, Utility and Methodology in the Muscular Assessment. *Rev. Int. De Med. Y Cienc. De La Act. Física Y El Deporte* **2010**, *10*, 620–629.
39. Orchard, J.; Seward, H. Epidemiology of Injuries in the Australian Football League, Seasons 1997-2000. *Br. J. Sports Med.* **2002**, *36*, 39–44. [CrossRef] [PubMed]
40. Bordalo-Rodrigues, M.; Rosenberg, Z.S. MR Imaging of the Proximal Rectus Femoris Musculotendinous Unit. *Magn. Reson. Imaging Clin. N. Am.* **2005**, *13*, 717–725. [CrossRef] [PubMed]
41. Scurr, J.C.; Abbott, V.; Ball, N. Quadriceps EMG Muscle Activation during Accurate Soccer Instep Kicking. *J. Sports Sci.* **2011**, *29*, 247–251. [CrossRef] [PubMed]

Disclaimer/Publisher's Note: The statements, opinions and data contained in all publications are solely those of the individual author(s) and contributor(s) and not of MDPI and/or the editor(s). MDPI and/or the editor(s) disclaim responsibility for any injury to people or property resulting from any ideas, methods, instructions or products referred to in the content.

MDPI AG
Grosspeteranlage 5
4052 Basel
Switzerland
Tel.: +41 61 683 77 34

Bioengineering Editorial Office
E-mail: bioengineering@mdpi.com
www.mdpi.com/journal/bioengineering

Disclaimer/Publisher's Note: The title and front matter of this reprint are at the discretion of the Guest Editors. The publisher is not responsible for their content or any associated concerns. The statements, opinions and data contained in all individual articles are solely those of the individual Editors and contributors and not of MDPI. MDPI disclaims responsibility for any injury to people or property resulting from any ideas, methods, instructions or products referred to in the content.

www.ingramcontent.com/pod-product-compliance
Lightning Source LLC
Chambersburg PA
CBHW061552220926
51850CB00005B/318
* 9 7 8 3 7 2 5 8 6 6 3 0 4 *